DATE DUE

JAN 2 2 2007			
JUL 1 1 2007			
JAN 0 3 2008			
MAY 2 2 2012			

Demco, Inc. 38-293

CLINICAL
MANAGEMENT
OF
ARTICULATORY
AND
PHONOLOGIC
DISORDERS

THIRD EDITION

CLINICAL MANAGEMENT OF ARTICULATORY AND PHONOLOGIC DISORDERS

Mary E. Gordon-Brannan, Ph.D.

Professor Emerita
Portland State University

Curtis E. Weiss, Ph.D.

Private Practice

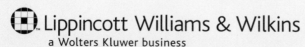 Lippincott Williams & Wilkins
a Wolters Kluwer business

Philadelphia · Baltimore · New York · London
Buenos Aires · Hong Kong · Sydney · Tokyo

Acquisitions Editor: Peter Sabatini
Managing Editor: Andrea Klingler
Marketing Manager: Mary Martin
Production Editor: Julie Montalbano
Designer: Terry Mallon
Compositor: Schawk
Printer: Courier Corporation-Westford

First Edition, 1980
Second Edition, 1987

Library of Congress Cataloging-in-Publication Data
Gordon-Brannan, Mary E. (Mary Ellen), 1943–
    Clinical management of articulatory and phonologic disorders / Mary E. Gordon-Brannan, Curtis E. Weiss.—
3rd ed.
        p. ; cm.
    Weiss' name appears first on the previous ed.
    Includes bibliographical references and index.
    ISBN 0-7817-2951-3 (alk. paper)
    1. Articulation disorders. 2. Speech therapy. I. Weiss, Curtis E., 1936– II. Title.
        [DNLM: 1. Articulation Disorders. 2. Voice Disorders. WV 500 G662c 2007]
RC424.7.W44 2007
616.85'5—dc22

                                                                                    2006003488

Dedication

This book is dedicated to Herold S. Lillywhite (1908–1999) for his unique expertise and coauthorship of the first two editions of this book. This dedication is also in recognition of his outstanding contributions to the profession of speech-language pathology as demonstrated by the awarding of honors to him from the Oregon Speech-Language and Hearing Association, the American Speech-Language-Hearing Association, and the American Cleft Palate Association. His spirit lives on in this book.

Preface

The third edition of *Clinical Management of Articulatory and Phonologic Disorders* is a major revision of the second edition, which was last published in 1987. Although numerous advances have occurred in the practice of speech-language pathology, the disorder area of articulation/phonology continues to be a prominent one in our profession. It is also often one of the earliest areas of disorder studied in an undergraduate or graduate program. Its relevance for preparation and intervention is clearly seen when a student becomes a clinician; a significant portion of the caseload will include articulatory/phonologic disorders.

In addition to the "articulatory/phonologic"-only clients, nearly all other types of communication disorders will involve speech sound deviations. Caseloads in most settings—schools, medical facilities, private speech-language and hearing clinics, private practice, and college and university settings—include clients with articulatory/phonologic disorders. Thus, there is a continuing need in the field of communication disorders for thorough, practical, and contemporary information devoted to the study of articulation and phonology.

FOCUS OF THE TEXT

In recognition of such a need, this book focuses on speech sound development and disorders and their management. As with the earlier editions, our intent is to discuss articulation/phonology and associated disorders thoroughly and, at the same time, keep the material as uncluttered, direct, and pertinent as possible. Emphasis is placed on the many approaches and techniques of treatment embodying the latest reliable information from research findings and clinical practice available in the field. We provide current information about articulatory/phonologic disorders while not abandoning older research, assessment tools, and treatment methods that are still relevant today.

The word *clinical* was purposely included in the title to emphasize to clinicians, regardless of settings, the importance of assuming a clinical approach or philosophy in assessment and treatment. To us, the term denotes the concepts of thoroughness and individuality essential to success in all settings. Clinical management, as used in this book, implies *optimum treatment* of all clients with articulatory/phonologic disorders in all possible settings rather than management of clients only in a "clinical" setting. We continue to believe in an eclectic approach and thus have presented information about numerous assessment tools and treatment approaches and techniques.

FEATURES

To reiterate, our goal in this book is to provide a comprehensive review of information relevant to articulatory/phonologic disorders. Each chapter begins with a new list of the **Objectives** for the chapter and concludes with a **Summary**. **Questions** framed in boxes appear before each major section to guide the reader's attention to the main points, and the **Review Questions** at the end of each chapter reemphasize the main points presented. Finally, a **Glossary** is provided at the end of the book to assist the reader with terminology. Boldface on terms within the text indicates that these words appear in the glossary. When these words are introduced for the first time, they are in boldface, but not thereafter.

ORGANIZATION

The first four chapters provide the backdrop for the study of speech sound disorders. In Chapter 1, we introduce the topic by demonstrating the significance of speech sound disorders and the impact they may have upon an individual's life. In Chapter 2, recognizing that it is probably a review for most students, we briefly identify and describe the speech processes, the articulators, the English phonemes, and a distinctive features system, and we discuss the acoustical and perceptual aspects of speech. Chapter 3 covers the phonological system and phonological development, including the motor and linguistic aspects of the sound system, phonological acquisition theories, components of the phonological system, and typical stages of phonological development. This information is important because it reflects the expectations at various stages of the speech of children and adults. Chapter 4 addresses dialectic speech variations through discussion of the major dialects of the United States, bilingualism and second language acquisition, the American Speech-Language-Hearing Association's position on working with individuals with dialect variation and those acquiring English as a second language, critical issues related to assessment of culturally and linguistically diverse populations, and intervention issues for limited English proficient children and adults.

The remainder of the book deals more directly with speech sound disorders. Chapter 5 provides information about the nature of articulatory/phonologic disorders, including classification systems, etiologies, and related factors and characteristics. The last five chapters deal with the actual management of speech sound disorders. Chapter 6 comprehensively presents information about the assessment and diagnosis of articulatory/phonologic disorders. Chapter 7 describes how to transition from assessment to intervention for individuals with articulatory/phonologic disorders. In this chapter, we discuss the need for treatment, factors to consider in selecting a treatment approach and specific targets, and some related guidelines for the treatment process. Chapters 8 and 9 present a wide variety of treatment approaches for individuals with articulatory/phonologic disorders. Chapter 8 describes treatment approaches that are characterized as phonetically or motorically based; that is, they focus on individual speech sounds, whereas Chapter 9, in contrast, describes treatment approaches that have a linguistic or phonological base and focus on speech sound patterns. Of course, there is considerable overlap among these approaches. Each treatment approach is described thoroughly in terms of what the clinician does to implement them. The last chapter, Chapter 10, provides tips for implementing treatment by describing four structural modes for treatment sessions, speech sound elicitation procedures, descriptions of various types of generalization, and guidelines and methods for carryover.

NEW TO THIS EDITION

In this edition, we have added contemporary information and issues; deleted sections from the previous edition that input from our readers indicated was only marginally relevant or useful; and added additional material on phonological acquisition theories, phonological development, dialectic variations of speech sound production, and treatment approaches and techniques. Replacing the second edition's chapter on treatment of special populations is a new inclusive approach that addresses the articulation/phonological treatment of individuals across all types of disabilities whenever relevant throughout the book. Our intent is to provide practical information on articulation/phonological management based on the various suggestions we have received from practicing clinicians, university professors, and students nationwide. We are grateful for these suggestions, encouraged by the responses received, and excited that this third edition is published by Lippincott Williams & Wilkins. We hope that our response to the many individuals who took the time to send us suggestions for this new edition has resulted in a relevant and functional book for its readers.

Finally, we also believe it important to communicate the professional underpinnings of this work. We bring to this book a depth and breadth of education and experience, covering a combined total of more than 75 years of working in clinical settings, doing research, supervising student clinicians, and teaching in the field of communication and its disorders. Combined, we have had experience as speech-language pathologists in public schools and private and university clinics, medical schools and as professors in clinical, academic, and research environments. As coauthors, we have striven to effectively combine our experience and expertise to bring students, instructors, supervisors, and practicing clinicians practical information about the assessment and treatment of articulatory/phonologic disorders based on a foundation of knowledge about the anatomy and physiology of articulation, theories of speech sound acquisition, and typical phonological development.

Mary Gordon-Brannan
Curtis E. Weiss

Acknowledgments

We are pleased to present this third edition and want to acknowledge those who have helped in various ways to bring it to fruition. Special recognition and acknowledgment are extended to Kathi Hoffer for writing the chapter on dialectic variations, which provided us with much-needed expertise in this area. Thanks also to Frank Bender for contributing the sample IEP in Appendix H. Sincere gratitude and appreciation are extended to Barbara Hodson, Hal Edwards, and Rhea Paul, esteemed professionals in the field, for their mentorship of the lead author. Their continued support and encouragement strongly influenced the completion of this project.

Similarly, we are grateful to Joan McMahon, Ellen Reuler, and Maxine Thomas, all of whom are local colleagues and friends who gently prodded us to continue writing and who provided positive reinforcement along the way. We especially want to acknowledge the excellent assistance given by Linda Napora and John Butler, formerly of Lippincott Williams and Wilkins, who began this writing project with us and expertly guided our efforts. Additional acknowledgments to the publisher must include Andrea Klingler, current associate managing editor, who worked closely with us during the last year to bring our book to completion.

Of special importance, we are indebted to the countless students and clients who guided us along the way as we taught and learned from these experiences during our careers. Likewise, we are indebted to the many professors and practicing clinicians who offered their constructive comments in recent years so that we could produce this edition. Finally, a warm thanks goes to Steve Brannan, husband and colleague, and Sharyn Weiss, wife and associate, who generously gave their input and support during all stages of this work.

Mary Gordon-Brannan
Curtis E. Weiss

Contents

CHAPTER 1

Significance of Articulation and Phonology and Their Disorders

"Only the feet that move in order dance. Only the words that move in order sing."

—Alfred Noyes

CHAPTER OBJECTIVES

- Describe the importance of oral communication to functioning in today's society.
- Characterize the use of the speech mechanism for speech production.
- Elucidate the important role of articulation proficiency in successful oral communication.

- Describe the social-emotional, educational and occupational, and interpersonal effects of articulatory and phonologic disorders.

It has been said, "Every time you say a word, you perform a miracle." Yet those of us who use words so freely and so easily take them for granted, forgetting that oral communication probably is the most important and most complex of all human behaviors. Hulit and Howard (2002) have expressed it this way:

> Speech is so much a part of the human experience that we truly take it for granted, but it is a wondrous human gift. The next time you engage in a conversation with one or more people, consider the speech chains that connect speakers and listeners. Marvel at the speed involved in the sending and receiving of messages. Notice how quickly speakers become listeners and listeners become speakers in a ballistic communication give-and-take that defies understanding (p.12).

Why is oral communication important to functioning in today's society?

IMPORTANCE OF ARTICULATION TO ORAL COMMUNICATION

Oral communication is important because it is the primary means for interacting with others, for expressing feelings and ideas, for venting anxieties and frustrations, for making requests and demands, for controlling the behavior of others, for learning about the world (by commenting and asking questions, for example), for providing information, and for enabling one person to find out what another person is perceiving and thinking. Concisely stated, "speech . . . allows brains to connect" (Hulit & Howard, 2002, p. 12). Oral communication is complex because it involves understanding and the use of abstract, arbitrary symbols; uses many different combinations of **phonemes**, **morphemes**, words, and phrases; integrates millions of neurons, nerve fibers, and multiple synaptic connections of the neurologic system; and simultaneously encompasses most of the bodily systems in its feedback functions.

Oral communication is complex from another standpoint and, because of this, it is quite unstable as a human process. The speech structures have more basic, biologic functions. All of the organs used in the process of oral communication have a more demanding priority than producing speech, or indeed of hearing and processing it as well. That priority is the preservation of the human organism in the face of any kind of threat, be it real or imagined, overt or covert. Thus, the communication process may be altered or stopped temporarily or permanently by illness, physical threat, psychological trauma, or many other conditions that may occur. The secondary nature of oral communication has been called an *overlaid* or *assumed* function.

In large measure, this is true even though there is a strong claim made by nativist language theorists (Chomsky, 1957, 1965; Dale, 1972; Lenneberg, 1967) and others that an innate capacity for development of language exists in the human being at birth—that it is biologically or genetically based in humans. Among other features, these theorists point to small, but important, differences in the structure and function of the organs used for speech that are not found in other animals. Because muscles of the tongue and lips are more highly developed and agile, the human being can alter **respiration** to produce speech by a different interplay of muscles than for normal breathing without speech. Hulit and Howard (2002) agree with Hocket (1960) that productivity of speech is a unique characteristic of human communication. Humans can produce utterances they have never heard nor said before. Hulit and Howard (2002) concluded that "the productivity or creativity of language gives human speakers a communicative power that is not shared by any other animal" (p. 9). Humans can be creative because of their symbol-producing brains that accommodate the learning of language.

It is difficult to disagree with any of the preceding, but the viewpoint does not alter the fact that the speech mechanism is, first and foremost, a vegetative mechanism with priority always given to the biologic function when a choice must be made. It may be that the finer muscle development of the articulators and the ability to alter respiration for speaking are results of learning to speak rather than causes. Even though humans seem to possess an innate capacity for language development, oral communication must be learned and taught. The fact that humans can accomplish this incredible feat, using organs designed biologically for other functions, approaches the miraculous.

The idea that the learning of language emanates from both innate capacity and environmental influences is in concert with the viewpoint of social interactionist language theorists, which holds that language development results from some combination of biologic/genetic and environmental factors (Bates & MacWhinney, 1987; Chapman et al., 1992; James, 1990). Thus, it seems "that both the child's internal abilities and resources (for content and form [including phonology]) and the social opportunities of the surrounding environment (use) are important in the acquisition of language" (Gelfer, 1996, p. 18). It is hypothesized that through this process, children learn the rules of communication and language, including phonological rules, and thus attain the ability to create unique utterances and sentences they have never heard nor said before (Hulit & Howard, 2002).

The development of this distinctly human attribute has been described from various viewpoints. Scholars, scientists, and clinicians have marveled, theorized, studied, experimented, and conjectured for centuries about the emergence, intricacies, and complexities of oral communication (e.g., Bates & MacWhinney, 1987; Chapman et al., 1992; Chomsky, 1957, 1965, 1981; Compton, 1970; Fillmore, 1968; Gleason, 2005; Hulit & Howard, 2002; Ingram, 1989; McLaughlin, 1998; Piaget, 1962). They have been intrigued, frustrated, and often awed by the potential power of language to effect both positive and negative changes. Oral communication is an invaluable asset for those persons who have mastered it, but it is an enormous liability for those who have not. This unstable, "borrowed" achievement shapes human behavior that is, in turn, shaped by it. Communication offers freedom for great achievement, but it is also a heavy responsibility for personal and social conduct, and proficiency in it (or lack thereof) can mean success or failure for the individual.

The anatomic and neurophysiologic mechanisms that mediate perception, respiration, **phonation**, **resonation**, and **articulation** help to make oral expression possible (Zemlin, 1998). Articulation is the principal vehicle for conveying meanings, thoughts, ideas, concepts, and attitudes through sounds, words, phrases, and sentences. An oversimplified definition of articulation is the adjustments and movements of the speech structures and **vocal tract** necessary for modifying the breath stream for producing the phonemes and prosodic-linguistic features of speech. Psycholinguistic literature suggests that **phonology** is the mastery of phonological rules and contrastive features that govern the perception and production of speech; that is, the readily distinguishable speech mechanism adjustments that produce different speech sounds.

Articulatory and phonologic disorders, commonly thought to be the most treatable of communication disorders, may also be the most commonly underestimated types of communication disorders regarding the ease of remediation. Not only are these disorders a frequently occurring type of communication disorder, but they also are variable across etiologic modalities. For example, articulatory disorders associated with **cleft palate** are quite different from articulatory disorders associated with **cerebral palsy**. **Misarticulations** associated with **apraxia of speech** present a completely different articulation pattern than those associated with lateral **distortions** of **sibilants**. The treatment approaches likewise are different.

As with any deviation of human behavior, generalizations about articulatory/phonologic disorders should be made with caution, if at all. What initially might appear to be a "simple" articulatory disorder may prove to be an exceedingly difficult articulatory/phonologic disorder to remediate. The common interdental **lisp** may be common because it is not readily amenable to treatment as a result of its possible multiple etiology. The functional articulatory disorder may turn out to be organically based, requiring multidisciplinary assistance. Knowledge of the anatomy and neurophysiology of speech, phonetics, acoustics, phonology, scientific method, and learning theory is an indispensable requisite if the clinician is to treat articulatory and phonologic disorders successfully.

Perhaps certain types of articulatory and phonologic disorders are quickly and effectively remedied, but just as certainly, there are those that may not be alleviated with present-day techniques. The challenge to the student, the future clinician, remains—to master the science and art of clinically assessing and treating persons who have articulatory or phonologic disorders. Implicit in this challenge is the need for creating, developing, and exploring new, different, and hopefully more efficient and effective diagnostic and treatment strategies and techniques.

If articulation and phonology are deficient, oral communication is impaired. The extent to which oral communication is impaired depends on several variables, including the person who has the impairment. No two persons with a similar speech disorder may experience the same degree of disability. Likewise, one listener may be unaware of the presence of an articulatory disorder, whereas another may be quite aware of the disorder and may be highly distracted by it. A third person may ask, "So what if articulation is defective. Haven't we all seen and heard teachers, movie stars, community leaders, and politicians with defective articulation?" Such different attitudes may also exist among those persons who have deviant articulation. However,

clinical experience shows that most adolescents and adults with articulatory/phonologic disorders are acutely aware of, and bothered by, their deviant speech.

> What three areas of one's life might be affected by articulatory/phonologic disorders?

EFFECTS OF ARTICULATORY AND PHONOLOGIC DISORDERS

The effects of an articulatory disorder may not be readily apparent to the listener, but they could have far-reaching repercussions on the person's social–emotional well-being, occupation, and of course, interpersonal relations. As Van Riper and Emerick (1990) so aptly stated, "We who have spoken so much so easily and for so long find it hard to comprehend the remarkable miraculous nature of speech—this peculiarly human tool" (pp. 2–3). Have we taken communication for granted? Other communication disorders may be equally devastating, but the fact that articulation constitutes a large percentage of all communication disorders makes it the cause of much human distress and suffering. Because articulation is so visible and audible, it invites judgments and penalties by listeners that are out of proportion to the severity of the actual deviation. It has always been so. A biblical account (Judges 12:5–6) illustrates such a judgment and resulting penalty. The Gileadites had captured the fords of the river Jordan to prevent the Ephraimites from crossing over to Ephraim. The account says, "And it was so, that when one of those Ephraimites which had got away said, 'Let me go over' that the men of Gilead said to him, 'Are you an Ephraimite?' If he said, 'Nay' then they said to him, 'Say now "Shibboleth,"' and he said 'Sibboleth,' for he was not able to give it the right sound. Then they took him and put him to death there by the Jordan. And there were forty and two thousand Ephraimites put to death at that time" (King James version). Modern man does not exact such severe punishment on others because of the inability to articulate a word correctly, but many less severe and sometimes devastating penalties are exacted.

This leads to a discussion of the potential social–emotional, occupational and educational, and interpersonal difficulties emanating from the presence of articulatory/phonologic disorders. Obviously, none of these areas is mutually exclusive because all of them deal with communication and other similar aspects of human behavior. For these reasons, one area cannot be affected without affecting the other areas; however, they will be considered separately here.

> What are some potential adverse social–emotional effects of articulatory/phonologic disorders?

Social–Emotional Effects of Articulatory and Phonologic Disorders

Beginning in childhood, the person with deviant articulation or phonology may experience unfavorable comments, teasing, ostracism, exclusion, labeling, and frustration (Van Riper & Erickson, 1996). Such experiences may result in a low sense of personal worth with the accompanying attitudes of feeling different, incompetent, stupid, socially inept, or disliked. As these unfavorable attitudes continue to develop, they may affect academic performance and behavior. The person with atypical articulation may begin to "play the part" of an atypical person. Grades may begin to drop, and disruptive behavior may become commonplace.

Some instances of truancy and delinquency may have their roots in atypical articulation development, and evidence exists of a higher prevalence of communication disorders among prisoners (Bountress & Richards, 1979; Sample, Montague, & Buffalo, 1989; Taylor, 1969; Wagner, Gray, & Potter, 1983). Sample et al. (1989) reviewed six studies and compared the prevalence of communication disorders among prisoners with those of nonprisoners. Although there was a wide range (2.9–28.5%) of prevalence figures in these six studies, the mean prevalence rate of articulatory disorders was 16%, in comparison to an estimated prevalence figure of 3% in nonprison populations. In their study of incoming prisoners in Arkansas, Sample et al. also found elevated prevalence figures for all categories of communication disorders, except for stuttering, including a rather high prevalence of 12.56% for articulatory disorders. At variance with these findings, Crowe, Byrne, and Henry (1999) reported prevalence figures of speech-only disorders in a maximum security prison in Mississippi to be comparable to or somewhat lower than prevalence among the general population. Nonetheless, Crowe et al. (1999) speculated, based on case histories of their prison clients, similar case reports from others, and the relatively high prevalence of communication disorders in some inmate populations that there might be a direct or indirect cause–effect relationship between communication disorders and antisocial behavior. As with nonprison populations, articulation is often found to be the disorder in question.

Recent literature based on past research findings has reported on the high relationship between communication disorders and emotional or behavioral disorders in children and adolescents (e.g., Brinton & Fujiki, 1993; Cantwell & Baker, 1991; Prizant et al., 1990; Prizant & Meyer, 1993). For example, Hummel and Prizant (1993) noted that the rate of co-occurrence of speech, language, and communication disorders and emotional or behavioral disorders in children and adolescents is 50 to 70% in various settings, "including public schools, community speech and language clinics, and inpatient and day treatment psychiatric settings" (p. 217). As early as 1960, Trapp and Evans found that children with articulatory disorders demonstrate anxiety levels commensurate with the severity level of their speech disorder. It is Prizant and Meyer's (1993) contention that communication is important in the development of self-image and sense of self, and thus, children with communication disorders are at risk of not developing a sense of self, a sense of emotional well-being, or both. The exact relationship between social–emotional impairment and communication difficulties is not clear, but many emotional and behavioral disorders may be a result of communication disorders.

If social–emotional problems develop because of deficient articulation, then speech-language pathologists have a great responsibility for alleviating such disorders early in a child's life. From the standpoint of social–emotional well-being, safety, protection of society, and simple economics, preventing articulation problems and successfully treating them early in life would seem to be the best clinical approach (Weiss & Lillywhite, 1981).

It is almost ironic that unacceptable speech potentially causes unacceptable social–emotional adjustment, which in turn is treated through effective speech. Psychoanalysis and certain other forms of psychiatric intervention rely on effective speech for treating clients whose problems may have stemmed from disordered speech early in life. The fact that deficient articulation may no longer be present in adulthood tends to minimize the relationship, or at least the awareness of a relationship, between disordered articulation and social–emotional problems. Disordered articulation as a cause of adjustment problems may be obscured or not even considered when it is not present at the time the psychological problem becomes manifest. Determining cause and effect of human psychopathology is not easy. Behavioral scientists would be the first to admit that making an accurate differential diagnosis relative to etiology is a challenging and complex task. More research is needed to determine the effect that disordered articulation has on social–emotional adjustment. The cumulative effects of a mild, not to mention severe, articulatory disorder on psychosocial development may be surprising.

> What are some potential adverse educational and occupational effects of articulatory/phonologic disorders?

Educational and Occupational Effects of Articulatory and Phonologic Disorders

Communication skills are important for students to be successful in school. This concept is supported by research that shows that teachers perceive students with speech and language disorders as poorer performers in the classroom than their normal peers (Bennet & Runyan, 1982; Cornick & Thomas, 1986; Ebert & Prelock, 1994). Thus, it appears that communication disorders, including articulatory and phonologic disorders, have a potentially negative effect on educational achievement.

The average person is capable of successfully performing thousands of different jobs. This statement, however, presupposes that the person has normal oral communication skills. The presence of a speech disorder can significantly reduce the number of job possibilities. After all, how many occupations do not require intelligible articulation? Even if the actual job has a low communication demand, the potential employee with deficient articulation may

not be able to speak well enough during the interview to avoid rejection. It is still true that many people, including employers, associate disordered or different speech with ignorance, incompetence, and even lack of intelligence. In this highly verbal society, persons may be judged, or misjudged, more by their type of speech than by any other factor or combination of factors.

As Van Riper and Erickson (1996) and Weiss, Gordon, and Lillywhite (1987) have pointed out, the amount and kind of penalty encountered by those who have communication disabilities depend on seven factors. These factors are listed in Table 1.1 and are described as follows:

1. *Articulation demand*: The more a person with a communication disability has to talk, the greater the potential penalty.
2. *Offsetting personal assets*: The more positive behaviors and attributes present in an individual, the less that person may be bothered by deficient articulation and the less the penalty.
3. *Overprotection*: The greater the overprotection, the more vulnerable that person becomes to penalty from the speech disability.
4. *Sensitivities, maladjustments, or attitudes of listeners*: The more distracted listeners are by disordered articulation, the greater the penalty. The worst penalties come from persons who are most sensitive about some difference of their own; that is, deviant articulation.
5. *Attitudes of a speaker who is disabled*: A negative attitude by the speaker is often transferred to and assumed by the listener, potentially resulting in greater penalty.
6. *Vividness or peculiarity of speech disorder*: The more unusual the speech is in terms of acoustic, physiologic, and cosmetic distortion, the greater the penalty.

TABLE 1.1

Factors Influencing the Degree of Disability of Persons with Communication Disorders

Articulation Demand
Offsetting Personal Assets
Overprotection
Sensitivities, Maladjustments, or Attitudes of Listeners
Attitudes of a Speaker Who Is Disabled
Vividness or Peculiarity of Speech Disorder
Degree of Unintelligibility

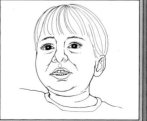

7. *Degree of unintelligibility*: The more unintelligible the speech, the greater the penalties. The penalties are great when persons listen, but cannot understand.

These disabling effects may assume different severity levels depending on the person with disordered articulation, the situation, and the overall environment. Regardless of the assets and potential the person may have, when articulation is deficient, the penalties imposed by society or self-imposed penalties will present barriers that interfere with self-actualization.

> What are some potential adverse interpersonal effects of articulatory/phonologic disorders?

Interpersonal Effects of Articulatory and Phonologic Disorders

Different societies and cultures have different value systems. Some cultures stress physical attributes, some emphasize material possessions, some place high premiums on educational achievements, and some regard artistic accomplishments highly. A large segment of the U.S. population considers articulate communication important; thus, disordered articulation in this society is one of the more serious disabilities a person can have. Van Riper and Erickson (1996) presented several autobiographic testimonies of persons affected by communication disorders. The poignant experiences these persons related emphasize the effect that disordered communication can have on interpersonal relations.

Their testimonies included experiencing various covert and overt penalties (Fig. 1.1). Many persons with typical speech may not be cognizant of the types and extent of penalties that are faced daily by persons with communication disabilities.

Oral communication abilities have been shown to affect social interactions as early as preschool age. Rice, Sell, and Hadley (1991) found that, in a preschool classroom, children with articulation impairments initiated interactions with peers less frequently than did their normal speech and language peers. These children also used shorter responses and nonverbal responses more often. Along the same lines, the preschoolers with articulation impairments responded less frequently to peer initiations and were ignored more often by peers who initiated interactions with them (Hadley & Rice, 1991). The researchers concluded that "peer interaction difficulties may be concomitant consequences of early speech and language impairments" (Hadley & Rice, 1991, p. 1308). Such experiences may well have an adverse effect on the development of social interaction skills of children with speech disorders.

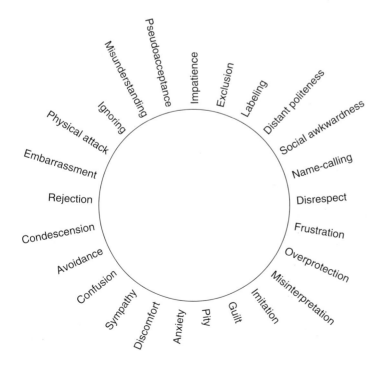

FIGURE 1.1 Penalties associated with articulatory/phonologic disorders.

Even mild articulatory disorders result in negative attitudes from peers toward persons with one or more misarticulations (Crow Hall, 1991; Freeby & Madison, 1989; Madison, 1992; Silverman, 1976; Silverman & Falk, 1992; Silverman & Paulus, 1989). In one study, fifth and sixth graders judged two students with misarticulated /r/ sounds more negatively on **intelligibility** and some personality factors, as compared to two students with no articulation errors (Freeby & Madison, 1989). Crow Hall (1991) likewise found that fourth and sixth graders rated fellow students with /r/ errors and with /s/ and /z/ errors more negatively on semantic differential scales than students with no misarticulations. Similar results occurred for a high school student with an /r/ misarticulation who was rated by high school sophomores, as well as for a college student who was rated by college freshmen and sophomores (Silverman & Falk, 1992; Silverman & Paulus, 1989). Similar perceptions of adult speakers with mild misarticulations have been found with adult listeners judging adult speakers (Mowrer, Wahl, & Doolan, 1978; Silverman, 1976). Examples of semantic descriptions of individuals with mild articulatory disorders are "frightened," "nervous," "tense," "more isolated," "less employable," and "less friendly."

Penalties experienced by persons with communication disabilities vary according to the seven factors contributing to disabling conditions described earlier. People use various ways, usually with good intentions, to penalize others whose behavior deviates from their own standards or from what is generally considered acceptable. As pointed out previously, almost any type of communication disorder may stimulate penalizing behavior by a typical speaker toward one with deviant speech. There are two characteristics of deficient articulation that attract the most attention and thereby draw the most penalties: (1) conspicuousness of the articulatory disorder and (2) degree of unintelligibility (Weiss, 1982). Either one may result in the person experiencing several overt and covert penalties (Fig. 1.1).

Many children and some adults attach labels, usually negative ones, to persons who exhibit any kind of behavior that they do not understand or that is considered to be different, such as disordered articulation. The child with a pronounced lateral lisp, a conspicuously misarticulated /r/, or unintelligible speech may be labeled, teased, and sometimes ridiculed. During the early years, this can be quite direct and persistent. During adolescence and adulthood, labeling may be more subtle and less obvious, but either way, it can be devastating.

When a handy label cannot be found or when name-calling does not seem to fit, mocking imitation of the different speech often occurs, resulting in embarrassment, frustration, or other discomfort in the individual with the disorder. An interdental lisp, for example, invites imitation, and the **substitution** or /w/ for /r/ or /l/, such as in "witto wed widing hood," can hardly be resisted. In fact, many parents and others often find it so difficult to resist that they also imitate the articulation errors, much to the detriment of the child. It should be noted that this kind of imitation is different from imitating and stimulating an infant's baby sounds or babbling, which is desirable in helping the child learn to talk (Hulit & Howard, 2002; Weiss & Lillywhite, 1981). Imitation that can be cruel and damaging is that which occurs after a child is past the stage when a sound should be used correctly, but for some reason is not. Ridicule of this kind by a parent, sibling, classmate, or other person can have a long-lasting negative influence on the child's communication development and emotional health.

Other forms of unfavorable attention, although less direct and sometimes more esoteric, can be equally damaging. Some of these are anxiety, overprotection, pity, and condescension. Parents, in particular, may show undue anxiety and may sometimes overprotect the child with a speech problem. Fortunately, all public schools now have clinical services for children with speech disabilities, and the speech-language clinician often will facilitate attitudes at home that are as advantageous as possible for the child with a speech problem. More difficult still is trying to control the penalties of pity and condescension, because these may be exhibited covertly by anyone and at any time or place. It is essential to help the child learn to react in a mature, rational manner toward such attitudes.

Impatience, avoidance, rejection, and exclusion—characteristics that may be exhibited at times by children or adults—are difficult to control. A surprising number of parents, other adults, and sometimes teachers may show impatience at not being able to understand a child with a severe articulation problem. They may misunderstand and misjudge the child. Such a penalty only reinforces the child's feelings of inadequacy and amplifies the effects of the disorder. Avoidance, rejection, or outright exclusion is more likely to be used by children. Fortunately, these drastic behaviors are not exhibited in most cases, but the child with **dysarthria**, apraxia of speech, or a severe phonologic disorder who cannot be understood or who may even sound and look somewhat grotesque to peers when trying to speak quite possibly will be avoided, rejected, or excluded from games, conversations, clubs, and parties. When negative behaviors reach such proportions, the results can be serious and lasting.

The child with a speech disorder who suffers from unfavorable experiences may react in any number of ways. Embarrassment and frustration may be the most common reactions and perhaps the least serious. Feelings of guilt and shame may also occur, especially when the child has been teased or ridiculed at home or at school or has been made to feel inadequate because of the speech problem. In the very young child, confusion may result and the entire process of communication development may be seriously disrupted or delayed.

The most effective safeguard for the child is to prevent articulatory disorders from occurring or from developing further, but this may not always be possible. However, many of the penalties can be avoided or reduced in number and severity by an awareness, understanding, and acceptance of the speech problems by parents, teachers, and others most directly involved with the child. The surest and most efficient way to eliminate negative experiences altogether when articulatory and phonologic disorders are present is to have the problems treated at the earliest opportunity by a certified speech-language pathologist.

From this thought, we will discuss the many etiologies, intervention approaches, and overall clinical management of articulatory/phonologic disorders among those persons who need, although sometimes seemingly do not want, the professional help of speech-language pathologists.

SUMMARY

For most individuals, oral communication is important for functioning effectively in society, especially in the United States. Deficient articulation and phonology results in impaired communication. There are social–emotional, occupational and educational, and interpersonal effects of disordered articulation and phonology. Several penalties result from deviant articulation and phonology, a frequently occurring disorder of communication. The degree and type of penalty a particular affected person experiences depends on seven factors: (1) articulation demand, (2) offsetting personal assets, (3) overprotection, (4) sensitivities, maladjustments, or attitudes of listeners, (5) attitudes of the speaker with a communication disorder, (6) vividness or peculiarity of the speech disorder, and (7) degree of unintelligibility. The most effective safeguard against articulatory and phonologic disorders is prevention or early intervention, and whenever possible, keeping the disorder from becoming worse.

REVIEW QUESTIONS

1. Why is oral communication considered important for functioning optimally in today's society?

2. What is meant by the concept that the speech structures produce speech as an *overlaid function*?

3. What two factors contribute to the development of language?

4. What is a definition of articulation?

5. What is the relationship between articulatory/phonologic disorders and antisocial behavior?

Between articulatory/phonologic disorders and emotional and/or behavioral disorders?

6. What seven factors affect the amount and kind of penalty that individuals with communication disabilities experience?

7. How might others perceive individuals with articulatory and phonologic disorders?

8. How might inadequate oral communication skills affect interactions of preschoolers?

CHAPTER 2

The Speech Mechanism and the Phonetic System

"Death and life are in the hands of the tongue."

—Proverbs

CHAPTER OBJECTIVES

- Briefly review the anatomy and physiology of the four speech processes, including respiration, phonation, articulation, and resonation.
- Characterize the role of the neurological and auditory systems in the articulation process.
- Identify and describe the movable and immovable articulators.

- Characterize the vowels, diphthongs, and consonants of the American English phonetic system.
- Describe a **distinctive feature** system for English phonemes.
- Briefly address acoustic and perceptual aspects of speech.

The answers to three questions are critical to an understanding of speech:

1. What is speech?
2. How is speech produced?
3. What are the sounds of speech?

The first question may be answered in several ways. Speech is the phonological component of an established oral communication system; a series of individual phonemes intricately blended and sequenced to form words; a vehicle for conveying language; an element of resonance and language; a composite of arbitrary symbols produced by structures and muscles not originally intended for communication; and vocal tract movements or adjustments, **air turbulence**, constriction, or interruption of the breath stream (Perkins, 1977). Speech may also be viewed as a learned behavior, social phenomenon, novel response, oral gesture, and a means of establishing interpersonal rela-

tions, maintaining emotional homeostasis, and manipulating human behavior (Simon, 1957). Speech is unique because of its late ontogeny, because it is exclusive to human beings and different from other forms of human behavior, and because it uses a symbol system. In this book, speech, articulation, and phonology are used interchangeably to include the production and perception of speech sounds in meaningful units and their rules mediated by the bodily systems and the structures referred to as the articulators. This chapter focuses on the phonetic system, i.e., the sounds used in speech production, preceded by a review of the processes involved in speech production and a description of the structures and functions of the speech mechanism.

What are the four basic processes involved in the production of speech?

THE SPEECH PROCESSES

The speech mechanism involves two basic components: the anatomic structures and the physiologic functions of the innervation and other bodily systems. Because these bodily systems were innately intended to provide life-sustaining functions, the speech mechanism can be considered a "borrowed" mechanism, one that is inextricably superimposed on the existing biologic functions. Use of these different systems in oral communication clearly implicates speech as an *overlaid* function making articulation vulnerable to any condition that threatens the welfare of the human organism. Articulation also is subservient to less serious interferences. For example, regardless of the importance of ongoing communication, when the basic biologic need to cough or sneeze occurs, the speaker's eloquent articulation ceases abruptly to make way for the disruptive cough or sneeze. This sharing of functions further underscores the extraordinary and complex nature of the speech mechanism so that the difficulty involved in trying to review simply and concisely the anatomy and physiology of articulation can be appreciated readily. A simple explanation is not possible because articulation is not a simple process. It is sufficient to state that the neurophysiology of speech continues to mature until about 12 years of age, even though articulation itself changes spontaneously very little after 7 years of age when all of the phonemes are usually mastered.

Eleven interrelated systems in the body participate in mediating speech (Zemlin, 1998). Obviously, some systems are more closely involved than others in the development and production of speech. Nevertheless, integration of all the systems of the human body is essential for normal speech to occur. The systems are listed in Figure 2.1. The skeletal, articular, and digestive systems provide the structures of the speech mechanism while the vascular, nervous, respiratory, and muscular systems provide the functional aspects of the speech mechanism. In essence, these seven systems constitute the anatomic and physiologic systems necessary for speech production. The remaining four systems assist with the emotional, prosodic, pragmatic, and other nonverbal aspects of speech.

Traditionally, in speech science, the 11 body systems are condensed to four to six (depending on the speech scientist you cite) primary, but overlapping, functional systems involved in oral communication generally referred to as speech *processes*. Four basic processes of speech production include:

1. *Respiration* provides the energy source for speech production and comprises the lungs; bronchi; trachea; larynx; air passageways of the pharynx, nose, and sometimes the mouth; rib cage; diaphragm; and associated structures (Fig. 2.2).
2. *Phonation* is the process of producing sound by the vocal folds of the larynx and provides the sound source for all speech sounds except for **voiceless** consonants (Fig. 2.3).
3. *Articulation* shapes the speech sounds. The movable and immovable articulators are within the vocal tract. (Note: The articulators are described later in this chapter.)
4. *Resonation* is the process of modifying the **voiced** breath stream by amplifying and damping certain frequency components of the speech sounds. The three resonating cavities are the pharyngeal, oral, and nasal cavities (Fig. 2.4).

Two other systems involved in speech production are the auditory and neurological systems. *Audition* (hearing) provides feedback to the speaker regarding the speech produced in addition to being the important mechanism for hearing the speech of others. The central (brain and spinal cord) and peripheral (cranial, spinal, and peripheral nerves) *nervous* systems are involved in speech perception and production. The cerebral hemisphere of the brain is the ultimate center of all neural activity and is the controlling system for articulation. Because the auditory and neurological systems are so important to the acquisition, development, production, and perception of speech, some discussion of them seems warranted.

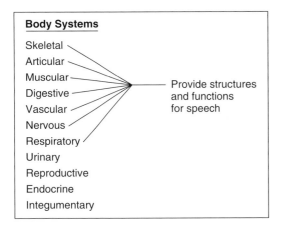

Body Systems

Skeletal
Articular
Muscular
Digestive
Vascular   Provide structures
Nervous   and functions
Respiratory   for speech
Urinary
Reproductive
Endocrine
Integumentary

FIGURE 2.1   The 11 systems of the human body.

What does the neurological system contribute to articulation?

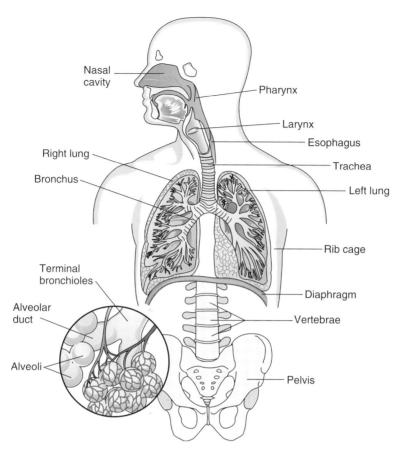

FIGURE 2.2 A schematic drawing of the anatomic parts of the respiration system.

Neurological System of Articulation

Composed of the brain and spinal cord, the central nervous system (CNS) is the highest-level nervous system and the one that controls the overlapping movements of the articulators. The cortex of the brain consists of billions of highly specialized nerve cells and many neural pathways that connect the two hemispheres of the brain, one part of the CNS with other parts of the CNS, and two points within parts of the brain. The excitation of nerve cells and aggregates of nerves within certain parts of the brain eventually provides innervation to the articulators and other structures necessary for speech production.

Closely related to the neurology of articulation are four areas of the brain cortex involved in oral communication: (a) posterior communication center (including Wernicke's area), (b) anterior communication center (Broca's area), (c) auditory cortex, and (d) motor cortex (Fig. 2.5). The posterior center re-

ceives and interprets oral communication while the anterior center formulates and programs the motor speech movements and expressive language. These two communication centers are connected by a bundle of nerve fibers called the *arcuate fasciculus*. A lesion of the anterior communication center can result in apraxia of speech or in Broca's aphasia, while a lesion of the posterior communication center can cause a problem in auditory processing or in Wernicke's aphasia. The lower part of the motor cortex has motor control over the articulation structures.

Functionally, the brain has been described as a symbolic receiver and transformer (Perkins, 1977) because it receives and transforms sensory-motor experiences into ideational symbols called *language*. As the highest level of neuromuscular integration, the brain is also capable of telling articulators when, where, and how to move (Carpenter, 1983; Gardner, 1975; Minifie, Hixon, & Williams, 1973; Zemlin, 1998). Weighing a mere 2.8 to 3.1 pounds, it is capable of performing a magnitude of truly remarkable functions, one of which is articu-

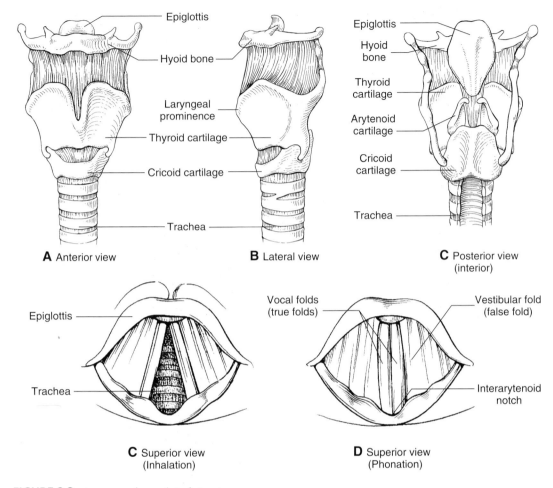

A Anterior view   **B** Lateral view   **C** Posterior view (interior)

C Superior view (Inhalation)   **D** Superior view (Phonation)

FIGURE 2.3   Larynx and associated structures.

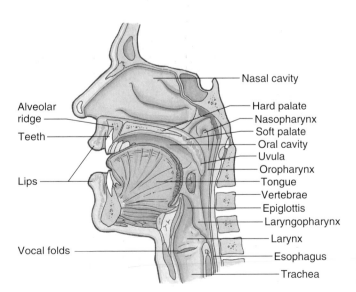

FIGURE 2.4   Vocal tract, including the nasal, oral, and pharyngeal cavities, and articulation structures.

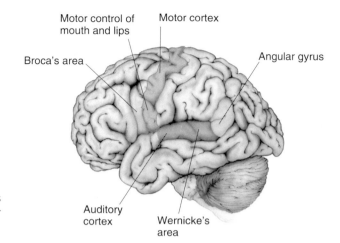

FIGURE 2.5 Key components of the speech and language systems in the left hemisphere. In the frontal lobe, Broca's area lies next to the area that controls the mouth and lips in motor cortex. Wernicke's area, on the superior surface of the temporal lobe, lies between auditory cortex and the angular gyrus.

lation. However, as remarkable as it is, the brain still cannot perform articulation functions without help from the peripheral nervous system, specifically the cranial nerves.

A major motor pathway descending from the cortex to the brain stem (corticobulbar) connects with the cranial nerves of the peripheral nervous system that innervate the head, face, neck, and laryngeal structures and thus move the articulators. Another major motor pathway descends from the cortex but connects with the spinal cord (corticospinal) and the spinal nerves that serve the trunk and extremities, including the respiration muscles that supply the energy for speech production (Seikel, King, & Drumright, 2005; Zemlin,

1998). A lesion to the upper part of the motor pathway in the cortex can result in spasticity of muscles, whereas a lesion to the lower part of the motor pathway can result in flaccidity of muscles. Both types of involvement can be symptomatic of motor speech disorders commonly known as dysarthria. The 12 paired cranial nerves (referred to by names and by Roman numerals) follow complicated pathways from their origins at the base of the brain to peripheral structures of the head, face, and neck (including all of the articulators). Seven of the cranial nerves are intimately involved in speech production. Table 2.1 identifies these seven cranial nerves and their speech functions.

TABLE 2.1

Cranial Nerves Involved in Speech Production and Their Functions

Number	Name	Speech Function
V	Trigeminal	Motor to mastication muscles (mandible) and tensor veli palatini of soft palate; sensory to face, mouth, upper and lower jaws, tongue, nasopharynx, and nasal cavity
VII	Facial	Motor to facial muscles; sensory to tongue and soft palate
VIII	Vestibulocochlear (acoustic)	Sensory for hearing
IX	Glossopharyngeal	Motor to pharynx; sensory to pharynx, tongue, and soft palate
X	Vagus	Motor to pharynx, larynx, and tongue; sensory to pharynx, larynx
XI	Accessory (spinal accessory)	Motor to pharynx, larynx, and soft palate
XII	Hypoglossal	Motor to tongue

Why is hearing important to speech development and production?

Audition

The auditory mechanism consists of the outer ear, middle ear, inner ear, cranial nerve VIII, neural pathway to the temporal lobe, and the auditory cortex (Fig. 2.6). This mechanism has several parts that function together in perceiving sound. Speakers perceive themselves somewhat differently than do listeners because of differing modes of sound transmission. When speaking, some sound vibrations pass through the bones of the face and skull (and the outer ear and middle ears into the inner ear), whereas the listener perceives the sound vibrations coming only through the outer and middle ears into the inner ear. However, self-perception of speech does not seem to affect how one speaks or learns to speak.

Most would agree that speech is learned or stimulated largely through the sense of hearing— absent, of course, any hearing loss or **auditory perceptual** problems. Maintenance of normal speech may be related more to **tactile** and **kinesthetic** feedback. The hearing mechanism then is important to self-monitoring of speech, which involves auditory recognition and discrimination of distinctive and other features of speech. As such, it plays an integral role in oral communication.

Where are the articulation structures located?

ARTICULATORS

Because the speech structures are simultaneously responsible for speech and resonance characteristics and because resonator adjustments are an unavoidable consequence of speech movements, speech and resonance are considered inseparable aspects of oral communication. The articulators are structures located in the vocal tract; that is, the pharyngeal, oral, and nasal cavities. Figure 2.4 schematically illustrates the articulators. The active or movable articulators move to contact the passive or immovable articulators that serve as the point of contact (Table 2.2). The primary movable articulators include the lips, mandible (lower jaw), tongue, and soft palate or **velum**, while the immovable articulators include the **alveolar ridge**, hard palate, teeth, and nose. The cheeks and pharyngeal cavity contribute to the articulation of speech sounds as well. Although not an articulator per se, the larynx as a vocal tract cavity and sound generator is directly involved in the production of every voiced phoneme. The pharynx (throat) functions primarily as a resonator.

Which structures comprise the movable articulators?

Movable Articulators

The most important and most active articulator is the tongue. It fills a large part of the oral cavity and is the primary modifier of oral cavity configurations. At-

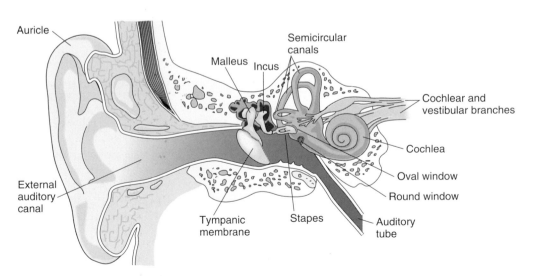

FIGURE 2.6 Anatomy of the ear.

TABLE 2.2

Movable and Immovable Articulators

Movable Articulators	Immovable Articulators
Tongue	Alveolar ridge
Lips	Hard palate
Mandible	Teeth
Soft palate	Nasal cavity
Cheeks *	
Larynx **	
Pharynx *	

*Often not listed as an articulator, but does play a role in articulating speech sounds.

**Traditionally not considered an articulator.

tached only on one end, it is involved in the production of the phonemes and in resonation. The basic biologic functions of the tongue are tasting, chewing, and swallowing. The tongue (Fig. 2.7A, C) may be divided into tip, blade, dorsum, body, and root. Its two distinct functional parts are the anterior two thirds and the posterior one third. The tongue consists of four intrinsic muscles (superior and inferior longitudinal, transverse, and vertical), which change the shape of the tongue and are more important to **consonant** production, and four extrinsic muscles (genioglossus, hyoglossus, palatoglossus, and styloglossus), which move the tongue within the oral cavity and are important to vowel production (Fig. 2.7C). These intrinsic and extrinsic muscles function in concert to produce speech.

A restricting factor in tongue mobility can be the **frenulum** (lingual frenum), a slip of connective tissue attached to the anterior undersurface of the tongue (Fig. 2.7B). If the frenulum is attached too far forward or too near the tip of the tongue, **ankylglossia** (or tongue-tie) is the result. Attached appropriately, the frenulum provides control and stability of the tongue for speech and vegetative purposes.

Because the tongue is the most important articulator, its malfunction (because of paralysis, injury, or atrophy, for example) can result in severe articulatory disorders. Cranial nerve XII (hypoglossal) is primarily responsible for **lingual** function in speech. This nerve provides motor functioning of all intrinsic and extrinsic tongue muscles except the palatoglossus that is supplied by cranial nerve XI (accessory) (Seikel et al., 2005; Zemlin, 1998). Cranial nerve V (trigeminal) provides tactile feedback from the anterior two thirds

of the tongue to the brain, and cranial nerve IX (glossopharyngeal) provides general sensory information from the posterior one third of the tongue.

The lips are made up mainly of the orbicularis oris muscle and a composite of other muscles of the mid and lower face. These insert into the orbicularis oris, including the buccinator, risorius, levator labii superior, levator labii superior alaeque nasi, zygomatic major and minor, depressor labii inferior, mentalis, depressor and levator anguli oris, incisivus labii superior and inferior, and platysma muscles (Seikel et al., 2005; Zemlin, 1998). The action of the orbicularis oris is to close the mouth and pucker the lips. The other muscles variously function to retract the lips, elevate the upper lip, elevate the corners of the mouth, depress the lower lip, depress the corners of the lips, and protrude the lower lip. The lips are primarily responsible for the production of /p/, /b/, /m/, and /w/ and are partially responsible for /f/, /v/, and other consonants and vowels requiring varying degrees of lip movements (including lip-rounding, lip protrusion, and lip retraction) and for the cosmetic aspects of facial expression. Because of their mobility, involvement of the lips has to be quite extreme before articulation is affected, such as in lip paralysis or severe scarring from trauma or surgical repair. Motor innervation of the lips is by cranial nerve VII (facial) and sensory is through cranial nerve V (trigeminal).

The lower jaw (or mandible) is involved in articulation and resonance. As the only movable bony articulator, excluding the hyoid bone, the mandible can increase and decrease the size of the oral cavity and can facilitate tongue elevation by narrowing the vertical dimension of the mouth. By altering the size and shape of the oral cavity, the mandible also plays a role in resonation. Although lateral movements of the mandible are also possible and necessary for mastication (chewing) and deglutition (swallowing), these movements, mediated by the pterygoid muscles, are not necessary for articulation. The masseter, temporalis, lateral and medial pterygoid, digastricus, geniohyoid, and mylohyoid muscles are responsible for mandibular movements (Seikel et al., 2005; Zemlin, 1998). Innervation is provided primarily by cranial nerve V.

The *soft palate* or velum begins at the end of the hard palate and extends backward to the pharynx, terminating at the uvula. It completes the back portion of the roof of the mouth and the floor of the nasal cavity and is the only movable structure in the roof of the mouth. It is the site of contact for back-of-mouth phonemes—/k/, /g/, and /ŋ/—and adds the final component for adequate **velopharyngeal closure** necessary for all phonemes except the three nasal sounds. It contains the following

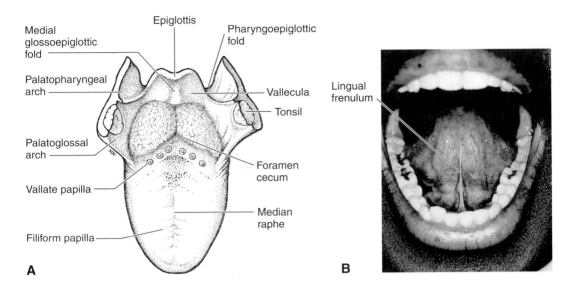

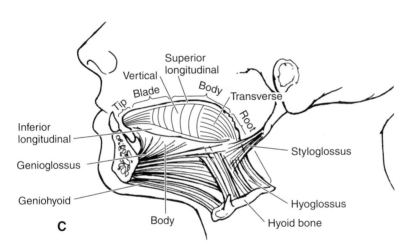

FIGURE 2.7   (A) Anterior two thirds and posterior one third of the tongue. **(B)** Frenulum of the tongue. **(C)** Functional parts of the tongue and its intrinsic and extrinsic muscles.

muscles: levator veli palatini, tensor veli palatini, palatoglossus (or glossopalatine), palatopharyngeus (or pharyngopalatine), and muscularis uvulae (Seikel et al., 2005; Zemlin, 1998). Damage to the soft palate or nerves that innervate it can be devastating to the production of any oral speech. Motor innervation is provided by cranial nerves V, X (vagus), and XI, and sensory by cranial nerve IX.

Two of the soft palate muscles form the pillars of fauces, which are curtains of muscle and mucosa partially separating the oral cavity from the pharyngeal cavity. The anterior pillars are made up primarily of the palatoglossus muscles; posterior

pillars are made up of the palatopharyngeus muscles. The fauces are located on either side of the oral cavity at the back of the mouth, forming the posterior border of the oral cavity. They function primarily in resonation, but probably also influence the articulation of back vowels and velar consonants through velopharyngeal movement and control. Their mesial movement during phonation, in addition to the movement of the lateral pharyngeal walls is important in achieving velopharyngeal closure (Hall, 1994). Located between the anterior and posterior fauces on each side are the palatine tonsils, commonly called the tonsils (when they have not been removed or are completely atrophied as in most adults).

An important movable vocal tract cavity in the production of sounds is the pharynx. This tubelike structure is surrounded by muscles and can be divided into the laryngopharynx (or hypopharynx), oropharynx, and nasopharynx (or epipharynx). The nasopharynx is the narrowest part of the pharynx and is the site of velopharyngeal closure. The pharynx functions in modifying resonance and in assisting with speech sound production. This structure serves as a variably sized resonating cavity and as an articulator for closing off the nasal cavity, with the help of the soft palate, for all but the three nasal phonemes—/m/, /n/, and /ŋ/. Velopharyngeal closure is sphincteric (circular) in nature. When the pharynx is incapable of such sphincteric closure, then speech will probably be characterized by nasal airflow on pressure consonants and **hypernasality** on vowels. Interestingly, children have greater intra-oral breath pressures than adults for production of pressure consonants (Bernthal & Beukelman, 1978). In both cases, articulation is affected because the oral–nasal airflow balance is disturbed. Muscles that provide the functional capability for the pharynx include the superior, medial, and inferior constrictors, salpingopharyngeus, palatopharyngeus, stylopharyngeus, cricopharyngeal, and thyropharyngeal (Seikel et al., 2005; Zemlin, 1998). The pharyngeal tonsils, more commonly called adenoids, situated in the nasopharynx may also contribute to velopharyngeal closure in children. Sensory and motor innervation is provided by cranial nerves IX, X, and XI.

As noted above, the anatomy and physiology of the velopharyngeal mechanism is important in the normal production of phonemes. Except for three sounds (/m/, /n/, /ŋ/) in which the **velopharyngeal port** is open, the mechanism is variably closed for all of the other phonemes in English. The key word here is variably, because the mechanism is differentially closed (or perhaps more appropriately, differentially open) for different sounds and for different articulation contexts. By listening to oneself with a listening tube or stethoscope, different degrees of nasal resonance can be perceived during the production of different phonemes and phonemic contexts suggesting that the velopharyngeal mechanism is not completely closed for nonnasal sounds. The **fricatives**, **affricates**, and **plosives** tax the velopharyngeal mechanism the most because these phonemes require the most continuous intra-oral air pressure.

Because the muscles of the pharynx and velum must function synergistically to achieve velopharyngeal closure, their coordination is essential to normal articulation and resonance. Even when the muscles of the pharynx or of the velum are functioning well, the acoustic outcome may not be normal articulation and resonance unless both muscle groups are functioning in synchrony. Velopharyngeal closure occurs as the result of the velum moving up and back, the lateral pharyngeal wall moving medially, and the posterior pharyngeal walls moving anteriorly.

Generally considered part of the soft palate, the uvula is not important to velopharyngeal closure or articulation, except perhaps in producing a "uvular trill" and has been implicated in snoring. Innervation is by cranial nerve XI.

Although not directly involved in articulation, the cheeks add stability to the sides of the oral cavity, mainly by the buccinator muscles, and they contribute to the cosmetic aspects of facial expression in speech. To a minimal degree, the cheeks contribute to resonation. The buccal cavity (space between the lateral teeth and cheek) is involved in oral resonance when the mandible is lowered and in high-pressure consonant production; it also contributes to the distortion heard in lateral sibilant sound distortions (Seikel et al., 2005). In persons who have undergone a laryngectomy, the cheeks may play a major role whenever buccal speech is taught. Motor innervation is by cranial nerve VII and sensory innervation by cranial nerve V.

The larynx is primarily considered the sound source, but in a sense, it functions as an articulator by producing the voicing feature of several consonants and all vowels and diphthongs. Normal production of /h/ and atypical use of **glottal stops** among some speakers with articulatory disorders and with repaired cleft palate are other examples of the larynx functioning as an articulator. Also, some English dialects use the larynx as an articulator of glottal stops. Motor innervation is by cranial nerves IX and X and sensory innervation through cranial nerve X.

Which structures comprise the immovable articulators?

Immovable Articulators

Located directly behind the upper front teeth is a rough, bony surface (rugae) of the maxillary dental arch known as the alveolar ridge. It is this immovable structure that is involved in some front-of-mouth consonants, including /t/, /d/, /n/, /l/, /s/, and /z/. These sounds are produced by the tongue tip making contact with part or most of the alveolar ridge. The alveolar ridge is a common place of articulation and the preferred place of lingual contact during rest and while swallowing. Structural deviations, resulting from clefts or other damage to the alveolar ridge, can cause articulation problems with the phonemes mentioned above. Sensory innervation of its mucosa is provided by cranial nerve V.

Located immediately behind the alveolar ridge is the hard palate, or roof of the mouth, that separates the nasal cavity from the oral cavity and extends from the alveolar ridge to the soft palate. It is lined with mucosa and serves as a passageway for the oral breath stream. The hard palate and the tongue are directly involved in the production of /ʃ/, /ʒ/, /tʃ/, /dʒ/, /r/, and /j/. The hard palate can be narrow, wide, high, or low. Any of these conditions, if excessive or cleft, may adversely affect articulation. Sensory innervation of the mucosa of the hard palate is also provided by cranial nerve V.

Contributing to the cosmetic as well as the articulation aspects of speech are the teeth. The upper and lower teeth are housed within the maxillary and mandibular dental arches and are used for masticating and provide an articulation surface for the production of various speech sounds. The teeth may be deciduous or permanent, depending on the age of the person. The number and alignment of teeth vary widely among individuals. The average number of deciduous teeth is 20, and the average number of permanent teeth is 32, which includes the incisors, cuspids, bicuspids, and molars. The teeth are important in the production of /f/, /v/, /θ/, and /ð/, and they help to produce the friction quality of the fricative sounds because of the breath stream passing over the cutting edges of the incisor teeth. As with the lips, the teeth are not indispensable to essentially normal articulation in many persons because of their ability to compensate for dental malocclusions and other dental deviations (Bernthal & Bankson, 2004). Other persons, however, may not be able to compensate adequately so that their articulation can be adversely affected by severe dental abnormalities. Sensory innervation of the teeth is provided by cranial nerve V.

The nose (or nasal cavity) provides the air passageway for production of /m/, /n/, and /ŋ/. It also serves as one of the resonating cavities for speech. Divided by a septum, the nasal passageways on either side must be unobstructed for normal articulation and resonance. Sensory innervation of the mucosa of the nose is provided by cranial nerve V.

Compare and contrast the terms *phones*, *phonemes*, and *allophones*.

ARTICULATORY PHONETIC SYSTEM

Almost 50 sounds in General American English comprise our phonetic system according to the broad transcription or phonemic classification. However, the number will vary from regional dialect to regional dialect, from phonetician to phonetician, from discipline to discipline, from classification system to classification system, and, in some cases, from speaker to speaker. These sounds, or speech **segments** as they are also called, are traditionally indicated by symbols of the International Phonetic Alphabet (IPA), although other symbol systems have been used (Edwards, 2003). The current version of the IPA symbols appears in Appendix A.

Phones refer to sounds produced by the human vocal tract without regard to a particular language, whereas a phoneme is an "abstract speech sound found in the phonological system of a particular language" (Edwards, 2003, p. 374). A phoneme is a family, class, or group of phonetically similar sounds. Phonemes are the smallest, nonmeaningful perceptible unit of oral language. This is not to be confused with the term *morpheme*, which is the minimal unit of meaningful speech in a particular language. Phonemes contrast with one another to differentiate the meaning of spoken words. Thus, a phoneme, or segment, is semantically distinctive. It denotes meaning, which is the key word in this explanation. Contrasting pairs or minimal pairs are good examples of how one sound can change the meaning of otherwise similar words, such as *pat* and *bat*. In this example, /p/ and /b/ are two different phonemes because they signal different meanings. Unlike phonemes, **allophones** are noncontrastive or nondistinctive; they do not change the meaning of a word. Thus, allophones are variant forms of phonemes—variations in pronunciation of a phoneme such that they remain part of the phoneme family, as is the case in which an **aspirated** /k/, **unaspirated** /k/, and unreleased /k/ are all acceptable allophones of the phoneme /k/ in the English language. Another illustration of how sounds vary even though meaning does not change is the phenomenon that an aspirated /p/ and an unreleased /p/ in *top* are both perceived by the listener to be the same word, even though /p/ is pronounced differently. To reiterate, when a change in meaning occurs because of the way the sound is produced, the sound or segment of that production is contrastive or distinctive. When no change in meaning occurs, a noncontrastive or nondistinctive feature is indicated, as in the examples of allophones just cited. Technically speaking, no two sounds or pronunciations are exactly alike, although they may seem to be because our auditory discrimination abilities do not perceive the subtle allophonic variations as differences.

Phonetics may be described as the "study of speech sounds, their form, substance, and perception," and phonemics is the study of speech sounds within a language (Edwards, 2003, p. 374). Phonetics may also be considered the motoric aspect of articulation, whereas phonemics is the linguistic aspect of articulation, which further complicates the problem of trying to discuss articulation as a process separate from language.

The following basic considerations are important to the discussion of our phonetic system (Judson & Weaver, 1965):

- Speech sounds are produced by structures that are part of the vegetative system.
- Speech sounds are perceived by the auditory mechanism.
- Speech sounds are symbol units.
- Speech sounds are learned.
- Speech sounds are influenced by forces that work to produce variation, such as duration, rate, and stress.
- Speech sounds are influenced by forces that work to prevent variation such as auditory, tactile, and kinesthetic or **proprioceptive** feedback.

These considerations lay the foundation for analyzing and describing phonemes, allophones, and phones. However, caution should be used in generalizing from isolated speech samples such as phonemes, syllables, and isolated words to contextual speech. Also, speech movements really cannot be described as specific events or as containing exact articulator placements for individual sounds, especially in consideration of concepts such as overlapping movements (Shohara, 1939 as cited in McDonald 1964a), **assimilation** (Stetson, 1951), **abutting consonants** (McDonald, 1964b), **coarticulation** (Winitz, 1969), and **ellipsis** (Tiffany & Carrell, 1977). The fact that articulation is a dynamic and variable function including both segmental (referring to individual sounds) and **suprasegmental** (referring to **prosody**) features cannot be overlooked. All of these characteristics of speech, along with speech perception by the listener as well as by the speaker, must be considered in the development and use of speech.

The contributions of descriptive linguistics, psychology, anthropology, sociology, phonetics, psycholinguistics, and, of course, speech-language pathology toward understanding the contemporary concepts of articulation are immeasurable. In this section, the American English phonetic system is reviewed mainly from the standpoint of the anatomy and physiology, perception, and use of each sound— 14 vowels, 4 diphthongs, and 25 consonants. Often, the IPA is used to symbolize the different sounds in our language, and it is reasonably adequate to record and describe the sounds of all the dialects related to English. Table 2.3 lists the phonetic symbols and key words for the phonemes described in this section. Table 2.4 shows the frequency of occurrence of the English phonemes, which is especially useful information when selecting which phonemes to target in treatment. The authors describe the speech sounds of English while being mindful that sounds vary from dialect to dialect and from phonetic context to phonetic context.

What are the characteristics of vowels?

Vowels

Vowels are speech sounds produced by a mostly unobstructed vocal tract with the only contact being between the tongue and the gum ridges in the oral cavity. They form the nucleus of nearly all syllables and have characteristic vocal tract configurations. Phoneticians use 14 to 16 distinct vowels to represent American dialects (Edwards, 1986; Edwards, 2003; Garn-Nunn & Lynn, 2004; Small, 2005).

Identification and description of vowels are complicated by the following:

- There are no "pure" vowels.
- They are very similar to diphthongs.
- They are the combined result of the coupling of the articulation–resonation system.
- Their features vary depending on whether a system of narrow or broad transcription is used.
- Not every vowel symbol used in the IPA is a distinctive vowel; some are considered allophones of other vowels.
- Vowels, as well as the other phonetic classes, contain considerable arbitrariness, which is necessary to maintain uniformity.
- There is no "preferred" standard of pronunciation in this country.
- Articulation varies continually, depending on suprasegmental features such as stress, rate, and duration.
- They are influenced by coarticulation.

Vowels are described primarily by tongue height (vertical tongue placement) and tongue advancement (horizontal tongue placement). Lower

TABLE 2.3

Vowel, Diphthong, and Consonant Symbols and Key Words

Vowel	Key Word	Diphthong	Key Word	Consonant	Key Word
/i/	eat	/aɪ/	ice	/p/	pie
/ɪ/	it	/aʊ/	out	/b/	boy
/e/	ate	/ɔɪ/	boy	/t/	tie
/ɛ/	ebb	/ju/	use	/d/	do
/æ/	at			/k/	key
/ʌ/	up			/g/	go
/ə/	about			/f/	feet
/ɜ˞/	earth			/v/	vote
/ɚ/	butter			/θ/	thick
/u/	soon			/ð/	that
/ʊ/	hook			/h/	home
/o/	oat			/s/	sew
/ɔ/ *	caught			/z/	zoo
/ɑ/, /a/,/ɒ/ *	cot			/ʃ/	shoe
				/ʒ/	beige
				/tʃ/	chew
				/dʒ/	jump
				/m/	my
				/n/	nice
				/ŋ/	thing
				/j/	yet
				/w/	wet
				/hw/ **	which
				/l/	low
				/r/	row

*Dependent on dialect; **becoming nonphonemic.

jaw positioning is related to tongue height—the lower the tongue in the oral cavity, the lower the mandible. Secondary vowel characteristics include tension of the speech musculature and lip rounding/unrounding. Tense vowels generally are longer in duration and are produced with more muscular tension as compared to lax vowels. Figure 2.8 illustrates approximate tongue positions for all vowels except the unstressed r-colored vowel /ɚ/ (Bloodstein, 1979). Table 2.5 describes additional characteristics of vowels. The features of voicing and **continuant**/noncontinuant need not be included because all vowels are voiced and continuant. All vowels, along with **diphthongs** and **semivowel** consonants, are further classified as **sonorants**. Thus, vowels may be described as having maxi-

mum vocal tract constriction toward the front, middle, or back of the mouth; with the tongue assuming positions of varying height (high, mid, or low); with lip positions ranging from neutral to rounded to retracted; with the speech muscles assuming varying degrees of tenseness and laxness; and with the lower jaw position ranging from near approximation (neutral position) with the upper jaw to moderately lowered. Conceptually, 14 vowels are placed on the vowel quadrilateral representing their articulatory placements relative to where the tongue is in closed approximation to the palate (Fig. 2.9). By definition, **cardinal vowels** include the high, mid, and low front and back vowels; they are also called *anchor* vowels (Edwards, 2003). A brief discussion of these 14 vowels follows.

TABLE 2.4

Frequency of Occurrence of All Phonemes

Overall Ranking	Vowels and Diphthongs			Consonants		
	Phoneme	Rank	%	Phoneme	Rank	%
1	/ə/	1	20.12			
2	/ɪ/	2	14.44			
3				/t/	1	12.77
4				/n/	2	11.46
5	/æ/	3	9.44			
6	/i/	4	8.49			
7				/r/	3	8.32
8				/l/	4	7.69
9				/s/	5	7.47
10	/ɑ/	5	6.99			
11	/ɛ/	6	6.85			
12				/d/	6	5.65
13	/aɪ/	7	5.50			
14	/o/	8	4.95			
15				/z/	7	4.90
16				/m/	8	4.74
17				/ð/	9	4.61
18				/k/	10	4.30
19	/ju/	9	4.0			
20	/e/	10	3.95			
21				/w, hw/	11	3.6
22				/b/	12	3.48
23				/h/	13	3.26
24				/v/	14	3.17
25	/ɚ/	11	2.90			
26	/ʌ/	12	2.87			
27				/f/	15	2.86
28				/p/	16	2.35
29.5	/aʊ/	13	2.20	/ŋ/	17	2.20
31				/j/	18	2.01
32.5	/ɔ/	14.5	2.00			
32.5	/ʊ/	14.5				
34	/u/	16	1.60			
35				/g/	19	1.57
36	/ɝ/	17	1.50			
37				/θ/	20	0.97
38				/ʃ/	21.5	0.88
39				/dʒ/	21.5	0.88
40				/tʃ/	23	0.63
41	/ɔɪ/	18	0.20			
42				/ʒ/	24	0.16

Source: Edwards, H. T. (2003) Applied phonetics: The sounds of American English. (3rd ed.) Clifton, NY: Delmar Learning.

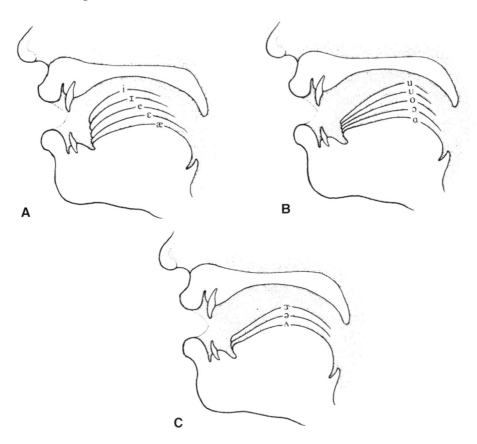

FIGURE 2.8 Approximate tongue positions for the vowels. **(A)** Front vowels. **(B)** Back vowels. **(C)** Central vowels. (Reprinted with permission from Bloodstein, O. (1979). Speech pathology: An introduction. Boston, MA: Houghton Mifflin)

> Which five vowels are identified as the front vowels and how do they differ from one another in their production?

Front Vowels /i/, /ɪ/, /e/, /ɛ/, and /æ/

/i/ as in *heat* is classified as a high front, tense vowel, being the highest tongue-positioned front vowel. It is sometimes called the *long e*. It is tense and produced with considerable tongue-hard palate constriction. The lips are slightly parted and unrounded or perhaps slightly retracted. The jaws are nearly in approximation. /i/ is considered a cardinal vowel because of the high front position on the vowel quadrilateral and may be diphthongized as /iɪ/or /iə/. It is generally acquired without difficulty.

/ɪ/ as in *hit*, the next highest tongue-positioned front vowel, is classified as a lower-high front, lax vowel and is sometimes referred to as the *capped-i* or *short-i*. The lips are unrounded or retracted and slightly parted. It is a lax vowel produced with constriction between the tongue and front part of the hard palate, and the jaw is lowered slightly. It is the second most frequently occurring vowel. Its production may be unstable in those with phonologic disorders (Stoel-Gammon & Herrington, 1990) and often presents a problem for persons learning English as a second language (Edwards, 2003).

/e/ as in *wait* is classified as a mid front, tense vowel and is produced with mid-high tongue position and somewhat parted and unrounded lips. It may be referred to as the *long a*. It is a tense front vowel that has less tongue-hard palate constriction and a lower jaw position than /ɪ/. It is considered a cardinal or anchor vowel for the mid-front position on the vowel quadrilateral. In American English, this sound tends to be diphthongized in stressed syllables as /eɪ/, which functions as an allophone of /e/ and thus is not phonemic. It is the least frequently occurring front vowel, but is typically acquired without difficulty.

TABLE 2.5

Features of Vowels

Place	Vowel	Articulatory Posture	Voicing	Tension	Duration	Constriction
Front of mouth (tongue shifted forward)	/i/	Tongue high, lips slightly parted	Yes	Tense	Long	Considerable
	/ɪ/	Tongue lower, lips parted more	Yes	Lax	Short	Considerable
	/e/	Tongue lower, lips parted more	Yes	Tense	Long	Some
	/ɛ/	Tongue lower, lips parted more	Yes	Lax	Short	Little
	/æ/	Tongue lowest, lips parted more	Yes	Lax	Short	Little
	/a/	Tongue low and slightly farther back, lips parted	Yes	Lax	Short	Little
Middle of mouth (central)	/ʌ/	Mid-tongue mid-high, lips parted	Yes	Tenser than /ə/	Long	Some
	/ə/	Mid-tongue mid-high, lips parted	Yes	Laxer than /ʌ/	Short	Some
	/ɝ/	Tongue retroflexed or "humped," lips rounded	Yes	Tense	Long	Considerable
	/ɚ/	Tongue retroflexed or "humped," lips rounded	Yes	Lax	Short	Considerable
Back of mouth (tongue shifted back)	/u/	Back of tongue high, lips rounded	Yes	Tense	Long	Considerable
	/ʊ/	Back of tongue lower, lips rounded	Yes	Lax	Short	Considerable
	/o/	Back of tongue lower, lips rounded	Yes	Tense	Long	Some
	/ɔ/	Back of tongue lower, lips rounded	Yes	Lax	Short	Little
	/ɑ/	Back of tongue lowest, lips parted	Yes	Lax	Short	Little
	/ɒ/	Back of tongue lowest, lips rounded	Yes	Lax	Short	Little

Adapted with permission from Weiss C. E, Lillywhite H. S. (1981). Communication disorders: A handbook for prevention and early intervention. (2nd ed. St. Louis, MO: Mosby.

/ɛ/ as in *bet* is classified as a low-mid front, lax vowel, sometimes referred to as *epsilon* or *short e*. Tongue and jaw positions are slightly lower than for /e/. The lips are parted a little more and are unrounded. It causes frequent difficulty for persons who are nonnative English learners and for some persons with severe phonologic disorders (Edwards, 2003).

/æ/ as in *bat* is classified as a low front, lax vowel produced with the tongue in the lowest position of all the front vowels. It is referred to as *ash*, *short a*, or *flat a*. The lips are parted considerably with no lip rounding or lip retraction. The jaw is lower than for the other front vowels such that the tongue seldom touches the upper teeth. It is one of the cardinal vowels, representing the low front position on the vowel quadrilateral. Its frequency of occurrence is third among all vowels and diphthongs. It presents a problem for some with severe phonologic disorders and for nonnative English speakers (Edwards, 2003).

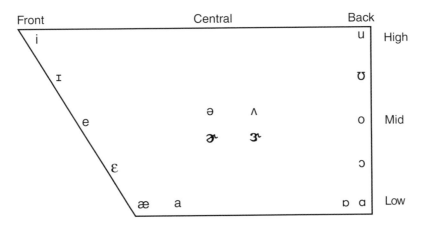

FIGURE 2.9 Vowel quadrilateral.

> What are considered the four central vowels and how are they differentiated from one another?

Central Vowels /ʌ/, /ə/, /ɝ/, and /ɚ/

Although there seems to be much variation in their production, the central vowels tend to be produced with the highest part of the tongue and the major vocal tract constriction occurring near the middle of the mouth, hence the name central vowel. Phoneticians typically include four central vowels in order to differentiate between the stressed and unstressed features (Edwards, 1986; Edwards, 2003; Small, 2005).

/ʌ/ as in *cup* has also been described as a back vowel by some phoneticians; however, it is typically classified as a mid-to-back central, lax vowel, although it is tenser than /ə/ (Edwards, 2003; Heffner, 1952). It is sometimes called the *caret, short u,* or *upside-down v*. Because it is the stressed counterpart of the neutral schwa /ə/ vowel, /ʌ/ appears only in stressed syllables in words. Maximum tongue-hard palate constriction is near the middle of the oral cavity, both vertically and horizontally. The tongue may be shifted back slightly, the lips are unrounded and apart, and the jaw is lowered a little for this sound. It seems to be less accurately produced than front and back vowels, according to Stoel-Gammon and Herrington (1990) and can be a confusing vowel for nonnative English speakers (Edwards, 2003).

/ə/ as in *about* is classified as a mid central, lax vowel. It has been the subject of disagreement among phoneticians because its features are not readily distinctive. This symbol represents the unstressed counterpart of /ʌ/ which occurs only in

unstressed syllables in words and is often referred to as *schwa* or the *neutral vowel*. It is of similar tongue height as its stressed counterpart, but has less muscle contraction in the tongue root. The lips are unrounded and parted somewhat, and the jaw is lowered slightly. It is the most commonly occurring vowel and sometimes causes difficulty for children with severe phonologic disorders and for nonnative English speakers (Edwards, 2003).

/ɝ/ as in *heard* is a mid central r-colored, tense vowel and is used only in stressed syllables. It is called the *stressed schwar,* the *reversed hooked epsilon,* or the *rhotic* or *r-colored vowel*. The sound is produced with great variability. Vertical tongue position is mid to mid-high, depending on the speaker and the speech context. The lips are slightly rounded and parted, and the jaw is lowered slightly. It is the symbol used in stressed syllables and should not be confused with consonant liquid /r/. It is misarticulated frequently by persons with phonologic disorders and can be problematic for nonnative English speakers.

/ɚ/ as in *better* is the unstressed counterpart of /ɝ/ and is thus classified as a mid central r-colored, lax vowel. A common label for /ɚ/ is *unstressed schwar* or *hooked schwar*. It is more lax than /ɝ/ and is produced with primary constriction of the vocal tract in the middle of the mouth, both horizontally and vertically. The lips are apart and slightly rounded, and the jaw is depressed slightly. This symbol is used only in unstressed syllables. It is produced almost identically as its stressed counterpart except with less tongue-root tension. Tongue position for articulating this sound and its stressed counterpart is retroflexed or bunched depending on the speaker and/or phonetic context (Wood, 1974). One point is certain: this vowel and the other two members of the /r/ family are among the most difficult sounds (both vowels and consonants) to learn, which accounts for their commonly being misarticulated by children and adults alike. Because of their frequency of occurrence, their misarticulation can cause a very conspicuous articulation deviation. Misarticulation is also difficult to correct in many persons.

Which vowels are considered back vowels and how are they different from one another in their production?

Back Vowels /u/, /ʊ/, /o/, /ɔ/, and /ɑ/

The last group of vowels, five in all, are those produced toward the back of the oral cavity, logically called the back vowels. They are generally produced by retracting the body of the tongue, which causes maximum linguapalatal constriction of the vocal tract toward the back of the mouth. With the exception of /ɑ/, the vowels are produced with lip rounding. As a group, they are the least frequently used of the vowels (Edwards, 2003).

/u/ as in *boot,* the highest tongue back position, is classified as a high back, tense, rounded vowel produced with the primary tongue-palate constriction high toward the back of the mouth. The tongue is raised toward the soft palate, the lips are rounded and narrowly parted, and the jaw is almost closed. It is a cardinal vowel, representing the high back position on the vowel quadrilateral. It is generally acquired without difficulty.

/ʊ/ as in *book* is produced with the tongue somewhat lower than for /u/, although it is still classified as a high back, lax, rounded vowel. It is referred to as *upsilon, capped-u,* or *flying u.* It is made with the lips apart and rounded, and the jaw is lowered slightly. It sometimes presents problems for persons with severe phonologic disorders and for nonnative English speakers (Edwards, 2003).

/o/ as in *boat* is a mid back, tense, rounded vowel. Vertical position of the tongue is near the middle and the jaw is lowered slightly more than for /ʊ/. It may be called the *long o* or the *closed o.* It is a cardinal vowel for the mid back position on the vowel quadrilateral. This vowel may be diphthongized as in /oʊ/ in some stressed syllables and, as such, functions as an allophone of /o/ and thus is not phonemic. It is generally acquired without difficulty.

/ɔ/ as in *bought* is a mid-low back, lax, rounded vowel, although some phoneticians characterize it as tense (Ladefoged, 2001; Small, 2005). It is sometimes called the *open-o or reversed c* vowel. The lips are apart, rounded, and protruded, and the jaw is lower than for the preceding back vowels.

Because of regional dialects, many American English speakers do not use this vowel, and consequently have difficulty discriminating it from other low back vowels (Edwards, 2003). It is easily acquired by children whose dialect uses it.

/ɑ/ as in *cot,* the lowest back vowel, is classified as a low back, lax (unrounded) vowel. The tongue is retracted and on the floor of the mouth. The jaw is lowered as much as for any other vowels, and the lips are widely parted and unrounded. Some phoneticians describe it as tense and others as lax (Edwards, 1986; Edwards, 2003; Ladefoged, 2001; Small, 2005). It is considered a cardinal vowel, representative of the low back position on the vowel quadrilateral. Speakers of some dialects use /ɑ/ instead of /ɔ/; thus, discriminating between this vowel and /ɔ/ can be challenging for some listeners. /ɒ/, the lip rounded version of /ɑ/, is used by speakers of some dialects, as is also the case for /a/, which is a low front vowel (slightly behind /æ/). Essentially /ɑ/, /ɒ/, and /a/ function as allophones.

What characterizes diphthongs in contrast to vowels?

Diphthongs

Features of four diphthongs are included in the following discussion (Fig. 2.10). Some phoneticians regard two others, /eɪ/ and /oʊ/, as distinctive diphthongs; however, because these are really allophonic variations of /e/ and /o/, we will not categorize them as separate diphthongs. Some phoneticians also consider vowel plus /r/ combinations to be diphthongs and transcribe them as **offglides** (/ɪɚ/, /ɔɚ/, /ɛɚ/ or /ɪɝ/, /ɔɝ/, /ɛɝ/, etc.) rather than as /ɪr/, /ɔr/, /ɛr/, and so on. Here, we are transcribing these combinations with the nonsyllabic /r/ when the combination represents one syllable, whereas /ɚ/ and /ɝ/ are used in combination with vowels when representing two syllables (for example, /haɪr/ for *hire,* and /haɪɚ/ for *higher*).

By definition, a diphthong is "two vowels produced consecutively in the same syllable by moving the articulators smoothly from the position of one to the other so that together they serve as the nucleus of the syllable" (Edwards, 2003, p. 369). Three of the diphthongs are considered offglides ("a transition from a vowel of longer duration to one of shorter duration"), and one is an **onglide** ("a transition from a preceding sound into a vowel of longer duration") (Edwards, 2003, p. 373). Physiologically, there is a shifting of articulator positions either upward or toward the back or

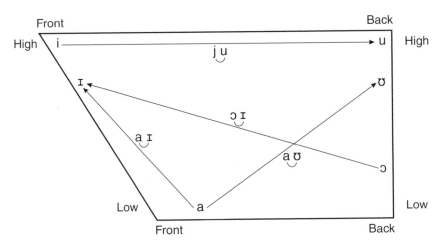

FIGURE 2.10   Vowel quadrilateral showing the placement of diphthongs.

front of the oral cavity, and phonetically they are symbolized by approximations of two-vowel phonemes (Fig. 2.10). All the diphthongs are typically acquired early and only present difficulty for children with severe phonologic disorders. With the possible exception of /ju/, the diphthongs are not challenging for nonnative English speakers (Edwards, 2003).

If vowels can be described as having resonance, then diphthongs can be described as having resonance shifts or changes resulting from a shift or adjustment of the vocal tract structures. Thus, all diphthongs are continuants and are of similar duration—relatively long. Two distinct vocal tract constrictions occur for each diphthong. The reader is cautioned that other publications may include other systems of classification and different terminology. Nevertheless, one should always be more concerned with the sound features and consideration thereof than with terminology. A brief discussion of the diphthongs follows.

> What two vowels comprise each of the three onglide English diphthongs?

Onglide Diphthongs /aɪ/, /aʊ/, and /ɔɪ/

/aɪ/ as in *pie* is an approximate combination of /a/ and /ɪ/; it is approximate because no diphthong is an exact replication of any two vowels. The tongue glides smoothly and quickly from a low, central (or front or back, depending on the phonetician) position to a high, front position, and the jaw moves from a moderately lowered position to a slightly more raised position producing a resonance change. Vocal tract

constriction occurs at two different places. The lips are unrounded. Because the tongue is raised from one position to another, this diphthong and all the other diphthongs produced by a raising of the tongue for the second part of the sound are called rising diphthongs. It is the most frequently occurring diphthong.

/aʊ/ as in *cow* is described as resembling a combination of /a/ and /ʊ/. The tongue shifts from a low, central (or front or back, depending on the phonetician) position to a high, back position. The lips move from a neutral position to a moderately rounded position, while the jaw moves from a wide open position to a nearly approximated position with the upper jaw.

/ɔɪ/ as in *toy* is a resonance change caused by articulator and vowel tract constriction shifts from a mid back vowel /ɔ/ to a high front vowel /ɪ/. The lips change from a slightly rounded position to a neutral position. The tongue moves upward and forward, and the jaw likewise moves upward for this rising diphthong. It is the least frequently occurring English vowel and diphthong and the next to last of all the sounds.

Offglide Diphthong /ju/

/ju/ as in *use* is the offglide diphthong. It is not a rising diphthong because the tongue moves from a high front position (/i/) to a high back position /u/. The lips move from a neutral or slightly retracted position to a rounded position, although some speakers round their lips during the production of the /j/ component. The jaw maintains a relatively stationary position.

> What categories are used for classifying consonants?

Consonants

Perhaps, with the possible exception of foreign dialects, the consonants are of more concern to the diagnostician and clinician of articulatory disorders than are the vowels and diphthongs. This is because most children and adults with articulatory/phonologic disorders have more difficulty with consonants than with vowels, with the sole exception of the stressed and unstressed "vocalic r" sounds /ɝ, ɚ/.

In this section, 25 consonants are discussed in terms of:

- Place of articulation (where the sound is made)
- Manner of articulation (how the sound is made)
- Laryngeal activity (vibration or no vibration of vocal folds)
- Degree of vocal tract constriction (amount of interruption of breath stream)
- Tension of speech musculature (whether muscles are relatively tense or lax).

Additionally, the developmental stage of acquisition for each consonant is generally characterized as:

- Early developing—3 to 4 years
- Middle developing—4.5 to 5.5 years
- Late developing—6 to 7 years.

Frequency of occurrence for consonants is shown in Table 2.4.

Consonants are sounds produced by partially or completely obstructing the vocal tract constriction that produces the syllabic pulses of speech. Consonants can be described as sounds produced by occluding (**stops** and affricates), diverting (nasals and laterals), obstructing (fricatives), and gliding articulator movements (glides) of the outgoing breath stream. An understanding of how each phoneme is made and how each one sounds is important in becoming a competent diagnostician and clinician of articulatory disorders. Understanding the movements required in producing speech sounds may also provide invaluable perceptual information to the clinician.

Some consonants are continuants, that is sounds that can be prolonged, and some are noncontinuants, that is sounds that cannot be prolonged. Stops and affricates are noncontinuants, while all other sounds, including vowels and diphthongs are continuant. Consonants can be divided into the two main categories of **obstruents** and sonorants. Obstruents are consonants produced with a completely or partially obstructed vocal tract; sonorants are sounds produced with a relatively open vocal tract, inclusive of vowels, diphthongs, and sonorant consonants. Sonorant consonants are further subdivided into the categories of **nasals**, which are sounds produced with

the air directed through the nasal cavity, and **approximants**, which include consonants that are produced with the airstream directed through the oral cavities with the articulators approaching one another, but not to the extent that air turbulence is produced. **Strident** is a subcategory that refers to obstruent consonants produced by "directing the airflow against a surface, such as the back of the upper teeth, so that considerable friction is produced" and includes some fricatives and the affricates (Edwards, 2003, p. 34). Sibilants, a subcategory of strident, include "hissing/hushing" sounds produced with mid- to high-frequency turbulence. In this book, the manner of consonants is categorized as follows:

- Stops—sounds produced with complete stoppage of the breath stream in the vocal tract with a buildup of air pressure behind the point of obstruction, sometimes with a sudden release of air pressure causing an explosive sound
- Fricatives—sounds produced with partial blockage of the breath stream forcing the airstream through a narrow channel with considerable intra-oral breath pressure causing turbulence or friction
- Affricates—sounds that begin as a stop and end as a fricative
- Nasals—sounds produced with a closed oral cavity and an open nasal cavity through which the airstream passes resulting in nasal resonance
- **Liquids**—generic term for /l/ and /r/, consonants that are produced with no friction
- **Glides**—sounds produced with a continued motion of the articulators providing a rapid transition to or from a vowel

Table 2.6 displays place, manner, and voicing features for the consonants.

What characterizes stop consonants and what are the place and voicing features of each of the six stops?

Stops /p/, /b/, /t/, /d/, /k/, /g/, (/ʔ/)

When producing stops, the airstream is completely obstructed momentarily in the vocal tract. The air is sometimes, though not always, released suddenly with an "explosion," thus stops are also called plosives and **stop-plosives**. All of these sounds are obstruents and noncontinuants.

/p/ as in *pal* is categorized as a **labial** (lip)—or more specifically **bilabial** (both lips)—voiceless stop that requires complete obstruction of the voiceless outgoing breath stream and muscular

TABLE 2.6

Traditional Phonetic Classification System of Consonants: Place, Manner, and Voicing Features

Place		Stop Voiceless	Stop Voiced	Fricative Voiceless	Fricative Voiced	Affricate Voiceless	Affricate Voiced	Nasal Voiceless	Nasal Voiced	Glide Voiceless	Glide Voiced	Liquid Voiceless	Liquid Voiced
Labial	Bilabial	/p/	/b/						/m/	/hw/	/w/		
	Labiodental			/f/*	/v/*								
Alveolar		/t/	/d/	/s/**	/z/**				/n/				/l/
Palatal	Alveopalatal					/tʃ/**	/dʒ/**						
	Linquapalatal (Postalveolar)			/ʃ/**	/ʒ/**						/j/		/r/
Dental (interdental or linguadental)				/θ/	/ð/								
Velar		/k/	/g/						/ŋ/				
Glottal		/ʔ/		/h/									

* Strident

**Strident and sibilant

tension, primarily of the closed lips. At the same time, the velopharyngeal port is also closed, enabling the breath stream to be trapped and built up inside the mouth without escaping through the nose before the lips are parted quickly to allow the release of the air. Depending on the phonetic context, this and other stops may be produced with aspiration (audible airflow), without aspiration (inaudible airflow), or without release (unreleased). It is released with aspiration—exploded—in initial word position and stressed syllables, unaspirated in **clusters**, e.g., /sp/, and often unreleased in word final position. For /p/, the jaw is slightly lowered and the tongue is in the neutral position when this sound is produced in **isolation**. In contextual speech, the tongue and jaw positions are influenced by preceding and subsequent sounds. All stops are noncontinuants; that is, they cannot be prolonged indefinitely (as can fricatives). This sound is early developing. /p/ and its **cognate** /b/ can be taught by actually holding the client's lips together while impounding the air and suddenly releasing them. A mirror can be useful in teaching these sounds.

/b/ as in *bat* is the voiced cognate of /p/ and thus is categorized as a labial voiced stop. It is produced similarly except the larynx is in vibration and is produced with less aspiration than its cognate. Similar to /p/, it is often unreleased in word final position and is an early developing sound.

/t/ as in *to* is an **alveolar sound**, or more specifically a **lingua-alveolar** (tongue tip-alveolar ridge), voiceless stop. It requires complete obstruction of the breath stream and muscular tension, primarily of the tongue. It is the most frequently occurring consonant sound in spoken English. As with most of the consonants, the velopharyngeal port is closed in varying degrees. This sound is made by momentarily holding the tip and blade of the tongue against the alveolar ridge with the lateral margins of the tongue contacting the contiguous teeth or alveolar ridge or both in order to impound the breath stream completely. Breath pressure thus is built up inside the mouth and suddenly released by quickly pulling the tongue tip and blade away from the alveolar ridge, producing the sound. The lips are in a neutral, slightly parted position, and the jaw usually is lowered a little as the sound is produced. As with the other voiceless stops, /t/ can be produced with aspiration, without aspiration, and unreleased, depending on the phonetic context. When in **intervocalic** position (between vowels), this sound may be produced as a **tap** (/ɾ/) or **flap** that seems to be a pronunciation somewhere between a /t/ and /d/. It is voiced and is

a rapid movement of the tongue tip to contact the alveolar ridge and is returned to the floor of the mouth along the same path (Ladefoged, 2001; Small, 2005). It is an early developing sound. A tongue depressor can be helpful in elevating the client's tongue tip for production of this sound and its cognate.

/d/ as in *do* is classified as an alveolar voiced stop and is the voiced cognate of /t/. It is made the same way except it requires vibration of the vocal folds. It also has more lax speech musculature producing less aspiration than its voiceless counterpart. This is quite typical for all voiceless stops. Similar to /t/, it is often unreleased in word final position and may be produced as a tap intervocalically. It is generally acquired early.

/k/ as in *cat* or *kite* is a **velar** or linguavelar (tongue-soft palate) voiceless stop that requires complete, momentary constriction of the vocal tract. It includes muscular tension and, of course, considerable aspiration. This sound is made with the back of the tongue sealing off the breath stream by contacting the soft palate, back molars, and posterior gum ridge. These movements are preceded by a closing of the velopharyngeal mechanism, which enables a buildup of air pressure behind this point of obstruction. The back of the tongue is then lowered suddenly to permit the rushing of air through the mouth and the accompanying release of the sound. The tip of the tongue and lips are apart and in a relatively neutral position. As with the other voiceless stops, /k/ can be produced with aspiration, without aspiration, and unreleased. This sound is acquired relatively early, but is misarticulated more frequently than the other voiceless stops. An effective way of teaching this sound and its cognate /g/ is to depress and stabilize the anterior part of the tongue with a tongue depressor or gloved finger, if you dare, while the client attempts to produce the sound with the posterior part of the tongue.

/g/ as in *go* is classified as a velar voiced stop and is the voiced cognate of /k/. It is made similarly except that the vocal folds are in vibration and the speech musculature is more lax, producing less aspiration. It is often unreleased in word final position and in some clusters. It is acquired relatively early and is misarticulated more frequently than the other two voiced stops.

/ʔ/ is a glottal voiceless stop consonant that is not a phoneme in American English, but is considered a phoneme by some non-American English speakers. It is mentioned here because sometimes it is used in American English. It is produced by momentarily stopping the breath stream at the level of the vocal folds, resulting in a buildup of air pressure below them. When the air is released, an audible noise occurs. This sound sometimes functions as an allophone for the phonemic stops and sometimes is used to release vowels in stressed syllables. Generally, it is considered a misarticulation when used as a substitute for another sound.

What characterizes the fricative consonants and what are the place and voicing characteristics of each of the nine fricatives?

Fricatives /f/, /v/, /θ/, /ð/, /h/, /s/, /z/, /ʃ/, and /ʒ/

Fricatives are phonemes having a distinct "friction" sound caused by the airstream passing through a narrow opening such that the breath stream is only partially blocked. With the exception of /θ/ and /ð/, these sounds are also classified as stridents, and the last four plus /tʃ/ and /dʒ/ comprise the subcategory of sibilants because of their "hissing" quality resulting from mid-to-high frequency air turbulence. All fricatives are continuants and obstruents.

/f/ as in *fun* is a labial, or more specifically **labiodental** (lip-teeth), voiceless fricative and a strident. The speech musculature is tense, and the degree of breath stream constriction is considerable. The tongue is in a neutral position, and the velopharyngeal mechanism is closed. The fricative is produced by closing the velopharyngeal port, lowering the jaw slightly, raising the lower lip and drawing its inner border backward against the cutting edges of the upper front teeth, and forcing air through this light constriction between the lower lip and upper teeth. The tongue is not involved in the articulation of this fricative. This sound is sometimes difficult to discriminate from /θ/ and /s/ because of its similar high frequency and low intensity components. It is an early developing sound. This sound and its cognate /v/ can be taught with the aid of a mirror. The Young and Hawk (1938) motokinesthetic approach of actually manipulating the articulators has been effective in teaching these two sounds.

/v/ as in *very* is a labial (labiodental) voiced fricative and is the voiced cognate of /f/. It differs in production in that it requires laryngeal activity and less tension and is produced with less airflow. Because these cognates are readily visible, they have certain advantages in remediation if they are misarticulated. This sound is mastered late in speech sound development and creates difficulty for persons with phonologic disorders and for nonnative English speakers (Edwards, 2003).

/θ/ as in *thin* is a **dental**, **interdental**, or **linguadental** (tongue-teeth) voiceless fricative. It is referred to as the *voiceless-TH-sound* or *theta*. The lips are in a parted, neutral position, and the sound is made by closing the velopharyngeal port, lowering the jaw slightly, lightly placing the flattened tip and blade of the tongue on the cutting edges of the upper front teeth between the upper and lower teeth, and forcing the breath stream through the space between the tongue and teeth. Some persons produce the sound by placing the front of the tongue on the back of the upper front teeth, creating air turbulence between the tongue blade and back of the teeth. Because it has the least intensity of all the speech sounds, it is difficult to perceive. This sound is late developing and often presents a challenge for those with phonologic disorders and for nonnative English speakers (Edwards, 2003).

/ð/ as in *this* is a dental voiced fricative that is the voiced cognate of /θ/. Its features differ only in voicing and more lax musculature. It is referred to as the *voiced-TH* or *eth* sound. Although it occurs more frequently than /θ/ and has more intensity, it is a difficult sound to perceive. As with /θ/, it is acquired late in speech development and presents difficulty for persons with phonologic disorders and those learning English as a second language (Edwards, 2003).

/h/ as in *high* is a glottal (larynx) voiceless fricative. It occurs only in word-initial and word-medial positions, not in word-final and syllable-final positions. The articulators are relatively inactive, except for the necessary postures for the sound to follow in contextual speech. This fricative is made by lowering the jaw slightly, closing the velopharyngeal mechanism, and forcing voiceless air through the slightly **adducted** glottis and tensed vocal tract until it produces an audible friction noise at the level of the glottis or in the oral cavity (Edwards, 2003). Because it is so influenced by sounds that immediately follow it in speech (assimilation), its features are difficult to specify. It usually is coarticulated with the vowel that it follows. It has no cognate and is an early developing sound that can present difficulties for some nonnative speakers (Edwards, 2003).

/s/ as in *say* and *cent* a strident and is the first of the four fricatives that are also sibilants (discussed later). It is described as an alveolar voiceless fricative having tense speech musculature and considerable vocal tract constriction. It is produced by closing the velopharyngeal port and placing the tongue blade and tip behind the upper front teeth (or, for some persons, with the tip down and behind the lower front teeth) near the alveolar ridge with the lateral margins contacting the contiguous teeth or gums or both. The tongue blade assumes a narrow groove at the midline necessary for producing a "hissing" sound. The lips are apart and neutral, and the lower jaw is almost in approximation with the upper jaw. The perceived sound is the result of the breath stream being forced through the narrow lingua-alveolar orifice and the cutting edges of the upper front teeth. This sound and its voiced cognate /z/ are important sounds in English because they occur frequently (fifth and seventh of the consonants) and because they serve important grammatic functions for plurals; possessives; and third person singular, present-tense verb morphemes (Edwards, 2003). Yet, it is a problem encountered frequently in the caseloads of speech-language pathologists. Furthermore, deciding when this sound has been articulated acceptably by a client is not always easy for the clinician; perhaps developing a clinical philosophy of relative acceptability for /s/ and /z/ might be more useful and realistic. /s/ can be taught by instructing the client to produce /t/ lightly and prolonging it. The final sound should approximate /s/; similarly, producing /d/ should approximate /z/. /s/ is acquired during the middle stages of speech development and typically is not problematic for nonnative English speakers.

/z/ as in *zoo* and *is* is an alveolar (lingua-alveolar) voiced fricative. It is classified as a strident and sibilant and is the voiced cognate of /s/. Its features differ in the voicing and more lax musculature. Clinicians quite commonly do not spend clinical time working on /z/ when both it and /s/ are misarticulated. Instead, some correct both sounds by working only on /s/. However, others have found that treatment is more efficient when both sounds are targeted simultaneously. It is a later developing sound and is frequently misarticulated by individuals with phonologic disorders.

/ʃ/ as in *shoe* and *sugar* is a **palatal**, postalveolar—or more specifically, linguapalatal (tongue-hard palate)—voiceless fricative and is classified as a strident and sibilant. It is called the *esh*, *stretched-S*, or the *SH* sound (Edwards, 2003). Some phoneticians use the symbol /š/, which is sometimes called *s wedge*. It is produced by closing the velopharyngeal port and elevating the flattened tip, blade, and body of the tongue so that the blade nearly touches the alveolar ridge. The sides of the tongue contact the contiguous teeth and gums of the hard palate, and the tongue is broadly grooved in such a way that the breath stream must pass centrally down the tongue and out of the mouth, rather than past the lateral margins of the tongue as in /l/. The tongue is grooved somewhat broader than for /s/, resembling placement for /tʃ/.

The jaw is lowered slightly, and the lips are typically rounded. This sound is the loudest of the sibilants and fricatives. /ʃ/ and its cognate /ʒ/ are commonly misarticulated in persons who also have an interdental or lateral lisp affecting /s/ and /z/. /ʃ/ can be taught by having the client assume the tongue position for /t/ and gently lowering the tongue tip from the alveolar ridge and prolonging the sound. Softly prolonging /d/ can be used as an approximation for teaching /ʒ/. The sound is acquired during the middle stages of development and causes difficulty for individuals with phonologic disorders, although typically not for nonnative English speakers (Edwards, 2003).

/ʒ/ as in *treasure* and *azure* is a palatal voiced fricative that is the voiced cognate of /ʃ/ and thus is also a strident and sibilant. It is sometimes referred to as the /ɛʒ/ *sound*. Some phoneticians transcribe it as /ž/ and refer to it as *z wedge*. It is produced similarly to its cognate except for voicing and laxer speech musculature. It is the least frequently occurring sound (Table 2.4) and never occurs in word-initial position in English. It is a later developing sound and causes difficulty for persons with phonologic disorders and nonnative English speakers (Edwards, 2003). However, it is seldom targeted in treatment because it occurs so infrequently in spoken American English.

> What characterizes the affricate consonants and what is the place and voicing features of each of the two affricates?

Affricates /tʃ/ and /dʒ/

The affricates are noncontinuant obstruent sounds that are also considered stridents and sibilants. Production of these sounds begins with a stop and ends with a fricative.

/tʃ/ (/č/) as in *chew* is a palatal (alveopalatal) voiceless affricate. When the /č/ symbol is used, it may be called the *c wedge*. It has been described as a blending of the voiceless lingua-alveolar stop-plosive /t/ and the voiceless palatal fricative /ʃ/. In addition to being an affricate, it is considered a noncontinuant strident and sibilant. Its production includes complete obstruction or constriction of the breath stream and tension of the speech musculature, mainly the tongue. The velopharyngeal mechanism is closed, and the lips are slightly rounded or neutral. During its production, the jaw is lowered slightly. This sound is made by obstructing the breath stream with the tongue tip and blade at the alveolar ridge similar to the production of /t/, except that the tongue is spread more widely. The margins of the tongue are in contact with the contiguous teeth and gums. The tongue is released by retracting and grooving it into the position of /ʃ/ rather than lowering it suddenly as in /t/, resulting in a combination of explosion and friction noise. /tʃ/ is a middle developing sound and presents difficulty for both children with phonologic disorders and nonnative English speakers (Edwards, 2003). Because of the physiological similarity between /ʃ/ and /tʃ/, clinicians commonly teach /tʃ/ by instructing the client to assume the position for /t/ and to relax and lower the very tip of the tongue. Another way of achieving /tʃ/ is to have the client position the tongue for /t/ while the clinician creates a groove on the tip of the client's tongue by pushing it down slightly with a toothpick. It can also be taught by having the client produce /t/ and /j/ in rapid succession.

/dʒ/ (/ĵ/) as in *just* and *angel* is a palatal (alveopalatal) voiced affricate and is the voiced cognate of /tʃ/. It is sometimes called the *j wedge* when transcribed as /ĵ/. It is made similarly except that the vocal folds are vibrating and the speech musculature is laxer, producing less aspiration. This sound may be described as a blending of the stop /d/ and the fricative /ʒ/. Similarly to /tʃ/, it is a middle developing sound and presents a problem for persons with phonologic disorders and nonnative English speakers (Edwards, 2003). This sound can be taught similarly as /tʃ/, except /d/ is used as the initial target position rather than /t/.

What characterizes the nasal consonants and what are the place features for each of the three nasals?

Nasals /m/, /n/, and /ŋ/

Nasals, along with liquids and glides are also called sonorants or semivowels. It should be noted that vowels and diphthongs are also considered sonorants. The three nasal consonants have in common the prominent features of resonance or vowel-like quality, complete oral tract obstruction, and nasal airflow. All of these nasals are continuants and voiced with no voiceless cognates. They also are assimilated frequently with vowels that are in juxtaposition. Resonance occurs in the nasal as well as in the oral and pharyngeal cavities during the production of nasal consonants. Nasals are sometimes **syllabic**; that is, they function as the nucleus of syllables.

/m/ as in *me* is featured as a labial (bilabial) voiced nasal. Obstruction of airflow through the oral cavity is complete, and the speech muscles are quite lax. This sound is made by occluding the lips, opening the velopharyngeal port, and emitting the vocalized breath stream through the nose. The tongue remains in a neutral position, and the jaw is lowered slightly. However, if one were to produce it by occluding the nose, the result would be an approximation of /b/. In fact, /m/ along with /p/ and /b/ can be taught by holding the lips together and providing visual feedback with the use of a mirror. /m/ is acquired early in speech development.

/n/ as in *no* is an alveolar (lingua-alveolar) voiced nasal. The degree of airflow obstruction through the oral cavity is complete, and the speech muscles are rather lax. This sound is made by placing the tongue tip and blade on the alveolar ridge with the lateral margins of the tongue contacting the contiguous teeth and the gums and providing complete obstruction of oral airflow. The velopharyngeal mechanism is open, the jaw is lowered slightly, and the lips are slightly parted and are in a neutral position. The vocalized breath stream passes through the nasal cavity. A tongue depressor for elevating the tongue tip and blade and a mirror for visual feedback can be helpful in teaching this very common sound. It is acquired early and is the second most frequently occurring consonant in spoken English.

/ŋ/ as in *sing* is categorized as a velar (linguavelar) voiced nasal and is called the *Eng*, *hooked n, engwa*, or the *engma* sound. The vocal tract is completely obstructed, and the speech muscles are lax. It is produced by elevating the posterior part of the tongue body against the soft palate, back molars, and posterior gum ridge and emitting the voiced breath stream through the nose. The jaw is lowered slightly, and the lips are in a neutral position. A sound resembling /g/ is made when producing /ŋ/ with the nose occluded. By holding the anterior part of the tongue down and pushing the body and posterior part of the tongue back, the clinician can usually assist the client in producing /ŋ/. In English, this sound does not occur in word-initial position, but only in word-medial and word-final positions. Although it is generally mastered later than /m/ and /n/, it is still an early developing sound.

What characterizes the glide consonants and what are the place and voice features for each of the three glides?

Glides /j/, /w/, and /hw/

Glides, along with the nasals and liquids, comprise the category of semivowels. Additionally, the glides and liquids comprise the category of approximants, which are "speech sounds that are produced with the articulators in close approximation but not to the extent that turbulence is created" (Edwards, 2003, p. 368). The acoustic properties of the glides are the result of the articulator movements toward or away from the target position, rather than the position itself; it is the movement pattern that distinguishes these phonemes. In English, the two glides are considered onglides. They are always **prevocalic**, occurring only in word-initial and word-medial positions. There are no voiceless cognates for the approximants.

/j/ as in *yes* is classified as a linguapalatal voiced glide requiring little breath stream constriction and muscular tension. It is sometimes called the *yod* or *yat* and is produced as the tongue tip and blade move or shift to the position of the subsequent vowel while the vocalized breath stream passes over the elevated tongue. The jaw also shifts to a lower position, depending on the subsequent sound in contextual speech, contributing to the perceptible change in resonance, similar to that of diphthongs. The lips are apart and in a neutral position, and the velopharyngeal mechanism is closed. The sound begins in a high front position resembling /i/. The sound can be taught by first having the client prolong /i/ while abruptly lowering the mandible and tongue. It is acquired early in speech development.

/w/ as in *we* is classified as a bilabial voiced glide requiring limited breath stream obstruction and speech muscle tension. It is made by closing the velopharyngeal mechanism, rounding and protruding the lips moderately, and emitting the vocalized breath stream between the rounded lips. The jaw is lowered slightly, and the tongue begins in a high back position similar to /u/ and moves into the position for the sound to follow. The diphthong-like resonance change occurs because of the movement of the lips and jaw. Helping the client purse the lips, along with providing visual feedback, has proved successful in teaching this early developing sound.

/hw/ as in *when* is a bilabial voiceless glide, but is rapidly becoming extinct in spoken English. Some phoneticians use the symbol /ʍ/ and refer to it as the *inverted W*. It can be considered a cognate of /w/, varying mainly in aspiration, tension, and unvoicing. Because it is rarely aspirated, it has been deleted in the items on most formal articulation tests. The nonaspirated /w/ appears largely to have replaced it in conversational speech. If clinicians elect to teach this sound, they can do so in a similar manner as teaching /w/ with the exception of increasing the amount of oral airflow.

How are the two liquid consonants produced?

Liquid /l and /r/

Phoneticians have come to categorize /l/ and /r/ as liquids, although the term does not describe their manner of production. These liquids are also members of the semivowel and approximant categories and some phoneticians classify them as glides (Edwards, 2003). They do not have voiceless cognates.

/l/ as in *life* is classified as an aveolar (lingua-alveolar) voiced liquid. It is sometimes referred to as a semivowel, **lateral**, or glide and is the only lateral in the English language. It can also function as the nucleus of a syllable and, as such, is indicated by /l̩/. It requires little breath stream constriction and muscular tension. It is produced by closing the velopharyngeal port and elevating and holding the tongue tip against the alveolar ridge with its lateral margins not in contact with the contiguous structures. Other tongue positions are also used in producing allophonic variations of /l/. The breath stream passes on either side of the elevated tongue tip to produce this lateral sound. The jaw is lowered slightly, and the lips are apart and in a neutral position. This continuant is highly variable in terms of its production. The /l/ family probably should be taught two different ways. The releasing /l/ requires harder lingua-alveolar contact and faster release than the arresting /l/. In teaching both forms of /l/, the clinician may choose to stabilize the jaw with a wedge and actually assist the tongue elevation of the client. Some speech-language pathologists recommend not teaching the arresting /l/ because of the difficulty of teaching it in this position, because omitting final /l/ generally does not affect intelligibility, and because it often seems not to be perceived as omitted by laypersons. /l/ develops during the middle stages of speech sound development and presents problems to individuals who have phonologic disorders and who are nonnative English speakers (Edwards, 2003).

/r/ as in *read* is a Palatal linguapalatal voiced liquid. Some phoneticians consider the /r/ to be a glide because, in a sense, it functions as an onglide and an offglide. It is part of the /r/ family and "is probably the most variable of the speech sounds, based on the way it functions in the various dialects" of English (Edwards, 2003, p. 202). It is the third most frequently occurring consonant and is made in a similar way as the /r/-colored vowels /ɝ/ and /ɚ/. This sound is produced by raising the tongue toward the hard palate, while the velopharyngeal port is closed. It can be produced in two different ways, either retroflexed or centrally bunched. A retroflex production entails raising the tongue tip and curling it back toward the alveolar ridge or front of the hard palate. In the bunched or "humped" production, the tongue tip is lowered and the tongue blade is raised toward the palate. The lips tend to be slightly rounded, and the jaw is lowered slightly. These postures will vary according to the sound context and the individual speaker (Wood, 1974). /r/ is acquired during the middle and late stages of speech development. This consonant is one of the most frequently misarticulated sounds in the English language as well as one of the most difficult to correct. Both tongue placements for producing /r/—that is "retroflexed" and "humped back"—should be attempted before determining which is easiest for an individual client. Because the contour, width, and movement of the tongue have to be very precise to produce an acceptable /r/, exploring these three dimensions with the client is often necessary before an acceptable /r/ is achieved.

> How does one describe phonemes by using a distinctive feature system in contrast to a phonetic system that classifies sounds according to manner, place, and voicing?

DISTINCTIVE FEATURE SYSTEM

Another way of describing sounds is to use a distinctive feature system. Distinctive features are characteristics of sounds that are smaller units than phonemes. Each characteristic or feature is considered on a binary basis, being either present or absent (specified as "+" or "−," respectively) in a given phoneme with each phoneme then being described as a "bundle of features." Thus, each phoneme has a unique set of distinctive features, with no two phonemes having an identical set of features. Several distinctive feature systems have been developed over the years (Chomsky & Halle, 1968; Halle, 1964; Jakobson, Fant, & Halle, 1952; Jakobson & Halle, 1956; Singh & Polen, 1972; Singh & Singh, 1972), but there is still disagreement concerning the best set of distinctive features that should be used, if any. The system developed by Chomsky and Halle (1968) seems to be more widely cited. The distinctive features in their system are listed in Table 2.7, along with a description of the "+" feature rather than for the "-" feature.

Tables 2.8 and 2.9 use Chomsky and Halle's (1968) system to show the distinctive features for English vowels and consonants. As an alternative, a distinctive feature system that uses more traditional phonetic categories is included in Appendix B. Such a system may be more useful to a speech-language pathologist in determining need for treatment and in devising treatment plans for persons with articulatory/phonologic disorders.

SPEECH ACOUSTICS, PERCEPTION, AND PRODUCTION

The acoustic aspect of speech science allows classification of vowels and consonants as well as identification of the special factors and features involved in speech perception. Most of the data on the acoustics of speech concern intensity levels of speech and their spectra (frequency components over time), yet the acoustic energy of speech is very small (Denes & Pinson, 1993). In fact, our vocal folds use only a fraction of the energy from the breath stream, or about one twentieth of 1%. This energy is dispersed in all directions and varies greatly within and between speakers. Thus, it is not surprising that the intensity of telephone conversations varies over a range of about 100 to 1 (from 75 to 55 dB). Even someone who speaks at a normal conversational level has approximately a 700-to-1 range of intensities between the weakest and strongest speech sounds. Intensity variations from quiet to normal to loud speech range from 45 to 85 dB. Different productions of the same sound vary even though the differences may be imperceptible.

Speech energy is generated at frequencies from roughly 50 to 10,000 Hz with the greatest energy being between 100 and 600 Hz. Vowels are the strongest sounds, generating the most energy. This is partly why they convey more meaning or intelligibility (understandability) than most consonants. The strongest vowel is /ɔ/ as in *bought*, and the weakest vowel is /i/ as in *be*. As a group, the liquids and glides are the most intense of the consonants. The strongest consonant is /w/ as in *weed*, which is 126 times as intense as the weakest consonant /θ/ as in *think*. This might provide a major reason why all the other sounds are easier to perceive than /θ/ (Edwards, 2003).

The spectrum of speech, which specifies the frequency and intensity of each component of the speech wave, is important to intelligibility. It is a major factor enabling persons to perceive sounds as being recognizably different. The most important features of the vowel spectrum are frequencies and amplitudes of the different **formants** (peak reso-

TABLE 2.7

Description of Distinctive Features Specified by Chomsky and Halle (1968)

+ Feature	Description	Phoneme Classes	− Feature
Vocalic	Voiced and constriction in oral cavity does not exceed that used for the high vowels /i/ and /u/	Vowels, liquids	Nonvocalic
Consonantal	Obstruction in the midline region of the vocal tract	All consonants *	Nonconsonantal
Sonorant	Relatively open vocal tract that facilitates voicing and resonation	Vowels, liquids, glides, nasals	Nonsonorant or obstruent
Rhotic **	Vowels with /r/ coloring	/ɚ, ɝ/	Nonrhotic
Advanced **	Forward positioning of the tongue used in some diphthongs	/aɪ , aʊ/	Nonadvanced
Front **	Body of the tongue anterior to neutral position for vowels	Front vowels	Nonfront
Coronal (Acute)	Tongue blade raised above its neutral position /ə/	Dental, alveolar, and palatal consonants	Noncoronal (grave)
Anterior (Compact)	Obstruction located in front of the alveopalatal region used for /ʃ/	Labial, dental, and alveolar consonants	Nonanterior (diffuse)
High	Body of the tongue raised above its neutral position for /ə/	High vowels, velars, glides, sibilants	Nonhigh
Low	Body of the tongue lowered below its neutral position for /ə/	Low vowels, /h/	Nonlow
Back	Body of the tongue retracted from its neutral position for /ə/	Back vowels, velars, /w/	Nonback
Rounded	Lips are pursed	Back vowels except /ɑ/, /r/, /w/	Nonrounded
Distributed	Constriction extended for a considerable distance in vocal tract	Glides, affricates, /ʃ, ʒ/	Nondistributed
Nasal	Lowered velum with airstream passing through the nasal cavity	Nasal consonants	Nonnasal
Lateral	Lowered side(s) of midsection of the tongue allowing airstream to flow over the sides of the tongue	/l/	Nonlateral
Continuant	Incomplete constriction of airstream so airflow is not blocked through the oral cavity	Fricative, liquid, and glide consonants	Noncontinuant or stop
Tense	Considerable muscular contraction in root of the tongue	High and mid front and back vowels, /ʌ, ɝ/, voiceless consonants, /l, dʒ/	Nontense or lax
Voiced	Vocal folds vibrate	Vowels, voiced consonants	Nonvoiced or voiceless
Strident	Noisiness resulting from airflow against a surface or partial closure	Sibilants and labiodentals	Nonstrident

* Chomsky & Halle considered /h/, /w/, and /j/ nonconsonantal.

** Feature not proposed by Chomsky & Halle (1968), but rather by Edwards (2003) to differentiate among English vowels.

TABLE 2.8

Distinctive Features for Vowels of American English Specified by Chamsky and Halle (1968)

Features	Front					Central				Back				
	i	ɪ	e	ɛ	æ	ʌ	ə	ɝ	ɚ	ɑ	ɔ	o	ʊ	u
Vocalic	+	+	+	+	+	+	+	+	+	+	+	+	+	+
Consonantal	−	−	−	−	−	−	−	−	−	−	−	−	−	−
Sonorant	+	+	+	+	+	+	+	+	+	+	+	+	+	+
Rhotic	−	−	−	−	−	−	−	+	+	−	−	−	−	−
Advanced	−	−	−	−	−	−	−	−	−	−	−	−	−	−
Front *	+	+	+	+	+	−	−	−	−	−	−	−	−	−
High	+	+	−	−	−	−	−	−	−	−	−	−	+	+
Low	−	−	−	−	+	−	−	−	−	+	−	−	−	−
Back	−	−	−	−	−	−	−	−	−	+	+	+	+	+
Rounded	−	−	−	−	−	−	−	+	+	−	+	+	+	+
Tense	+	−	+	−	−	+	−	+	−	−	−	+	−	+
Voiced	+	+	+	+	+	+	+	+	+	+	+	+	+	+

* Feature proposed by Edwards (2003), but not used by Chomsky & Halle (1968).

nant frequencies). Analysis of these resonances and peaks has shown that speech is a continuously varying process and that the acoustic characteristics of speech vary with time (Denes and Pinson, 1993). These aspects of speech science certainly help one appreciate the dynamics of speech.

The chain of events that results in oral communication has been succinctly described by Denes and Pinson (1993):

> The movements of the vocal organs generate a speech sound wave that travels through the air between speaker and listener. Pressure changes at the ear activate the listener's hearing mechanism and produce nerve impulses that travel along the acoustic nerve to the listener's brain. In the listener's brain a considerable amount of nerve activity is already taking place, and this activity is modified by the nerve impulses arriving from the ear. This modification of brain activity, in ways we do not fully understand, brings about recognition of the speaker's message. We see, therefore, that speech communication consists of events linking the speaker's brain with the listener's brain. (pp. 3–4)

Denes and Pinson further remind us that, in a speaker–listener situation, there really are two listeners, not one, because the speaker is also engaged in self-listening while speaking.

Closely related to the acoustics of speech is speech perception. Several theories of speech perception have been postulated, one of which is the motor theory of speech perception. According to this theory, the listener perceives speech by matching the incoming signal against an internally generated signal resulting from subconsciously articulating the incoming speech sounds. However, this theory does not necessarily imply that the same neural mechanisms that control speech production also control speech perception; it also does not seem to explain all the facts of speech perception.

To transmit a thought orally, the speaker begins by selecting appropriate words and sentences (semantic level). Thus, oral communication begins with the occurrence of neural and muscular activity (physiologic level) and is terminated by the speaker with the generation and transmission of a sound wave (physical or acoustic level). This process is reversed by the listener. How the message is interpreted by the listener depends on several factors, including acoustic and nonacoustic input. First, the spectrum of the speech sound wave influences the perception of the incoming speech signals, including periodic (tonal) or aperiodic (noisy) sound waves, frequency components and their intensity, formant frequencies, formant transitions, duration of certain speech sound segments, and intensity of

TABLE 2.9

Distinctive Features for Consonants of American English (Chomsky & Halle, 1968)

Feature	Stops/Affricates								Fricatives									Nasals, Liquids, and Glides						
	p	b	t	d	k	g	tʃ	dʒ	f	v	θ	ð	s	z	ʃ	ʒ	h	m	n	ŋ	l	r	w	j
Vocalic	−	−	−	−	−	−	−	−	−	−	−	−	−	−	−	−	−	−	−	−	+	+	−	−
Consonantal	+	+	+	+	+	+	+	+	+	+	+	+	+	+	+	+	+	+	+	+	+	+	+	+
Sonorant	−	−	−	−	−	−	−	−	−	−	−	−	−	−	−	−	−	+	+	+	+	+	+	+
Coronal	−	−	+	+	−	−	+	+	−	−	+	+	+	+	+	+	−	−	+	−	+	+	−	−
Anterior	+	+	+	+	−	−	−	−	+	+	+	+	+	+	−	−	−	+	+	−	+	−	−	−
High	−	−	−	−	+	+	+	+	−	−	−	−	−	−	+	+	−	−	−	+	−	−	+	+
Low	−	−	−	−	−	−	−	−	−	−	−	−	−	−	−	−	+	−	−	−	−	−	−	−
Back	−	−	−	−	+	+	−	−	−	−	−	−	−	−	−	−	−	−	−	+	−	−	+	−
Rounded	−	−	−	−	−	−	−	−	−	−	−	−	−	−	−	−	−	−	−	−	−	−	+	−
Distributed	−	−	−	−	−	−	+	+	−	−	−	−	−	−	+	+	−	−	−	+	−	−	−	+
Nasal	−	−	−	−	−	−	−	−	−	−	−	−	−	−	−	−	−	+	+	+	−	−	−	−
Lateral	−	−	−	−	−	−	−	−	−	−	−	−	−	−	−	−	−	−	−	−	+	−	−	−
Continuant	−	−	−	−	−	−	−	−	+	+	+	+	+	+	+	+	+	−	−	−	+	+	+	+
Tense	+	−	+	−	+	−	+	−	+	−	+	−	+	−	+	−	−	−	−	−	−	−	−	−
Voiced	−	+	−	+	−	+	−	+	−	+	−	+	−	+	−	+	−	+	+	+	+	+	+	+
Strident	−	−	−	−	−	−	+	+	+	+	−	−	+	+	+	+	−	−	−	−	−	−	−	−
	p	b	t	d	k	g	tʃ	dʒ	f	v	θ	ð	s	z	ʃ	ʒ	h	m	n	ŋ	l	r	w	j

the signal (Denes & Pinson, 1993). Nonacoustic features that contribute to perception include type of phonology, vocabulary, syntax, prosodic features, and pragmatics used, as well as the context in which the speech signal is delivered (such as who is the speaker, what is the topic or environmental setting, etc.).

The many phonetic combinations found in contextual speech challenge one's understanding of these perceptual and productive phenomena of articulation. Each phonetic context has its unique perceptual and productive characteristics. Each speaker has unique articulators that result in much variability in the spectra of the speech produced. Realizing such a huge number of communication variations is almost incomprehensible. Yet, speech-language pathologists have somehow been remarkably successful in teaching clients acceptable articulation perception and production. And just how have they accomplished such commendable feats? One can only speculate, but they probably taught auditory discrimination, auditory memory, auditory conceptualization and other cognitive skills, self-monitoring skills, articulator placements, articulator movements, and other attending and imitative skills usually in a hierarchical order of difficulty and with ample appropriate **reinforcement**.

Although not all the data are in concerning how humans produce and perceive phonemes, enough clinical and scientific information is available to assist anyone who desires a better understanding of how articulation occurs. Before reviewing the information, one should remember several points. First, different persons prefer different ways of learning. Some prefer the auditory modality, some prefer the visual modality, some prefer auditory and visual modalities, and some prefer to learn experientially (and perhaps some prefer not to learn at all). Finding the preferred learning modality will help the clinician achieve success in treatment. Second, some individuals have comparatively sluggish motor coordination skills that nonetheless are within normal limits. Compensation and modification may need to be considered for them, such as talking a little slower or with less precision. Third, the articulators themselves are highly individualistic. Tongues of some persons seem relatively small in comparison with the size of their oral cavities. Some palates are high and narrow, and some are low and wide. Some teeth are quite large, long, and crowded; others are small, short, and spaced. These structural variations may be significant in some individuals just as functional variations may be. As an example, how can a person with

a slightly restricted lingual frenulum easily produce a retroflexed /r/? Might not a centrally elevated tongue body be a more desirable way of achieving an acceptable /r/? Fourth, what is the overall learning potential of certain individuals? Some learn rapidly, some less rapidly, and some have limited learning potential. Still others grasp the cognitive aspects of phoneme production but have difficulty carrying out the motoric movements. Fifth, closely allied with learning potential is motivation for learning. All clinicians have probably worked with potentially gifted clients who "couldn't care less" about mastering articulation. Unless clients can be motivated, acceptable articulation may never occur. These are some of the considerations underlying articulatory acquisition, but undoubtedly there are others.

To accomplish phoneme production of /z/, for example, the individual has to engage the anterior and supplemental communication centers that instruct the larynx, tongue, velopharyngeal muscles, and jaw to assume their proper positions. These motor impulses course down the motor pathway to the brain stem where they trigger cranial nerve nuclei of cranial nerves V, VII, VIII, IX, X, XI, and XII located at the base of the brain. Impulses traverse the respective cranial nerve pathways until they reach their destination—the articulators they innervate. These impulses activate the articulators to move into their correct positions for the production of /z/. Instantaneously, kinesthetic impulses from the movements of the articulators are sent to the base of the brain then to the posterior communication center for interpretation. In addition, the auditory impulses from the friction noise produced by the air flowing over the tongue go up through the bones of the face and skull, through part of the hearing mechanism, and to the posterior communication center. This is generally how an isolated phoneme is produced and perceived. Imagine the multiplicity of nerve impulses coursing to and from the respective communication centers during contextual speech. Fortunately, a speaker does not have to monitor consciously all of these neural activities and articulator movements. It seems that only when a phoneme, word, or sentence is misproduced does the conscious feedback or monitoring system become activated. In articulation acquisition, the complex functions of overlapping movements, ballistic movements, multiple articulation, and discrimination processing are not directly taught, at least not as discrete entities. Nevertheless, they somehow are learned by most individuals, perhaps in part through practice in hearing themselves and others speaking.

Finally, all of these neurologic, motoric, cognitive, and sensory activities are influenced additionally by the physical and psychological health of the individual. What other variables come into play when the speaker feels ill, exhausted, or depressed? Conversely, what happens to articulation when one is feeling exceptionally healthy, energetic, or elated? Or what happens to one's articulation when the emotional content abruptly changes? The factors that affect articulation are many and varied, but for normal articulation to develop, the following characteristics should be present:

1. All articulators are structurally normal.
2. Innervation of the articulators is intact.
3. Sensory feedback, including tactile, kinesthetic, and auditory, is normal.
4. The articulators are capable of functioning in a coordinated manner.
5. The articulators function in a cosmetically acceptable manner.
6. Ample motivation is present.
7. A sufficient number of articulation opportunities exist.
8. Articulation efforts are positively reinforced.

SUMMARY

Respiration, phonation, resonation, and articulation constitute the primary processes involved in speech production. Through the neurological system, these processes must interact and interrelate in a synergistic manner for normal speech to occur. Although speech production and perception place greater demands on some of these processes than on others, all systems must be basically intact for speech to develop and be used intelligibly. Respiration, if adequate for sustaining life, usually will provide an adequate energy source for setting the vocal folds into vibration and for transmitting their vibrations. Normal phonation requires normal functioning of the vocal folds, which includes normal laryngeal structures, innervation, and aero-dynamic function. Resonance relies on selective filtering or modification of the vocal tract cavities. These cavity configurations, along with the tonus of their walls, modify the laryngeal buzz into usually acceptable voice quality. Articulation, the last major process, includes the modification of the vocal tract through a partial or complete interruption of the flow of breath to produce the distinctively different sounds in the English language. These four processes work together with the innervation systems to mediate speech and, therefore, can be considered the anatomy and physiology of the speech mechanism.

The speech mechanism is used to produce phones. Speakers and listeners identify the phones as distinctive speech sounds or phonemes. Speakers produce allophones or variant forms of phonemes, depending on their phonetic context and dialect. The movable and immovable articulators are used to produce approximately 50 distinct phonemes in American English, including vowels, diphthongs, and consonants. Vowels are produced with an unobstructed vocal tract. Differing tongue positions are used to make the different vowels that are categorized as front, central, and back vowels. Diphthongs are a combination of two vowels made in rapid succession. Consonants are sounds produced with a partially or completely obstructed vocal tract. Traditionally, they are categorized by three parameters: (a) manner, (b) place, and (c) voicing. Speech sounds can also be described using a distinctive feature system in which each phoneme has a distinct bundle of features. There is much variability from speaker to speaker, phonetic context to phonetic context, and dialect to dialect in the way speech sounds are produced. When sounds are spoken, a speech sound wave is produced with certain acoustic features that can be displayed as sound spectra. In addition to nonacoustic features, this acoustic output allows the listener, and the speaker, to interpret the speech that is produced. In addition to the background information of anatomy and physiology of the speech mechanism and of the phonetic system for English speech sounds, the ways in which speech is acquired will be explored next.

REVIEW QUESTIONS

1. In what way is articulation an "overlaid" function? How might this affect articulation?

2. Identify and define the four basic speech processes. What anatomic structures are involved in each process? What two other bodily systems are involved in speech production?

3. Relate the need for an understanding of anatomy and physiology of speech to diagnosis and treatment of disordered articulation and phonology.

4. Which cranial nerves are involved directly in speech production and what roles do they play? What component of speech production would a lesion in each of these cranial nerves affect? What primary role do the spinal nerves play in speech production?

5. Where in the neurological system does the breakdown occur for apraxia of speech? For dysarthria?

6. Which bodily structures are the movable articulators? Which ones are the immovable articulators? Which is the most active and important articulator?

7. Define the following terms: phone, phoneme, allophone, and morpheme.

8. Compare and contrast the characteristics of vowels, diphthongs, and consonants.

9. What two primary characteristics describe American English vowels? What other characteristics are specified?

10. Fill in the vowels on a vowel quadrilateral. Which ones are the cardinal vowels?

11. What three primary phonetic characteristics traditionally describe consonants?

12. Describe the following manners of production for consonants: stop, fricative, affricate, nasal, glide, liquid, obstruent, sonorant, approximate, lateral, strident, sibilant, continuant, noncontinuant.

13. Describe the following place features for consonants: labial, alveolar, dental, palatal, velar, glottal.

14. What is the difference between a voiced and voiceless sound?

15. What are the two most frequently occurring vowels and diphthongs? The least frequently occurring? What are the two most frequently occurring consonants? The least frequently occurring?

16. Describe a distinctive feature system for speech sounds.

17. What is the most intense speech sound? The least intense?

CHAPTER 3

Phonological System and Development

"Hold fast the form of sound words."
—First Epistle to Timothy

CHAPTER OBJECTIVES

- Differentiate between the phonetic (motor) and linguistic (phonological) components of the sound system.
- Briefly describe phonological acquisition theories characterized as behaviorist, structuralist, generative phonology, natural phonology, nonlinear phonology, and optimality.
- Characterize the phonological system in terms of the phonemic inventory,

phonotactics, allophonic variations, and morphophonemics.
- Categorize and describe phonological deviations or processes.
- Describe the general stages of phonological development of children.
- Specify the general order of acquisition of consonants, vowels, word forms, and speech sound patterns.

Phonology is the study of the sound system of language and, as such, is considered a major component of language, along with **morphology** (word form), **syntax** (word order), **semantics** (word meaning), and **pragmatics** (functional usage). Phonology encompasses the formation or articulation of speech sounds as well as the linguistic knowledge of the sound system and sound patterns (Edwards & Shriberg, 1983). Often, the articulation part of phonology is referred to as the phonetic, motor, or mechanical component of speech production. It comprises the speech sounds that are produced, heard, and perceived as the result of movements of the articulators. On the other hand, the linguistic component of phonology is the formulation of sound sequences based on knowledge of the phonological system of our language that

involves knowing which phonemes are meaningful and using the rules of how these phonemes can be combined to form words.

Phonologic disorders affect both components described above; that is, the effect occurs at the articulation or phonetic level involving mastery of the motor ability and at the linguistic or phonological level involving the organizational aspects of the sound system. Speech-language pathologists need to be prepared to evaluate and intervene with phonologic/articulatory disorders at both of these levels.

What elements must a phonological acquisition theory explain for it to be considered adequate?

PHONOLOGICAL ACQUISITION THEORIES

Several theories of phonological acquisition have been devised over the years. This section highlights some of them and provides background knowledge about phonology. As specified by Stoel-Gammon (1991), a theory of phonological development must account for the following seven requirements to be considered adequate (p. 17):

- Account for the body of factual information gathered about phonological acquisition. To meet this requirement, the theory must account for *general patterns* as well as *individual differences* observed in order of acquisition of speech sounds, use of phonological strategies, and occurrence of phonological processes.
- Account for changes over time, including those that result in loss of a phonemic contrast and/or a decrease in phonetic accuracy and those that establish new phonemic contrasts and/or increase phonetic inaccuracy.
- Explain the role of input and account for the relationship between prelinguistic (babbling, for example) and linguistic development.
- Account for *phonetic* as well as *phonological* learning and be able to explain the mismatches that often occur between the two.
- Be consistent with one's understanding of speech perception and account for the relationship between perception and production in phonological acquisition.
- Be compatible with other theories of cognitive and general linguistic development and general learning theories.
- Make testable predictions regarding patterns of acquisition, error types, and possible individual differences.

No current theory is completely adequate to explain phonological development, although each theory does account for some required aspects. Generally, there are six major phonological acquisition theories with variations on the theme in each of the types of theories. Keeping other possibilities in mind, phonological theories can be categorized as:

- Behaviorist
- Structuralist
- Generative phonology
- Natural phonology
- Nonlinear phonology
- Optimality

These six types are briefly described in the sections that follow.

> Briefly characterize the behaviorist theory of phonological acquisition. Who were the developers of the theory?

Behaviorist Theory

Behaviorist theories (Mowrer, 1952; Olmstead, 1966, 1971) emphasize the role of reinforcement in speech acquisition (Ferguson & Garnica, 1975; Stoel-Gammon, 1991). Behaviorist theory necessitates the occurrence of imitating, practicing, experiencing, conditioning, and reinforcing behavior. Inherent in this theory is the need to communicate, with the child attending to and identifying with the caretaker. The process starts with the vocalizations of the caretaker being associated with primary reinforcers, including food, comfortable environmental conditions, and other things provided to meet the child's basic needs. Then, the child's own vocalizations become positively reinforcing to the child because of their similarity to the caretaker's vocalizations. The sounds produced more like the caretakers are selectively reinforced extrinsically by others and internally by the child.

> Briefly characterize the structuralist theory of phonological acquisition? Who was the early developer of the theory?

Structuralist Theory

The structuralist theorists (Jakobson, 1968, 1971; Jakobson & Halle, 1968 in Ferguson & Garnica, 1975) have postulated that universals exist in the acquisition of language in which the phonological development and systems of all languages are similar. They also contend that an invariant and innate order of stages of phonemic development in the learning of all languages exists, however the rate of progression through the stages of development is individual and variable. These universals apply to children and various languages as well as to aphasia in which the breakdown of the sound system proceeds in stages going in the opposite order to phonological development in children. Parenthetically, the latter contention regarding aphasia subsequently has not been borne out by empirical research (Ferguson & Garnica, 1975).

The sequence of stages is based on oppositions of sound classes or sound feature contrasts rather than on individual sounds. As the developing system becomes more complex, more sound contrasts occur. Phonemic development begins with the labial stage, in which vowel acquisition begins with a wide vowel (usually /ɑ/) and an anterior labial stop (usually /p/). Thus, the first contrast is between vowels and consonants. The next stage involves adding a nasal sound that contrasts to the oral stop for a nasal–oral contrast followed by a labial–alveolar contrast. Phonological development continues with the addition of sounds, such as fricatives, affricates, liquids, and velars, that provide contrasts to the existing system.

Another characteristic of the structuralist theory developed by Jakobson is that babbling and meaningful speech are distinct and independent, which means there is no relationship between babbling and speech—the concept of discontinuity theory (Ferguson & Garnica, 1975; Stoel-Gammon, 1991). However, researchers are accumulating data that do not support this hypothesis, but rather support the notion that **canonical babbling** and the first words uttered share many commonalities (Oller, 1980; Oller, Eilers, Bull, & Carney, 1985; Stoel-Gammon & Otomo, 1986; Vihman, Macken, Miller, Simmons, & Miller, 1985). It is thus likely that babbling is important in the acquisition of an adult phonological system. This latter contention is strongly supported by Kent (1990) who stated that production of canonical syllables during the babbling stage is significantly prognostic for later speech development.

Briefly characterize the generative phonology theory of phonological acquisition? Who were the developers of the theory?

Generative Phonology Theory

Generative phonology theory, most often associated with Chomsky and Halle (1968), posits that there is an explicit set of distinctive features from which phonemes are generated (Ferguson & Garnica, 1975). The underlying representation of a phoneme is its distinctive features. Various linguists have proposed several sets of features, and no consensus on a universal set exists.

In this theory, phonological rules are applied to the underlying representations to form the surface representations, a process called derivation. Phonological rules connect the knowledge component with the production component and convert underlying representations or the deep structure of a language to derive surface

structures. The rules specify the sound segments that change, how they change, and the conditions under which they change. Said another way, phonological rules describe what the underlying form (form that is not actually uttered) is, what form the speaker actually says (surface form) rather than the underlying form, and under what conditions the speaker produces the surface form. Phonologists write phonologic rules in the form of A → B / C_D that reads "input" or representation of one or more features (A) "becomes" (→) "output" (B) "in the context of" (/) "the phonetic environment" C_D). In other words, some representation of one or more features undergoes a change in some context (Ingram, 1997). According to Creaghead and Newman (1989), "the goal in writing a linguistic rule is to make it as general as possible so that it will cover the largest number of actual utterances while excluding those cases that do not fit the rule" (p. 30). Thus, these rules describe how the surface form is derived from the underlying form. AQ1

Another aspect of the generative approach is rule ordering, which means that "when two or more phonological rules exist, they have a fixed order in which they must be applied" (Ingram, 1997, p. 12). A last general concept of the generative theory is markedness, which refers to the characterization of phonological naturalness. Generally, speech sounds that are unmarked or less marked are those that are acquired earlier and occur in more languages of the world, whereas marked sounds are those that are acquired later and occur less frequently in different languages. For example, voiced obstruents are said to be more marked than voiceless obstruents. AQ2

The order of distinctive feature acquisition has been of recent research interest. For example, five levels of development were characterized by Dinnsen (1992) as follows:

- Level A—Inclusion of only vowels, glides, obstruent stops, and nasals with no voicing or manner distinction for obstruents and no non-nasal sonorants
- Level B—Addition of voice distinction among the obstruents, including voiced and voiceless stops
- Level C—Addition of fricatives and/or affricates
- Level D—Addition of one liquid (either /l/ or /r/)
- Level E—Inclusion of all sound classes and an extended distinction in either or both classes of liquids or obstruents

According to Dinnsen, this order of sound acquisition is applicable to both normal and disordered phonological systems.

Briefly characterize the natural phonology theory of phonological acquisition? Who was the early developer of the theory?

Briefly characterize the nonlinear phonology theory of phonological acquisition?

Natural Phonology Theory

The premise of the theory of natural phonology, introduced by Stampe (1969, 1979; Donegan & Stampe, 1979), is that the sound patterns of language "are governed by natural forces in human systems of vocalization and **auditory perception**" (Grunwell, 1997, p. 37). Rather than acquiring a phonological system, children begin with a set of innate and universal processes and learn to suppress those that do not occur in their home language (Stoel-Gammon, 1991). Said another way, children develop their speech sound system by modifying their innate or "natural" system of phonological processes as a response to listening to speakers of their language. According to Stampe (1979), "a phonological process is a mental operation that applies in speech to substitute, for a class of sounds or sound sequences presenting a common difficulty to the speech capacity of the individual, an alternative class identical but lacking in the difficult property" (p. 1). The idea is that children are limited physiologically in their ability to produce some sounds and thus use phonological substitutions, omitting sound features that are difficult to produce. When learning to talk, children attempt to match their pronunciations to the adult model but tend to simplify their speech sound productions. They change the innate phonological processes to match the adult form. As they develop, the innate system is modified gradually to develop into the adult system as they suppress, limit, and reorder phonological processes.

According to Edwards and Shriberg (1983), "some segments, sound classes, consonant and vowel systems, types of syllables and rules and processes are more natural than others" (p. 87). The more natural ones are those that are learned sooner by children and that appear in more languages. They give the examples that the most common or natural vowel system is /i,ɑ,u/, the most natural stop system is /p,t, k/, and the most common syllable type is CV (consonant followed by a vowel). A natural phonological process is defined as "a systematic sound change affecting an entire class of sounds or sound sequence . . . . Natural processes are generally said to be phonetically motivated—due to articulatory, perceptual, or acoustic factors, and to involve the simplification of a more complex articulation" (p. 91). Specific phonological processes or deviations are described in a later section of this chapter.

Nonlinear Phonology Theory

Nonlinear theory encompasses theories termed prosodic, autosegmental, metrical, and underspecification (Bernhardt & Stoel-Gammon, 1994, 1997). In this approach to describing phonological acquisition, separate levels of representation or tiers for various prosodic and segmental units are organized hierarchically. An example from Bernhardt and Stoel-Gammon appears in Figure 3.1, which shows word, foot, syllable, onset-rime, skeletal, and segmental (phoneme) tiers for the word *monkey*. In this case, the skeletal tier is a way to link the prosodic and segmental levels. In the nonlinear approach, segments composed of features are organized hierarchically rather than merely as bundles of features. Figure 3.2 from Bernhardt and Stoel-Gammon illustrates the hierarchical features (geometry) of the English phonemes. At this point, it is not important that the diagrams be understood fully. Rather, the diagrams are presented here to illustrate the concept of the hierarchical arrangement of varying levels of speech sounds as well as the proposed hierarchy of the features of phonemes.

Underspecification is a concept featured in nonlinear theory. "During speech production processing, some feature content is automatically supplied for output because of built-in redundancies in the phonological system" (Bernhardt & Stoel-Gammon, 1997, p. 165). These features are also said to be predictable; that is, to be the default. For example, in English, +sonorant implies +voice because all sonorants in English are voiced. Consequently, +voice is not specified in the underlying representation of nasals, glides, liquids, and vowels, and voicing is said to be the default when producing sonorants. On the other hand, +voice or -voice must be specified for the stops, fricatives, and affricates because English speakers produce voiced and voiceless obstruents. In these sounds, -voice is considered the default or underspecified feature and +voice is the nondefault or specified feature. Further, theorists propose that -continuant is the default feature for consonants and thus is the underspecified feature, whereas +continuant needs to be specified because it is the nondefault feature. The same phenomenon is true for place of articulation, which in nonlinear theories includes dorsal (velar), labial, and coronal articulation placements. According to Bernhardt and Stoel-Gammon, coronal (+anterior) is the default

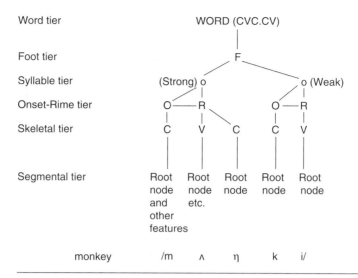

Word tier	WORD (CVC.CV)
Foot tier	F
Syllable tier	(Strong) o o (Weak)
Onset-Rime tier	O—R O—R
Skeletal tier	C V C C V
Segmental tier	Root node and other features Root node etc. Root node Root node Root node

monkey   /m   ʌ   ŋ   k   i/

FIGURE 3.1 Representation of the word *monkey* from the word level to the Root node link on the segmental tier. (From Bernhardt B., & Stoel-Gammon C. (1994). Nonlinear phonology: Introduction and clinical application. *Journal of Speech and Hearing Research 37,* 127. Copyright 1994 by American Speech–Language–Hearing Association. Reprinted with permission.)

Key: F = Foot. This is composed of a strong and weak syllable.
        o = Syllable
        O = Onset. This included all prevocalic consonants (C) in a syllable.
        R = Rhyme/Rime. This includes the vowel (V) and postvocalic
            consonants in a syllable.

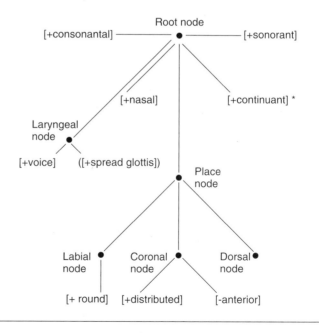

FIGURE 3.2 Feature geometry for English consonant system. (From Bernhardt B., & Stoel-Gammon C. (1994). Nonlinear phonology: Introduction and clinical application. *Journal of Speech and Hearing Research 37,* 127. Copyright 1994 by American Speech–Language–Hearing Association. Reprinted with permission.)

Note: Specified features are indicated with plus or minus values.
Labial, Coronal, and Dorsal nodes are considered monovalent; that is, to have only a plus value when present.
* Affricates are defined with branching structure of the feature [continuant]; that is, they have both a [-continuant] (stop) and [+continuant] (fricative) value.

(underspecified or predicted) place, whereas coronal (-anterior), labial, and dorsal are the specified or nondefault features. Generally, as children develop speech, they begin by producing the underspecified segment elements from the other tiers and gradually add specified features until the adult phonological system is acquired. For example, the default for syllable structure, one of the tiers in the hierarchy of units, is CV, whereas other syllable structures (e.g., CVC and CCVC) must be specified before appearing in speech production.

So far, specified and underspecified features have been described as though they were universal or language-specific. However, it is hypothesized that child-specific defaults exist as well. While it seems that most children (even those with disordered phonological development) tend to produce stops and nasals earlier than fricatives and liquids, there is more variability in the order of development of place features, with some children preferring labials and others having velars as a default rather than the universally expected coronal preference (Bernhardt & Stoel-Gammon, 1997).

> Briefly characterize the optimality theory of phonological acquisition?

Optimality Theory

Optimality theory represents the most contemporary group of theories being advanced and is aligned with connectionist theory put forth in cognitive psychology (Barlow & Gierut, 1999). As with other types of theories, the optimality approach posits that input (underlying representations) and output representations (surface structure) exist. With this approach, the speech is characterized both from a relational and independent framework, which is not true of the natural phonology approach that focuses on a relational analysis of the child's speech.

In optimality theory, constraints generate surface (output) representations, not rules. A constraint is defined as "a limit on what constitutes a possible pronunciation of a word" (Stemberger & Bernhardt, 1997, p. 211). Some constraints are more important than others and thus are ranked higher; others are not as important and sometimes can be ignored or violated. Each potential output is evaluated by all constraints at once, and the output that violates the fewest high-ranked constraints will be chosen as the optimal (or best) production of the word. Put another way, "the *optimal* pronunciation of the word does not violate the very

important constraints; it violates the least important constraints" (p. 215). Constraints are ranked, and the ranking differs in different languages and in different children. Two types of constraints are ranked: (1) faithfulness constraints ensure that output resembles input, and (2) output constraints specify that the output may not contain something or must contain something (Stemberger & Bernhardt). It should be noted that Barlow and Gierut (1999) described the second constraint slightly differently and identified the second type as markedness constraints that specify that output forms must be unmarked in structure. Nonetheless, these two types of constraints often are antagonistic or in opposition to one another. The rank order of constraints is denoted by » with the constraint to the left being more important than the constraint to the right. An example provided by Stemberger and Bernhardt (1997) for a child who uses coronals for velars is:

> Not(Dorsal) » Survived (Dorsal) » Not(Labial) » Not(Coronal)

The lowest-ranked constraint is not to use a coronal, whereas the highest-ranked constraint is not to use a dorsal; therefore, coronals are used in the production of words that contain velars (dorsals) in the input—the adult underlying form. It is theorized that, early in phonological development, markedness (or output) constraints are ranked higher than faithfulness; but, with maturation, faithfulness becomes higher ranked and thus, the adult sound system is gradually acquired (Barlow & Gierut, 1999).

None of the theories fully accounts for all aspects of phonological development, and the principles of each overlap with one another and are not mutually exclusive. Some of the theories stress the innate capacities of the speech learners, some focus on the external input and influences, and some incorporate both internal and outside factors. It is probable that acquisition of the sound system requires innate knowledge or capacity and external input from persons in the environment.

> What features describe the phonetic aspect of the phonological system? What features describe the phonological aspects?

PHONOLOGICAL SYSTEM

Phonology is concerned with all aspects of the system and production of speech sounds. The difference between two levels of analyses, that is, phonetic and phonological, was clearly described by Stoel-Gammon and Dunn (1985). Phonetic analysis of a sound system encompasses three aspects: (1) articulation or the way sounds are formed by the speech mechanism, (2) acoustic or physical components, and (3) psychological or the way sounds are perceived by the listener. The phonetic aspects of the sound system were described in Chapter 2. Phonological analysis of a sound system involves four aspects: (1) inventory of the phonemes in a particular language, (2) description of the patterns of the use of these phonemes, (3) description of the phonemes as produced in various phonetic contexts or the allophonic variations, and (4) description of morphophonemic alternation changes in sound patterns. These four components are presented in more detail below.

What is the phonemic inventory of a language?

Phonemic Inventory

A phoneme is a family of sounds perceived to be the same speech sound, and when a phoneme is changed, the meaning of the word is different. Each language has a unique set or inventory of phonemes with differing numbers of sounds. As children develop the phonological system of their language, they learn the sounds that are part of the language and have meaning to speakers and listeners of that language. In the case of English, depending on the phonologist or phonetician, there are approximately 14 vowels, 4 diphthongs, and 25 consonants. Other languages have different numbers of sound units, as well as different inventories of distinctive phonemes.

Define phonotactics and give examples of English phonotactic rules.

Phonotactics

Phonotactics refers to the rules for how sounds can be combined to formulate syllables and words (Edwards & Shriberg, 1983). For example, in English /ŋ/ does not occur in the initial position of words and the cluster of /tl/ does not occur as a blend at the beginning of syllables. Edwards and Shriberg provided the examples that, in English, as many as three consonants can release a syllable

and up to four can arrest a syllable so that the longest syllable possible in English is CCCVC-CCC as in the word *strengths* (/strɛŋkθs/). They further stated that the restrictions of phonemic combinations within a syllable do not necessarily apply to sequence restrictions between syllables in a word. For example, although /gm/ does not occur within a syllable, it can occur in abutting syllables within a word as in *pragmatic* (/prægmætɪk/). As these examples demonstrate, English and other languages place restrictions on where certain sounds can appear, on the possible combinations of sounds, on the number of consonants that can be combined in the initial and final positions of syllables, and on the possible order of the occurrence of the sounds. These rules involve the concept of patterning, which refers to the phenomenon that sounds with similar phonetic features in a given language follow the same patterns of usage and have similar allophones. As an example in English, the three voiceless stops (/p, t, k/) are all aspirated in the word-initial position before a stressed vowel.

What is meant by allophonic variations?

Allophonic Variations

An allophone is a variant of a phoneme that does not change the meaning. The most common example is the use of aspirated stop consonants in the initial position of syllables but unaspirated or unreleased stop consonants in the final position of syllables. English speakers identify these two forms as the same sound even though they are articulated slightly differently. The /t/ phoneme is aspirated in word-initial positions as in *top* and often unaspirated in word final position as in *pot*. Both forms of /t/ are perceived by English speakers as the /t/ sound.

Define morphophonemics and provide some examples as to how it affects sound usage.

Morphophonemics

Morphophonemics refers to the change in the sound structure of morphemes, the smallest units of meaning. Morphophonemic rules specify how sounds are produced in combinations of

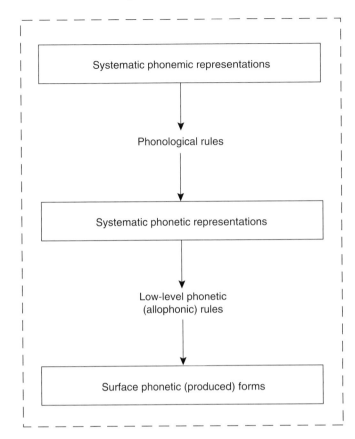

FIGURE 3.3 An expanded schematic representation of the phonological component of generative-transformational grammar. The level designated as the systematic phonemic level is said to be similar to the Bloomfieldian morphophonemic level. (From Edwards M. L., & Shriberg, L. (1983). *Phonology applications in communicative disorders (p. 72).* San Diego: CA: College-Hill Press. Reprinted with permission of original author.)

morphemes. For example, a rule specifies the way in which plural forms are to be produced such as /s/ in *cats*, /z/ in *bags*, and /əz/ in *dresses*. Figure 3.3 is a schemata illustrating the components of phonology as visualized and described by Edwards and Shriberg (1983).

> What are phonological processes or deviations?

PHONOLOGICAL PROCESSES OR DEVIATIONS

Important concepts for understanding phonological development (described in the next section of this chapter) are **phonological processes** or deviations. They involve speech sound patterns that differ from the way in which adult speakers of a language pronounce words and are used by children (and persons with phonologic disorders) as they develop their speech. These patterns are referred to as phonological processes or deviations, and they describe the differences or alterations between the sounds actually produced and the sounds present in

the adult standard production of words. The terms phonological processes and deviations are used interchangeably throughout this book. The concept of phonological processes has its roots in natural phonology theory, although many clinicians use it as a basis for describing how children simplify their productions of adult forms. Usually, these deviations simplify the sound production and are systematic modifications of a class of sounds or sound sequences. Another way of stating this is the spoken form deviates from the underlying or basic form and usually is easier to produce than the adult or target form. An example of a process is **stopping**, which is the substitution of stop consonants for nonstop sounds as in /tʌn/ for *sun*. Speech-language pathologists working with individuals who are phonologically disordered need to determine the phonological deviations used by individual clients that result in atypical phonological or articulation patterns. This analysis leads to the planning and implementing of effective intervention programs.

As mentioned earlier, most phonological deviations simplify the adult form, with the assumption that a basic form is the underlying phonological representation. A process changes the form, resulting in

TABLE 3.1

Categories and Examples of Phonological Deviations or Processes

	Categories of Phonological Deviations (Processes)		
Syllable Structure	Harmony or Assimilation	Feature Contrast or Substitution	Other
Syllable deletion (reduction) Example: /lɪdl̩/ → /lɪl/	Consonant assimilation labial Example: /bɔl/ → /bɔb/ velar - Ex: /tek/ → /kek/ alveolar - Ex: /tek/ → /tet/ nasal Example: /mus/ → /mun/	Fronting Example: /gʊd/ → /dʊd/	Articulation shifts Example: /θʌm/ → /fʌm/ Example: frontal lisp Example: lateral lisp
Final consonant deletion Example: /tɑp/ → /tɑ/		Backing Example: /ti/ → /ki/	
Coalescence Example: /sket/ → /tet/		Affrication Example: /ʃit/ → /tʃit/	Idiosyncratic
Epenthesis Example: /dɪg/ → /dɪgə/	Voicing prevocalic voicing Example: /ponɪ/ → /bonɪ/	Deaffrication Example: /pitʃ/ → /pit/	
Diminutization Example: /dɑl/ → /dɑli/	postvocalic devoicing Example: /dɔg/ → /dɔk/ prevocalic devoicing Example: /bɔɪ/ → /pɔɪ/	Palatalization Example: /sop/ → /ʃop/	
Doubling Example: /dɔg/ → /dɔdɔ/	postvocalic voicing Example: /pʌp/ → /pʌb/	Depalatalization Example: /mætʃ/ → /mæts/	
Glottal replacement Example: /bʊk/ → /bʊʔ/	Syllable reduplication Example: /pʌdl̩/ → /pʌpʌ/	Gliding Example: /ræt/ → /wæt/	
Metathesis Example: /bæskət/ → /bæksət/		Vowelization (vocalization) Example: /dɔr/ → /dɔʊ/	
Migration Example: /stɪk/ → /tɪks/		Denasalization Example: /noz/ → /doz/	
		Neutralization Example: using /d/ for all consonants	

a modified form that is the surface form or phonetic representation (Edwards & Shriberg, 1983). In other words, the basic form is the adult standard and the surface form is the sound pattern produced by the child or client. Various classification systems of phonological deviations or processes have been devised, but they share commonalities (Hodson, 2004; Hodson & Paden, 1991; Ingram, 1989; Khan, 1985; Lowe, 1994; Shriberg & Kwiatkowski, 1980; Weiner, 1979). The following classification system consolidates several others and divides phonological processes into four categories: (a) syllable structure, (b) assimilation or harmony, (3) feature contrast or substitution, and (d) other (Table 3.1).

> Define syllable structure phonological deviations. Identify and describe the phonological deviations of this type.

Syllable Structure

Syllable structure deviations are changes in the consonant/vowel (CV) makeup of the syllables of standard adult word forms. The modifications tend to go toward a CV construction. The number and/or sequence of vowels and consonants in the surface form differ from that in the adult standard form of the target word. For example, if the word *probably* (/prɑbəbli/) is pronounced as /prɑbli/, the CV makeup is changed from CCVCVCCV to CCVCCV, and thus the CV structure of the syllable has been changed. This is the case for all the types of syllable structure deviations described here. The four most common syllable structure processes are (a) **weak syllable deletion**, (b) **cluster reduction**, (c) deletion of final consonants, and (d) **glottal replacement** (Weiner, 1979). These and other syllable structure deviations are described below. It is important to note that all of these processes, except glottal replacement, **migration**, **metathesis**, and initial consonant deletion, have been noted in the speech of typically developing children and are thus considered developmental phonological processes.

Syllable Deletion

Syllable deletion, sometimes referred to as syllable omission or syllable reduction, occurs when one or more syllables of a multisyllabic word is omitted. Two examples are saying /tɛ fon/ for *telephone* and /laɪn/ for *lion*. In these cases, the CV structure changes respectively from CVCVCVC to CVCVC and CVVC to CVC. A subtype is weak syllable deletion that describes omission of an unstressed syllable in a multisyllabic word. This deviation is also referred to as unstressed syllable deletion. Examples are /teto/ for *potato* and /nɑnɑ/ for *banana*. In both of these cases, the CV structure is changed from CVCVCV to CVCV. Syllable deletion typically occurs during the first 50-word stage of expressive language development. It should be noted that weak syllable deletion is a speech sound pattern that continues to be used by adult speakers of a language and is usually not an appropriate target for speech treatment of either children or adults. However, targeting two- and three-syllable words is appropriate for children with phonologic disorders who almost exclusively use one-syllable words.

Final Consonant Deletion

Final consonant deletion or omission of final consonants occurs when the final **singleton** consonant in a word or syllable is omitted. This deviation sometimes is referred to as open syllable. Examples include /bo/ for *boat* and /mɑ/ for *mop*. In these two examples, the CV makeup of the words is changed from CVC to CV.

Initial Consonant Deletion

Initial consonant deletion or omission of initial consonants occurs when the initial singleton consonant in a word or syllable is omitted. Examples include /ot/ for *coat* and /e/ for *say*. In these examples, the CV makeup of the words is changed from CVC to VC and CV to V, respectively. Initial consonant deletion is considered an atypical or nondevelopmental phonological deviation.

Cluster Reduction

A cluster is defined in this book as two or more abutting consonants, regardless of whether the consonants appear in the same syllable or in two different syllables. Thus, the term *cluster* is more inclusive than the term **blend**, which refers to two or more abutting consonants appearing in the same syllable. To avoid confusion, some phonologists (Hodson, 2004; Hodson & Paden, 1991) prefer to use the term *consonant sequence omission* rather than cluster reduction, contending that it is a more inclusive term because they define cluster as two contiguous consonants in the same syllable. However, not all phonologists place this restriction on the term *cluster* (e.g., Bankson & Bernthal, 1990a, 1990b; Khan & Lewis, 2002). Cluster reduction is the deviation in which one or more consonants comprising a consonant cluster is omitted. The deleted consonant can be a sonorant or an obstruent. Examples are /tet/ for *skate* and /bek/ for *break*. In these two cases, the CV structure is changed from CCVC to CVC. When all consonants in a cluster are omitted, the deviation may be labeled cluster omission as in /in/ for *green*.

Coalescence

Coalescence has been described in two different ways. First, this deviation has been characterized as the replacement of two consonants with a different consonant that contains phonetic features of the two target consonants of a cluster (Hodson, 2004; Hodson & Paden, 1991). Examples include /fok/ for *smoke* in which /f/ has the stridency feature of /s/ and the labialness of /m/, and /ten/ for *plane* in which the /t/ has the alveolar placement of the /l/ and the stop manner of the /p/. In both examples, the syllable structure changed from CCVC to CVC.

The term *coalescence* has also been applied to syllables of multisyllabic words such that a speaker produces a multisyllabic word with fewer syllables than the underlying form with segments from both syllables being retained (Khan, 1982). Examples provided by Khan include /mɛn/ for *melon*, which contains /mɛ/ from the first syllable and /n/ from the second syllable, and /ræʃ/ for *radish*, which contains /ræ/ from the first syllable and /ʃ/ from the second syllable. Both types of coalescence result in a change in the structure of the syllable. The first type, coalescence of consonants of a cluster, is also a form of cluster reduction; the second type, coalescence of syllables, is a form of syllable deletion.

Epenthesis

Epenthesis refers to the addition of a sound to a word. The addition is often a vowel, often /ə/, although consonants are sometimes added as well. Added vowels commonly occur between two consonants of a consonant cluster and after a final voiced stop. An example of the first case is /bəlæk/ for *black*, and of the second case, /mʌdə/ for *mud*. The syllable structure changes from CCVC to CVCVCV and CVC to CVCV, respectively. Sometimes, it seems that the latter case results from articulatory intervention in which a final voiced stop is targeted. An example of adding a consonant is /fwʌn/ for *fun* with the syllable structure changed from CVC to CCVC. Adding a consonant to form a cluster generally is an atypical or nondevelopmental pattern.

Diminutization

Diminutization is the deviation of adding an /i/ or /ɪ/ or consonant plus /i/ or /ɪ/ to the end of a word. The resulting word is considered an immature speech pattern ("baby talk") and typically occurs during the first 50-word stage of language development. This pattern is also a form of epenthesis. Examples include /hæti/ for *hat* and /dɑgi/ for *dog*.

Doubling

Doubling is a deviation described by Stoel-Gammon and Dunn (1985) as repeating a word, usually a monosyllabic word, resulting in a multisyllabic word. Examples of doubling are /bɑbɑ/ for *ball* and /bæbæ/ for *bad* in which the syllable structure is changed from CVC to CVCV. This deviation is also a form of epenthesis. Although different, this deviation is similar to the process of **reduplication**, which can occur in multisyllabic words. It is categorized as a harmony or assimilation process and is described next.

Glottal Replacement

Glottal replacement is the process of substituting a glottal stop for a consonant. This deviation can be classified as a feature contrast or substitution pattern. However, a glottal stop is not a meaningful or distinctive phoneme in the English language or most dialects and thus is treated as an omission for purposes of classification as to deviation type. Weiner (1979) hypothesized that it serves as a marker for an omitted consonant. Research has not shown this deviation to occur frequently in the speech of the typically developing child (Khan, 1982). It should be noted that /ʔ/ is a distinctive phoneme in some other languages and a few English dialects. Use of glottal stop by American English speakers is not considered a typical deviation, but rather an atypical or nondevelopmental one. This deviation occurs with some frequency in children with cleft palate as they attempt to stop the airflow before it reaches the oral and nasal cavities or as a substitution for sounds they are unable to produce. Examples of glottal replacements are /fɪʔɪŋ/ for *fishing* and /bæʔ/ for *bath*.

Metathesis

Metathesis is the pattern of transposing or reversing consonants in a word. Although the CV structure of the word does not change per se, the sequence of the consonants changes, thus, it is regarded in this book as a syllable structure deviation. Frequently cited examples include /æmɪnʊl/ for *animal* and /ɛfələnt/ for *elephant*. This pattern is atypical or nondevelopmental and occasionally is used by persons with apraxia of speech.

Migration

Migration involves the movement of a phoneme from one position in the word to another position. Examples include /puns/ for *spoon* with the /s/ moving to the end of the word and /pəsgɛtɪ/ for *spaghetti* with the /s/ sound moving from the beginning of the first syllable of the word to the end of the first syllable. In the first example, the syllable structure changes from CCVC to CVCC and from CCVCVCV to CVCCVCV in the second example. This deviation is atypical or nondevelopmental, sometimes occurring in persons with apraxia of speech.

Define assimilation or harmony phonological deviations. Identify and describe the phonological deviations that are of this type.

Assimilation or Harmony Deviations

The second major category of phonological deviations is assimilation or **harmony** deviations in which a sound or syllable is changed to become more similar to another sound or syllable in the word. Thus, in these deviations, the sounds or syllables of a word become more alike. The influence of one sound or syllable upon other sounds or syllables in a word can be from left to right or from right to left. **Progressive assimilation** occurs when a sound in a word is influenced by a preceding sound; that is, a later sound in the word is changed. **Regressive assimilation** occurs when a sound is influenced by a later sound so that an earlier sound in the word is changed. Assimilation can be contiguous (influencing sound is adjacent to the changed sound) or noncontiguous (influencing sound is not next to the changed sound). Assimilation occurs even when the influencing phoneme is omitted in the production (Hodson, 2004; Hodson & Paden, 1991). Several types of assimilation appear in the speech of children that can be classified as consonant, voicing, and syllable assimilation or harmony. Most of these deviations have been noted in children who are developing speech normally. Throughout this book, the terms *harmony* and *assimilation* are used interchangeably when referring to phonological deviations.

Consonant Assimilation or Consonant Harmony

Various forms of consonant assimilation occur in progressive and regressive forms, including labial assimilation, velar assimilation, alveolar assimilation, and nasal assimilation. Labial assimilation occurs when a nonlabial sound is changed to a labial in the presence of a labial sound either preceding or following the affected consonant in the adult standard production of the word. An example of progressive labial assimilation is /bop/ for *boat* and of regressive labial assimilation is /wʌm/ for *thumb*. Velar assimilation occurs when a nonvelar consonant is replaced by a velar consonant in the environment of a velar consonant in the target word. An example of progressive velar assimilation is /koŋ/ for *comb* and of regressive velar assimilation, /gɔgi/ for *doggie*. Alveolar assimilation refers to the case when a nonalveolar sound is changed to an alveolar consonant in the presence of an alveolar sound in the adult standard production of the word. Examples of progressive and regressive alveolar assimilation are /dɔdi/ for *doggie* and /tæt/ for *cat*, respectively. If a child produces /tæ i/ for *candy*, alveolar assimilation is being used even though the alveolars of /n/ and /d/ are omitted in the surface form. Nasal assimilation occurs when a nonnasal sound is replaced by a nasal sound in the presence of a nasal sound in the target word. An example of progressive nasal assimilation is /non/ for *nose* and of regressive nasal assimilation is /nʌni/ for *sunny*. These are the most frequently reported types of consonant assimilation in terms of place and manner of articulation. However, other types of manner harmony also occur, including stop assimilation and fricative assimilation, which operate in a similar way as the assimilation deviations just described (Weiner, 1979).

Voicing Assimilation or Harmony

Voicing deviations are not always considered assimilation processes, but rather are simply categorized as voicing phonological deviations. The authors of this book, however, have chosen to consider them assimilation processes. Two types of voicing assimilation are commonly reported, including prevocalic voicing and final consonant devoicing. Prevocalic voicing refers to voicing an unvoiced consonant when it precedes a vowel. What seems to be happening is the voicing of the vowel influences the voicing feature of the preceding consonant. Examples include /bɪg/ for *pig* and /dæg/ for *tag*. Voicing errors occur in blends as well. An illustration is producing /gwim/ for *cream*. **Postvocalic** devoicing is changing a voiced obstruent at the end of a word to a voiceless obstruent. It is hypothesized that this occurs because of the silence following the word and thus is an assimilation of the silence (Ingram, 1989). Reportedly, it is the most frequent type of voicing alteration occurring in adults and developing children often in conjunction with a slight vowel prolongation (Hodson, 2004; Hodson & Paden, 1991). Examples include /pɪk/ for *pig* and /bis/ for *bees*.

The other two possibilities of voicing errors, such as prevocalic devoicing and postvocalic voicing, occur infrequently and are considered atypical or nondevelopmental patterns. Prevocalic devoicing is the deviation in which a voiced consonant sound that precedes a vowel is changed to a voiceless consonant, theoretically because of the influence of the silence following the preceding word. Examples include /pin/ for *bean* and /tet/ for *date*. Similarly, postvocalic voicing occurs when a voiceless sound following a vowel is produced as a voiced sound, presumably influenced by the preceding voiced vowel. This is the rarest form of voicing alteration (Hodson & Paden, 1991). Saying /piz/ for *peace* and /bæg/ for *back* are two illustrations of postvocalic voicing.

Syllable Harmony or Assimilation

Reduplication is a syllable harmony or assimilation deviation in which all or part of a syllable is repeated. Reduplication can occur in complete and partial forms. Examples of complete reduplication are /wɑwɑ/ for *water* and /bɑbɑ/ for *bottle*. Examples of partial reduplication include /dɑdɪ/ for *doggie* and /nudu/ for *noodle*. This deviation tends to occur in the speech of young children who have an expressive vocabulary of 50 or fewer words.

Define feature contrast or substitution phonological deviations. Identify and describe the phonological deviations of this type.

Feature Contrast or Substitution Processes

A third group of phonological processes are feature contrast processes (Weiner, 1979) or substitution processes (Ingram, 1989; Stoel-Gammon & Dunn, 1985). These deviations involve replacing one sound by another sound without being influenced by the surrounding phonemes. The substitutions generally are of one class of phonemes replacing another class of phonemes. These deviations affect liquids, stops, fricatives, affricates, nasals, and glides, and most of them occur in the speech of typically developing children.

Stopping

Stopping has been described in slight variations by phonologists. Hodson and Paden (1991) defined it as a substitution of stops for continuants. Khan (1982) described it as substitution of stops for fricatives and affricatives. Edwards and Shriberg (1983) indicated that stopping refers to fricatives, affricates, liquids, and glides being replaced by stops. Bankson and Bernthal (1990a, 1990b) described it as stops replacing fricatives, affricates, and liquids. Although many phonologists consider substituting stops for affricates to be stopping, Hodson (2004) indicated that such substitutions should not be classified as stopping because affricates already contain a stop component. Rather, they prefer to describe the replacement of an affricate with a stop as **deaffrication** (described below). Stopping is a commonly used process, particularly for fricatives (Hodson & Paden, 1991). Examples include /kɪt/ for *kiss*, /du/ for *zoo*, and /tʌni/ for *funny*.

Fronting

Fronting refers to the replacement of a target phoneme with another phoneme that is articulated anteriorly to the target sound. Technically, fronting occurs in any instance in which the place of articulation in the surface form is produced farther forward in the oral cavity than in the adult standard production. However, at least one phonologist specifies that when assessing children, fronting is identified only when an anterior consonant replaces a posterior consonant (Hodson, 2004). Velar fronting is a common type in which alveolars are substituted for velars. Examples of velar fronting include /dem/ for *game* and /taʊ/ for *cow*. Palatal fronting also occurs when a palatal sound is replaced by an alveolar or labial. Palatal fronting has also been called **depalatalization** (described below). Examples include /tip/ for *sheep* and /dzʌmp/ for *jump*. Fronting occurs much more frequently

than the corollary process of backing except in children born with a cleft palate.

Backing

Backing occurs when a target sound is replaced with another sound whose place of articulation is posterior to it; it also has been described as a posterior consonant replacing an anterior consonant (Hodson, 2004). Examples include /ko/ for *toe* and /hit/ for *seat*. This deviation seldom occurs and thus is considered an atypical or nondevelopmental deviation. In an attempt to stop the airflow, children with cleft palate may use the phonological deviation of backing.

Affrication

Affrication occurs when a stop component is added to a continuant consonant, most commonly a fricative. In other words, a nonaffricate becomes an affricate. Examples include /tsʌn/ for *sun* and /tʃo/ for *show*.

Deaffrication

Deaffrication is the process of replacing an affricate with a nonaffricate; that is, changing an affricate to a continuant or a stop. Examples are /ʃɛr/ or /tɛr/ for *chair* and /zʌmp/ or /dʌmp/ for *jump*. During typical speech development, children may use both patterns of affrication and deaffrication as they are sorting out the differences between affricates and fricatives (Hodson & Paden, 1991).

Palatalization

Palatalization occurs when a sound is produced as a palatal rather than as a nonpalatal. Some preschoolers may use this pattern while sorting out the contrast between alveolars and palatals (Hodson & Paden, 1991). Examples include /ʃup/ for *soup* and /toʒ/ for *toes*.

Depalatalization

Depalatalization is the opposite of palatalization in that a palatal consonant is replaced by a nonpalatal. Two examples are /mæs/ for *mash* and /dzæm/ for *jam*. Some phonologists call these phonological deviations palatal fronting.

Gliding

Gliding refers to the use of a glide (/w, j/) for another consonant. Gliding occurs frequently on prevocalic liquids (/r, l/) in singletons and clusters, and sometimes on fricatives. Gliding of fricatives occurs primarily in children with deviant phonology and thus is characterized as an atypical pattern, whereas gliding of liquids is typical during speech development. Examples of gliding include /wen/ for *rain,* /jɪtl̩/ for *little*, and /gwin/ for *green*.

Vocalization or Vowelization

Vocalization, also called **vowelization**, is the deviation in which a vowel is substituted for a syllabic consonant (/l̩, ɜ˞, ɚ, m̩, n̩, ŋ̍/). Examples include /bɑdo/ for *bottle* and /kaʊ/ for *car*.

Denasalization

Denasalization, not to be confused with hyponasality (introduced in Chapter 2), occurs when a nasal is replaced by a nonnasal sound, often a stop that has the same articulation placement, such as a **homorganic** stop. This process occurs more frequently in word-initial and medial positions than in word-final position (Weiner, 1979). Examples include of /dak/ for *knock* and /spok/ for *smoke*.

Neutralization

Neutralization occurs when several different phonemes are replaced by one sound. This process may appear on vowels *and* consonants. Vowels are often replaced with /ʌ/, /ə/, /ɑ/ (Weiner, 1979). One cannot predict the consonant that will replace a particular group of sounds because different speakers show different preferences. For example, the authors observed a child who replaced all prevocalic fricatives and affricates with /j/ such that *sun* was pronounced as /jʌn/ and *juice* as /ju/, whereas another child used /g/ for the consonants pronouncing *shoe* as /gu/ and *truck* as /gʌ/. Both children were essentially unintelligible.

> Identify and describe other phonological deviations.

Other Processes

Articulation Shifts

Some deviations have been labeled articulation shifts in which minimal shifts occur in place of articulation, while the manner and voicing features do not change (Hodson, 1986a). These processes are commonly thought of as typical developmental misarticulations and, as Hodson indicated, these shifts alone seldom affect intelligibility, although they may be distracting. One type of articulation shift is substitution of anterior stridents /f, v, s, z/ for /θ, ð/. It should be noted that the substitution of /f/ for /θ/ especially in the final position, is standard in many Black English dialects. Examples include /fɪŋk/ for *think* and /maʊf/ or /maʊs/ for *mouth*. A second type is sibilant distortions, including frontal and lateral lisps. A frontal lisp is the production of /s/ and /z/ and sometimes the other sibilants (/ʃ, ʒ,

tʃ, dʒ/) with a protruded tongue or with the tongue placement being too far forward. In a lateral lisp, the air is emitted laterally between the upper and lower teeth rather than medially for the production of sibilants.

Idiosyncratic Patterns

Individual children sometimes use deviations that are unique to their phonological system. Several examples have been cited in the literature, some of which were described earlier in the chapter. Table 3.2, developed by Lowe (1994), illustrates and describes 15 of the more frequently mentioned **idiosyncratic** processes. These phonological processes are considered atypical or nondevelopmental deviations. It is important that speech-language pathologists be cognizant of the potential of a client using idiosyncratic processes so that effective, efficient clinical programs can be developed for individuals.

> What is meant by the idea that a difference between the child's production and the adult standard might be the result of multiple deviation patterns?

Multiple Processes or Deviations

Children frequently apply more than one phonological deviation or process when producing a single word, rather than using only one pattern per word. For example, /kʌb/ for *glove* results from cluster reduction, velar fronting, and stopping. Another example is the use of cluster reduction, gliding, vowelization, and partial reduplication when producing /waʊwʊ/ for *flower*. It is necessary to analyze the nature of the phonological systems of individual clients if effective intervention programs are to be developed.

> Distinguish between independent analysis and relational analysis of children's speech.

PHONOLOGICAL DEVELOPMENT

Stoel-Gammon and Dunn (1985) succinctly characterized language development as follows:

> Babies begin to coo and babble shortly after birth. They produce identifiable words around their first birthday and short sentences around their second

TABLE 3.2

Unusual/Idiosyncratic Phonologic Processes

Process	Definition
Atypical Cluster Reduction	Deletion of the member that is usually retained Example: play → /le/
Initial Consonant Deletion	Deletion of word-initial consonant or cluster so that the initial sound is a vowel Example: shoe → /u/, star → /ɑr/
Medial Consonant Deletion	Deletion of intervocalic consonants Example: beetle → /bio/
Backing of Stops	Replacement of front consonants by phonemes made posterior to the target phonemes (typically velars) Example: toe → /ko/
Apicalization	Labial replaced by an apical (tongue tip) consonant Example: bow → /do/
Glottal Replacement	Substitution of a glottal stop for consonant usually in medial or final position Example: bat → /bæʔ/
Backing of Fricatives	Replacement of fricatives with fricatives that are made in a more posterior position Example: suit → /ʃut/
Medial Consonant Substitutions	Replacement of intervocalic consonants with one or more phonemes Example: butter → /bʌja/
Denasalization	Substitution of nasal consonants by a homorganic, nonnasal Example: no → /do/
Devoicing of Stops	Replacement of a voiced stop with a voiceless phoneme (usually a stop) in word-initial position Example: daddy → /tædi/
Fricatives Replacing Stops	Substitution of a fricative consonant for a stop consonant Example: bat → /bæs/
Stops Replacing Glides	Substitution of a stop consonant for a glide Example: yellow → /dɛlo/
Metathesis	Reversal of position of two sounds; the sounds may or may not be adjacent Example: most → /mots/
Migration	Movement of a sound from one position in a word to another position Example: soap → /ops/
Sound Preference Substitutions	Replacement of groups of consonants by one or two particular consonants Example: /s/, /z/, /ʃ/, /tʃ/, /dʒ/ → /t/

From Lowe, R. J. (1994). *Phonology. Assessment and intervention applications in speech pathology (p. 110)*. Baltimore: Williams & Wilkins. Reprinted with permission.

birthday. By the age of five, they have acquired a vocabulary of about 2,000 words, can produce syntactically complex sentences, and can accurately pronounce most of the sounds of their language; they are, in essence, well on their way to full mastery of the structural and pragmatic aspects of one of the most complex communication systems we know—human language. (p. 1)

This discussion will focus on what has actually been observed in children as they acquire their speech sounds and patterns from infancy through approximately 8 years of age. Phonological development will be considered from the perspectives of individual phoneme acquisition, distinctive features, and phoneme classes and syllable structures.

Phonological acquisition data have been collected through widely varying procedures by various researchers since 1931. Some data have come from spontaneous speech productions, while others have been from single-word elicitations, and still others from imitated productions. The data have been analyzed in two different ways: (a) independent analysis and (b) relational analysis. In independent analyses, the child's system is described without comparison to the adult system and can include: (a) an inventory of phonemes classified by word position and articulation features, (b) an inventory of syllable and word shapes used, and (c) sequential constraints on phoneme usage. On the other hand, in relational analysis, the child's productions are compared to the adult standard relative to speech sound segments, features, rules, and phonological processes. Both types of data are presented here after a brief description of the general stages of phonological development.

> Identify and characterize six stages of phonological development.

Stages of Phonological Development

Phonological development has been described as a series of stages or steps leading to adult phonological systems. As described by Stoel-Gammon and Dunn (1985), four general stages of phonological development occur from the ages of 0:1 (years:month) to 8:0. Other researchers have added two other stages extending to 16:0+ (Hoffman & Norris, 1989; Ingram, 1989). Ingram, who is widely cited in the literature, described six stages of phonological development that correspond with Piaget's cognitive and linguistic stages. Obviously, the age levels associated with each stage are only guidelines and the stages overlap rather than being discrete developments. Before proceeding with a more traditional discussion of phonological development, we begin with a review of the phonological stages and Piaget's stages of cognitive development that correspond to each (Ingram, 1989). Because it has become a classic characterization of phonological development, Ingram's table showing concomitant stages of development for cognition, phonology, and linguistics appears in Table 3.3.

Stage 1: Prelinguistic (0:1–1:0)

Stages 1 and 2 of phonological development occur during Piaget's first cognitive stage, the sensorimotor period (birth to 18 months of age). During this time, children develop systems of movements and perception. They explore objects and learn about their properties and functions, develop preverbal vocalizations (babbling) and perceptual skills, and begin the processes of simplifying speech use.

Children communicate through crying and gestures (reflexive vocalizations) that may not be as important to speech development as the nonreflexive vocalizations (vocal play). Imitative abilities also increase. Perceptual and discrimination abilities are present during infancy (Gleason, 2005; Kuhl, 1994; McLaughlin, 1998). During phonological Stage 1, the infant produces reflexive and nonreflexive vocalizations, some of which are speech-like. These vocalizations are characterized as prelinguistic because they do not have stable sound-meaning relationships. During the end of this period, speech-like vocalizations or babbling predominate. Stage 1 is described more fully in the Babbling section.

Stage 2: First Words (1:0–1:6).

During phonological Stage 2, Piaget's cognitive stage continues to be the sensorimotor period. Meaningful speech production emerges ending with an expressive vocabulary of about 50 words. The syllable structure of these words is characterized as simple, such as CV, CVC, and CVCV. Consonants produced are primarily stops, nasals, and glides. The words seem to be produced as whole units rather than as words composed of individual phonemes or sounds.

Stage 3: Phonemic Development (1:6–4:0)

Piaget's cognitive Stage 2, the period of concrete operations (1.5 to 4 years of age), includes the onset of symbolic representation, symbolic play, and the concepts of past and future. The phonological stage that corresponds to this cognitive stage is the occurrence of single morphemes. During phonological Stage 3, word productions no longer are whole-word units, but rather are comprised of phonemes. The inventory of speech sounds is increased, and misarticulations of most sounds nearly disappear by 4 years of age. The number of different sound classes, phonemes, and syllable structures increases, and phonological patterns become more complex with consonant clusters and multisyllabic words being added to the speech repertoire. Although many children substitute one sound for another, the typical 4-year-old produces most phonemic contrasts correctly at least some of the time. During this telegraphic linguistic stage, the child gradually discontinues applying some phonological processes (Ingram, 1989).

Stage 4: Stabilization of the Phonological System (4:0–8:0).

In cognitive Stage 3, the intuitional subperiod (4 to 7 years of age), children rely on immediate perception to solve various tasks. They also begin to

TABLE 3.3

Piaget's Cognitive Stages of Development with Approximate Ages and the Grammatical and Phonological Stages That Correspond to Each

Piaget's Stages	Linguistic Stages	Phonological Stages
Sensori-motor period (0:0–1:6) Development of systems of movements and perception. Child achieves notion of object permanence.	1. Prelinguistic communication through gestures and crying. 2. Holophrastic stage. Use of one-word utterances.	1. Prelinguistic vocalization and perception (birth–1:0). 2. Phonology of the first 50 words (1:0–1:6).
Period of concrete operations (1:6–12:0) Preconcept subperiod (1:6–4:0) The onset of symbolic representation. Child can now refer to past and future, although most activity is in the here and now. Predominance of symbolic play.	3. Telegraphic stage. Child begins to use words in combinations. These increase to point between 3 and 4 when most sentences become close to well-formed, simple sentences.	3. Phonology of single morphemes. Child begins to expand inventory of speech sounds. Phonological processes resulting in incorrect productions dominate until around age 4 when most words of simple morphological structure are correctly spoken.
Institutional subperiod (4:0–7:0) Child relies on immediate perception to solve various tasks. Begins to develop the concept of reversibility. Child begins to be involved in social games.	4. Early complex sentences. Child begins to use complements on verbs and some relative clauses. These early complex structures, however, appear to be the result of juxtaposition.	4. Completion of the phonetic inventory. The child acquires production of troublesome sounds by age 7. Good production of simple words. Beginning use of longer words.
Concrete operations subperiod (7:0–12:0) Child learns the notion of reversibility. Can solve tasks dealing with conservation of mass, weight, and volume.	5. Complex sentences. Child acquires the transformational rules that embed one sentence into another. Coordination of sentences decreases, v. the increase in complex sentences.	5. Morphophonemic development. Child learns more elaborate derivational structure of the language; acquires morphophonemic rules of language.
Period of formal operations (2:0–16:0) Child learns the ability to use abstract thought. Can solve problems through reflection.	6. Linguistic intuitions. Child can now reflect upon the grammar quality of his speech and arrive at linguistic intuitions.	6. Spelling. Child masters ability to spell

From Ingram, D. (1989). *Phonological disability in children* (2nd ed.). San Diego, CA: Singular Publishing Group, Inc. Reprinted with permission.

develop the concept of reversibility and to become involved in social games. The corresponding phonological stage is the completion of the phonetic inventory. During phonological Stage 4, children complete acquisition of the adult system as reflected by stabilization of the production of the sounds that were variably produced and acquisition of the remaining phonemes. They learn the production of all troublesome sounds by age 7 and show good production of most simple words and some longer, more difficult words. Additionally, they gain more understanding of the phonemic system as they begin to read and write.

Stage 5: Morphophonemic Development (7:0–12:0)

Piaget's cognitive Stage 4 is referred to as the concrete operations subperiod (7 to 12 years of age). During this period, children learn the concept of reversibility and learn to solve tasks dealing with conservation of mass, weight, and volume. At the same time during phonological Stage 5, phonological development continues as they acquire morphophonemic rules and a more elaborate derivational structure of the language. Children learn how to spell and read, use vowel shifts, and apply contrastive stress for differentiating compound words from noun phrases such as *blackboard* from *black board*. Morphophonemic alterations are learned, such as changes between *electric* and *electricity* in which the final /k/ in *electric* becomes /s/ in *electricity* (Ingram, 1989). Thus, phonological acquisition is not complete by age 7 years as has been traditionally thought. It continues until 12 years of age and perhaps even longer when mastery of spelling is considered. However, sound production of the approximately 50 sounds in the English language usually is mastered by 7 years of age.

Stage 6: Spelling (12:0–16:0+)

The last cognitive Stage 5 is the period of formal operations (12 to 16 years). During this time, children learn the ability to use abstract thought and to solve problems through reflection. The phonological counterpart is mastery of spelling ability. During phonological Stage 6, spelling skills are acquired and perfected (Hoffman & Norris, 1989; Ingram, 1989).

Babbling

As described earlier, the first stage of phonological development is considered prelinguistic. Babbling, which dominates infant vocalizations during the later phases of the prelinguistic stage, seems to function as a transition between early vocalizations and meaningful speech.

The prelinguistic stage consists of two categories of vocalizations:

- Reflexive vocalizations, such as cries and coughs, that are automatic responses to internal and external stimuli
- Nonreflexive vocalizations, such as cooing and babbling that are voluntary vocal activities (Oller, 1980; Stoel-Gammon & Dunn, 1985; Vihman, 2004).

The prelinguistic stage of acquisition is divided into five phases (Oller, 1980; Stoel-Gammon & Dunn, 1985; Vihman, 2004). Again there is considerable overlap between the phases, but new behavior is added at each successive level. The associated age ranges are merely guidelines as individuals differ relative to the timeline (Fig. 3.4).

- *Phase 1: Phonation (0:0–0:1).* Reflexive vocalizations dominate in the first phase. Some of these sounds are described as "quasi-resonant nuclei," meaning they have limited resonance, such as speech sounds produced with a relatively closed mouth. They give the impression of being syllabic nasal sounds.

- *Phase 2: Cooing (0:2–0:3).* During the second babbling (or gooing) phase, velar and uvular consonant-like and back vowel-like sounds are produced. "Primitive syllables" may be perceived, but they lack the timing elements of CV syllables characteristic of meaningful speech.

- *Phase 3: Expansion (0:4–0:6).* Vocal play is predominant in the third phase with a wide variety of productions, including squeals, yells, bilabial trills, friction noises, and vowels. Some CV sequences are produced, but they tend to be slow and irregular in timing and thus are not truly canonical syllables. The infants now seem to have increasing control over their vocal mechanisms.

- *Phase 4: Reduplicated Babbling (0:7–0:9).* The fourth phase is the beginning of canonical babbling in which CV syllables are produced with a true consonant and a fully resonant vowel. During this time, the same CV syllable is repeated. Sounds produced are primarily stops, nasals, and glides with place of articulation being primarily labial and alveolar. Velar sounds have declined dramatically. The vowels typically are lax.

- *Phase 5: Variegated Babbling (0:10–1:0).* During the last phase of prelinguistic development, CV syllables are produced with various consonants and vowels. Also, these variegated syllables are produced with adult-like prosody.

Production of canonical CV syllables is believed to be important to later phonological development. Canonical syllabic forms are characterized as those "obeying timing restrictions of natural languages" (Oller et al., 1985, p. 48). Spectrographic analysis of canonical syllables show regular syllable timing, short formant transitions, high-frequency energy, and nasal resonances in these vocalizations. Quasi-resonant syllables do not have these same features. Auditory input seems to be critical for frequent, repetitive canonical babbling because quantitative and qualitative differences have been found between infants who are normally hearing and those who are hearing impaired (Maskarinec, Cairns, Butterfield, & Weamer, 1981; Oller et al., 1985; Stoel-Gammon & Otomo, 1986). Normally hearing infants with Down syndrome show speech patterns similar to typically developing infants during the first 15 months of life, but they show considerable delay in the onset and development of meaningful speech (Smith & Oller, 1981).

Characterize the sequence of acquisition of consonants and vowels as children acquire the English sound system.

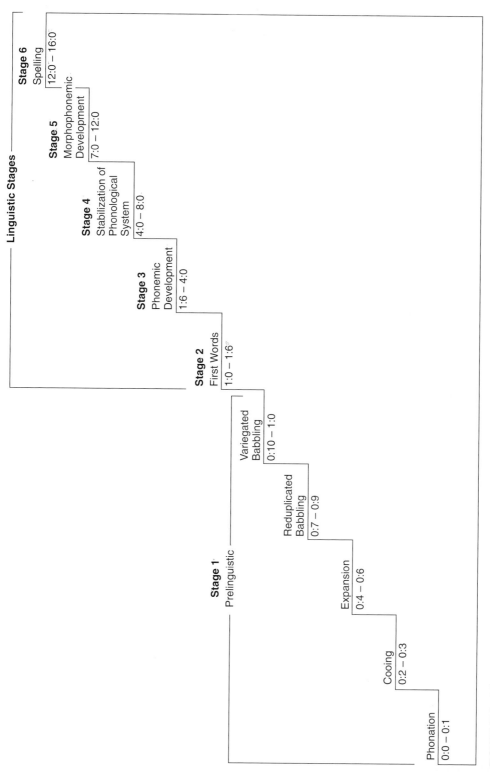

FIGURE 3.4 Schematic representation of stages of phonological development, including prelinguistic stages.

Individual Phoneme Development

Consonants

A few studies on consonant acquisition have looked at the use of consonants in both words and non-words uttered by young children (Robb & Bleile, 1994; Stoel-Gammon, 1985, 1987; Vihman et al., 1985; Vihman, Ferguson, & Elbert, 1986). Speech acquisition longitudinal data on 33 young subjects, aged 1:3 to 2:0 has been collected by Stoel-Gammon (1985, 1987). The data came from spontaneous speech samples produced by children who used 10 to 50 different identifiable words during an hour-long data collection session; consequently, some subjects were not used at the younger age levels. Stoel-Gammon contended that spontaneous speech is a more appropriate method for these younger subjects because they often do not respond to single-word elicitation or imitation procedures. She used independent analysis to describe the sound inventories of her subjects. As expected, the mean number of phonemes used increased with age (Tables 3.4 and 3.5). The inventory of initial sounds was always larger than the final sound inventory. Initial sound inventories were composed mostly of stops, nasals, and glides (/h, w/) that are voiced and anterior. By 24 months, voiced and voiceless velars and voiceless fricatives were added. Final sound inventories primarily included voiceless stops and alveolar phonemes, with /r/ being added at 24 months. In the 1987 study, the data were also analyzed relationally by computing the percentage of consonants correct for the 2-year-olds with a resultant mean of 70% (range of 43–91%).

Useful descriptive information also emanated from Robb and Bleile's (1994) study of the speech

TABLE 3.4

Syllable-Initial Consonant Inventories Organized by Age Level from Three Different Studies

	Consonant Phonemes in Inventories (n of Subjects)		
Age in Years: Months	Robb & Bleile (1994) (60% or More of Subjects)	Stoel-Gammon (1985) (50% or More of Subjects)	Dyson (1988) (50% or More of Subjects)
0:8	d t k m h (3)	—	—
0:9	d m n h w (3)	—	—
0:10	b d t m n h (3)	—	—
0:11	d m n h (4)	—	—
1:0	b d g m h (4)	—	—
1:1	b d g m h l (5)	—	—
1:2	b d g t k m n h w l (7)	—	—
1:3	b d g n h w (6)	b d h (7)	—
1:4	b d h w j l (7)	—	—
1:5	b d g p k m n h w (7)	—	—
1:6	b d m n h w (7)	b d m n h w (19)	—
1:7	b d g p t k m n h f s (5)	—	—
1:8	b d g p k m n h s w (6)	—	—
1:9	b d g t k m n h w (3)	b t d m n h (32)	—
1:10	b d g p t k m n s z w (4)	—	—
1:11	b d g p t k m n h s w j (4)	—	—
2:0	b d p t k m n h s w (3)	b t d k g m n h w f s (33)	p b t d k g f s h m n w j l (10)
2:1	b d g p t k m n h f s ʃ w j dʒ (3)	—	—
2:5	—	—	p b t d k g f s h m n w j l (10)
2:9	—	—	p b t d k g f s h m n w j l (10)
3:3	—	—	p b t d k g f s h m n w j l r (10)

TABLE 3.5

Syllable-Final Consonant Inventories Organized by Age Level from Three Different Studies

Age in Years: Months	Consonant Phonemes in Inventories (n of Subjects)		
	Robb & Bleile (1994) (60% or More of Subjects)	Stoel-Gammon (1985) (50% or More of Subjects)	Dyson (1988) (50% or More of Subjects)
0:8	t m h (3)	—	—
0:9	m h (3)	—	—
0:10	t m h s (3)	—	—
0:11	m h (4)	—	—
1:0	m h (4)	—	—
1:1	h s (5)	—	—
1:2	h s (7)	—	—
1:3	n h (6)	none (7)	—
1:4	t h (7)	—	—
1:5	t h s (7)	—	—
1:6	t h s (7)	t (19)	—
1:7	t k m n h s (5)	—	—
1:8	d t k h s (6)	—	—
1:9	k n h s (3)	t n (32)	—
1:10	t k s (4)	—	—
1:11	t k h s r (4)	—	—
2:0	t k n s (3)	p t k n r s (33)	p t d k tʃ ʔ f s ʃ m (10)
2:1	d p t k m n h f s l r (3)	—	
2:5	—	—	p t d k tʃ ʔ f s ʃ m ŋ ' (10)
2:9	—	—	p t k ʔ f s z m n ' (10)
3:3	—	—	p t d k ʔ f v s z ʃ m n ŋ r ' (10)

samples over a 12-month period of seven children, aged 8–14 months at the beginning of the study and 19–26 months at the end of the study. The findings showed that: (a) the number of consonants in their sound inventories increased over time; (b) the number of consonants used in the initial position was greater than in the final position; (c) stops and nasals came in earlier than fricatives; and (d) bilabial, alveolar, and glottal place of articulation predominated and came in earlier than velars. The overall results are similar to Stoel-Gammon's (1985) study except that more consonant types were used at the younger ages possibly because all nonreflexive utterances were included in the data, not just recognizable words. More specific data regarding consonant acquisition patterns appear in Tables 3.4 and 3.5. While the summary of the findings shown in Table 3.6 are for children aged 8–25

months are from the Robb and Bleile study, they are in general agreement with other studies. This type of normative information on consonant production in both words and nonwords is useful for assessing toddlers because there is evidence that children under 19 months of age use nonwords in more than 50% of their utterances (Robb, Bauer, & Tyler, 1994; Robb & Bleile, 1994).

The phonetic inventories of slightly older children were collected by Dyson (1988) who conducted a quasi-longitudinal study on a group of young children (tested at mean ages of 2:0 and 2:5) and an older group (2:9 and 3:3). Their phonetic inventories that were produced in words are shown in Tables 3.4 and 3.5.

The approach typically used in collecting consonant acquisition normative data is relational analyses; that is, comparison of the child's sounds

TABLE 3.6

Summary of Major Findings of a Longitudinal Study of Consonant Inventories of Young Children

Area of Analysis	Findings
Syllable-Initial Consonants	
8–16 months	Approximately six consonants
	Mostly voiced consonants
	Predominantly oral and nasal stops
	Predominantly bilabial, alveolar, and glottal
17–25 months	Approximately 10 consonants
	Voiced consonants dominate, but voiceless consonants occur
	Greater variety of consonants within oral and nasal classes
	Modest increase in the number of fricatives
	Velar consonants become more common
Syllable-Final Consonants	
8–16 months	Approximately two consonants
	Mostly voiceless consonants; voiced consonants are nasals
	Predominantly oral and nasal stops, as well as fricatives
	Primarily alveolars and glottals with some bilabials
17–25 months	Approximately five consonants
	Voiceless consonants continue to dominate, but voiced consonants become more common
	Nasals, oral stops, and fricatives are predominant
	Bilabials, alveolars, velars, and glottal are predominant
Frequency of Occurrence of Manner Classes	
8–25 months	Oral stops occur most frequently
	Frequency of nasal consonants declines near the eleventh month
	Frequency of fricatives and affricates, liquids, and glides is low and relatively constant
Frequency of Occurrence of Place Classes	
8–25 months	Alveolars and labials occur most frequently
	Velars and glottals occur much less frequently

From Robb, M. P., & Bleile, K. M. (1994). Consonant inventories of young children from 8 to 25 months. *Clinical Linguistics & Phonetics, 8,* 304. Reprinted with permission.

to the adult standard. Earlier as well as later studies of phonological development have focused on establishing group norms for correct production of individual phonemes and consonant clusters. Table 3.7 presents a summary of data from eight representative studies relative to the expected age levels for development of individual phonemes, and

Table 3.8 describes some of the characteristics of these studies. Perusal of the data shows that the order of acquisition of individual sounds is fairly consistent across the studies, but a range of age levels exists among the studies as to when specific sounds are found to be acquired. Presumably, this is because of different data collection procedures,

TABLE 3.7

Age Levels for Phoneme Development According to Eight Studies

Phonemes	Wellman et al. (1931)	Poole (1934)	Templin (1957)	Sander (1972)	Prather et al. (1975)	Arlt et al. (1976)	Irwin et al. (1983)	Smit (1990)
m	3	3.5	3	before 2	2	3	1.5	3
n	3	4.5	3	before 2	2	3	2	3–3.5
h	3	3.5	3	before 2	2	3	2	3
p	4	3.5	3	before 2	2	3	3	3
f	3	5.5	3	3	2–4	3	3	3.5–5.5
w	3	3.5	3	before 2	2–8	3	2	3
b	3	3.5	4	before 2	2–8	3	1.5	3
ŋ		4.5	3	2	2	3	3	7–9
j	4	4.5	3.5	3	2–4		3	4–5
k	4	4.5	4	2	2–4	3	3	3.5
g	4	4.5	4	2	2–4	3	3	3.5–4
l	4	6.5	6	3	3–4	4	3	5–7
d	5	4.5	4	2	2–4	3	3 and 6	3–3.5
t	5	4.5	6	2	2–8	3	3	3.5–4
s	5	7.5	4.5	3	3	4	3	7–9
r	5	7.5	4	3	3–4	5	3	8
tʃ	5		4.5	4	3–8	4	3 and 6	6–7
v	5	6.5	6	4	4	3.5	3 and 6	5.5
z	5	7.5	7	4	4	4	3	7–9
ʒ	6	6.5	7	6	4	4	3	
θ		7.5	6	5	4	5	4	6–8
dʒ			7	4	4	4	3	6–7
ʃ		6.5	4.5	4	3–8	4.5	3	6–7
ð		6½	7	5	4	5	not by 6	4½–7

From Creaghead, N. A., Newman P. W., & Secord, W. A. (1989). *Assessment and remediation of articulatory and phonological disorders (p. 47).* (2nd ed.). Columbus, OH: Merrill Publishing Company. Adapted with permission.

varying criteria, and individual differences among the subjects. The data from these studies came from single-word productions except for the norms reported by Irwin and Wong (1983) who used spontaneous speech samples. Arlt and Goodban (1976) used word imitations. With the exception of the Irwin and Wong (1983) and the Smit, Hand, Freilinger, Bernthal, and Bird (1990) studies, each phoneme was represented in each relevant position only once. In contrast, the other researchers used various stimuli to elicit the words spontaneously when possible; however, delayed or immediate imitation was implemented when the **stimulus** did not spontaneously elicit the target word from the child being tested. The most recent normative study of

speech sound acquisition was conducted by Smit and associates (1990). Criteria for acceptable responses were either correct or marginally correct sound productions allowing for variants that might occur in adult forms and/or that are acceptable allophones. Thus, their response criteria were probably less strict than those of other studies. In addition to presenting data at the 90% criterion, they reported percentages of correct responses for each target phoneme and consonant cluster in each position tested for each of 10 age groupings (Appendix C1). The percentage of correct production by each age group for each phoneme was calculated by Irwin and Wong (1983) for their 100 subjects. These data appear in Appendix C2.

TABLE 3.8

Subjects, Stimuli, and Criteria for Mastery Used in Cross-Sectional Studies of Speech Sound Development

Study	n	Ages in Years	Stimuli	Criterion
Wellman et al. (1931)	204	2–6	Pictures Questions	75% in three positions
Poole (1934)	140	2.6–8.5	Pictures Objects Questions	100% in three positions
Templin (1957)	480	3–8	Pictures	75%
Prather et al. (1975)	147	2–4	Pictures	75% in two positions
Arlt & Goodban (1976)	240	3–6	Word repetition	75% in two positions
Irwin & Wong (1983)	100	1.5–6	Spontaneous speech with toys, books, questions	75%
Smit et al. (1990)	947	3–9	Photographs	90%

From Creaghead, N. A., Newman P. W., & Secord, W. A. (1989). *Assessment and remediation of articulatory and phonological disorders (p. 47)*. (2nd ed.). Columbus, OH: Merrill Publishing Company. Adapted with permission.

The criteria for considering a sound acquired is rather high for these studies, ranging from 75% in two word positions to 100% for three positions. Therefore, Sander (1972) reanalyzed the Wellman, Case, Mengert, and Bradbury (1931) and the Templin (1957) data to determine the customary age of production, which is the age at which 51% of the children at a given age level produced the sound correctly in at least two positions. In Figure 3.5, the customary age is compared with the 90% criterion level, which shows a considerable difference in the norms. For example, the customary age for /s/ is 3 years while the 90% criterion age level is 8 years of age. A difference for each consonant is at least 1.5 years. Grunwell (1987) compiled some of these same phoneme acquisition data and displayed it according to Ingram's (1989) developmental stages (Table 3.9).

Kenney and Prather (1986) examined the consistency of productions of nine phonemes that are frequently misarticulated, including /θ, r, l, s, ʃ, tʃ, f, t, k/). Subjects ranged in age from 2.5 to 5 years. Their productions improved with increasing age. The phonemes ranked as follows from most to least frequently misarticulated: /r/, /θ/, /l/, /ʃ/, /tʃ/, /s/, /f/, /k/, and /t/. Consistency of production varied by word position for some of the sounds, but not for /k/, /s/, and /t/.

Vowels

The acquisition of vowels has seldom been considered in normative studies, however some longitudinal and cross-sectional vowel acquisition data have been collected using both independent and relational analysis (Otomo & Stoel-Gammon, 1992; Pollack, 1991). The vowel phonetic inventories of four children longitudinally collected at 15, 18, 21, 24, and 36 months of age appear in Table 3.10 (Selby, Robb, & Gilbert, 2000). These figures reflect independent analyses of the vowels actually produced in babbling and in speech without analyzing the accuracy of the vowels used. Seemingly, they reflect the motor or articulation capabilities of the children. As expected, the number of vowels used increased as the children became older. The corner vowels were produced early. By 36 months, all vowels were produced including /ɝ/. Tense and lax vowels are used throughout the age levels from 15 to 36 months as is the case for both front and back vowels. Davis and MacNeilage (1990) followed the vowel productions of a 14-month-old female for 6 months. During the ages of 14–28 months, she used all vowels in both babbling and speech. (Note: /ɝ/ was not included in the study.)

Relational data in which the children's vowel productions are assessed as to accuracy when compared to the adult target have been collected by a few investigators. The most complete data available on correct vowel production were collected by Irwin and Wong (1983). The spontaneous speech of their subjects, aged 1:6 to 6:0, had high percentages of correct vowel production. Table 3.11 shows that, except for the rhotic vowels, the vowels and diphthongs were produced correctly more

Age Level

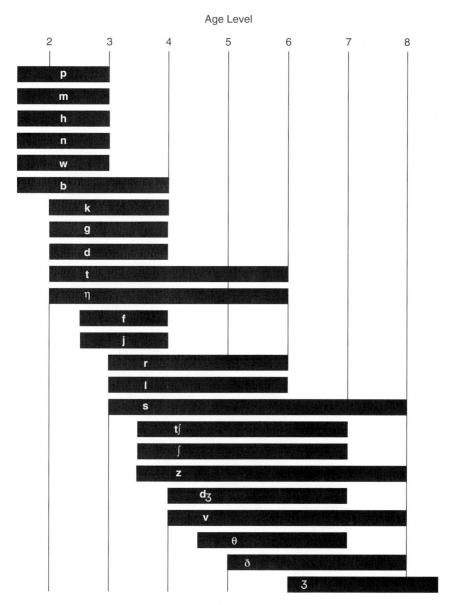

FIGURE 3.5 Average age estimates and upper age limits of customary consonant production. The solid bar corresponding to each sound starts at the median age of customary articulation and stops at an age level at which 90% of all children are customarily producing the sound (Templin, 1957; Wellman et al., 1931). (From Sander, E. (1972). When are speech sounds learned? *Journal of Speech and Hearing Disorders, 37,* 62. Copyright 1972 by American Speech–Language–Hearing Association. Adapted with permission.)

than 85% of the time from 2 years of age. Developmental level stages of vowel acquisition as proposed by Stoel-Gammon and Herrington (1990) are shown in Table 3.12. These levels were derived from their review of the literature, but are not entirely in agreement with results from other studies. However, they do provide a useful guideline.

Other studies have looked at vowel acquisition of a few (hopefully representative) young children.

The vowel productions of two children whose vowel usage was analyzed over a 2-month period (aged 1:10–2:0 and 2:0–2:2) used inaccurate vowel productions when compared to the adult target (Bleile, 1989). The young girl in the Davis and MacNeilage (1990) quantitative case study was 57% correct in her vowel usage in speech, with /u/, /o/, /i/, and /ɪ/ being produced correctly at least 75% of the time. The most frequent errors occurred

TABLE 3.9

Profile of Phonological Development—Phonological System

Stage VII (4:6<)	Stage VI (4:0–4:6)	(3:6–4:0)	Stage V (3:0–3:6)	Stage IV (2:6–3:0)	Stage III (2:0–2:6)	Stage II (1:6–2:0)	Stage I (0:9–1:6)
m n ŋ	m n ŋ		m n ŋ		m n (ŋ)	m n	Labial Lingual
pb td tʃ dʒ kg	pb td tʃ dʒ kg		pb td kg		pb td (kg)	pb td	Nasal
fv θð sz ʃ	fv sz ʃ		f s		w h	w	Plosive
w l r j h	w l (r) j h		w (l) j h				Fricative
							Approximant

From Grunwell, P. (1987). *Clinical phonology (p. 31).* (2nd ed.). Baltimore, MD: Williams & Wilkins. Adapted with permission.

on /ɜ˞/, /ɛ/, /ə/, all of which were incorrect at least 70% of the time. Otomo and Stoel-Gammon (1992) investigated the unrounded vowel productions of young children over an 8-month period when the subjects were 22, 26, and 30 months of age. Generally, the corner vowels /i/ and /ɑ/ were mastered early and /ɪ/ and /ɛ/ were the least accurately produced throughout the study.

> What is the general order of acquisition of distinctive features of the phonologic system?

Distinctive Feature Development

A few research efforts have been directed toward sound acquisition in terms of distinctive features. The distinctive feature system devised by Chomsky

TABLE 3.10

Group Vowel Inventory at Each Age Interval Based on 75% Occurrence Across Four Children

Age (months)	Inventory	Size
15	ɑ, ɪ, ʊ, ʌ	4
18	ɑ, i, u, ʊ, ʌ, ɔ, æ	7
21	ɑ, i, ɪ, ɛ, u, o, ʌ, ɔ	8
24	ɑ, i, ɪ, ɛ, e, u, o, ʌ, æ	9
36	ɑ, i, ɪ, ɛ, e, u, ʊ, o, ʌ, ɔ, æ, ɜ˞	12

From Selby, J. C., Robb, M. P., & Gilbert, H. R. (2000) Normal vowel articulations between 15 and 36 months of age. *Clinical Linguistics & Phonetics, 14,* 260. Reprinted with permission.

and Halle (1968) or a modified form of it has been used (Table 2.7). Irwin and Wong (1983) did a distinctive feature analysis of their sound acquisition data and noted that even at age 1:6, 18 of the 26 distinctive features were at least 90% correct. The feature most frequently in error was +strident. At 2 years of age, only two features were less than 90% correct; at 3 years, one feature; and none beyond 4 years.

A different approach is to look at distinctive feature development through implicational laws as explained by Dinnsen, Chin, Elbert, and Powell (1990):

> The occurrence of a particular phonetic distinction in an inventory necessarily implied the occurrence of certain other distinctions in that inventory. Thus, the presence of a distinction characteristic of one level implied the presence of all the distinctions characteristic of simpler levels. (p. 32)

They developed a five-level model or hierarchy of phonological complexity that they contended corresponds to phonological development in "normal" children (Fig. 3.6). For example, nasals, stops, and glides emerge early and these appear in the simplest level (Level A), but fricatives, affricates, and liquids are acquired later in levels C–E. Using this system, phonological development is viewed as the "acquisition of contrasts rather than of specific sounds" (p. 36). These complexity levels can be applied to both typical and disordered development. Additionally, Dinnsen et al. hypothesized that this hierarchy applies to other languages as well.

> What word shapes and phonological deviations do young children use in their speech productions?

TABLE 3.11

Percentage of Correct Usage of Vowel-Like Sounds by Age

Sounds	Phonemes	Age in Years				
		1.5	2	3	4	6
Vowels	/i/	76	96	100	97	100
	/ɪ/	73	84	99	96	98
	/e/	46	89	100	97	100
	/ɛ/	35	89	100	98	100
	/æ/	50	96	100	99	99
	/ɝ/	2	45	100	92	95
	/ɜ/	—	—	100	100	—
	/ɚ/	3	27	99	87	94
	/ə/	60	86	100	84	99
	/ʌ/	73	99	100	99	99
	/ɑ/	81	97	100	98	100
	/ɔ/	53	97	100	98	100
	/o/	58	91	100	97	99
	/u/	59	99	100	87	99
	/ʊ/	77	93	100	100	100
Subtotal		61	91	100	96	99
Diphthongs	/aɪ/	47	98	100	99	100
	/aʊ/	62	99	100	99	100
	/ɔɪ/	60	97	100	96	100
	/ɪu/	40	100	—	67	—
Subtotal		49	98	100	99	100
Syllabics	/n̩/	0	73	100	—	100
	/l̩/	27	50	100	93	100
	/m̩/	0	—	—	—	100
Subtotal		25	56	100	93	100
Total		59	91	100	96	99

From Irwin, J., & Wong, S. (1983). *Phonological development in children: 16 to 72 months (p.158)*. Carbondale, IL: Southern Illinois University Press. Reprinted with permission.

TABLE 3.12

Stages of Acquisition of Vowels as Characterized by Stoel-Gammon and Herrington (1990)

Early Development	Middle Development	Late Development
/i, u, o, ɑ, ʌ/	/æ, ʊ, ɔ, ə/	/e, ɛ, ɪ, ɝ, ɚ/

Phoneme Classes and Syllable Structures

Research into developmental aspects of phoneme classes and syllable structures generally falls into two types of analyses: independent and relational.

Independent Analyses

Some researchers who have investigated syllable and word structure found that the first structures to emerge are CV and reduplicated CVCV, followed by CVC. Next, consonant clusters and

Level A: [syllabic]

             [consonantal]

             [sonorant]

             [coronal]

                ↑

Level B: [voice]

                ↑

Level C: [continuant]

             [delayed release]

                ↑

Level D: [nasal]

                ↑

Level E: [strident]

             [lateral]

FIGURE 3.6   Implicational hierarchy of phonetic features. (From Dinnsen, D., Chin, S. B., Elbert, M., & Powell, T. W. (1990). Some constraints on functionally disordered phonologies: Phonetic inventories and phonotactics. *Journal of Speech and Hearing Research, 33,* 33. Copyright 1990 by American Speech–Language–Association. Reprinted with permission.)

unreduplicated multisyllables emerge, with the first bisyllables being a combination of monosyllables already used, such as CVCV and CVCVC (Pollock & Schwartz, 1988). By the age of 2 years, children are using several VC word structures.

All 33 of the 2-year-old subjects in a study of their spontaneous speech used CV structures; 97% used CVC, 79% used CVCV, and 67% used CVCVC (Stoel-Gammon, 1987). Further, more than half of the 2-year-olds produced consonant clusters (58% of the children used consonant clusters in the initial position, 30% in the medial position, and 48% in the final position). The characteristics of the spontaneous speech of a typical 2-year old is illustrated in Figure 3.7. In a longitudinal study of these same children (followed from 15–24 months of age), Stoel-Gammon (1985) investigated their phonetic inventories and generally found that:

- Stops, nasals, and glides emerge early before fricatives and liquids
- Anterior sounds precede posterior ones
- Sounds with the same place and manner features usually occur in initial position before final
- Voiced stops occur in initial position before voiceless stops, but voiceless stops occur before voiced stops finally
- /r/ usually appears in final position first

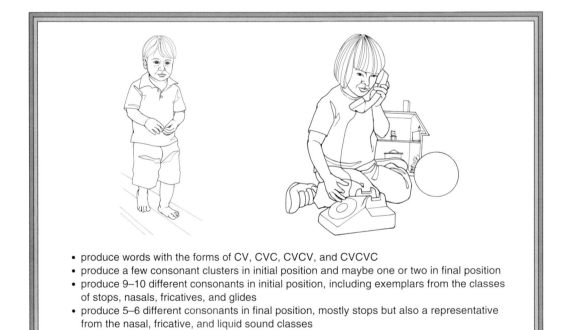

- produce words with the forms of CV, CVC, CVCV, and CVCVC
- produce a few consonant clusters in initial position and maybe one or two in final position
- produce 9–10 different consonants in initial position, including exemplars from the classes of stops, nasals, fricatives, and glides
- produce 5–6 different consonants in final position, mostly stops but also a representative from the nasal, fricative, and liquid sound classes
- match the consonant phomenes of the adult word with 70% accuracy

FIGURE 3.7   Phonological characteristics of a typical 2-year-old (Stoel-Gammon 1987).

Overall, Stoel-Gammon noted individual differences in terms of age of onset of speech, but found regular patterns in the order of emergence of sounds and sound classes that also reflect continuation of prelinguistic vocalization patterns.

Word shapes and consonant cluster usage was investigated by Dyson (1988) in a quasi-longitudinal study. The mean number of different clusters produced in the initial position ranged from 4.5 to 10.7 for the youngest and oldest groups, respectively, and from 4.2 to 7.7 in final position. There was no consistent pattern in the emergence of clusters because different subjects used different clusters; however, all children used at least four different clusters with /fw/ being the most frequently occurring (Table 3.13). Dyson concluded that, when they were compared with normative data on younger and older subjects, these children were "filling in the gaps in phonetic inventory and word-shape development" (p. 92). Table 3.14 presents the word shapes used by these children in their spontaneous speech. The following developments for these 2- to 3-year-olds were summarized this way:

- Word-initial and word-final inventories are becoming more balanced in number of segments used.
- Voiced stops are emerging word finally.
- The word-final fricative /s/ is used; and /v/, /z/, and /ʃ/ are emerging.
- Voiceless affricates are beginning to appear in both word positions.

- A wide variety of consonant clusters appears word initially and word finally.
- Most words are closed monosyllables, but two-syllable words of various types make up more than 10% of the samples.

The percentage of occurrence of various word forms produced by older subjects (3- to 6-year-olds) was explored by Shriberg, Kwiatowski, Best, Hengst, and Terselic-Weber (1986). As with the younger groups of children, the most frequent type was CVC followed by CV structures and various other monosyllabic word forms. All age groups studied also used two- and three-syllable words (Table 3.14).

Relational Analyses

Using phonological process analysis, several studies have compared child productions of words to the adult target. Because different phonological deviations are studied by various researchers, it is not feasible to compare the results directly. However, developmental trends can be gleaned from the combined results. The speech of 60 typically developing children at three age levels ranging from 1.5 to almost 2.5 years was analyzed by Preisser, Hodson, and Paden (1988). The results appear in Table 3.15, which shows that the most frequently occurring phonological processes were cluster reduction and liquid deviations (omission of liquid sound, gliding, and vowelization) and the least frequent was prevocalic (syllable-initial) obstruent

TABLE 3.13

Word-Initial and Word-Final Clusters Used in Two or More Adult Lexical Items

Younger Group				Older Group			
M Age 2:0		M Age 2:5		M Age 2:9		M Age 3:3	
Initial	Final	Initial	Final	Initial	Final	Initial	Final
(ts)	(ts)	(fw)	ts	(fw)	(ts)	(fw)	ts
fw	(ŋk)	(bw)	(ps)	(kw)	(ps)	(kw)	(ps)
					(nts)	(bw)	(ns)
					(ŋk)	(tr)	(ntʃ)
						(sp)	(ŋk)
						(st)	
						(sn)	
						(sl)	

Note: Segments in parentheses represent transitional segments used twice by only 4 of 10 children or used once by 6 or more children.

From Dyson, A. (1988). Phonetic inventories of 2- and 3-year-old children. *Journal of Speech and Hearing Disorders, 53*, 89–93. Copyright 1988 by American Speech–Language–Hearing Association. Reprinted with permission.

TABLE 3.14

Mean Percentage of Each Word Shape Examined in 2- to 6-Year-Olds

Word Shape	Mean Percentage (Rank Order by Type)				
	Younger Group*		Older Group*		Older Group**
	2:0	2:5	2:9	3:39	3–6 years
CVC	40.2	38.3	40.2	33.9	30.6
	(1)	(1)	(1)	(1)	(1)
CV	21.6	17.6	20.1	16.6	22.6
	(2)	(2)	(2)	(3)	(2)
Other Monosyllable	13.2	16.3	12.5	21.3	10.5
	(3)	(3)	(3)	(2)	(5)
Two-Syllable Word	12.7	14.2	12.0	14.5	13.5
	(4)	(4)	(4)	(4)	(3)
VC	7.1	7.7	9.0	8.5	12.5
	(5)	(5)	(5)	(5)	(4)
V	4.8	5.1	5.7	4.5	9.0
	(6)	(6)	(6)	(6)	(6)
Three-Syllable Word	0.4	0.7	0.4	0.7	1.3
	(7)	(7)	(7)	(7)	(7)

* Dyson, A. (1988). Phonetic inventories of 2- and 3-year-old children. *Journal of Speech and Hearing Disorders, 53,* 89–93.

** Shriberg, L. D., Kwiatkowski, J., Best, S., Hengst, J., & Terselic-Weber, B. (1986). Characteristics of children with phonologic disorders of unknown origin. *Journal of Speech and Hearing Disorders, 51,* 140–160.

omission. It is particularly interesting to note that by the age of 2:5, none of the phonological processes studied occurred at a mean frequency above 30%. The mean frequency of occurrence of phonological deviations decreased by more than 50%, going from 55% to 22%. Thus, considerable development occurs during this 1-year period such that speech production becomes more similar to that of adults.

A longitudinal study of 2-year-olds over a 7-month period investigated their use of 10 phonological processes (Dyson & Paden, 1983). By the end of the study, these children were using fronting, stopping, and final consonant deletion less than 10% of the time (Table 3.16). Gliding, which occurred primarily on liquids, was present in almost 50% of the possible occurrences, and cluster reduction occurred 30% of the time. Dyson and Paden (1983) hypothesized that final consonant deletion will be the first process to be suppressed and that gliding will be the last one to be suppressed. They also noted that "suppression is not a clear-cut, steadily advancing progression . . . [and that] the majority of instances showed vacillation

among several strategies . . . . [and] these children experimented with several strategies for producing a particular segment" (p. 16). They concluded that the period from 2 to 3.5 years is one during which children are experimenting with different strategies to produce the adult model.

The phonological processes used by 3-, 4-, and 5-year-olds were investigated by Haelsig and Madison (1986). As expected, the overall percentage of occurrence of phonological processes decreased with age (Table 3.17). Velar assimilation, prevocalic voicing, gliding of fricatives, affrication, and denasalization were rarely used by any of the subjects. None of the processes occurred more than 13% of the time in the 5-year-old group, and weak syllable deletion was the only process occurring more than 15% of the time in the 4.5-year-old group. The greatest reduction in phonological process usage occurred between 3 and 4 years of age, although there is much individual variation.

The frequency of occurrence of phonological processes was looked at in a group of older children, including 3- to 6-year-olds (Shriberg et al., 1986).

TABLE 3.15

Phonological Process Percentage-of-Occurrence Means and Standard Deviations for Three Chronological Age Groups (N = 20 per Group)

Phonological Process	1:6–1:9 M	1:10–2:1 M	2:2–2:5 M
Omissions			
Cluster reduction	93	76	51
Postvocalic obstruent	45	13	4
Syllable reduction	43	10	3
Prevocalic obstruent	14	7	3
Class Deficiencies			
Liquid deviation	91	75	64
Stridency deletion	56	41	23
Velar deviation	45	23	14
Nasal/glide deviation	49	23	11
Average	55	34	22

From Preisser D. A., Hodson B. W., Paden E. P. (1988) Developmental phonology: 18–29 months. *Journal of Speech and Hearing Disorders, 53,* 127. Copyright 1988 by American Speech–Language–Hearing Association. Adapted with permission.

TABLE 3.16

Decrease in Percentage of Occurrence of Five Processes, from First to Eighth Testing of 2-Year-Olds

Phonological Process	% First Testing	% Eighth Testing
Gliding	53.8	47.9
Cluster Reduction	49.6	30.2
Fronting	15.6	9.5
Stopping	13.7	9.3
Final Consonant Deletion	10.6	4.4

From Dyson, A., & Paden, E. (1983) Some phonological acquisition strategies used by two-year-olds. *Journal of Childhood Communication Disorders, 7,* 6–18. Copyright 1983 by The Council for Exceptional Children. Adapted with permission.

TABLE 3.17

The Frequency of Occurrence of Phonological Process Errors by Age

Process	3:0	3:6	4:0	4:6	5:0
Gliding liquids	48	55	24	12	0
Weak syllable deletion	38	37	27	28	13
Glottal replacement	38	31	8	8	6
Cluster reduction	30	18	10	15	7
Labial assimilation	30	14	14	4	2
Vocalizations	28	40	26	6	1
Deletions of final consonants	22	15	6	10	5
Stopping	14	21	8	6	0
Fronting	10	9	6	0	1
Alveolar assimilation	8	25	8	2	2
Final devoicing	6	0	1	0	0
Denasalization	6	8	0	0	0
Velar assimilation	5	2	0	0	0
Prevocalic voicing	2	8	0	0	0
Gliding of fricatives	1	8	0	2	2
Affrication	0	5	0	0	0

From Haelsig, P. C., & Madison, C. L. (1986). A study of phonological processes exhibited by 3-, 4-, and 5-year-old children. *Language, Speech, and Hearing Services in Schools 17,* 109. Copyright 1986 by American Speech–Language–Hearing Association. Reprinted with permission.

Most of the singleton consonants were produced correctly, and most of the consonant clusters were either correctly produced or produced with distortions. The most frequently occurring phonological processes, in order of percentage of occurrence, were stopping, cluster reduction, liquid simplification, and palatal fronting, although all of these occurred less than 20% of the time.

Other researchers have explored the course of development of specific sound classes and/or processes. For example, palatal and velar fronting in 31- to 54-month-old children was found to occur in about a fourth of the 2.5 - to 3-year-olds and in 3.5% of the 4- to 4.5-year-olds (Lowe, Knutson, & Monson, 1985). Interestingly, velar fronting occurred more frequently, and palatal fronting never occurred in the absence of velar fronting.

From their review of the literature, Stoel-Gammon and Dunn (1985) reported that some phonological deviations disappear by the age of 3 years, while others persist beyond the age of 3 years. The processes expected to disappear by 3 years and those that persist are included in Table 3.18. Shriberg and Kwiatkowski (1980) reported that all phonological processes disappear from the phonological systems between the ages of 1.5 to 4 years with a few residual occurrences persisting after that time. Finally, a useful summation of the use of phonological deviations was developed by Grunwell (1987) and appears in Figure 3.8.

TABLE 3.18

Phonological Processes That Are Expected to Disappear and to Persist Beyond 3 Years of Age

Processes Suppressed by 3 Years of Age	Processes Persisting Beyond 3 Years of Age
Unstressed syllable deletion	Cluster reduction
Final consonant deletion	Epenthesis
Doubling	Gliding
Diminutization	Vocalization
Velar fronting	Stopping
Consonant assimilation	Depalatalization
Reduplication	Final Devoicing
Prevocalic voicing	

From Stoel-Gammon, C., & Dunn, C. (1985). *Normal and disordered phonology in children.* Baltimore, MD: University Park Press. Adapted with permission.

> What is the usefulness of normative data of phoneme acquisition in the provision of services to children who have articulatory/phonologic disorders?

Contributions and Limitations of Phoneme-Oriented Acquisition Data

The first efforts to provide normative information about phonological development resulted in phoneme-oriented acquisition data. Such information was needed for assessment and intervention for children with articulation disorders. These norms provide valuable guidelines for the clinician. However, as Smit (1986) pointed out, the normative data collected by various researchers differ, so it is difficult for clinicians to know which data to use in making diagnostic and treatment decisions.

A major limitation to the phoneme-oriented data is the criteria used to indicate what is normal and not normal. In order for the production of a phoneme to be considered correct, it had to be produced completely correctly. Distortions, substitutions, and omissions were given the same weight, with all such misarticulations being scored as incorrect. Obviously, omissions represent a greater deficiency than substitutions and distortions; and substitutions, greater than distortions. One gets the impression that sometimes acceptable allophonic productions were counted as incorrect, such as the production of intervocalic /t/ (Templin, 1957).

A second problem with the criteria is the level set in terms of the percentage of subjects who must produce a sound correctly in order for it to be considered developmentally stable or acquired. Researchers tended to set 75% and 90% criterion levels, which means that, for a sound to be considered developmentally acquired, 75% or 90% of the subjects needed to produce it correctly in the one stimulus word used to elicit the sound in a certain position or in two of the three word positions. Many of the phoneme-oriented articulation test norms use the 90% criterion level for specifying the acquisition age level, quite a stringent criterion. If 9 of 10 children are uttering the sound correctly at that age, then many younger children are also correctly producing the sound. Data showing progression of phonological development is more useful than the set criterion levels.

Often, only the phoneme-oriented criteria are used in client selection and in target selection, which can present a problem. Other factors need to

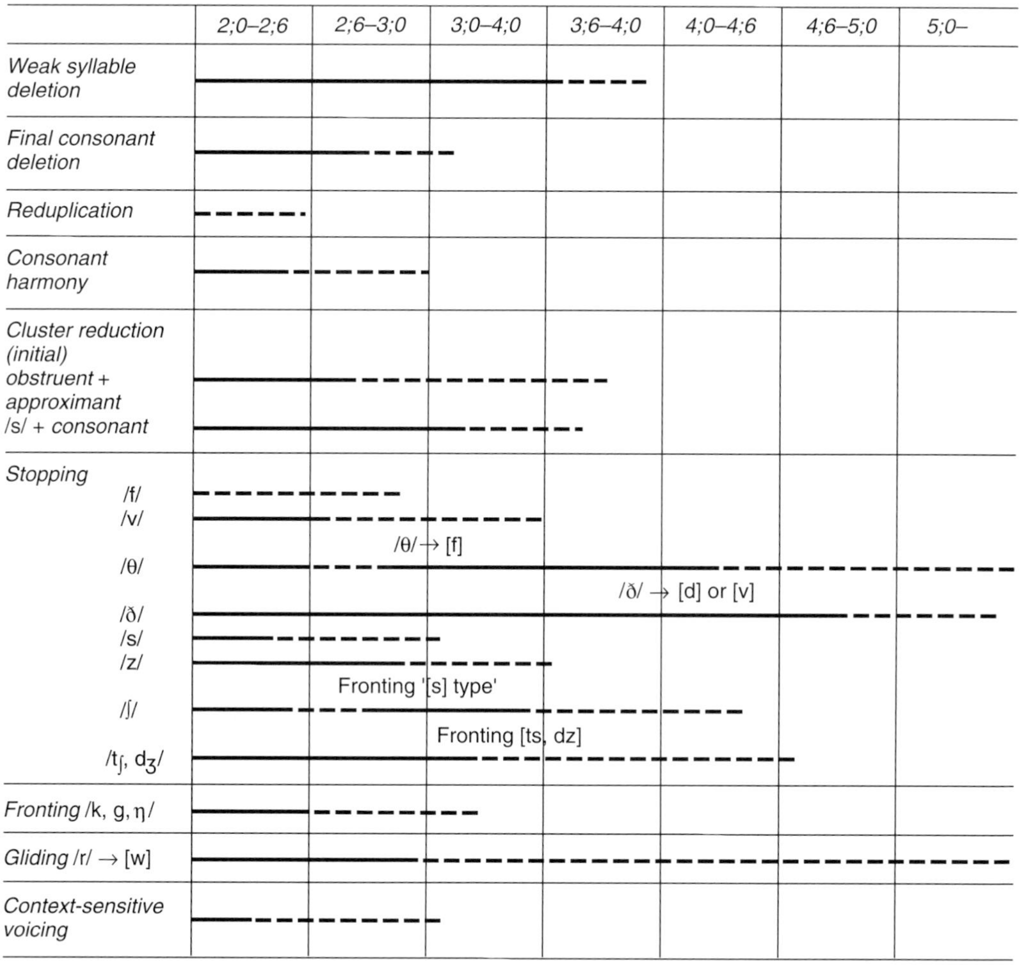

	2;0–2;6	2;6–3;0	3;0–4;0	3;6–4;0	4;0–4;6	4;6–5;0	5;0–
Weak syllable deletion							
Final consonant deletion							
Reduplication							
Consonant harmony							
Cluster reduction (initial) obstruent + approximant /s/ + consonant							
Stopping /f/ /v/ /θ/ /ð/ /s/ /z/ /ʃ/ /tʃ, dʒ/							
Fronting /k, g, ŋ/							
Gliding /r/ → [w]							
Context-sensitive voicing							

Annotations within the Stopping section: /θ/ → [f]; /ð/ → [d] or [v]; Fronting '[s] type'; Fronting [ts, dz].

FIGURE 3.8 Chronology of phonological processes. (From Grunwell, P. (1987). *Clinical phonology.* (2nd ed.). Baltimore: Williams & Wilkins. Reprinted with permission.)

be considered in such decisions, especially the types of errors and the degree of intelligibility. This is becoming more critical now that intervention is occurring more often with younger and younger children.

SUMMARY

Phonology is the study of the sound system of language, which includes the phonetic and linguistic components. Over the years, several theories have been devised to describe how the sound system is acquired by children. Each of the theoretical approaches helps to explain the development of the sound system, but none is completely adequate. The phonological system of a language can be described by its phonemic inventory, phonotactic rules, allophonic sound variations, and morphophonemics. In the process of developing their speech, children often use phonological deviations in their speech productions. Children with articulatory/phonologic disorders use some of these deficient, as well as atypical, patterns in their speech. As children acquire the sound system, they progress through stages of speech development, including prelinguistic utterances (such as cooing and babbling), first words, phonemic development, stabilization of the sound system, morphophonemic development, and spelling. Generally, vowels (with the exception of the rhotic vowels) are acquired early. Consonants tend to be acquired in a sequential order, beginning with the anterior stops, nasals, and glides progressing to alveolar and velar stops and nasal and palatal glide, and ending with the palatal fricatives and affricates and liquids. The first word forms are CV structures that gradually expand to include more complex CV structures (such as VC, CVC), words containing consonant blends, and two or more syllable words.

An integral part of providing service to persons with articulatory/phonologic disorders is an awareness and understanding of the phonological system. In this chapter, theoretical, descriptive, and developmental aspects of phonology were discussed, and the importance of understanding the speech sound system in intervening with individuals with speech problems was underscored. Even though additional information is needed (and is coming), the current state of phonological science is adequate to provide the speech-language pathologist with some helpful clinical data. Implicit in the existing data is the need to identify typical and deviant phonological patterns and to assign a hierarchical significance to them so that subsequent intervention can be facilitated.

REVIEW QUESTIONS

1. Differentiate between the phonetic (motor) and linguistic (phonological) components of the speech sound system.

2. Describe, in one or two sentences each, the essence of the following phonological acquisition theories: (a) behaviorist, (b) structuralist, (c) generative phonology, (d) natural phonology, (e) nonlinear phonology, and (f) optimality.

3. Compare phonotactics, allophonic variations, and morphophonemics and give some examples of rules in the English language for each of these aspects of the phonological system.

4. Define phonological deviations or processes.

5. What are four categories of phonological deviations? Describe frequently occurring deviations of each type, such as cluster reduction, velar assimilation, and stopping.

6. Identify and describe the six stages of phonological development.

7. Identify and describe the four stages of prelinguistic verbalizations.

8. Describe the general sequence of speech development in terms of the acquisition of vowels, consonants, distinctive features, and C/V word shapes.

9. Which phonological processes are suppressed or lost early in phonological development? Which ones are retained longer? Which ones generally do not occur in normal development?

10. Why, as a speech-language pathologist, is it important to know what characterizes typical phonological development?

CHAPTER 4

Dialect Variations of Speech Sound Production

Kathleen Hoffer

"I have always felt that the action most worth watching is not at the center of things but where edges meet. I like shorelines, weather fronts, international borders. There are interesting frictions and incongruities in these places, and often, if you stand at the point of tangency, you can see both sides better than if you were in the middle of either one. This is especially true, I think, when the apposition is cultural."

—Fadiman, 1997 (p. *viii*)

CHAPTER OBJECTIVES

- Describe the characteristics and prevalence of major dialects of the United States.
  - American English dialects—Southern, Eastern, Mainstream American English (MAE) or General American English (GAE)
  - African American Vernacular English (AAVE) dialect
  - Latino dialects
  - Asian American dialects
  - Middle Eastern American dialects
- Describe major concepts related to bilingualism and second-language acquisition.
- Explain the American Speech-Language-Hearing Association's position on working with individuals with dialect variation and those acquiring English as a second language.
- Identify critical issues related to articulation and phonological assessment of culturally and linguistically diverse (CLD) populations.
- Describe goals and strategies for intervention related to accent modification and articulation or phonological remediation with limited English-proficient children.

Speech-language pathologists in a rapidly diversifying culture encounter individuals from ethnic, cultural, and linguistic backgrounds very different from their own. This chapter is designed to help today's speech-language pathologists understand those differences, know their scope of practice as specified by the American Speech-Language-Hearing Association, identify possible speech disorders, and develop treatment plans that are culturally relevant.

The sound system or phonology used during speech, although generally defined as a component of form, also has an impact on the linguistic domains of content and use. How individuals speak informs others of their place of origin, educational status, language proficiency level, social class, ethnicity, health status, emotional state, and group identity. In the famous musical *My Fair Lady,* Professor Henry Higgins transforms Eliza Doolittle, a poor flower girl who worked on the streets of London, into an aristocratic lady able to fool European royalty by merely changing her dialect from cockney to the King's English, with, of course, some training in proper etiquette befitting a person of the upper class. Changing a person's speech alone may well affect one's self-image, interpersonal skills, and ultimately one's view of the world, and certainly others' perceptions.

We are not likely to encounter an Eliza Doolittle, but we can consider some very real possibilities, real people, real backgrounds (only the names have been changed) and real speech–language differences . . . or disorders?

- Luisa is a 10-year-old girl who recently arrived in the United States with her parents. She came from Guadalajara, and her parents were trained professionals. Her mother was a pharmacist, and her father was a construction contractor. None of them had studied English, but all were well educated. Luisa had done well in school and had just passed the fourth grade. The parents have begun studying English as a Second Language (ESL) in a local church program and are making rapid progress. Luisa has just started fifth grade at her local school. She speaks fluent Spanish, but only a few words of English. As the school speech-language pathologist, what is your role?
- Mei is a graduate student from China in a university program majoring in Music. She can read and write English well, but she has more difficulty with pronunciation, even after several years of ESL. Should she enroll in the University Speech and Hearing Clinic to work on her accent?
- Jose is a 9-year-old Filipino boy with a repaired cleft lip and palate who was born and raised in the United States. He continues to have intermittent hypernasality with some misarticulations despite several years of intensive speech intervention. What cultural considerations must

the speech-language pathologist keep in mind in working with the family and in making recommendations for further intervention?
- Tyrone is a 6-year-old African American child attending a mostly white school in the Northwest. His parents use an African American dialect of English when speaking with each other and the children at home. His first grade teacher has referred him for a speech-language evaluation at school. What should the assessment process include, and what would be goals for intervention?
- Yusef is a middle-aged man from the Middle East who has resided in the United States for 5 years. He was trained as an engineer in his country, but has had difficulty finding a job in the United States and is driving a taxi to earn a living. He wants to improve his accent in spoken English. What would be an appropriate approach to treatment, and what special cultural issues may be critical?

These are likely characters and scenarios that a speech-language pathologist may encounter. This chapter offers insight into working with such individuals. It surveys current information on dialects of the United States, describes features of the sound systems that result from a native language influencing English speech production, explores the prevalence of diverse cultures in the United States, and highlights cultural considerations in assessment and intervention.

What are the main dialects of American English?

DIALECTS

A **dialect** is a variation of language spoken by a group of speakers specific to a geographic region, socioeconomic factors, class, ethnicity, and/or educational background. The differences between dialects of a language may be semantic, syntactic, morphologic, pragmatic, and/or phonologic. Many people may find it necessary to **code-switch** between two dialects. For instance, an African American may speak Mainstream American English (MAE; also referred to as Standard or General American English) in a professional or educational setting, but switch to African American Vernacular English (AAVE) in the home with family and friends, as a dialect can have a unifying effect for groups of speakers. People who are able to speak two dialects effectively and code-switch appropriately are considered **bidialectal.**

An individual's form of speech is referred to as an **idiolect**. An idiolect is similar to a speech fingerprint that can identify speech patterns peculiar to one individual only. Such speech printing is currently used for voice recognition in computer work and security systems. Each person is able to recognize the voice of friends within seconds on the telephone, identifying them by their idiolect. Individuals may use different **registers** within their own idiolect for interacting in different situations with people of different status. For example, one might speak differently to parents, bosses, colleagues, partners, children, and pets by varying intonation, voice quality, vocabulary, rate, complexity, and articulation. How people speak not only identifies them as individuals and to what group they belong, but it displays their emotional state (through loudness, vowel duration, pause time, and pitch variation), their general health (through hoarseness, denasality, and breathiness), their level of self-confidence (through loudness, clarity, and word attack), and their perception of their own relative status within a group.

Most languages of the world have several dialects. Historically, when dialects have been separated geographically or politically for long periods, separate languages eventually evolve. The line between separate dialects and different languages is not always a clear, decisive division. For example, although Chinese has one writing system, it comprises nine mutually unintelligible languages and their subdialects, with Mandarin being the most popular language (Lehman, 1973). However, some linguistic historians would posit that Chinese was originally one language and the current "languages" are mere dialects of the original Chinese language.

All dialects of a language are inherently equal in their capacity to express linguistic codes representing human thought and emotion. However, societies historically and universally bestow greater prestige on certain dialects, so people tend to grant higher status to the dialect of the most influential, powerful, or dominant group, as evidenced by Oxford English, Parisian French, High German, and Castilian Spanish. These high status dialects are generally the basis for the literary language of the country. Regional dialects are used in literature only to convey special dramatic elements, such as Mark Twain's use of Southern and African American English in his book *The Adventures of Huckleberry Finn* (1884).

Jim . . . looked at me steady without ever smiling and says: "What do dey stan' for? I's gwyne to tell you. When I got all wore out wid work, en

wid de callin' for you, en went to sleep, my heart wuz mos' broke bekase you wuz los', en I didn' k'yer no' mo' what become er me en de raf'. En when I woke up en fine you back ag'in, all safe en soun', de tears come, en I could 'a' got down on my knees en kiss yo' foot, I's so thankful. En all you wuz thinkin' 'bout wuz how you could make a fool uv ole Jim wid a lie." (p. 111)

According to Edwards (2003), the most common dialects in the United States are:

- Eastern American English, with subdivisions of New England, New York City, and Middle Atlantic Western
- Southern American English, with subdivisions of South Central, Southern, and Appalachian
- General American English (GAE), also referred to as Mainstream American English (MAE) or Standard American English (SAE is less popular because it implies that other forms are nonstandard), with subdivisions of Pacific Northwest, Pacific Southwest, Central Plains, and North Central
- African American Vernacular English (AAVE), also referred to as Black English or Ebonics.

Table 4.1 illustrates the phonological characteristics of the major American English dialects.

Other examples in the evolution of language and its changes are **pidgin** and **Creole**. A pidgin is an abbreviated language form that occurs when a dominant culture needs to communicate for trade purposes with a second subjugated culture. The process begins with a simplification of the dominant language phonologically, syntactically, and semantically (as one simplifies his or her speech when addressing someone who does not understand English, for example). The pidgin may be short-lived and die out when the need ceases, or it may evolve into a language of the community. This abbreviated language gains complexity and incorporates some aspects of the subjugated language. When a new generation of speakers grows up using the pidgin as its native language, a Creole language has been born. Creoles used in the United States today include Hawaiian, Haitian, Louisiana French, and Gullah. For information on the phonological attributes of each of these Creoles, refer to Iglesias and Goldstein (1998).

To determine the nature and extent of a speech disorder, a person's phonological system and resultant articulation of sounds must be evaluated and compared to speakers of the same language subgroup. Clinicians need to realize that the use of a dialect is not substandard speech production. Rather, it is a language difference, not a language disorder.

TABLE 4.1

Dialect Variations in American English

Characteristics	Standard American English (SAE, MAE, or GAE)	African American Vernacular English (AAVE) or Black English (BE)	Southern American English	Eastern American English
Regions	Spoken in the Great Lakes to Pacific region, used in media	Spoken in the South and in African American communities across the United States	Spoken south of the Ohio River, includes Appalachian English and Ozark English	Spoken in mid-Atlantic, New York City, and New England
Consonant clusters	Consonant clusters, each consonant produced	Cluster reduction, e.g., tes/test, kol/kold/, /potɛkt/protɛkt/ Syllable reduction in unstressed multisyllablic words, e.g., baut/əbaut	Epenthesis, sometimes vowel or /g/ may be inserted in cluster, e.g., gostɪs/gosts	Each consonant produced
Interdental consonants	Interdental sounds used, i.e., /θ/ and /ð/	t,f/θ, initial, medial, and final, respectively, e.g., tæŋk/θəŋk, nʌfɪŋ/nʌθɪŋ, tuf/tuθ; d,v/ð initial, medial, and final, respectively, e.g., dæt/ðæt, brʌvɚ/brʌðɚ, bæv/bæð	May be same as in AAVE for initial substitutions (stopping of fricative) t/θ d/ð	Same as SAE
Liquids	Production of liquids, /r/ (retroflex) and /l/ (produced as an alveolar in prevocalic position and slightly back as postvocalic)	Omitted in word final position, e.g., kɑ/kɑr, tu/tul	Postvocalic /r/ is often vowelized, e.g., iʌ/ir	Epenthesis of postvocalic /r/, e.g., aidɪɚ/aidɪə
Glide /w/	/w/ produced in word initial position	/w/ omitted in word initial position, e.g., ʌz/wʌz	Same as SAE	Same as SAE
Vowels and diphthongs	All vowels and diphthongs of SAE produced	Vowel lengthening preceding final stops	/ɔ/ used	/ɔ/ used as in law and dog
	Distinction between /ɑ/ and /ɔ/ minimized	Vowel nasalization precedes nasal, which is then omitted	Diphthongs become lengthened vowel, e.g., ai→ɑː as in fɑː/fair	Broad "a" used, /a/ as in ant/ænt

Note: "/" = "in place of"

When an individual comes from a bilingual community in which two languages are spoken (or from a bidialectal community in which two dialects are used), the speech norms from each subgroup must be used as the basis for comparison. In this context, the clinician can determine whether the person truly has a disordered sound system or whether that sound system replicates that of the community. It is also important to determine the degree of relative proficiency in each language or dialect because the sound system of the individual may be in a transitional state of second-language acquisition.

Possible language subgroups in the United States also include variations in English resulting from the influence of other prevalent languages. **Linguistic interference** occurs when a person's underlying linguistic patterns of the first language are applied incorrectly to a second language. At the phonological level, this phenomenon is referred to as a **foreign accent**. The major non-English languages that are commonly spoken by immigrants to the United States and may influence the production of English are, in order of prevalence, Spanish, Chinese, French, German, Tagalog, Vietnamese, and Italian, as illustrated in Table 4.2 (U.S. Bureau of the Census, 2000).

When a native Spanish speaker learns English, the sound systems of the two languages may clash, resulting in linguistic interference. Certain sounds in English are not used at all in Spanish and vice versa. In addition, different dialects of Spanish such as Mexican, Puerto Rican, Cuban, and Castilian Spanish have phonological variations. Sometimes, the individuals may have spoken an Indian language as their first language, so their Spanish is influenced by that language as well, especially those who have immigrated from southern Mexico, Central America, or areas of South America with large Native American populations. These possible influences are critical to keep in mind during an evaluation of speech sound production in English. A clinician must also possess knowledge of the phonology of the native language to predict proba-

ble error patterns in production of sounds and intonation in English. For information on phonological influences on English in Latino, Asian, and Middle Eastern speakers, see Table 4.3.

The terms **accent reduction** and **accent modification** have been applied to treatment for adults who are native speakers of a language other than English and wish to improve their speech production of English. Reduction or modification implies that something is wrong with an accent, although many would consider an accent rather charming and interesting. Accent *training* may be a more appropriate term for the individual who is attempting to keep the original accent but learn a new one (MAE, for example) and basically become bidialectal. If the speaker's speech production is so deviant as to impair communication in social interactions and the person has studied English for several years without major progress in acquisition of the English phonological system, then a speech disorder may be present. Some individuals may choose to work on their accent for academic or professional reasons. Training actors in producing various accents and dialects also may fall within a clinician's scope of practice.

> How has the attitude toward diversification of American society evolved?

TABLE 4.2

Percentage of U.S. Population (Over 5 Years of Age) Speaking English Only and Languages Other Than English in the Home

Language Spoken	Number of Speakers	Percentage of Population
Population over 5 years of age	262,375,152	100.0%
English only	215,423,557	82.1%
Other languages	46,951,595	17.9%
Spanish	28,101,052	10.7%
Chinese	2,022,143	0.8%
French	1,643,838	0.6%
German	1,383,442	0.5%
Tagalog	1,224,241	0.5%
Vietnamese	1,009,627	0.4%
Italian	1,008,370	0.4%

From the U.S. Bureau of the Census. Statistical abstract of the United States, 2000. (120th ed.). Washington, DC: Author.

THE DIVERSIFICATION OF AMERICAN SOCIETY

Since the mid-1960s, the multicultural fabric of our society has been embraced as a societal ideal by many Americans, despite opposition. The critical importance of respecting cultural differences and maintaining mutual understanding, cooperation, and compassion has become especially poignant for Americans since the attacks of September 11, 2001. As we work to understand how the world perceives the United States, we are called upon to rise above negative stereotyping and become a model of cultural and linguistic diversity—not to make immigrants melt away their past, their cultures, their religious beliefs, and their languages, but rather to embrace the beauty and richness inherent in a multicultural society. Many have moved away from the *melting pot* analogy that blended, mixed and altered the individual elements and are moving toward a *salad bowl* notion of diverse, separate, and interesting components maintaining their color, texture, and individuality.

The Immigration and Nationality Act of 1965 opened the doors of the United States by establish-

TABLE 4.3

Common Errors in English Resulting from Influence of Other Languages

Standard American English	Spanish-Influenced English	Chinese-Influenced English	Middle Eastern-Influenced English
As produced by native adult speakers	As produced by native Spanish speakers speaking English as a second language	As produced by native speakers of Chinese, speaking English as a second language (may be similar to other Asian language native speakers)	As spoken by Middle Eastern individuals speaking English as a second language
Consonant clusters	Epenthesis used to maintain CVCV morphologic structure, e.g., ɛstɑp/stɑp	Epenthesis or consonant deletion	Epenthesis or consonant deletion
Interdentals /θ, ð/	No interdentals used in Spanish except for Castilian, which has a frontal lisp modeled after King Ferdinand's lisp, e.g., tɪn/θɪn, dæt/θæt	/t/ or /s/ used for /θ/ /d/ or /z/ used for /ð/	θ→s, initial, e.g., sɪn/θɪn θ→t, medial, final, e.g., bæt/bæ θ ð→z, initial
Sibilants /s,z,ʃ/ Affricates /tʃ,dʒ/	/z/ doesn't exist in Spanish z→s, e.g., su/zu Dentalized /s, ʃ,tʃ/ are same sound (allophones, thus are used interchangeably in English, e.g., tʃɪp/ʃɪp, ʃɚʃ/tʃɚtʃ /s/ is often omitted in postvocalic position in certain dialects, such as Puerto Rican	May use /s/ and /ʃ/ to substitute for similar English sounds or clusters	/s,z/ used correctly in English, but may have difficulty with affricates, substituting /ʃ/ for /tʃ/, e.g., mʌʃ/mʌtʃ and /ʒ/ for /dʒ/, e.g., ʒok/dʒok
Labiodentals /f,v/	Spanish has a bilabial fricative /β/ that is often substituted for the English /v/	/v/ → /b/, initial, medial, e.g., bɛri/vɛri	/v/→/f/, final, e.g., faif/faiv /v/→/w/, e.g., wɛri/vɛri
Alveolar stops /t,d/	Dentalized	May be deleted in word final position	Glottal stop may be substituted
Liquids /r,l/	Trilled /ɹ/ or tap /ɾ/ substituted for /r/	/r,l/ is one phoneme in Chinese, so are often used interchangeably when speaking English, or /r/ may be omitted	/r/ may be trilled or tapped
Glides /w, j/	Pharyngeal fricative /x/ may be substituted for the glides	/w/→ /v/, e.g., vɚk/wɚk	
Vowels and diphthongs	Vowels may be simplified to /ɑ,e,i,o,u/	Reduced vowel length Difficulty with production of /ɛ,æ, ɪ,ɔ,ʌ/	Difficulty with producing /ɔɪ,i, æ/
Other phonological processes	Final consonants limited in Spanish to /s,n,l,r,d/, so other consonants and consonant clusters are difficult in word final position	Only two final consonants in Mandarin (n, ŋ) Cantonese allows for final /m,n, ŋ,p,t,k/ Problems with syllabic stress, may cause telegraphic, clipped speech. Syllable deletion may occur	Uvular fricatives and pharyngeal fricatives may be used for English fricatives

Note: "/" = "in place of"

ing regional quotas, which began a new wave of immigration, primarily from Asia and Latin America, rather than from Europe as had been the case with earlier immigration movements. The increase in ethnic and linguistic diversity in the United States is even greater than had been predicted in the 1980s. Not only has immigration increased, but the birthrates among immigrant groups have remained high. According to the U.S. Bureau of the Census (2000), the "minority" population was estimated at 87 million, but has increased by 90% over the past two decades. The fastest growing ethnic groups in the United States during the 1990s were the Latino population (58% increase), Asians (48% increase), Native American and Alaska Native (26% increase), African American (16% increase), and Pacific Islander (9% increase). Predictions are that by the year 2050, approximately one half of the U.S. population will be culturally and linguistically diverse, and by 2020, half of the children attending public schools will come from culturally and linguistically diverse (CLD) backgrounds.

Numerous challenges face speech-language pathologists who provide services to CLD students. First and foremost, a clinician must become culturally competent. Cultural competence entails increased sensitivity, knowledge, and understanding of those from diverse backgrounds to be more effective in service delivery to a multicultural population. Clinicians must also be familiar with concepts related to bilingualism and second-language acquisition. University programs in speech, language, and hearing have begun to develop curricula to prepare graduate students to work with individuals from backgrounds very different from their own. However, many professionals who graduated before this became a primary concern tend to lack such preparation. The American Speech-Language-Hearing Association (ASHA) declared multicultural issues to be one of its focused initiatives in 2001, and it continues to develop and disseminate resources for professionals to increase their cultural competency. ASHA also encourages recruitment of CLD students for graduate programs. Additional barriers to providing appropriate, culturally competent services, identified by Roseberry-McKibbin (2002), include:

- Limited empirical research on bilingualism in individuals with disorders
- Paucity of bilingual, bicultural speech-language pathologists
- Time limitations on assessment, because assessing a CLD child requires nearly twice as much time (6 hours) as a monolingual child (3.5 hours) (Langdon, 1992)

- Limited availability of appropriate special education and ESL materials for assessment and intervention

---

What is ASHA's position on dialects?

ASHA POSITIONS ON MULTICULTURAL ISSUES

ASHA Position on Dialects

Since the early 1970s, ASHA has demonstrated interest in multicultural issues such as differentiating dialect from disorder, nonbiased assessment of CLD populations, culturally appropriate interventions, and effective teaching strategies for ESL. The association has wrestled with scope of practice for accent and dialect training as well as for ESL. Position papers have been written and rewritten to define and refine the speech-language pathologist's role in working with CLD populations.

ASHA's technical report titled *American English Dialects* (2003) addressed the importance of dialect being viewed as a neutral term: " . . . no dialectal variety of American English is a disorder or a pathological form of speech or language" (p. 45). However, separate from dialect use, a CLD individual may have a speech or language disorder. It is critical for the speech-language pathologist to have the following competencies in order to differentiate dialect from a true disorder:

- Recognition of dialects as rule-governed
- Knowledge of linguistic features of the dialect used by the client
- Familiarity with nonbiased assessment to include knowing sources of test bias, alternative administration, and scoring of standardized tests
- Experience in using informal assessment strategies, such as observation, interviewing, and language sampling
- Ability to analyze test results using knowledge of dialect as the basis.

Traditionally, speech-language pathologists have served only those with identified disorders, but the speech-language pathologist may provide elective services as well to those who have no disorder but who wish to gain proficiency in the MAE dialect. This would entail adding another dialect to the CLD individual's repertoire, creating a bidialectal individual. There is no intent to replace an individual's first dialect, only to add the option of using the MAE dialect for appropriate contexts.

The speech-language pathologist must have a complete understanding of current attitudes toward the use of different dialects in the local community, an awareness of the cultures involved, and a sensitivity to the historical perspective. It would be helpful for the speech-language pathologist to have supervised instruction and experience in methods of accent training, which involves intonation training and direct work on specific phonemes and phonological patterns.

> What is ASHA's position on working with ESL in school settings?

ASHA Position on Working with ESL in the Schools

ASHA's Multicultural Issues Board (1998) offered guidelines for the many speech-language pathologists in the schools who have been requested to provide services to children learning English as a second language. If the child has a communication disorder, the speech-language pathologist needs special training in culturally and linguistically appropriate assessment and intervention, including first- and second-language acquisition. The policies of the local school district, along with state and national guidelines, should be reviewed with regard to procedures and service delivery for students with limited English proficiency (LEP). ASHA (1989) specified additional guidelines for bilingual speech-language pathologists.

For children acquiring English as a second language in a normal manner, the question of whether a speech-language pathologist should teach ESL has arisen in numerous school districts struggling to provide appropriate services with limited numbers of trained personnel. ASHA consistently has stated that ESL instruction be provided only by trained, knowledgeable professionals who have had specialized training in second-language acquisition theory and ESL methodology. If speech-language pathologists have not had specialized training, they should collaborate with ESL instructors in the preassessment, assessment, and intervention stages. If no ESL instructor is present in a district, speech-language pathologists should provide ESL only when they possess the requisite skills; otherwise, they must limit their involvement to consulting with teachers and parents and maintaining an advocacy role.

> What is ASHA's position on dialect of a speech-language pathologist?

ASHA Position on Dialect of Speech-Language Pathologists

ASHA (1998) tackled the complex issue of dialect variation in speech-language pathologists who were providing clinical service to persons with communication disorders. ASHA maintains that members may not discriminate against persons who speak with a nonstandard dialect in educational programs, employment, or service delivery. However, the clinician must have the necessary diagnostic and clinical skills and be able to model required treatment targets. In addition, the clinician may not have limited English proficiency.

ASHA encourages speech-language pathologists and audiologists to demonstrate nondiscriminatory behaviors in their professional lives by showing an active acceptance of linguistic diversity, displaying cultural competence, and celebrating the diversity that enhances so many lives. There may be a distinct advantage in hiring culturally and linguistically diverse professionals, given the rapid diversification of American society.

ASSESSMENT AND INTERVENTION: ARTICULATION AND PHONOLOGY

Language acquisition follows universal norms, with minor variations that depend on language and culture. Most societies expose young children to two languages or dialects early in life, although monolingualism prevails in the United States. When children acquire two languages before the age of 3, they are considered simultaneous bilinguals. These children reach developmental milestones in each language at approximately the same age as monolingual children. Some children may evidence phonological interference patterns, with the phonological rules of one language influencing the production of the other language. Ray (2002) reviewed phonological development patterns reported by numerous researchers (Fantini, 1978; Genesee, 1989; Holm & Dodd, 1999; Leopold, 1970; Vihman, 1985; Volterra & Taeschner, 1978; Yavas, 1995). Although the studies were not in total agreement, there seems initially to be one phonological system used by the child for the two languages, with separation into two phonological systems occurring between 2 and 3 years of age (Vihman, 1985).

Successive bilingualism refers to learning one language in the home and later learning another language in another setting, such as a preschool or school. The level of proficiency in each language depends on the duration and extent of exposure to the language and attitudes toward the languages as well as other intrapersonal and interpersonal variables. The author once evaluated a 3-year-old boy from a Spanish-speaking home who was attending a local Head Start program. He already had realized that English was the higher-status language in his community, and he informed his mother he did not want to speak Spanish anymore, and in fact wanted her to speak only English to him. The preschool teachers then began to work toward raising the status of Spanish in the classroom, with an eventual positive outcome. Attitudes toward languages can be developed at a very young age.

> What is a culturally and linguistically appropriate way to assess and treat preschoolers from diverse backgrounds?

Assessing and Treating Preschoolers

Young children with multiple misarticulations and unintelligibility who are not keeping pace with developmental norms in the areas of speech and language, despite normal development in other domains, are generally considered to have a phonologic disorder. The use of a phonological approach to assess and remediate highly unintelligible children was investigated by Hodson and Paden (1991). This phonological cycles approach was found to be effective and required fewer years of treatment than the traditional articulation approach. The *Hodson Assessment of Phonological Patterns* (HAPP-3, Hodson, 2004) and the *Assessment of Phonological Processes—Spanish* (App-Spanish Hodson, 1986b) are of high interest to preschoolers, because they are allowed to manipulate and name common objects and pictures. Protocols facilitate rapid transcription of the child's productions. Results can be analyzed for percentage of occurrence rates in the phonological processes of syllable reduction, singleton consonant deletions, consonant sequence reductions, sonorant deficiencies, and obstruent deficiencies. Additionally, results can provide insight about the presence of glottal replacement, substitution processes (fronting, backing, palatalization, depalatalization, stopping, gliding, vowelization, affrication, deaffrication and vowel neutralization), assimilation processes, metathesis, migration, coalescence, reduplication, epenthesis, diminutization, voicing alterations, and minimal place of articulation shifts. Analyses provide the basis for

targeting certain phonological patterns during treatment, cycling through each pattern, moving from the most stimulatory to the least stimulatory pattern, and targeting two or more phonemes within each pattern. This is considered a cognitive–linguistic approach, based on developmental phonology theory and research, but it incorporates many aspects of traditional articulation treatment as well, such as establishing auditory and kinesthetic images, feedback, and self-monitoring.

The phonological cycles approach can be easily adapted to the needs and linguistic backgrounds of children from culturally and linguistically diverse backgrounds. The author had the opportunity to co-supervise, with Dr. Hodson, a graduate student clinician from Puerto Rico working with a 3-year-old Mexican American girl who was blonde and came from a Jewish family from Mexico City. Initial APP-Spanish testing indicated a profound phonological deficit, with most utterances consisting of *eta*. Spanish was the only language spoken in the home, so treatment was provided in Spanish using the cycles approach during a 2-year period. Consistent progress toward improving overall intelligibility in Spanish was noted.

Ray (2002) reported similar progress using a cognitive–linguistic approach with a multilingual 5-year-old boy who had been exposed to Hindi and Gujarati since birth and could be considered simultaneously bilingual in those two languages. He then began preschool at 4 years of age where only English was spoken, so he was also a successive bilingual. The parents reported that he had articulation problems across all languages. According to thorough testing, no **dyspraxia** or other language problems were evident. Before beginning intervention, two naturalistic speech samples for each language were obtained, transcribed by judges fluent in all three languages, and analyzed for presence of phonological processes, percentage of consonants correct, and speech intelligibility in different situations. The *Goldman-Fristoe Test of Articulation* (Goldman & Fristoe, 1986) was also administered, and phonological processes were identified using the Khan-Lewis protocol (2002).

English was chosen as the language of treatment, at the request of his parents. Remediation included reducing simplification patterns, using minimal pairs to learn phonological contrasts, and perceptual training, as well as a home treatment program used daily by the parents. Intervention lasted 5 months, and progress on the phonological processes was tracked monthly. Even though English was the language of treatment, generalization and an increase in overall intelligibility across all three languages occurred. Thus, it is not mandatory that all languages be treated, but it is essential to assess all languages spoken.

Ray (2002) concluded that phonological patterns from the first two languages, which have similar phonologies and lexicons, were applied to English speech production, indicating the extended use of a common phonological system. With successive bilingualism, the timing for separation of the phonological systems is apparently more variable. Ray (2002) provides this conclusion: "Developmental bilingual/multilingual phonology is a very complex matter and requires more information regarding its different aspects, including the importance of age, first language phonology, and how phonological patterns are acquired" (p. 313).

What about using a traditional articulation approach with preschoolers from culturally and linguistically diverse backgrounds? The traditional approach to articulation treatment, established by Charles Van Riper in the 1930s, includes identification of errors in speech production; establishment of correct productions at the sound, syllable, word, and phrase levels; generalization to connected speech in different settings; and maintenance. Perceptual training, also referred to as auditory discrimination or ear training, is a hallmark of the traditional approach, and it requires that the child learn to hear and discriminate the sound before trying to produce the sound. This approach can be effective with preschoolers who manifest articulation errors in their native language, but are generally intelligible.

Again, it is essential that the speech-language pathologist possess a familiarity with the sounds of the child's native language or dialect and use a parent or informant from that language or dialect group to help with diagnosis. Standardized articulation procedures or tests exist in several languages that can be helpful in the identification process. These assessments include:

- *Assessing Asian Language Performance* (Cheng, 1991)
- *Medida Española de Articulación (Measurement of Spanish Articulation)* (Mason, Smith, & Hinshaw, 1976)
- *Spanish Articulation Measures* (Mattes, 1995)
- *The Spanish Preschool Articulation Test* (Tsugawa, 2000)

Generally accepted assessment practices require administration of a standardized test, but informal assessment techniques may need to be used for languages not covered by existing test materials. Such techniques, which should involve the participation of a native speaker, may include naming of objects, repetition of short phrases, estimates of intelligibility by informant and parents, and evaluation of **stimulability**. Lists of sound repertoire, omissions, substitutions, distortions, and additions can then be formulated. When the child is also acquiring English, these results should be compared to English productions. A traditional articulation treatment plan would then be developed if overall intelligibility is above 70%. For less intelligible children, a phonological treatment approach may be more appropriate.

> What are culturally competent assessment and intervention practices for articulation and phonology treatment in the public schools?

Culturally Competent Assessment and Intervention Practices in the Schools

A comprehensive approach to speech and language assessment is preferable in working with all children, but it is essential in accomplishing a least-biased assessment for a culturally and linguistically diverse student. Notice the use of the term *least-biased* rather than *nonbiased*. Some bias exists in any assessment, but the priority is to attain a least-biased level. By being culturally competent, knowledgeable about first- and second-language acquisition, gaining information on local language norms, researching the phonologies of languages and dialects involved, and using a comprehensive approach and a multidisciplinary team, bias should be minimal. The general goals of assessment include:

- Determining whether a speech-language disorder (or merely a difference) exists
- Deciding on the severity level of the disorder, such as whether it warrants intervention
- Providing a direction and basis for appropriate treatment methodology

However, because cultural and linguistic issues add complexity, additional questions must be answered before evaluating, as suggested by Ortiz and Garcia (1988):

1. Has a *pre-referral process* been followed to include:
   - Is the student experiencing communication problems that interfere with academic progress or social interactions?

- Do perceptions of teachers, parents, and aides agree?
- Have systematic efforts been made to identify the problem source(s) and has any corrective action been taken?
- Have difficulties persisted over time?
- Have other programming alternatives been used?

2. Has a *referral protocol* been followed to include:
- Have school and medical records been checked?
- Does the referral source often refer a certain type of child?
- Has the teacher documented and tried alternative methods in the classroom?
- Have other classroom placements been tried, such as bilingual or ESL?
- Is the assessment team familiar with the child's cultural and linguistic background?
- Is socioeconomic level a possible factor?
- Have remedial programs been tried for a sufficient period?

Given the nature of second-language acquisition, additional time of exposure to the second language sometimes can significantly alter speech production. Roseberry-McKibben (2002) outlined the stages of second-language acquisition for normally developing children:

1. *Interference* or transfer, in which rules of the first language are applied to the second language. This is especially true for phonological patterns and more so with older students than younger ones, who tend to have a more flexible phonological system.
2. *Fossilization*, in which specific idiosyncratic errors in the second language remain despite a high level of proficiency.
3. *Interlanguage*, in which a transient, evolving set of rules is developed by the speaker for using the second language with inconsistent error patterns.
4. *Silent period*, during which students may just listen to the new language for 2–6 months, without speaking the language.
5. *Code switching*, in which there is constant mixing of the two languages in conversation as is typical in most bilingual communities, but may be used because of lack of competence in one language (Langdon, 1992).
6. *Language loss*, in which a common happening (such as skill in the second language) increases, the first language becomes vulnerable, especially when the first language is viewed as having lower status.

Two other major concepts related to bilingualism also should be mentioned, because they are critical for serving children in the public schools. Cummins (1992) determined that the acquisition of basic interpersonal communication skills (BICS) requires approximately 2 years of exposure to a language. With BICS, a person can carry on a conversation, follow directions, go shopping, eat at a restaurant, and function well in a highly contextual, "cognitively undemanding" situation. To reach that next level of linguistic functioning in a contextually reduced, cognitively demanding situation such as understanding a lecture, reading a textbook, or taking a standardized test, one would need an addition 5 to 7 years of exposure to language to reach cognitive academic language proficiency (CALP).

The common underlying proficiency model proposed by Cummins (1992) states that having a solid foundation in the first language allows a person to achieve a similar level of proficiency in the second language, but if that first language is limited by switching too soon to the second language, students may have more difficulty learning a second language and may suffer long term cognitive effects and later academic delays. According to Cummins, efforts should be made to support students in becoming bilingual and biliterate and in developing high levels of proficiency in both languages.

Let's return to our first case study about Luisa.

Luisa, a 10 year old, had recently arrived from Mexico. She had been successful in school through the fourth grade, but after her arrival here she refused to speak in her new English-only classroom. The teacher immediately referred her for a speech and language evaluation. What would be an appropriate response to the teacher? What is your role as a speech-language pathologist?

Luisa may be going through a silent period while learning English. She is so new to this situation, but given her earlier academic success and her parents' high level of education, she probably just needs time to adjust and to have an advocate who will make sure she gets ESL assistance and that her classroom instruction has visual cues and incorporates methods of comprehensible input.

(Krashen, 1992)

Assessment of Culturally and Linguistically Diverse (CLD) Students in the Schools

Federal and state legislation over the past 25 years regulates the evaluation and remediation of CLD children, requiring testing in the student's primary language, educational programs in the primary language, nondiscriminatory testing, informed parental consent in the primary language, use of alternative forms of assessment, individualized education plans (IEPs), least-restrictive environment for instruction, and due process for parents to object to or appeal their child's evaluation and IEP. Assessment reports are required to include possible effects of socioeconomic factors, environmental deprivation, and cultural differences that may impact academic progress, but a disorder must exist separate from these factors and cannot be the result of such disadvantages. For detailed information on legislation, review Moore-Brown and Montgomery (2001).

When all factors have been considered and the referral for further speech-language assessment appears warranted, the child study team should continue with special education testing procedures. The school already should have acquired a home language survey from the family and a written permission-to-test form, in the native language signed by the parents. Schools should also have tested the student's language proficiency in the first and second language. Next, an extensive case history using an ethnographic interviewing approach should be completed with the parents, knowledgeable relatives, or caregivers using an interpreter as needed (Mattes & Omark, 1991; Roseberry-McKibben, 2002; Westby, 1990). For an excellent and thorough resource on training interpreters, refer to Langdon and Cheng (2002). After establishing rapport with the family, the interviewer gathers information on early development, in comparison to other children in the family, as well as prenatal care, birth history, early feeding patterns, behavior problems, health issues, and any special concerns the family may have regarding the child. Information on patterns of language use in the home environment is helpful in determining language dominance and proficiency in different situations.

It is the responsibility of clinicians to become well informed with regard to the culture, but they must also become an authority on the phonology of the native languages or dialects of children in the school. Figure 4.1 shows the comparative phonology of Spanish and English used for assessing children who speak Spanish as a first language.

In focusing on speech and articulation, information is also needed on babbling, first words, phrases, oral motor skills, sensory issues related to feeding, clarity of speech in the native language, intelligibility estimates by the parents, extent of ear infections, and explorations of the parents' perceptions of problematic sounds for the child. Efforts should also be made to determine the dialect of the parents, adequacy of their speech model, and history of their language.

Ideally, the assessment with the child should take place over time as the child becomes more comfortable with the examiner, the room, and the interpreter, as well as with performing academic tasks with the examiner. Language testing, which is beyond the scope of this chapter, usually should be screened as part of a speech evaluation. Formal and informal measures should be used in the assessment process. If an articulation/phonology test exists in the native language of the child, it should be administered. A standardized articulation or phonology test, such as the *Arizona Articulation Proficiency Scale-3* (Fudala, 2000), *Goldman-Fristoe Test of Articulation-Second Edition* (Goldman & Fristoe, 2000), or HAPP-3 (Hodson, 2004), should also be administered if the child speaks some English. In addition, a spontaneous speech sample in the native language, consisting of 150 to 200 words, should be obtained in a naturalistic, play setting. Speech should be recorded and transcribed phonetically, with the assistance of a native speaker/interpreter/informant. If the child speaks more than one language, spontaneous speech samples for each language should be obtained in a similar fashion. An oral motor examination should be performed to assess structure and function of the oral motor mechanism. Diadochokinetic rates should be measured for 1 to 3 syllable repetitions. Once the errors are determined, stimulability for correct sound production with practice and repetition should be evaluated. Misarticulations or phonological deficits must be confirmed in the native language to be diagnosed as an actual speech disorder. When the misarticulations only exist in English but the child's native language articulation is good, the problem is one of second-language acquisition and should be dealt with by the ESL teacher or classroom teacher, not the speech-language pathologist.

Let's return to our third case study about Jose.

Jose, a 9-year-old Filipino boy, has a repaired cleft lip and palate but continues to have misarticulations and some hypernasality. As a speech-language pathologist, you have deter-

COMPARISON OF SPANISH AND ENGLISH PHONOLOGY

I. Word and syllable structure: English   CVC, CCVC, CVCC, VC
    Spanish   CV, CVCV, VCV, VC
II. Final consonants are limited in Spanish to /s, n, l, r, d/.
III. Consonant blends are common in English, e.g. *strength*
    In Spanish, /s/ clusters allowed, but must be preceded by /e-/, thus adding one syllable. e.g. *espiritu*
IV. Spanish has 19 consonants, 5 vowels and 2 semi-vowels; English has 24 consonants, 11 vowels, and 2 semi-vowels. (One written English vowel may be pronounced in five different ways, but is produced consistently as one sound in Spanish.)
V. Spanish sounds not used in English include trilled /r/, tap /r/, /ñ/, /x/ and frontal/dental productions of /d, t, n, l/.
VI. English consonants not used in Spanish - /z, v, θ, ð, dʒ, w, ŋ, ʒ/.
VI. Dialects (Puerto Rican, Mexican, Castilian) vary in their productions of /s/, /r/, /j/, /x/.

CONSONANT CHART – English

	Bilabial	Labiodental	Interdental	Alveolar	Palatal	Velar	Glottal
Stops	p b			t d		k g	ʔ
Fricatives		f v	θ ð	s z	ʃ ʒ		h
Affricates					tʃ dʒ		
Nasals	m			n		ŋ	
Glides (Semi-Vowels)	(ω)				j	w	
Liquids				l ɾr			

CONSONANT CHART – Spanish (Mexican)

	Bilabial	Labiodental	Interdental	Alveolar	Palatal	Velar	Glottal
Stops	p b			t̪ d̪		k g	
Fricatives	β	f	(θᶜ)	s	(ʃ) (ʒ^SA)	χ ɣ	h
Affricates					tʃ		
Nasals	m			n̪	ɲ		
Glides (Semi-Vowels)					j	w	
Liquids				l̪ ɾr	(R^PR)		

C   - Castilian
SA - South American
PR - Puerto Rican

FIGURE 4.1   Comparison of Spanish and English phonology (compiled by K. Hoffer).

mined that his speech problems are structural, with dentition interfering with sibilant production and possible fistulae permitting some nasal airflow. You recommend that he see a craniofacial team for orthodontic, plastic, and oral surgery evaluation, and possible surgery. You inform the parents, but they believe he should just continue to work harder in treatment and he'll get better. What is your next step?

The parents may be worried about medical intervention and may lack medical insurance, but they would not admit this to "save face." It may be necessary to back off and just refer him to a local orthodontist, explaining again how the dental structures and possible fistulae are interfering with clear articulation. You may need to help the family seek funding through special programs. Later, a referral to a regional hospital with a craniofacial team might be more acceptable.

Intervention for Culturally and Linguistically Diverse (CLD) Students in the Public Schools

One way schools have sought to reduce expenditures at a time of shrinking educational budgets is to streamline special education and focus on full inclusion for students with special needs. Minimal special services are available, but the least restrictive environment for all students is guaranteed. Likewise, bilingual programs and ESL programs have been reduced, with CLD children transferred out of existing programs as soon as they acquire BICS. Responsibility for teaching multiculturalism falls on the shoulders of the classroom teacher, who is already overwhelmed with larger classes, fewer aides, more students with special needs, and more CLD children. The speech-language pathologist is a helpful resource for the classroom teacher and may become an ESL advocate, a collaborator in teaching using methods of comprehensible input, and a source of critical information on first- and second-language acquisition, as well as a provider of information to teachers on the cultures and languages of the local community.

After a CLD student has been evaluated and has qualified for special speech and language services, the speech-language pathologist assists in the formulation of the IEP. In addition to the goals related to the student's disorder, the following information should be included:

- Need for instruction in the first language
- Specified language of instruction for each objective
- Need for ESL instruction
- Degree of inclusion in the regular classroom

The IEP should be translated into the parents' language and should incorporate their concerns and suggestions. In fact, all written notices to the parents should be translated and followed up with a phone call. Home programs should be developed to support speech-language treatment goals and improve generalization. Regular communication with the parents to monitor progress and provide feedback is highly desirable. Let's return to our fourth case study about Tyrone.

Tyrone, a 6-year-old African American boy, has been referred by his first grade teacher because his speech is hard to understand. AAVE is spoken by his parents at home, although they do speak MAE in their professional lives. The parents expressed some concern that they also have difficulty understanding Tyrone and that his AAVE even has some misarticulations. An assessment by the speech-language pathologist was done, after research was performed regarding characteristics of AAVE and appropriate tests to use. Tyrone's language development was found to be within the average range, but he had sibilant and liquid distortions as well as cluster reduction in initial and final positions. It was determined that his speech production was not AAVE, but was in fact a mild articulatory disorder. What would be appropriate goals for intervention?

Tyrone was enrolled in a small group pullout for speech-language treatment. His misarticulations were targeted directly, and he responded well to treatment. The clinician encouraged him in his acquisition of the two dialects, AAVE and MAE. His parents supported this approach and worked with him at home daily.

WORKING WITH YOUTH AND ADULTS ON SECOND-DIALECT LEARNING

The instruction of a second dialect differs from second-language instruction. Dialect is a variation within a language. Differences between dialects may be reflected in all linguistic domains—phonologic, morphologic, syntactic, semantic, and pragmatic. It is not necessary that the entire language be taught; often, only the points of variation need to be covered. The general goal in second-dialect instruction is to create a bidialectal individual who can function effectively in MAE and maintain the native dialect for purposes of cultural identity and community cohesion. Taylor (1986) characterized the traditional approach to second-dialect instruction as a failure:

> The teaching of standard English to all learners is an implicitly and explicitly stated goal of the American school. Yet the national performance

of the American school in teaching Standard English to nonstandard English speakers is dismal. On almost every reported measure at the national or state level, children from nonstandard English speaking communities achieve lower competency levels in the language of education than children who come from standard English speaking communities. (p.156)

He noted the methodologies used are not culturally based and show a lack of awareness on the part of teachers. Taylor proposed an alternative approach with three prerequisites:

- Alteration of teacher attitudes toward nonstandard dialects
- Increase of teacher knowledge on second-dialect instruction
- Familiarity with ASHA guidelines, developed in the late 1970s, regarding Standards for Effective Communication programs, which includes definitions and information on components of the communication process, communication competence, aspects of effective assessment and instruction, necessary support systems, and effective program evaluations. (p. 183–186)

Taylor proceeded to thoroughly describe one model program that had proved effective in combining a structural linguistic approach with functional communication—"ACCPT: A Cultural and Communicative Program for Teaching Standard English as a Second Dialect." For a complete description of this program, see Taylor (1986), p. 160–175.

Accent Training with Adults

Speaking a nonstandard dialect may have a negative impact on employability. Although, according to the Civil Rights Act of 1965, it is illegal to discriminate against a person for reasons of national origin, race, gender, or religion, many employers refuse to hire individuals with a significant accent when that accent interferes with the individual's ability to perform a job. In April 1990, the U.S. Court of Appeals in San Francisco ruled "that such a refusal is allowed only if an essential part of the job involves speaking to the public" (*San Francisco Chronicle*, April 17, 1990). Research has found that people speaking other than the MAE dialect were offered lower paying jobs and more temporary placements than those who spoke Standard American English (Terrell & Terrell, 1983). Historically, in most countries of the world, many have regarded any dialect other than the standard dialect as deficient. ASHA's position paper on social dialects (1983) states, "No dialectal variety of

English is a disorder or pathological form of speech or language" (p. 23). A speaker of a nonstandard dialect is not a candidate for speech services unless a disorder within the native dialect is present or if the person elects to acquire Standard American English as a second dialect. So, what is the process for assessing and providing services for this special adult population? Two cases introduced at the beginning of the chapter provide some insight.

Mei is a graduate student from China majoring in Music at a university. She can read and write English well, but has more difficulty with pronunciation, even after several years of ESL. Should she enroll in the University Speech and Hearing Clinic to work on her accent?

If Mei chooses to work on improving her accent, she qualifies for services by a speech-language pathologist. Many individuals who speak their first language well have difficulty in acquiring good pronunciation in English and need special, intensive services. An evaluation should be administered to determine problem areas in intonation and pronunciation of English. Goals and objectives can then be formulated and treatment pursued. Many university clinics offer speech and language services to enrolled students free of charge or for a small fee.

Yusef is a middle-aged man from the Middle East who has resided in the United States for five years. He was trained as an engineer in his country but has had difficulty finding a job in the United States, so he drives a taxi to earn a living. He wants to improve his accent in spoken English. What would be an appropriate approach to therapy, and what special cultural issues may be critical?

Here is a case in which employability has been affected by accent difficulties. Yusef would require a slightly more extensive evaluation to determine his actual knowledge of English and level of linguistic competence in several domains. An ethnographic interview should be completed for a fuller understanding of his perspective, background, and concerns. He may need ESL services before specific work on his accent begins. Explanations may need a religious interpretation. Pride, dignity, and honor are especially important to persons from the

Middle East, so matters related to any problem require great sensitivity. There may be a lack of understanding regarding speech and language issues. Thorough explanation of accents and second-language acquisition may be important. Repetition of major points with emphasis may be helpful. Having the assistance of a respected male member of the local Middle Eastern community or a local religious figure may be of value in the assessment process (and perhaps this person can help with interpreting as needed).

Many accent training programs have been developed over the past 30 years to assess and remediate adults who choose to participate in learning a second dialect or to improve their accent as the final stage of acquiring English. Ferrier (1991) focused her efforts on pronunciation training for university teaching assistants (TAs) whose students were having difficulty understanding when the TAs taught courses. Surveys had indicated that nearly one third of all TAs were foreign-born, with most coming from Asia. Linguistic interference patterns are often greatest when the two languages being spoken are not historically related. This can result in a significant accent, despite excellent academic knowledge of English (Cheng, 1989). Ferrier (1991) described the services provided by Northeastern University's speech and language department, working in conjunction with the English Language Center:

- *Screening*—Speech is evaluated through reading single words, stress in multisyllabic words, and intonation in sentences. Overall intelligibility ratings during the TAs' teaching in their classes were also assigned.
- *Orientation*—Information is given on the program, accent, phonetics, oral hygiene, impact of dentition on articulation, and cross-cultural differences.
- *Training*
  - Phase I—correct pronunciation of words and sentences. Visi-Pitch can be used for visual feedback in teaching vowel differences and troublesome consonants (such as /l/ and /r/)
  - Phase II—generalization to spontaneous speech, such as practice of lectures and social situations
- *Program Evaluation*—TAs complete evaluation form regarding their satisfaction with the program. Students in their classes also fill out a form on their comprehension of the TAs' lectures.

Copies of the screening test, remediation plan, data collection form, and classroom assessment are provided in Ferrier's article.

Sikorski (LDS & Associates) has marketed assessment materials, as well as training workbooks, cassettes, and seminars to improve communication in workplaces in which second-language speakers may be experiencing difficulty. Intonation training is an important component in acquiring native-like competence in a second language, and Sikorski's program focuses on mastering the intonation patterns of English before mastering the consonants, vowels, and special vocabulary. Other major accent training programs include David Stern's (1992) *The Sound and Style of American English*, Arthur Compton's *Pronouncing English as a Second Language (P-ESL) Program*, and Audio-Forum's extensive listing of audio and videocassette programs for English as a Second Language, which includes pronunciation guides directed toward native speakers of different languages.

In working with accent training, always keep in mind that the client does not have a disorder or cognitive impairment, only a language difference. The following guidelines are suggested (Mayr-McGaughey, personal communication, 1995):

- Research the phonology, syntax, semantics and pragmatics of the client's language.
- Provide explanations for each activity, with visuals, workbooks, modeling, phonetic symbols, and mirrors.
- Place a strong emphasis on self-monitoring by using a tape recorder and having the person judge self-productions.
- Move from isolated sound to word to phrase immediately.
- Avoid constant correction on first production, but listen together to tape and correct the productions at that point.
- Have client keep a notebook on problem sounds, words, phrases, or idioms heard during the week.
- Use activities and materials that are relevant to the life experience and goals of the client.
- For generalization, observe client outside the clinic in real-life situations and interactions. Provide specific feedback to the client back in the clinic.
- Arrange small-group interactions for clients to practice learned skills with others and to focus on accent.
- Practice telephone conversations.
- Refer for additional services as needed (ESL, tutors, community groups).

SUMMARY

Given the nature of our increasingly diverse society, the American English language and speech reflects that diversity with its many variations, which include numerous regional, ethnic, and social class dialects, as well as dialects resulting from the influence of other languages, most notably Spanish and Chinese because of recent immigration patterns. In the field of speech-language pathology, clinicians may be called upon to work with those from other cultures and other linguistic backgrounds in a variety of settings including homes, preschools, clinics, hospitals, public schools, and geriatric settings. This chapter has presented the basics of developing culture competence to serve the CLD population effectively at different ages with different problems in different settings.

Most importantly, clinicians must be able to distinguish a speech/language disorder from a speech/language difference. Children or adults with language disorders in their native language qualify for speech and language services. Individuals who choose to learn a second dialect may also be served electively. The collective goal should be to create a society more tolerant of differences by embracing the concept of bilingualism and multiculturalism.

REVIEW QUESTIONS

1. What is the difference between a dialect, language, pidgin, and Creole? Give an example of each.

2. Are any dialects substandard? Explain why or why not.

3. What is the problem with the term *accent reduction*?

4. Describe the major dialects of American English.

5. What sounds in American English seem to be most influenced by other languages?

6. Define cultural competence. Explain barriers to providing culturally competent services in the field of speech-language pathology.

7. What is the position of ASHA on working with individuals with dialects and accents?

8. Should a speech-language pathologist in the schools work with ESL instruction?

9. If a speech-language pathologist speaks a nonstandard dialect, what does ASHA recommend?

10. Name assessment instruments appropriate for assessing Spanish-speaking preschoolers' articulation and phonology.

11. What has research shown about carryover from one language to another when the phonological cycles approach is used?

12. In the schools, a careful pre-referral and referral process should be followed before speech-language assessment is administered. Describe the elements of this process.

13. Name and describe six stages in the second-language acquisition of typically developing children.

14. Explain BICS and CALP.

15. What other informal measures are necessary when testing articulation? How are these modified for use with a child from another language background?

16. What does the speech-language pathologist need to know about the phonology of the client's native language?

17. Describe the components of an accent training program.

CHAPTER 5

Types and Potential Etiological Factors of Articulatory/Phonologic Disorders

"That is not good language that all understand not."

—Proverbs

CHAPTER OBJECTIVES

- Identify "labels" used for speech sound disorders.
- Identify the factors involved in making a diagnosis of articulatory/phonologic disorder.
- Describe the categorizations and types of articulatory/phonologic disorders.

- Identify potential etiological factors of articulatory/phonologic disorders: structural, physiologic and neuromuscular, sensory/perceptual, cognitive, hereditary, psychosocial and environmental, personal, linguistic and academic, and other speech areas.

W hat is the preferred label for speech sound disorders? Terminology has changed over the years, and speech-language pathologists continue to be perplexed as to what to call this group of communication disabilities (Fey, 1992; Hulit & Howard, 2002; Shriberg, 1982, 1997). In about 1920, the term *dyslalia* was replaced by *articulation disorder,* which was used until the 1980s. However, during the 1970s, clinical researchers began to analyze speech sound errors phonologically, and during the 1980s, clinicians and researchers began to use the term *phonologic disorders* more widely. During the 1990s and presently, there is no consistent use of the terms *articulation* and *phonology.* Some use articulatory disorder and phonologic disorder synonymously; some differentiate among *articulatory, phonologic,* and *combined articulatory/phonologic* disorders; some use the term *phonologic disorder* for all speech sound disorders with the rationale that phonology encompasses both the motor and linguistic aspects of the sound systems. Finally, some use the term *articulatory/phonologic disorders* as this book does. Articulatory/phonologic disorders can be

defined simply as speech sound(s) produced and used at variance with the linguistic community usage or age-level expectations. Later in this chapter, articulatory disorders and phonologic disorders are differentiated.

> What factors are considered when making a diagnosis of articulatory/phonologic disorders?

WHAT CONSTITUTES AN ARTICULATORY/PHONOLOGIC DISORDER?

As pointed out in Chapter 3, misarticulations occur normally during the early stages of speech development. Thus, when some articulation errors occur at certain age levels, the child is not considered to have an articulatory/phonologic disorder. Rather, use of such speech sound patterns is characteristic of typical speech acquisition. When do misarticulations or phonological deviations constitute a disorder? It is not easy to decide whether a given individual should be regarded as having an articulatory/phonologic disorder. Some research has shown that speech sound development continues until approximately 9 years of age with additional development of allophonic and prosodic levels occurring up to 12 years (Shriberg & Austin, 1998). For example, at least one study showed that acquisition of phonemes, that is, spontaneous correction of misarticulations without speech treatment, sometimes continues until the fifth grade (Bralley & Stoudt, 1977), and another found that articulation continues to develop until the fourth grade (Roe & Milisen, 1942). Nevertheless, it is generally agreed that by the second grade or by 7 to 8 years of age, most children have acquired normal articulation and basic phonological patterns as compared to adult standards (Table 3.7). When misarticulations are regularly present after the expected age of acquisition or when phonological development is behind the expected norms, the speech sound system is considered deficient.

As alluded to earlier, probably the most critical variable in determining whether articulation or phonology is deficient is the child's speech sound production as compared to normative data relative to the age at which specific phonemes are acquired and at which phonological deviations are suppressed (refer to Chapter 3). When a child's errors are atypical for the age level, they are considered an articulation delay or disorder. Standardized articulation/phonological testing results are helpful when the norms are for children of the same linguistic community. It is critical to make such comparisons with typical adult phoneme production patterns in the client's own linguistic community rather than with Standard American English patterns. Additional factors to consider when making a diagnosis include:

• Number of errors
• Consistency of errors
• Types of errors
• Types of phonological deviations (processes)
• Conspicuousness of errors (either auditory or visual)
• Ease of imitating correct production of misarticulated sounds (stimulability)
• Speech intelligibility (ability to be understood)
• Views held by the individual and others regarding the speech problem

One important variable mentioned in this list is intelligibility, which is affected by several articulation/phonological characteristics including the number of misarticulated sounds, consistency of misarticulations, the frequency with which misarticulated sounds occur, type(s) of misarticulations, and type(s) of phonological deviations. Intelligibility is also influenced by suprasegmental factors, such as prosody, voice characteristics, loudness, and fluency, and contextual/linguistic features (Gordon-Brannan, 1994). Obviously, the more unintelligible the speech is, the greater the severity of the problem and the greater the need for articulation treatment.

What terms are used to describe various types of articulatory/phonologic disorders?

TYPES OF ARTICULATORY AND PHONOLOGIC DISORDERS

Differentiate between an articulation/ phonological delay and a disorder.

Delay Versus Disorder

Speech-language clinicians often differentiate between use of an immature phonological system and a deviant system; that is, a delay versus a disorder. In a delay, the individual is following a normal sequence of development, but at a slower rate. For example, a 5-year-old who is speaking as a typically developing 3.5-year-old is exhibiting an articulation/phonological delay. Conversely, in a disorder, the person is using an atypical developmental pattern. Examples of disordered articulation include a 4-year-old who produces /s/ and /z/ correctly, but misarticulates the earlier developing stops; a 7-year-old who laterally distorts the sibilants (note that frontal sibilant distortions are typical patterns); or a 5-year-old who backs alveolars to velars. For purposes of efficiency, the term *disorder* will be used in this book for both delay and disorder, realizing that the diagnostician should try to differentiate between an articulation/phonological delay and an articulatory/phonologic disorder for most effective clinical management. In any case, it is obviously important to understand and know what characterizes typical articulation and phonological developmental errors/patterns as well as errors/patterns seen in persons with speech sound disorders.

> Differentiate between an articulatory/
> phonologic disorder that is phonetically
> based and one that is phonologically based.

Phonetic Versus Phonologic

Another classification system dichotomizes speech sound disorders into the categories of phonetic (motoric or articulatory) disorders and phonologic (linguistic or cognitive) disorders. Phonetic errors are the result of difficulty in producing the sounds and sound sequences of the language; that is, of executing motoric movements for speech sound production. Phonological errors are the result of a difficulty in understanding and implementing the underlying linguistic rules for producing sounds and sound sequences; that is, of using speech sounds incorrectly in a given language even though the motoric movements can be executed adequately. Basically, phonetic or motor misarticulations occur on speech sounds that the speaker has difficulty producing or seemingly cannot produce, whereas phonological errors occur on speech sounds that the speaker can produce, but does not use the appropriate sound in a certain speech/language context. Examples of phonetic errors are sound distortions such as lateralized /s/ and /z/ or a seeming inability to produce /k/ and /g/. An example of a phonological error is when a child uses a t/s substitution and yet uses s/ʃ and ʃ/tʃ (Note: "/" means "in place of"). In the latter case, the speaker can produce /s/ and /ʃ/, but does not use these sounds in the appropriate place. Different treatment approaches have been developed for phonetic and phonological errors; therefore, it is important to differentiate between these two types of misarticulations. The task is made more difficult because many children with articulatory/phonologic disorders make both types of errors simultaneously.

> Describe the classification system devised
> by Shriberg and associates for child speech
> disorders.

Speech Disorders Classification System

A classification system for speech sound disorders has recently been proposed by Shriberg and colleagues (Shriberg, 1997; Shriberg & Austin, 1998; Shriberg, Austin, Lewis, McSweeny, & Wilson, 1997; Shriberg & Kwiatkowski, 1994; Shriberg, Tomblin, & McSweeny, 1999) and includes four major categories:

- Normal or normalized speech acquisition
- Developmental phonologic disorders
- Nondevelopmental speech disorders (first occur after 9 years of age)
- Speech differences that include those associated with cultural diversity and accent reduction

Note that two of these categories—normal speech acquisition and speech differences—are not speech disorders. *Child speech disorders* is the label recommended by Shriberg for the group of speech sound disorders occurring during the speech acquisition developmental period (birth to 9 years) encompassing two groups: (a) special populations for all child phonologic disorders of known etiologies and (b) developmental phonologic disorders for those with unknown etiologies. The schema for the system appears in Figure 5.1. It should be noted that this framework has been considerably expanded based on research completed in the years since its publication.

Three classifications for child speech disorders emanate from the major category of developmental phonologic disorder—speech delay, questionable residual errors, and residual errors and one from the normal or normalized speech acquisition category—normalized speech acquisition/speech delay. The speech delay classification can occur between the ages of 2:0 (years:months) and 8:11 for children who use age-inappropriate omissions or substitutions. Those classified as questionable residual errors are aged 6:0 to 8:11 and have one or more sound distortions or common substitutions (w/r, w/l, vowel/r, vowel/l, t/θ, θ/s, ð/z, vowel/ɝ,ɝ). Those categorized with residual errors (RE) are 9 years and older who continue to have speech sound errors with RE-A representing those who have histories of speech delay and RE-B for those who have no history of speech delay. Etiological categories include:

- Unknown etiology, possibly genetic
- **Otitis media** with effusion
- **Developmental apraxia of speech (DAS)**
- Developmental psychosocial involvement
- Special populations, including craniofacial involvement and cerebral palsy

Normalized speech acquisition/speech delay represents a status that falls somewhere between the two categories of normalized speech acquisition and speech delay and is considered subclinical. Children in this category, aged 2:0–8:11, may meet the criteria for questionable residual errors at 6 years, normalize at any age up to 8 years, or meet the criteria for residual errors at 9 years.

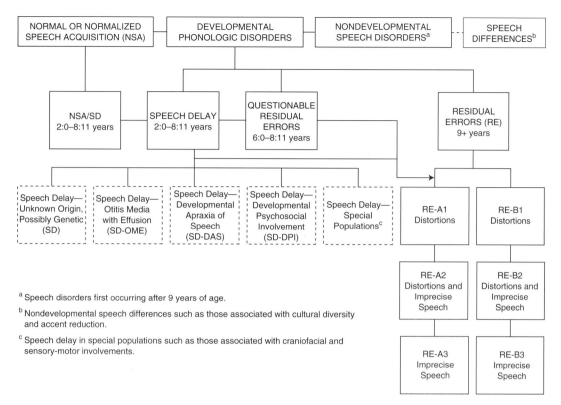

FIGURE 5.1   The speech disorders classification system developed by Shriberg and associates. (From Shriberg, L. D. (1997). Developmental phonological disorder(s): One or many? In B. W. Hodson & M. L. Edwards (Eds.). *Perspectives in applied phonology* (pp. 105–127). Gaithersberg, MD: Aspen Publishers. Reprinted with permission.)

Describe dyslalia, dysarthria, and apraxia of speech.

Dyslalia, Dysarthria, and Apraxia of Speech

A classic classification system includes three types that generally refer to etiological bases of the disorder. Two of these categories, dysarthria and **apraxia**, are widely used today, while the third one, **dyslalia**, is rarely used. Dyslalia, an old term, is defined as "defective articulation due to faulty learning or to abnormality of the external speech organs and not to lesions of the central (or peripheral) nervous system" (Wood, 1971, p. 11). Thus, it may be either a nonorganic or organic articulatory disorder.

Dysarthria is a motor speech disorder manifested as disorders of phonation, articulation, resonation, and prosody, singly or in combination, resulting from "weakness, paralysis, dyscoordination, primary and secondary sensory deprivation, and alteration in the tone of the speech musculature" because of impairment of the central nervous system, peripheral nervous system, and/or muscular system (Dworkin, 1991, p. 5–6). Dysarthria represents a group of motor speech disorders—rather than a single entity—involving one or more of the speech production parameters; that is, respiration, articulation, phonation, resonation, and prosody. Dysarthria results from impairment of any level of the neuromuscular system with both voluntary and involuntary movements being impaired. Seven types of dysarthria have been described: flaccid, spastic, ataxic, hypokinetic, hyperkinetic, mixed, and variable (Table 5.1). Many persons with dysarthria produce imprecise consonants, which compromises intelligibility.

Apraxia or dyspraxia of speech is a speech disorder characterized as an impairment in "planning, programming, and executing sequences of intentional movement for speech production" (Yorkston, Buekelman, Strand, & Bell, 1999, p. 73). The disorder is called, among other labels, **verbal apraxia** and **verbal dyspraxia**. Throughout this text, these terms are used interchangeably to refer to apraxia of speech. Apraxia of speech primarily affects articulation/phonology, and secondarily, there is "some disruption in prosody, although it is not

TABLE 5.1

Mayo Clinic Perceptual Classification of Dysarthria

Type	Perceptual Characteristics	Localization	Etiology	Neuromuscular Condition
Flaccid dysarthria	Breathy voice quality Hypernasality Imprecise consonants	Lower motor neuron	Viral infection (e.g., poliomyelitis), tumor, CVA, congenital conditions, disease (e.g., myasthenia gravis), palsies (e.g., bulbar, facial), trauma	Flaccid paralysis Weakness Hypotonia Muscle atrophy Fasciculations
Spastic dysarthria	Strained/strangled/harsh voice quality Hypernasality Slow rate Imprecise consonants	Bilateral upper motor neuron	CVA, tumor, infections (e.g., encephalitis), trauma, congenital conditions (e.g., spastic cerebral palsy)	Spastic paralysis Weakness Limited range of movement Slowness of movement
Ataxic dysarthria	Imprecise consonants Excess and equal stress Irregular articulatory breakdown	Cerebellar or cerebellar pathway lesion	CVA, tumor, trauma, congenital condition (e.g., ataxic cerebral palsy, Friedreich's ataxia), infection, toxic effects (e.g., alcohol)	Inaccurate movement Slow movement Hypotonia
Hypokinetic dysarthria	Monopitch Monoloudness Reduced stress Consonant imprecision Inappropriate silences Short rushes	Extrapyramidal system	Parkinson's disease, drug induced (e.g., reserpine or phenothiazine)	Slow movements Limited range of movement Immobility Paucity of movement Rigidity Loss of automatic aspects of movement Resting tremor
Hyperkinetic dysarthrias Predominantly quick	Imprecise consonants Prolonged intervals Variable rate Monoloudness	Extrapyramidal system	Chorea, infection, Gilles de las Tourette's syndrome, ballism sia (e.g., torticallis, or tardive dyskinesia)	Quick involuntary movements (e.g., myoclonic jerks, tics) Variable muscle tone
Predominantly slow		Extrapyramidal system	Athetosis, infection, CVA, tumor dystonia, drug induced, dyskinesia	Twisting and writhing movements Slow movements Involuntary movements Hypertonia
Mixed dysarthria Spastic-flaccid	Imprecise consonants Hypernasality Harsh voice quality Slow rate Monopitch Short phrases Distorted vowels Low pitch Monoloudness Excess and equal stress Prolonged intervals	Upper and lower motor neurons	Amyotrophic lateral sclerosis, trauma, CVA	Weakness Slow movement Limited range of movement

(continued)

TABLE 5.1 (Continued)

Mayo Clinic Perceptual Classification of Dysarthria

Type	Perceptual Characteristics	Localization	Etiology	Neuromuscular Condition
Spastic-ataxic-hypokinetic	Reduced stress Monopitch Monoloudness Imprecise consonants Slow rate Excess and equal stress Low pitch Irregular articulation breakdown	Upper motor neuron, cerebellar, extrapyramidal	Wilson's disease	Intention tremor Rigidity Spasticity Slow movement
Variable (spastic/ataxic/flaccid)	Variable (e.g., slow rate, harsh voice quality, irregular articulation breakdowns)	Variable (e.g., upper motor neuron, cerebellar, lower motor neuron)	Multiple sclerosis	Variable (e.g., spasticity, weakness, slow movement, limited range of movement inaccurate movement)
Others	Variable	Variable	Multiple CVAs, tumor, trauma, disease, etc.	Variable

Note: CVA = cardiovascular accident or stroke

From Darley, F., Aronson, A., & Brown, J. (1975) *Motor speech disorders.* (p. 13). Philadelphia, PA: W. B. Saunders. Copyright 1975 Elsevier Inc. Adapted with permission.

clear whether that disruption is primary to the disorder or a consequence of the impairment" (Yorkston et al., 1999, p. 73). Apraxia of speech is defined as "an impaired capacity to form vocal tract configurations and to make transitions between vocal tract configurations for volitional speech production in the absence of motor impairments for other actions using the same musculature" (Rosenbek, Kent, & LaPointe, 1984, p. 12). In other words, the person who is dyspraxic has difficulty positioning the articulators and sequencing the articulation movements for meaningful speech. Furthermore, the individual shows no difficulty with reflexive and volitional nonspeech movements, but has difficulty using the same musculature when producing meaningful phonemes and sequencing the movements to produce words. Many researchers consider apraxia of speech to be a motor speech disorder, but some argue that it is linguistically based (Air, Wood, & Neils, 1989; Rosenbek et al., 1984; Yorkston et al., 1999). Two forms of apraxia have been identified: acquired and childhood (or developmental). Acquired apraxia occurs after completion of speech and language development resulting from brain damage to, most commonly, Broca's area. In contrast, **childhood apraxia of speech (CAS)**, also labeled developmental apraxia of speech (DAS) or **developmental verbal dyspraxia (DVD)**, occurs while the child's speech and language are developing; a consistent neurological basis has not been identified (Air et al., 1989; Yorkston et al., 1999). Because CAS occurs while language acquisition is in progress, the disorder may have a more widespread linguistic effect.

Acquired apraxia of speech often occurs along with aphasia (and sometimes with dysarthria), and seldom occurs alone (Yorkston et al., 1999). Usually, auditory language comprehension is preserved. Apraxic speech is characterized as groping, off-target, and quite inconsistent articulation (Dworkin, 1991; McNeil, Robin, & Schmidt, 1997; Rosenbek et al., 1984; Yorkston et al., 1999). Generally, articulation errors increase as the complexity of the speech motor task increases with more errors occurring on clusters, fewer on singletons, and the least on vowels. There is more articulation breakdown on longer words, on imitative speech tasks than on spontaneous speech, on volitional-purposive speech than on automatic speech, on the most propositional words when reading, on later-developing sounds, and on less frequently occurring phonemes. More errors occur on initial consonants as compared to sitions. Speech sound substitution ␣re frequently than **omissions**, distor-␣␣␣**litions**. Most consonant substitutions ␣␣␣␣r two feature errors such that at least one feature is retained. Additionally, speech sound sequencing errors occur, that is, migration and metathesis, with anticipatory migration being the most frequent. Occasionally, sound repetitions occur as well as other types of dysfluency. Finally, the client may exhibit periods of error-free speech.

Clients with CAS have difficulty positioning and sequencing muscle movements specifically for speech production. This is manifest in difficulties in articulation and prosody. The specific symptoms vary from one client to the next, which makes it a difficult disorder to diagnose (Hall, Jordon, & Robin, 1993). Hall et al. (1993) completed a thorough review of the literature on childhood apraxia of speech and reported the following information, which is in general agreement with the symptoms described by Caruso & Strand (1999) and Yorkston et al. (1999). A summary of this information appears in Table 5.2. Generally, there is more difficulty with production of the later-developing sounds such that more errors occur on clusters, fricatives, affricates, and liquids. Consistent with this pattern, the developmental sequence tends to be similar to normal development, but at a much slower rate. The most frequent type of misarticulations in younger children with CAS involves omissions followed by substitutions, whereas older children use more substitutions and fewer omissions. They also use distortions and additions. Unusual errors such as additions, prolongations, repetitions of sounds and syllables, nonphonemic productions, voicing errors, and vowel and diphthong errors have frequently been reported. Children with CAS have difficulty sequencing phonemes and syllables, which is manifested in misarticulations of speech sounds that they can produce in less complex speech tasks, difficulty producing multisyllabic words and longer utterances, use of the phonological deviations of metathesis and reduplication (sometimes called *redundancies*), and difficulty with **diadochokinetic** tasks. Inconsistent and variable articulation is frequently mentioned in the literature as a characteristic of CAS. While research results have been inconclusive, according to Hall et al. (1993):

> . . . most children with DAS do exhibit some degree of inconsistency within their speech errors, dependent upon the complexity of the task being required of them. Inconsistencies may be particularly apparent when comparisons of the same task over several time periods are made and when repeated trials of the same speech task are required of the children. (p. 23)

Clients with CAS are often unintelligible, particularly so in conversational speech when the listener does not know the topic or context.

Groping articulation movements and silent posturing of the articulators are frequently present, which is noted especially after speech intervention is implemented (Hall et al., 1993). Groping is defined as an "active and ongoing series of movements of the articulators in an attempt to find the desired articulation position necessary for correct phoneme production" and silent posturing is a "static state of articulation position that occurs without sound production" (Hall et al., 1993, p. 38). Children with CAS have difficulty achieving and maintaining articulation configurations (Caruso & Strand, 1999; Yorkston et al., 1999). As with adults, children with CAS often exhibit prosody impairments although their nature varies from child to child. They also tend to use some dysfluencies. Many children with CAS present with **hypernasality**, hyponasality, or nasal air/sound emission that is frequently inconsistent and variable, which may be symptomatic of incorrect timing of velopharyngeal movements. This is consistent with Caruso and Strand's (1999) characterization of CAS. Finally, their progress in treatment tends to be quite slow, and those with severe CAS may never develop "normal" speech.

In CAS, articulation performance is influenced by context such that:

- Errors increase with increasing length of word or utterance
- Articulation breaks down more in sentences or conversational speech than in single words
- Errors increase with increasing phonetic complexity of the utterance
- Well-practiced utterances are produced or imitated more easily than unfamiliar utterances
- More errors occur in spontaneous production than in imitation, especially for new movement patterns (Caruso & Strand, 1999; Yorkston et al., 1999)

Oral apraxia is difficulty in performing nonspeech tasks using the articulation structures upon command or in imitation. Individuals with this impairment have difficulty voluntarily using the speech mechanism to complete nonspeech activities in the absence of structural or functional abnormalities of the articulators. Persons with acquired and childhood apraxia may demonstrate oral apraxia. It especially seems to be present in CAS (Hall et al., 1993; Yorkston et al., 1999).

What factors are involved in specifying severity level of impairment?

TABLE 5.2

Characteristics Frequently Occurring in Individuals with Childhood Apraxia of Speech (CAS)

Behavioral Categories	Characteristics
Articulation characteristics	Multiple speech sound errors
	Omissions—most common in younger children with CAS
	Substitutions—most common in older children with CAS
	Distortions
	Additions
	More difficulty with later-developing sounds (fricatives, affricates, liquids)
	Unusual errors
	Additions
	Prolongations
	Repetitions
	Nonphonemic productions
	Voicing errors
	Vowel and diphthong errors
Sound sequencing and timing characteristics	Metathetic errors (transposition of sounds and syllables)
	Reduplication (redundancy) errors
	Difficulty with particular sound sequences, even when the individual sounds are correct in isolation or CV combinations (sounds produced correctly in some sequences will be in error in other sequences of sounds)
	More difficulty with consonant clusters than singletons
	Nasal resonance problems
	Hypernasality
	Hyponasality
	Nasal emission
Movement characteristics	Difficulty imitating articulation configurations, especially for initial sounds
	Difficulty making movement transitions in and out of spatial targets
	Difficulty maintaining articulation configurations
	Groping movements of the articulators
	Silent posturing of the articulators
	Trial-and-error movement behavior
Disturbances in prosody	Slower rate
	Inappropriate or longer pauses
	Reduced stress variation
	Errors in syllabic stress
	Dysfluencies
Contextual changes in articulation proficiency	Errors increase with increasing length of word or utterance
	Repetition elicits better articulation performance than spontaneous production
	Sounds are more easily produced in single words than in sentences or conversation
	Errors vary with the phonetic complexity of the utterance
	Errors are inconsistently produced
Other factors	Receptive language performance superior to expressive language performance
	Presence of oral apraxia
	Slow progress in speech intervention

Adapted from Yorkston, K. M., Beukelman, D. R., Strand, E. A., & Bell, K. R. (1999) *Management of motor speech disorders in children and adults* (2nd ed.). Austin, TX: Pro-Ed, 1999. Adapted with permission.

Severity Levels

Severity of articulatory/phonologic disorders varies from mild to severe and from barely perceptible to the trained ear to completely unintelligible. Factors contributing to the severity level of a particular articulatory/phonologic disorder include: the number of misarticulated sounds; the consistency of misarticulations; the types of errors (typical or atypical; omissions, substitutions, distortions, additions); level of intelligibility; stimulability of the misarticulated sounds (ability to imitate the sound in error); normalcy of suprasegmental features (rate, intensity, stress, and rhythm); and the age of the person (Davis & Bedore, 2000; Perkins, 1977; Powers, 1971). Additional factors to be considered in determining severity are the prognosis for developing correct articulation and the probable amount of intervention needed for error correction. For example, a good prognosis means that the severity level frequently will be less than with a poor prognosis. Similarly, if years of treatment seem necessary for speech improvement, the problem is considered more severe than if the disorder will likely require less time to correct. Standardized testing results can provide guidance for assigning severity levels to a particular client. Suggested criteria for assigning severity levels based on standardized scores appear in Table 5.3.

Describe the types of misarticulations termed omissions, substitutions, distortions, and additions, as well as lisps.

Descriptions of Speech Sound Errors

Speech-language pathologists characterize speech sound errors as the particular phonological processes or deviancies, such as cluster reduction, gliding, or stopping, used by the client (refer to Chapter 3) and/or as descriptions of how individual phonemes are misarticulated. The most traditional system for labeling articulation errors is a description of how individual phonemes are misarticulated. The types of errors include: (a) omission, (b) substitution, (c) distortion, and (d) addition. An individual with articulation deviances may have one or a combination of these types of errors. For example, the same person may substitute /t/ for /k/, /f/ for /θ/, omit /l/ and /r/ in blends, and distort /s/ and /r/.

An omission is an articulation error in which a phoneme is not produced at a place where one should occur; for example, /kæ/ for /kæt/ in the word *cat* and /te/ for /ste/ in the word *stay*. Omissions are most common in the final position of words and occur less frequently in the medial position for most sounds. Initial consonants seldom are omitted with the exception of initial liquids and glides in some young children (Smit, 1993a). Omissions occur in two-element and three-element clusters in younger children; however, only rarely is an entire cluster omitted (Smit, 1993b). The number of omissions decreases with age; they appear more frequently in the speech of younger children and rarely occur in the speech of children ready for preschool. They are the greatest contributors to speech unintelligibility. Commonly, a hyphen (-) is used to indicate omissions such that -/t indicates that the /t/ sound is omitted.

A substitution is a misarticulation in which another phoneme replaces the correct phoneme, for example, /tet/ for /tek/ and /w ɛ d/ for /r ɛ d/. Substitutions are relatively common and typical in the speech of young children and are the most frequent type of articulation error in school-aged children, although the frequency of occurrence tends to decrease with age. The most common substitutions as reported by Byrne and Shervanian (1977) and Van

---

TABLE 5.3

Suggested Criteria for Assigning Severity Levels Based on Standardized Test Scores

Severity Level	Standard Deviation (SD)	Percentile	Standard Score (Mean = 100; SD = 15)
Normal	Within 1 SD	Above 16th percentile	85+
Mild	1–1.5 SDs below mean	8th–15th percentile	79–84
Moderate	1.5–2 SDs below mean	2nd–7th percentile	69–78
Severe	2–3 SDs below mean	Below 2nd percentile	Below 68
Profound	3+ SDs below mean	Beyond standard rating	Beyond standard rating

TABLE 5.4

Most Frequent Phonemic Substitutions

Substitution	Example
/w/ and /j/ for /l/	wæmp/læmp; jæmp/læmp
/w/ and /j/ for /r/	wɛd/rɛd; jɛd/rɛd
/θ/ or /t/ for /s/	bʌθ/bʌs; tʌn/sʌn
/ð/, /d/, or /s/ for /z/	ðu/zu; dibrə/zibrə; su/zu
/t/, /f/, or /s/ for /θ/	tʌm/θʌm; bof/boθ; tis/ti θ
/d/, /v/, /z/ for /ð/	dɪs/ðɪs; viz/ðiz; ziz/ðiz
/t/ or /g/ for /k/	tæt/kæt; gem/kem
/d/ or /k/ for /g/	do/go; kot/got
/b/ for /v/	bes/ves
/s/ or /tʃ/ for /ʃ/	tʃu/ ʃu; wɪs/wɪʃ
/l/ for /j/	lɛs/jɛs

Riper and Erickson (1996) are those shown in Table 5.4. Often, an earlier acquired sound is substituted for a later developing one, as illustrated by the substitutions of /w/ for /r/ and /t/ for /s/. Substitution errors are usually a change in one distinctive feature, such as place, manner, or voicing, not two or more features. The most frequent substitution involves the distinctive feature of place. Errors in the manner of production occur less frequently, and the least frequent feature error is voicing (Carrell, 1968; Winitz, 1975). Specific sound substitutions may be inconsistent from one production to the next as well as in the word position. Commonly, a substitution is denoted by identifying the substituted sound followed by a slash and the target sound such that t/k indicates that the /t/ sound is used in place of the /k/.

A distortion is an articulation error in which the standard phoneme is modified so that it is approximated, although incorrect. A distortion can be either visually or acoustically different, yet retain the basic characteristics of the target phoneme. Distortions occur more often than omissions in older children and adults and tend to be more consistent in usage than omissions and substitutions. The sounds most frequently distorted are the sibilants and the liquids. Diacritical marks are sometimes used to describe distortions.

An addition is a misarticulation in which a phoneme is added. For example, /bəlu/ for /blu/ and /wɪŋg/ for /wɪŋ/. This type of error occurs quite infrequently. In fact, the addition of the schwa (/ə/) within a consonant cluster is sometimes used as a remedial technique during the early stages of articulation treatment for eliciting clusters. Commonly, additions are denoted by identifying the target sound plus the added sound followed by a slash and the target such that fw/f indicates that the /w/ sound was inserted between the /f/ and the next sound as in producing *feet* as /fwit/.

Traditionally, misarticulations are further described relative to the position of sounds within a syllable or word. Three systems have been used: (a) initial, medial, and final; (b) prevocalic, intervocalic, and postvocalic; and (c) releasing and arresting. The first system considers misarticulations as they occur in a word, which can be at the beginning, such as /p/ in *put*; in the middle, such as /l/ in *below*; or at the end, such as /t/ in *hat*. Some criticism has been directed at this system because contextual speech really does not isolate phonemes in the initial and final word positions, with the exception of the first and last sounds in an utterance. More recently, consonant sounds have been described in relation to syllables in which they occur or in vowel contexts. Consonants can be described as occurring before (prevocalic), between (intervocalic), or after (postvocalic) a vowel or, alternatively, as starting (releasing) or ending (arresting) a syllable. Some recent elicited word tests assess words only in two positions—the releasing and arresting positions (i.e., initial and final positions). In contrast, articulation tests traditionally sample speech sounds in the three word positions of initial, medial, and final. All tests include clusters in the sampled words.

Because misarticulations frequently involve some or all of the sibilants /s/, /z/, /ʃ/, /ʒ/, /tʃ/, and /dʒ/, specific terminology is commonly used to describe substitutions and distortions of these phonemes. Speech-language pathologists thus need to be familiar with these terms. The term *lisp* refers to misarticulations of some or all of the sibilant sounds. Lingual, frontal, dental, and interdental lisps refer to substitutions and distortions in which the tongue is placed too far forward in the mouth so that it approximates the placement for /θ/ and /ð/. In a lateral lisp (**unilateral** or **bilateral**), the airstream is directed over one or both sides of the tongue rather than over the central portion of the tongue. In other words, the airstream flows between the upper and lower lateral teeth rather than between the upper and lower medial incisors. Nasal lisp involves direction of part or all of the airstream through the nasal cavity rather than through the mouth when producing sibilants. It may resemble a nasal fricative or a nasal "snort" or "snore." Strident lisp results in a high-frequency whistle or hissing sound caused by grooving the tongue tip too much or by the breath stream passing between the tongue and a hard surface such as that of dentures or other intra-oral appliances. The last type of sibilant error is the occluded or dentalized lisp. This lisp is characterized as having essentially no sibilant quality, so that /s/ and /z/ would be perceived more like /t/ and /d/ substitutions. This misarticulation results from occluding the breath stream in the oral cavity, usually by placing the tongue too far forward or not allowing for a narrow, grooved passageway for the breath stream to pass between the tongue and alveolar ridge. A malocclusion such as a closed bite or overbite can cause excessive anterior tongue crowding and a resultant occluded lisp.

Rhoticism indicates errors of the /r/ family. Lalling has been used to indicate misarticulations of /l/ and /r/ and possibly other tongue-tip consonants. Another term used to describe distortions of alveolars is **dentalization**, which refers to errors caused by placing the tongue too far forward so that it erroneously contacts the front teeth, notably on the alveolars. It is to be noted that the terms *rhoticism* and *lalling* are not widely used by speech-language pathologists today.

Some generalizations have been made about the types of errors. Misarticulations seldom occur on vowels and, conversely, are noted most frequently on consonants. This pattern is consistent with the sequence of speech development in that vowels are acquired before consonants. The most frequently misarticulated sounds are /s/, /z/, /θ/, /ð/, /tʃ/, /dʒ/, /r/, /l/, /ʃ/, /ʒ/, and /v/. These phonemes are the later appearing ones, and thus, are presumed to be the more difficult ones to produce in terms of neuromuscular coordination and precision. Errors occur most frequently on fricatives and affricates, often on liquids, less often on stops, and least frequently on nasals and glides. Consonant clusters also are frequently misarticulated. Generally, the fewest misarticulations are produced in the initial position and more in the medial position, with most occurring in the final position. There seems to be a progression in development from omissions to substitutions and sometimes on to distortions, with distortions being closer to correct articulation. One might say, then, that omissions are more severe errors than substitutions and that substitutions are more severe than distortions, which also follows a progressive diminution in the number of distinctive feature errors.

What are organic articulatory/phonologic and nonorganic (functional) disorders?

POTENTIAL ETIOLOGICAL FACTORS OF ARTICULATORY AND PHONOLOGIC DISORDERS

The systems for classifying articulatory and phonologic disorders have been presented, so the discussion now moves to the potential etiological factors of articulatory/phonologic disorders. Clearly, a certain level of neuromuscular development is necessary for accurate speech sound production. Integrity of the speech structures and their function is necessary for normal speech production. Other factors, however, are also required. Normal speech sound development and production involves both physical characteristics and capacities as well as perceptual, cognitive, and environmental influences. Byrne and Shervanian (1977) explained:

> Not all infants are born with the same capacity for mastering a language. In addition, each environment will interact with whatever capabilities the infant brings to it. The varying forces of capacity and environment shape the quality and quantity of language and speech development. (p. 18)

This concept of two influences on articulation/phonological development has led to dichotomizing etiology into organic and nonorganic (or functional) causes. Traditionally, the term *functional* has been used as a common synonym for any articulatory disorder for which no cause is apparent or that is assumed not to have a physical cause; they are labeled by default because there is no obvious organic basis. Thus, etiologies are classified as organic, nonorganic, or mixed. Organic causes are those in which there is a known structural, physiologic, neuromuscular, sensory, or cognitive deficit in the vocal tract or related structures. Conversely, a nonorganic cause is one in which there are no obvious signs of structural, physiologic, neuromuscular, sensory, or cognitive deficits. Mixed causes include both organic and nonorganic factors.

When attempting to determine causation, diagnosticians must keep in mind that many articulatory/phonologic disorders are not readily classifiable as purely organic or nonorganic; thus, they are not categorized in that way here. In some cases, the diagnostician can identify the etiology of an articulatory/phonologic disorder; however, in many cases, one cannot say with certainty what the actual cause is, but rather may make a professional judgment as to plausible causal factors. Additionally, there may be multiple etiological factors involved in a particular case; thus, looking for a multiplicity of causal factors rather than determining the exact cause is recommended. Much of the following information on etiological factors comes from studies based on: (a) descriptions of persons with speech sound disorders, (b) correlational studies of factors related to persons with articulatory disorders, and (c) comparisons of characteristics of persons with articulatory/phonologic disorders to persons without such disorders. Thus, one cannot conclude that these related factors are the cause of articulatory/phonologic disorders, but that they are somehow associated with speech sound disorders and potentially contribute to the development of misarticulations. Table 5.5 lists factors that may be related to the development of articulatory/phonologic disorders.

> Describe potential structural, physiologic, and neurological etiological factors of articulatory/phonologic disorders. Give some specific examples of potential causes.

Structural, Physiologic, and Neurological Factors

Logically, structural (or anatomical) and physiologic deviations of the face and oral cavity contribute to the etiology of articulatory disorders, although articulation errors do not invariably result from such deviations. Also, degrees of abnormality vary from minimal to gross, likely influencing the amount of impact on speech sound production (Peña-Brooks & Hegde, 2000). Structural and physiologic anomalies are often of a developmental nature, even though some result from trauma, surgery, or disease.

Over the years, children with functional articulatory disorders have been compared with children who are normal speakers relative to structural and physiologic differences of the articulators. Generally, research findings have not shown palate, tongue, and lip measurements to be related to articulation skills (Dworkin & Culatta,1985; Fairbanks & Green, 1950; Fairbanks & Lintner, 1951; Fletcher & Meldrum, 1968; McEnery & Gaines, 1941). Similarly, in a carefully conducted recent study, no notable differences were found on oral mechanism examinations between normally articulating children and those who have articulatory disorders (Dworkin & Culatta,1985). Nonetheless, according to Bloomer (1971), deformities of mouth opening, including small mouth opening; facial deformity, including asymmetrical or partially missing facial structures; lingual deformities, including

macroglossia (too large a tongue), **microglossia** (too small a tongue), or **glossectomy** (removal of the tongue); and nasal deformities, including deviated nasal septum or hypertrophied turbinates, may contribute to articulation/resonance resource deficits. The structure and function of specific articulators have been explored in research studies. The following findings are from those studies:

Lips

Structural deviations of the lips do not seem to compromise articulation abilities (Bernthal & Bankson, 2004; Peña-Brooks & Hegde, 2000). Even though surgical repair of clefts of the lips can result in a relatively immobile upper lip, this anatomical deviation generally does not result in misarticulations for most individuals. Even ablative surgery for cancer resulting in a shortened, immobile upper lip does not seem to result in speech problems (Bloomer & Hawk, 1973). Instead, speakers compensate for the deviation and produce acceptable labial consonants.

Teeth

Malocclusions (dental and jaw alignment irregularities) may contribute to misarticulations, although impaired articulation is not a necessary consequence of all malocclusions nor is a malocclusion present in all articulatory disorders (Bernthal & Bankson, 2004). Malocclusions are classified as Angle's Class I, Class II, and Class III (Fig. 5.2). Class I is **neutroclusion**, in which the dental arches are aligned properly, but some individual teeth or groups of teeth are misaligned. Class II is **distoclusion**, in which the mandible and mandibular teeth are retruded so that their position relative to the maxillary teeth is posterior. Class III is **mesioclusion**, in which the mandible and mandibular teeth are protruded so that their position relative to the maxillary teeth is anterior. Other terms are also used to describe deviant dentition. For example, **open bite** occurs when the central and lateral incisors of the maxilla (upper jaw) do not cover the mandibular (lower jaw) incisors, while closed bite occurs when the maxillary incisors overlap the mandibular incisors more than one third of the mandibular teeth. Overjet occurs when the upper incisors are too far anterior relative to lower incisors, and underbite occurs when the maxillary incisors are posterior to lower incisors. Crossbite is the case in which the lower teeth and upper teeth are not correctly aligned vertically with the lower teeth, which are either too far right or too far left of the upper teeth.

Some studies have shown a relationship between malocclusions and misarticulation. In one study, inferior adult speakers were shown to have

TABLE 5.5

Potential Etiological Factors of Articulatory/Phonologic Disorders

General Factors	Examples of Specific Conditions
Structural, physiological, neuromuscular	Dental malocclusions
	Short lingual frenum
	Partial or total glossectomy
	Insufficient velopharyngeal closure
	Cleft palate
	Removal of part of maxilla
	Tongue incoordination (poor diadochokinesis)
	Orofacial myofunctional disorders, including tongue thrust
	General motor incoordination
	Cerebral palsy
	Parkinson's disease
	Amyatrophic lateral sclerosis (ALS)
	Multiple sclerosis
	Huntington's disease
	Bell's palsy
	Myasthenia gravis
	Cerebral vascular accident
	Seizures
	Head injuries
	Infectious diseases, including encephalitis, meningitis
	Anoxia
	Metabolic disorders
	Neoplasm (abnormal growth)
Sensory/perceptual	Hearing loss (result of several causes)
	Fluctuating hearing loss (otitis media with effusion)
	Inadequate auditory perceptual skills, including poor speech sound discrimination
	Inadequate oral sensation/perception ability
	Visual impairment
Cognitive	Intellectual functioning below normal limits (result of several causes)
Heredity	Genetic factors
Environmental/psychosocial	Inadequate speech models
	Limited speech stimulation and motivation
	Inadequate/inappropriate reinforcement
	Emotional reaction to a traumatic experience
	Emotional reactions of others
	Psychosocial factors in the client (e.g., adjustment and behavioral problems, overly sensitive to others)
	Psychosocial factors in a parent (e.g., poorly adjusted, have higher standards)

(continued)

TABLE 5.5 (Continued)

Potential Etiological Factors of Articulatory/Phonologic Disorders

General Factors	Examples of Specific Conditions
Personal	Age
	Gender
	Sibling status including twins
	Socioeconomic status
Linguistic and academic	Other expressive language impairments
	Language comprehension deficits
	Poorer reading readiness skills
	Poorer reading skills
	Poorer spelling skills
	Deficient phonological awareness
Other speech	Stuttering disorder
	Voice disorders

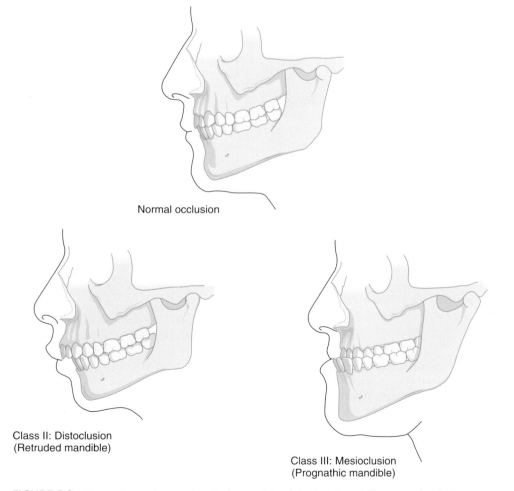

Normal occlusion

Class II: Distoclusion
(Retruded mandible)

Class III: Mesioclusion
(Prognathic mandible)

FIGURE 5.2 Illustrations of normal occlusion and Angle's Class II and Class III malocclusions.

more malocclusions, namely distoclusion and mesioclusion, than superior adult speakers, and they also tended to have one or more marked dental deviations (Fairbanks & Lintner, 1951). Luchsinger and Arnold (1965) reported that malocclusions are more frequently present in persons who lisp, whereas Bernstein (1956) found no higher rate of articulation problems in children with malocclusions except for those with open bite. In their study of the effects of missing teeth on articulation in young children, Bankson and Byrne (1962) noted a significant relationship between the absence of teeth and the misarticulations of /s/. Snow (1961) also found a higher percentage of misarticulated /s/ plus /f/, /v/, /θ/, /ð/, and /z/ among first grade children with missing teeth. Both studies reported that, even so, a number of children with missing teeth had normal speech. The results of these and other studies led to the conclusion that dental deviations occur more frequently in individuals with misarticulations, but they do not always result in articulatory disorders. "Most individuals learn to produce speech sounds correctly in spite of such deviations by using compensatory strategies," although dental anomalies may be a contributing factor in some persons (Peña-Brooks & Hegde, 2000, p. 179).

Tongue

A structural deviation frequently mentioned by laypersons is tongue-tie or ankyloglossia. This deviation is the result of a short lingual frenum or frenulum; that is, one that is attached too far forward on the undersurface of the tongue and restricts the range of tongue-tip movement. Ankyloglossia is seldom a significant factor; however, in rare instances, the following are indicators (Bloomer, 1971) that it may be a deterrent to correct articulation:

- Noticeably indented tongue-tip on protrusion
- Cannot contact the alveolar arch with tongue tip when the mandible is in normal vertical relationship to the maxilla for speech
- Cannot contact the angles of the mouth with the tongue tip
- Cannot produce alveolar and dental consonants

In these rare cases, consideration of a physician clipping the frenum may be in order.

Other tongue deviations have also been considered (Bloomer, 1971; Dworkin, 1978, 1980; Dworkin & Culatta, 1980, 1985; Johnson, Brown, Curtis, Edney, & Keaster, 1967; Leonard, 1994; Skelly, Spector, Donaldson, Brodeur, & Paletta, 1971). Except for a partially or entirely missing tongue (**aglossia**), correlating lingual deviations with articulation problems has not been fruitful. A tongue that is too large (macroglossia) or too small (microglossia) does not seem to be related to articulation skills. Speech intelligibility and articulation skills are compromised in persons with total or partial glossectomy (total or partial surgical removal of the tongue). The location and amount of the tongue that is removed has been shown to affect speech intelligibility. In a study of 50 speakers with varying degrees of glossectomy, misarticulations occurred most frequently on fricatives and plosives (Leonard, 1994). In three patients, speech intelligibility decreased over time as more of their tongues was surgically removed (Massengill, Maxwell, & Picknell, 1970). Patients with total glossectomy use compensatory mandibular, labial, buccal, and palatal movements, while patients with partial glossectomy use the remainder of the tongue to produce speech (Skelly et al., 1971). Those with tongue-tip removal use more articulation adaptations than those with unilateral tongue removal.

Tongue incoordination could be a causative factor in some cases, although this is not easily determined because of the extensive compensatory abilities of the tongue in some persons. Oral diadochokinetic tasks have been used to examine physiology of the articulators. Oral **diadochokinesis** is defined as the rapid repetition of antagonistic speech movements, more appropriately called maximum articulator movement abilities. The occurrence of tongue incoordination as an etiological factor has been supported by studies showing that individuals with articulatory disorders perform diadochokinetic tasks more slowly than normally articulating speakers (Dworkin, 1978, 1980; McNutt, 1977; Weiss, 1968). In two studies, children with frontal lisps were found to have significantly less tongue strength and slower diadochokinetic rates than speakers with normal articulation (Dworkin, 1978, 1980); however, in another study, no differences in tongue strength and diadochokinetic rates were found between children with normal articulation and those with disordered articulation (Dworkin & Culatta, 1985). They also found no differences between the two groups on tongue strength measurements. Some have questioned the clinical usefulness of obtaining diadochokinetic performance information except in CAS and in children with delayed or unusual oral-motor development (Bernthal & Bankson, 2004).

Soft and Hard Palate

Another oral structure important to articulation is the palate. The importance of the soft palate or velum to normal resonance and the production of pressure consonants have been reported extensively

(Bzoch, 1997; Morley, 1970; Spriestersbach & Sherman, 1968). Most of the studies have dealt with soft palate physiology, even though structure and function are not easily separated. When the soft palate is too short, does not move far enough, or does not move as quickly or consistently as it should, articulation and resonance usually are impaired because of inadequate velopharyngeal closure. It is not uncommon for a person diagnosed as having congenital palatal inadequacy to have a shorter-than-average velum as part of the problem. Sometimes, congenital palatal inadequacy is the diagnosis following removal of the adenoids. Cleft of the soft or hard palate is a major structural anomaly that causes articulation and resonance problems. Inadequate velopharyngeal closure leads to: (a) misarticulations of the pressure consonants, such as fricatives, affricates, and stops that result from reduced intra-oral air pressure; (b) sound substitution patterns using /ʔ/ and more posterior placements, such as pharyngeal fricatives, for the consonants; (c) nasal emissions; and (d) hypernasality of vowels, diphthongs, and vocalic consonants.

Historically, different configurations of the hard palate, such as high, narrow palate or low palatal arch, have received attention concerning their importance to articulation, but there is limited research regarding the hard palate. As with most of the oral cavity structures, research generally has not shown an association between articulatory disorders and variations of hard palate configurations, unless the structural deviation is extreme, as in the case of cleft palate or removal of part of the maxilla (Dworkin & Culatta, 1985; Fairbanks & Bebout, 1950; Fairbanks & Lintner, 1951). Certainly, clefts of the hard palate and surgical removal of the hard palate affect articulation abilities. In the United States, clefts of the hard palate are usually closed early in a child's life so that articulation often is not compromised. In the case of surgical removal of part of the hard palate, prosthetic devices often are used to close the opening between the oral and nasal cavities, thus decreasing the affect on articulation (Sullivan, Gaebler, Beukelman et al., 2002).

Tonsils and Adenoids

One final structural composite that should be considered is the lymph tissue, better known as the tonsils and adenoids. Enlarged or hypertrophied tonsils can obstruct the oral passageway and cause "drag" on the soft palate, forcing the breath stream through the nose (Blakeley, 1972). Enlarged adenoids can occlude the nasal passageway and cause an inadequate amount of air to resonate in the nose. The resulting condition is known as hyponasality

or **denasality**. Conversely, when the adenoids contribute to velopharyngeal (veloadenoidal) closure because the soft palate may be contacting them to achieve closure, their removal (adenoidectomy) then may increase the pharyngeal space to the extent that the soft palate no longer makes contact with the back pharyngeal wall. The resulting condition is hypernasality (or excessive nasal resonance and airflow, as well as weak production of the pressure consonants). Neither the tonsils nor the adenoids should be removed without regard to their subsequent effect on articulation and resonance. Removing part of the adenoidal tissue rather than all of it is another viable consideration in treatment.

Tongue Thrust

Orofacial myofunctional disorders, including **tongue thrust** and **lip incompetence**, has been linked to articulatory disorders in some individuals (ASHA, 1989). Orofacial myofunctional disorder has been defined as "any pattern involving oral and/or orofacial musculature that interferes with normal growth, development, or function of structures, or calls attention to itself" (ASHA, 1993, p. 22). Tongue thrust involves "inappropriate or excessive lingual contacts against or between the teeth at rest or during vegetative or communicative functions" and lip incompetence is described as "a lips-apart resting posture or the inability to achieve a lips-together resting posture without muscle strain" (ASHA, 1993, p. 22). Tongue thrust can be obligatory (organic); that is, a forward tongue position at rest or forward tongue movement because of structural or physiological constraints, such as posterior airway obstruction from enlarged tonsils or adenoids, short mandibular ramus, or long soft palate; or transitional (functional or habit) (ASHA, 1989, 1993; Peña-Brooks & Hegde, 2000). An ad hoc committee of ASHA reviewed the literature on orofacial myofunctional disorders and concluded the following:

- Infants use a tongue thrust swallow.
- Tongue thrust swallow pattern changes from infancy to childhood.
- At some point in development, the tongue thrust swallow is no longer used and is considered a contributing and maintaining factor in lisping, malocclusion, or both.
- A forward resting tongue posture can lead to malocclusion.
- Tongue thrust and/or forward resting tongue position coexist with lisping in some individuals.
- Tongue thrust treatment may facilitate correction of lisps or dentalization of the alveolars.

Associated symptoms of the tongue thrust pattern includes lip-open, mouth-open breathing posture, and finger- or thumb-sucking habits. Over the years, etiology has been attributed to bottle nursing, delayed maturation, structural deviations (such as airway obstruction, enlarged tonsils, and large tongue), upper respiratory problems, genetic predisposition, psychoemotional factors, and of course, neuromuscular incoordination (such as tongue instability and jaw instability), allergies, and poor sensory awareness. Tongue thrusting and malocclusion have been reported in normal speakers as well as in speakers with disordered speech (Subtelny, Mestre, & Subtelny, 1964). In summary, tongue thrust may be a causative factor, although no conclusions can be made about the causal relationship between misarticulations and tongue thrusting. Several studies have shown the coexistence of tongue thrust swallow pattern and misarticulations of /s/ and /z/ and other alveolar sounds (ASHA, 1989; Fletcher, Casteel, & Bradley, 1961; Jann, Ward, & Jann, 1964; Mason & Proffit, 1974; Palmer, 1962; Powers, 1971; Wadsworth, Maul, & Stevens, 1998; Weiss, 1970). The ASHA (1991) position statement on oral myofunctional disorders indicates that providing tongue thrust treatment is within the scope of practice for speech-language pathologists with the appropriate training. In a review of 15 studies that investigated the effectiveness of tongue thrust therapy, Hanson (1994) reported that 14 of them showed the treatment to be effective in altering swallowing and tongue resting patterns. In many public schools, treatment for tongue thrust is not provided without a concomitant articulatory disorder.

General Motor Incoordination

General motor incoordination in the absence of a neuromuscular disorder has been postulated as a possible cause of articulatory disorders, but research results have been contradictory and inconclusive (Dworkin & Culatta, 1985; Powers, 1971; Weiss, 1968). Although it generally has been concluded that persons with deviant articulation do not consistently show poor general motor ability, perhaps it is an etiological factor in selected individuals.

Neuromuscular Factors

Neuromuscular problems involving the control of the speech mechanism often result in articulatory disorders. These deviances may occur in the cerebrum of the brain such as in the case of acquired apraxia of speech. Some impairments occur in other parts of the central nervous system and in the peripheral nervous system that innervate the speech mechanism. Damage can cause paralysis, **paresis** (partial or incomplete paralysis), or incoordination of the speech muscles. Examples of such impairment include cerebral palsy, Parkinson's disease, paralysis and paresis of the tongue, amyotrophic lateral sclerosis (ALS), and Bell's palsy. The muscles themselves are involved in myopathies such as muscular dystrophy. Causes of neuromuscular disabilities range across a wide spectrum of impairments, including hereditary malformations, prenatal injuries, metabolic and toxic disturbances, tumors, traumas, seizures, infectious diseases, demyelinating diseases, muscular diseases, and vascular impairments. They can occur prenatally, in infancy, during childhood, and during adulthood.

Two major types of neuromuscular problems confronting speech-language pathologists are dysarthria and apraxia (described earlier). Dysarthria is more appropriately termed *dysarthrias* because there are a number of different dysarthric patterns, depending on the site of the lesion. It is a common motor speech problem among persons with cerebral palsy and post-stroke, but may result from any damage to the central or peripheral nervous systems and muscular systems that affect speech. The primary manifestation of this disorder is involvement of the speech musculature that impairs the motoric ability for both vegetative and speech functions, including respiration, phonation, and resonation as well as articulation. Some of the most prominent speech deviations reported among the dysarthrias are hypernasality, imprecise production of consonants, breathiness, monopitch, reduced or excessive stress, monoloudness, variable rate, prolonged intervals, distorted vowels, and harsh vowel quality (Darley, Aronson, & Brown, 1975). These symptoms obviously vary among the types of dysarthria (Table 5.1).

Dyspraxia or apraxia of speech (or verbal dyspraxia) is also a neurological speech problem; however, the nature of this problem is not one of paralysis or paresis, but rather of programming the articulators for speech production. Unlike dysarthria, muscle weakness and incoordination are absent and vegetative functions may be essentially normal. Dyspraxia may be present in anyone at any age, but it is commonly found among post-stroke patients and is characterized by an inability or difficulty in performing speech acts voluntarily. Also, verbal dyspraxia and dysarthria may be present in the same person (LaPointe & Wertz, 1974). Dyspraxia also can occur in children (as detailed earlier).

Describe potential sensory/perceptual etiological factors of articulatory/phonologic disorders. Give some specific examples of potential causes.

Sensory/Perceptual Factors

Hearing Impairment

Certain sensory/perceptual deficits can cause articulatory disorders. There is no question that auditory sensory problems are significant etiological factors (e.g., Churchill, Hodson, Jones, & Novak, 1988; Miccio, Gallagher, Grossman, Yont, & Vernon-Feagans, 2001; Paden, Matthies, & Novak, 1989; Shriberg, 1997; Shriberg, Friel-Patti, Flipsen, & Brown, 2000b). Hearing loss, depending on the severity and age of onset, can impair a person's ability to perceive sounds, including speech sounds. When the loss occurs during the period of speech acquisition, the child likely does not acquire normal articulation and oral language. Logically, the more severe the hearing loss, the more impaired the speech will be. Well-documented evidence suggests that there is a relationship between moderate to severe hearing loss during infancy and later speech problems (Paden, Novak, & Beiter, 1987; Roberts, Burchinal, Koch, Footo, & Henderson, 1988). Obviously, the type, degree, age of onset, and age of detection of the hearing loss will affect the type and degree of the articulation problem.

The terms *hearing impairment* and *hearing loss* refer to a hearing problem. Hearing impairments can be described as deaf or congenitally deaf, deafened or adventitiously deaf, and hard of hearing.

Deaf refers to severe or profound hearing loss (greater than 80 dB in the better ear) occurring before acquisition of speech such that the child is unable to understand and learn speech naturally by hearing, while *deafened* refers to severe hearing loss after speech has been acquired. *Hard of hearing* refers to auditory abnormality in which sufficient hearing sensitivity remains to permit oral communication, usually with the assistance of amplification, but may interfere with articulation learning and production especially when it is present in the infant or young child. Hearing losses often are classified as to their severity level as shown in Table 5.6.

Hearing impairment is generally categorized into three types, based on the site of the lesion. Sometimes, a fourth category, **central auditory processing disorder (CAPD)**, is also recognized. This type "refers to lesions in the brain that produce real but sometimes subtle symptoms . . . . CAPDs prevent many sufferers from taking advantage of their full hearing potential" (Martin & Noble, 2002, p. 329). One category is a **conductive hearing loss** in which the pathology occurs in the outer or middle ear as a result of an obstructed external ear, perforated eardrum, atypical ossicular chain, otitis media with effusion (fluid in the middle ear), otosclerosis, and so forth. The hearing loss in this type is mild or moderate and is usually treatable. In a **sensorineural hearing loss**, the lesion occurs in the inner ear, in the cochlea, or in cranial nerve VIII as a result of heredity, noise pollution, toxic effects from drugs, maternal and viral infections, diseases, injury, and so forth. These losses vary in severity level from moderate to profound and are typically permanent and may be progressive. Persons with a sensorineural hearing loss usually hear sounds in a distorted way, even with

TABLE 5.6

Severity Levels of Hearing Loss

dB	Degree of Handicap	Ability to Hear Speech
<0–14	None	Normal
15–25	Minimal	Difficulty with faint speech
26–45	Mild	Frequent difficulty with normal speech
46–65	Moderate	Frequent difficulty with loud speech
66–85	Severe	Speech may be heard with amplification
>86	Profound	May not use hearing for communication

Adapted from Hall BJ, Oyer HJ, Haas WH. Speech, Language, and Hearing Disorders: A Guide for the Teacher. 3rd Ed. Boston: Allyn & Bacon, 2001. Copyright © 2001 by Pearson Education. Adapted with permission of the publisher.

amplification (Martin & Noble, 2002). Generally, the more severe the hearing loss, the greater the distortion will be. For example, if the loss is prominent in the higher frequencies, then misarticulations of the unvoiced, high frequency fricatives often result. Children who are deaf usually have vowel and consonant misarticulations. For example, they tend not to distinguish between voiced and unvoiced consonants; to omit, distort, and substitute consonants and sometimes vowels; to nasalize vowels; and to misarticulate diphthongs. A third type of auditory impairment is mixed hearing loss, in which the individual has a combination of conductive and sensorineural hearing problems. Children with significant hearing losses tend to exhibit numerous speech errors (Table 5.7). Persons who become deafened tend to misarticulate low intensity, high frequency sounds (/s/, /ʃ/, /tʃ/, /f/, and /θ/) and produce final consonants with little energy (Calvert, 1982).

Recently, the relationship between articulation skills and fluctuating hearing loss (otitis media with effusion) because of repeated middle ear infections in infants and young children has been explored (e.g., Churchill et al., 1988; Miccio et al., 2001; Paden et al., 1989; Petinou, Schwartz, Mody, & Gravel, 1999; Shriberg, 1997; Shriberg et al., 2000a). Children with this type of loss often experience some degree of mild to moderate fluctuating conductive hearing loss with average thresholds of 25 dB HL (Petinou et al., 1999).

> Unlike other more severe and stable hearing losses (e.g., sensorineural), a transient loss may compromise the stability and consistency of the speech signal the child receives. Consequently, experience with an inconsistent auditory signal may interfere with the establishment of complete and stable linguistic representations of the ambient language. (p. 352)

Although some of the methodologies used have been questionable and the data conflicting (Roberts & Clarke-Klein, 1994), results of several studies indicate that there is a significant relationship between

TABLE 5.7

Misarticulations Commonly Associated with Hearing Loss

Type of Misarticulation	Specific Misarticulations
Omissions	Final consonants
	Consonant clusters
	Initial consonants
	/s/ in all positions
Substitutions	Voiced consonants for voiceless consonants
	Nasal consonants for oral consonants
	Vowel substitutions
	Low feedback substitutions (substitution of sounds easily perceived with tactile and kinesthetic feedback for those less easily perceived, such as /w/ for /r/)
Distortions	Distortions of stops and fricatives
	Imprecise production of vowels
	Prolongation of vowels
	Hypernasal vowel production
	Production of first or second vowel in diphthongs with inappropriate duration
Additions	Additions of vowels between consonants in clusters
	Insertion of breath before vowels
	Aspirated release of final stops
	Diphthongization of vowels

Calvert, D. R. (1982). Articulation and hearing impairments. In N. Lass, J. Northern, D. Yoder, & L. McReynolds (Eds), *Speech, Language and Hearing. Volume 2*. Philadelphia: PA: Saunders; Peña-Brooks, A., & Hegde, M. N. (2000). *Assessment & treatment of articulation & phonological disorders in children.* Austin, TX: Pro-Ed.

early fluctuating hearing loss and later speech development (Churchill et al., 1988; Miccio et al., 2001; Paden et al., 1987, 1989; Shriberg et al., 2000a). Many children with articulatory/phonologic disorders have a history of middle-ear involvement (Shriberg, 1997; Shriberg & Kwiatkowski, 1982a; Shriberg & Smith, 1983). Conversely, in a longitudinal study, no significant relationship was shown between otitis media during the first 3 years of life and later articulation/phonological deficiency (Roberts et al., 1988). Thus, it must be noted that not all children with histories of otitis media have clinically significant articulatory/phonologic disorders. Factors to consider include age of onset of otitis media, whether or not there is an associated conductive loss, magnitude and duration of the losses, frequency of the otitis media episodes, and environmental factors. Paden et al. (1987) found four specific factors to be predictive of the need for articulation/phonological intervention for young children (18 to 36 months of age):

1. Presence of velar deviations
2. Presence of cluster reduction
3. Lack of improvement in articulation 4 months after insertion of tubes
4. Time period of 6 months or more between initial diagnosis of otitis media and significant remission of this condition

Auditory Perception

Inadequate auditory perceptual skills may be a cause of articulatory disorders. This kind of deficiency is not to be confused with deficient auditory acuity or sensitivity (hearing loss). One may have normal hearing acuity, yet perceive speech sounds in an atypical manner; for example, out of sequence, reversed, or without recognition. The label used to describe these kinds of nonacuity-related hearing problems is auditory perceptual disorder.

Speech sound discrimination is an auditory perceptual skill that has been investigated frequently. Clinically, speech sound discrimination refers to the ability of individuals to detect differences between two speech sounds. Interestingly, infants can perceive differences between many speech sounds of their language by the time they are 1 year old, although they do not perceive all phonemic contrasts when they begin to say words (Bernthal & Bankson, 2004).

It seems logical that when an individual cannot discriminate speech sounds, speech acquisition would be impaired. Thus, **auditory discrimination** abilities of children with speech sound errors has been investigated with the result that studies have not consistently supported such a premise. Research

on the relationship between articulation deficiency and speech sound discrimination is conflicting and inconclusive. Whereas some researchers have found significant differences in speech sound discrimination abilities between normal speakers and speakers with articulatory disorders, others have not found significant differences (see literature reviews conducted by Bernthal & Bankson, 2004; Peña-Brooks & Hegde, 2000; Weiner, 1967; Winitz, 1984, 1989). Differences in results may be attributed to differences in discrimination tasks, ages of the subjects, and varying degrees of articulation deviancy. Some studies involved testing general discrimination abilities, while others involved phoneme-specific discrimination abilities. Most have examined discrimination abilities of external stimuli, such as the ability to discriminate speech sounds of other speakers, while some looked at discrimination of internal stimuli or self-discrimination, such as determining whether their own productions are correct or incorrect.

In the early studies on discrimination abilities, general discrimination was investigated; that is, the ability to detect the differences between a large number of speech sounds in a variety of phonetic contexts. In other words, children were asked, without regard to their own misarticulations, to indicate whether two words or syllables are the same or different. Later studies explored phoneme-specific discrimination abilities. In these studies, the children were asked to discriminate between the correct and incorrect productions of the speech sounds they misarticulate. In these studies, external speech sound discrimination was investigated, meaning that the task for the children was to make judgments about the speech productions of another person or of tape-recorded productions of one's own speech—external self-discrimination. In one study, approximately 70% of the children with misarticulations discriminated between the correct and incorrect speech sound productions of the sounds they misarticulated (Locke, 1980). Other studies have had similar results (Bernthal & Bankson, 2004; Peña-Brooks & Hegde, 2000). Thus, it appears that most children with misarticulations are able to discriminate the sounds they misarticulate from other sounds when produced by others, although some children with misarticulations demonstrate poor speech sound discrimination abilities for the sounds they misproduce. On the other hand, there seems to be a relationship between articulation proficiency and internal discrimination, including the task in which children make judgments about their own productions (Aungst & Frick, 1964; Lapko & Bankson, 1975; Wolfe & Irwin, 1973).

One other line of research has been conducted; namely, the effect of discrimination training on production of speech sounds. Again, the results have been inconclusive with some studies showing that discrimination training results in improved articulation (Jamieson & Rvachew, 1992; Rvachew, 1994; Rvachew, Rafaat, & Martin, 1999) and **self-monitoring** results in improved articulation (Koegel, Koegel, & Ingham, 1986; Koegel, Koegel, Van Voy, & Ingham, 1988). Yet, others have not shown such an impact of discrimination training (Gray & Shelton, 1992; Shelton, Johnson, & Arndt, 1977; Williams & McReynolds, 1975; Winitz & Bellerose, 1967). In summary, there appears to be a relationship between speech sound discrimination and speech sound production, but the nature of this association is unknown. It may be that: (a) poor discrimination abilities lead to misarticulations, (b) deficient articulation skills lead to poor discrimination abilities, or (c) some other factor results in poor discrimination abilities and deficient articulation. Difficulties in achieving carryover may or may not relate directly to lack of adequately developed speech discrimination skills. In the meantime, more pertinent research on speech discrimination should be undertaken. It is probably prudent to include **self-evaluation** and/or **speech perception training** in treatment for clients who show auditory perceptual deficiencies.

Oral Sensation/Perception

Oral sensation/perception provides the sensory feedback from oral cavity structures to the brain. Logically, these sensations would seem important in the development and maintenance of articulation. Considerable research was conducted using a variety of techniques in the 1960s and 1970s, including two-point discrimination (awareness of two points being touched rather than one), oral form recognition (**oral stereognosis**), and the effects on speech of anesthetizing the oral structures. Typically, in oral form recognition tasks, a plastic form is placed in the mouth and the subject is required to match it to a drawing of the form or to identify the shape of the form. This ability improves with age through adolescence (Bernthal & Bankson, 2004). Some research results have indicated that children with articulation errors tend to have more difficulty with oral form recognition (Ringel, House, Burk, Dolinsky, & Scott, 1970), but others have not shown a significant difference (Arndt, Elbert, & Shelton, 1970). McNutt (1977) found that children with /r/ misarticulations had greater difficulty with oral form perception than speakers with no articulation errors; however, this was not the case for children who misarticulated

/s/. A different approach to investigating the relationship between oral stereognosis and articulation was taken by Locke (1968), who found that normal speakers who had high form-recognition scores were better able to produce two German consonant sounds than normal speakers with low form-recognition scores. Two studies explored the effect of training in oral form recognition on the articulation skills of children with misarticulations. Results were conflicting with one study showing improved articulation (Wilhelm, 1971) and the other not showing improvement (Shelton, Willis, Johnson, & Arndt, 1973). In anesthetization studies on adults, the speakers tended to use imprecise articulations or misarticulations, although the speech remained intelligible (Gammon, Smith, Daniloff, and Kim, 1971; Prosek & House, 1975; Scott & Ringel, 1971). From their review of studies on the relationship between oral sensory function and articulation learning, Bernthal and Bankson (2004) concluded that "information concerning oral sensory function has not been shown to have clinical applicability" (p.164). In summary, research in this area has not demonstrated a clear relationship between oral sensation/perception and articulation.

Visual Acuity

One final sensory/perceptual factor that may be related to speech acquisition is visual acuity. Although little research has been done in this area, there is a higher incidence of articulation errors in persons who are blind (Powers, 1971). Because formation of one third of the speech sounds is visible, inability to see them could cause a delay in their acquisition.

> Describe cognitive etiological factors of articulatory/phonologic disorders.

Cognitive Factors

Cognitive variables are related to articulatory/phonologic disorders when intelligence falls below normal limits. Intelligence quotients of persons within the normal range do not seem to be correlated to articulation development. Persons below the normal range of intellectual functioning demonstrate a higher prevalence of articulation errors than do persons within the normal range. Individuals who are developmentally delayed (mentally retarded) usually demonstrate deficits in all areas of speech and language development. The pattern of articulation development often is similar to that of typically developing persons, but occurs to that of typically developing persons, but occurs at a delayed rate. However, just as in those who have normal cognition, some persons with lower cognitive function demonstrate unusual phonological patterns. Children with developmental delays tend to omit consonants and to be inconsistent in their articulation errors (Shriberg & Widder, 1990). Individuals who are developmentally delayed may never catch up, depending on the degree of mental retardation. Sometimes, problems resulting from neuromuscular deficiencies are present as well.

Mental retardation is defined by the American Association on Mental Retardation (AAMR, 2002) as follows:

> Mental retardation is a disability characterized by significant limitations both in intellectual functioning and in adaptive behavior as expressed in conceptual, social, and practical adaptive skills. This disability originates before the age of 18. (p. 1)

Similarly, it is defined by IDEA (U.S. Department of Education, 1997) as:

> . . . significantly subaverage general intellectual functioning existing concurrently with deficits in adaptive behavior and manifested during the developmental period that adversely affects a child's educational performance. (34 C. F. R., Sec. 300, 7[b][5])

The current favored method for determining the nature and extent of needed educational and related services for students who are developmentally delayed is the Supports Intensity Scale (Thompson, Bryant, Campbell et al., 2003). Data collected include:

- Frequency—how often the student needs supports for each targeted activity
- Daily support time—amount of time that should be devoted to supporting the student during a typical day
- Type of support—nature of supports the student needs to engage in a particular activity (Turnbull, Turnbull, Shank, & Smith, 2004, p. 235)

However, this new system is not yet being used universally (Turnbull et al., 2004). Rather, most states continue to use the 1983 classification system of the American Association on Mental Retardation (AAMR), which functionally classified individuals into four groups (Table 5.8).

Etiological factors of mental retardation fall into four broad categories:

- Biomedical—factors that relate to biological processes, such as genetic disorders or nutrition
- Social—factors that relate to social and family interaction, such as stimulation and adult responsiveness

TABLE 5.8

1983 American Association on Mental Retardation (AAMR) Classification System

Classification	Educational Classification	IQ Range	Characteristics
Mild	Educable	50–55 to 70.	Can usually master basic academic skills, whereas adults at this level may maintain themselves independently or semi-independently in the community.
Moderate	Trainable	35–40 to 50–55.	Can usually learn self-help, communication, social, and simple occupational skills, but only limited academic or vocational skills.
Severe	Severely/multiply handicapped	20–25 to 35–40	Require continuing and close supervision, but may perform self-help and simple work tasks under supervision.
Profound	Severely/multiply handicapped	Below 20 or 25	Require continuing and close supervision, but some may be able to perform simple self-help tasks. They often have other disabilities and require total life-support systems for maintenance.

TABLE 5.9

Causes of Mental Retardation from Timing Factors

Prenatal	Perinatal	Postnatal
Chromosomal disorders	Premature labor	Head injuries
Metabolic disorders	Meningitis at birth	Lead intoxication
Maternal malnutrition	Head trauma at birth	Child abuse and neglect

Turnbull, A., Turnbull, R., Shank, M., Smith, S. J. (2004). *Exceptional lives. Special education in today's schools* (4th ed.) Upper Saddle River, NJ: Pearson Education, Inc. © Pearson Education, Inc., 2004. Reprinted with permission.

- Behavioral—factors that relate to potential causal behaviors, such as dangerous (injurious) activities or maternal substance abuse
- Educational—factors that relate to the availability of educational supports that promote mental development of adaptive skills (AAMR, 2002, p. 126)

Etiologies are summarized in Table 5.9.

Describe potential environmental and psychosocial factors of articulatory/phonologic disorders. Give some specific examples of potential causes.

What is the evidence that genetic factors may play a role in the development of articulatory/phonologic disorders?

Heredity Factors

Often, speech-language pathologists note a tendency for a history of speech and language disorders in individuals with articulatory/phonologic disorders. Since the mid-1980s, the prevalence of articulatory/phonologic disorders in families has been systematically investigated to explore the hypothesis that, in some cases, there is a genetic basis for the disorder. Generally, research findings have supported the hypothesis that there is a higher prevalence of communication disorders in family members than in the general population (Felsenfeld, McGue, & Broen, 1995; Felsenfeld & Plomin, 1997; Lewis, Ekelman, & Aram, 1989; Shriberg & Austin, 1998; Shriberg & Kwiatkowski, 1994). Shriberg and Austin (1998) reported that perhaps as many as 60% of preschoolers with speech delay have unknown etiologies that are possibly genetically based. Results of twin studies have supported the idea that heredity is related to speech disorders. Articulation test scores were more closely associated in monozygotic (identical) twins than in dizygotic (fraternal) twins and siblings (Locke & Mather, 1987; Matheny & Bruggeman, 1973).

Environmental and Psychosocial Factors

Environmental and psychosocial factors are important in the development of normal articulation. In this light, one cause of deviant articulation may be inadequate speech models because children tend to imitate the articulation patterns heard. Parents, older siblings, babysitters, or other significant persons in the child's environment might provide poor speech models. The child may be in an environment in which little speech is used. Consequently, speech would seldom be heard, resulting in insufficient stimulation and modeling.

Another environmental factor is limited speech stimulation and motivation. For example, a child's wants may be anticipated or gestures accepted in the place of oral speech so that the child does not need to use speech to communicate needs and wants. This anticipation may be done by parents, siblings, and others. Similarly, parents usually are excellent interpreters. They often understand virtually everything the child who is unintelligible to others says; thus, the child really does not need to speak more intelligibly until associating with other children. In other instances, the child may be relatively isolated so that there is seldom a need to speak. In other situations, the child may be punished for incorrect articulations or not praised for good speech efforts and consequently choose not to speak. Although empirical data are not available regarding stimulation and motivation to speak intelligibly, clinical evidence indicates the importance of these factors in speech development.

A third environmental/psychosocial variable is inadequate or inappropriate reinforcement. If a child is not reinforced for accurate articulation or is reinforced for inadequate articulation, articulation errors may persist. When persons in the environment do not attend to or respond to the child's utterances and positively reinforce speech attempts, the child may choose not to speak in later situations. On the other hand, parents or others can be too tolerant of deviant speech and reinforce it; thus, the child will not attempt to alter misarticulations (Winitz, 1969). A child is reinforced for such errors by the listener who does not rephrase error-filled sentences and who acknowledges understanding of misarticulated words.

A child may stop developing articulation abilities or regress to more immature articulation patterns as a result of an emotional reaction to a traumatic experience. Examples are regression resulting from the birth of a sibling, hospitalization of a parent, or death of an important person in the child's environment. Articulation development may be impeded or stopped when a child undergoes a period of hospitalization, illness, or injury. Other similar situations can also adversely affect the child's articulation.

Anxiety, frustration, and discouragement on the part of others concerning the child's speech are etiological factors. Such emotional reactions to the person with disordered articulation of either organic or nonorganic etiology may result in the perpetuation of the disorder. Powers (1971) has summarized environmental influences very well:

> . . . it is obvious that the amount and kind of speech stimulation in the home is a powerful determinant of the child's articulation and language development. Certain environmental conditions and certain types of interaction between the child and his environment are necessary for the development of mature speech. To develop normal patterns of speech a child must hear normal patterns of speech, must have a need and desire to talk, must experience pleasure in hearing speech and in responding with speech, must have sufficient variety in his speech, and must be reacted to constructively by others. (p. 869)

Psychosocial factors, in either the child or parent, may influence articulation/phonological development. Winitz (1969) concluded from his review of studies that persons with articulation deficits have a greater proportion of adjustment and behavioral problems on nonstandardized personality inventories. At variance with Winitz, Powers (1971) found the results of studies on personality traits and adjustment to be inconsistent in their findings, with some showing a difference

between children with articulation deficits and normal speakers while others did not. In the examples of personality or psychologicalal differences, one wonders whether this difference is the cause or the result of the articulatory/phonologic disorder. Most probably, the relationship works both ways.

Researchers have also looked at psychosocial factors in parents. After reviewing the literature, Powers (1971) concluded that studies consistently showed a relationship between articulation skills and parental adjustment and attitudes. Some studies have shown that mothers of children with articulation deficits are more poorly adjusted, have less favorable attitudes toward their child, have higher standards, and are more critical. However, these findings are not consistently reported (Spriestersbach, 1956).

Shriberg and associates (1982a, 1986, 1994, 1997, 1998) conducted research on 178 children with speech delays, including functional articulatory/phonologic disorders, and collected information regarding potential psychosocial etiological factors using a rating profile. The researchers looked at the children's psychosocial behaviors and parent psychosocial inputs. These children were not compared to their normally speaking peers; rather, potential etiological factors were described for these children with speech delays. Some children with developmental speech delays were judged to have psychosocial needs. Two thirds were judged to be too sensitive or overly sensitive to others, more than 40% were described as being too concerned or overly concerned about others' feelings, and one third were seen to have psychosocial adjustment problems. Other psychosocial behavioral difficulties in these children were documented as well. Shriberg and colleagues also noted undesirable psychosocial characteristics in some of the parents of children with developmental speech delays, including being somewhat or considerably ineffective in behavioral management (27%), needing training in parenting (33%), overwhelmed by parenting responsibility (17%), and overly concerned about child's problem (17%). In summarizing their findings, Shriberg and Kwiatkowski (1994) stated:

> Parent reports and clinical judgments of parenting strategies suggest that significant external pressures are not prevalent in approximately 75% of children with developmental phonological disorders. No study to date has demonstrated that such variables are associated with the normal acquisition of speech. Rather, . . . these children are judged to experience internal pressures affecting their psychosocial adjustment . . . These descriptive data indicate that a significant number of chil-

dren with developmental phonological disorders experience psychosocial difficulties. (p. 1115)

In their etiological classification system, Shriberg and Austin (1998) classified approximately 7% of the children as speech delays with developmental psychosocial involvement. Finally, Shriberg (1997; Shriberg & Austin, 1998) cautioned that the developmental psychosocial involvement subtype of speech delay is the "most speculative."

In summary, some research findings have shown a relationship between articulatory/phonologic disorders and environmental/psychosocial factors, but the exact nature of personality traits and parental/home characteristics is unclear.

> How are the personal factors of age, gender, sibling status, and socioeconomic status related to articulatory/phonological skills?

Personal Factors

Personal factors, such as age, gender, sibling status, and socioeconomic status may affect the development of speech.

Age

As shown in Chapter 3, articulation and phonology abilities are related to age level until approximately 8 years of age. Children's articulation around the age of 4 years resembles that of adults and continues developing until the adult sound system is acquired, typically by 8 years of age. It is thus unlikely that an individual will outgrow an articulation/phonological delay after 8 or 9 years of age.

Gender

Gender is another variable that has been investigated. Since the 1920s, research results have shown that females have slightly better articulation skills than males; that is, they acquire speech sounds earlier than males. However, not all differences between males and females have been statistically significant (Dawson, 1929; Perkins, 1977; Templin, 1963; Winitz, 1969). The results of a recent large-scale normative study of mastery of speech sound acquisition showed similar results with girls tending to acquire sounds earlier up to 6 years of age (Smit et al., 1990). According to speech surveys, males also have a higher prevalence of articulatory/phonologic delays/disorders than females (Bernthal & Bankson, 2004; Hull,

Mielke, Timmons, & Willeford, 1971; Peña-Brooks & Hegde, 2000).

Sibling Status

Sibling status may be a factor related to articulation skills. Some research has shown that children without siblings, firstborn children, and children with greater age spacing between siblings have better articulation skills (Davis, 1937; Koch, 1956); however, other research has not supported these findings (Wellman, Case, Mengert, & Bradbury, 1931). The articulation skills of twins tend to be poorer than those of singletons. Occasionally, twins use unique speech patterns and words that are understood only by the twins themselves. These patterns are called **idioglossia** (twin speech, in lay terms). The differences in articulation skills might reflect differences in the frequency or quality of parental attention or of sibling interaction. In the preceding favorable circumstances, the parents spend more time with the child, providing a greater amount and better quality of speech patterns for imitation, especially during the formative years. In the cases of children from families having more than one child and smaller age spacing between siblings, the children probably spend less time with parents and more time with siblings, possibly resulting in greater exposure to lower level articulation models. Siblings also may not be as reinforcing. Although differences exist regarding sibling status, these differences seem to disappear rapidly after the child begins school.

Socioeconomic Status

Socioeconomic status has been investigated as a potential variable in the development and proficiency of articulation. Some research findings have shown that there is a higher incidence of articulation errors among lower socioeconomic levels (Powers, 1971; Templin, 1957; Weaver, Furbee, & Everhart, 1960; Winitz, 1969). According to Winitz, there is a low, positive correlation between articulation skills and socioeconomic status. His review of the literature showed that persons from upper socioeconomic levels provide a more favorable linguistic environment in that they model better speech patterns for the child to imitate and may be more reinforcing. They also tend to create more stimulation for speech development and provide a greater amount and better quality of articulation training. Yet, Everhart (1953, 1956) and Prins (1962) did not find a correlation between frequency of articulation problems and parental occupation. More recent research did not find a significant relationship between socioeconomic status and articulation skills (Smit et al., 1990). Thus, socioeconomic factors appear to have only a minor, if any, influence on articulation development and performance.

Finally, residing in a rural rather than in an urban area does not seem to affect speech development.

| How are linguistic and academic factors related to articulatory/phonologic disorders? |

Linguistic and Academic Factors

Phonology is one of the components of the larger system of language; consequently, researchers have explored the relationship between phonology and the other components of language—morphology, syntax, and semantics. The research literature has consistently shown that articulation/phonological impairments occur simultaneously with expressive language impairments (Bernthal & Bankson, 2004; Peña-Brooks & Hegde, 2000). In fact, from their review of the literature, Fey et al. (1994) estimated that 80% of children with phonological deficits show delays in grammar development and that 79% of children with specific language impairment also have phonological impairments. Others have estimated simultaneous occurrence percentages to be 60–80% (Tyler, Lewis, Haskill, & Tolbert, 2002; Tyler & Watterson, 1991) and 50–70% (Shriberg & Kwiatkowski, 1994). Concomitant problems in phonology and other language areas seem to be more prevalent in children with more severe articulation/phonological problems (Gross, St. Louis, Ruscello, & Hull, 1985), although this may not always be the case (Ruscello, St. Louis, & Mason, 1991). Some children (10–40%) with articulatory/phonologic disorders also have language comprehension deficits (Marquardt & Saxman, 1972; Shriberg & Kwiatkowski, 1994).

The relationship between phonology and other language domains has been investigated by looking at the effects of complexity upon expressive abilities. Generally, more articulation errors occur as syntax becomes complex (Panagos, Quine, & Klich, 1979; Schmauch, Panagos, & Klich, 1978). Similarly, more complex articulation patterns result in more grammatical errors (Panagos & Prelock, 1982). The association between phonology and grammar has also been investigated through treatment studies to determine the effects of targeting one area of deficit (for example, grammar) on the other area (for example, phonology). In two studies, phonological treatment resulted in improved syntax, and syntactic treatment resulted in improved phonology, although clients made the greatest gains in the area being treated (Matheny & Panagos, 1978; Wilcox & Morris, 1995). The results were partially supported by Hoffman, Norris, and Monjure (1990) and Tyler et al. (2002) who found that language treatment resulted in improved phonology and language, while phonology treatment resulted in improved phonology but not growth in language. These findings, however, were not supported by two other studies in that language-based intervention did not result in improved phonology for subjects with grammar and phonological deficits (Fey et al., 1994; Tyler & Watterson, 1991). There appears to be a significant relationship between phonology and the other domains of language, especially expressive morphology and syntax, but the exact nature of that association is undetermined. Implications of the findings of studies exploring the relationship are that there is a need to assess comprehensive and expressive language skills, as well as phonological skills, in children who have articulation/phonological impairments. Further, for most children with articulatory/phonologic disorders, treatment should be focused on phonological skills in order for improvement in this domain.

A final consideration concerns educational achievement. Over the years, researchers have investigated the relationship between phonologic disorders and educational problems, especially in reading and spelling. Early research findings were contradictory. While some earlier research did not show a relationship (Flynn & Byrne, 1970; Hall, 1938), other researchers reported an association between articulation performance and reading readiness, reading skills, and spelling (Fitzsimmons, 1958; Ham, 1958; Weaver et al., 1960; Winitz, 1969). Later research has tended to show a relationship between phonology, reading, spelling, and educational performance (Felsenfeld et al., 1995; Lewis & Freebairn-Farr, 1993). Furthermore, this relationship might also include linguistic variables. A child with an articulation problem will have, not uncommonly, a language problem as well as reading and spelling problems.

Recently, research findings have shown an association between phonologic disorders and deficient **phonological awareness** skills (Bird & Bishop, 1992; Hodson, 1994, 1997; Stackhouse, 1997; Webster & Plante, 1992). Phonological awareness "refers to rhyme, syllable and sound segmentation, manipulation, and blending" (Stackhouse, 1997, p. 158). It appears that poor phonological awareness skills are linked to reading and spelling problems; children with inadequate phonological awareness are at risk for academic difficulties (Ball, 1993; Catts, 1991; Clarke-Klein

& Hodson, 1995; Goldsworthy, 1996; Stackhouse, 1997; Swank & Catts, 1994). Thus, there is growing evidence that young children with severe phonologic disorders may have poor phonological awareness skills, which puts them at risk for later academic problems in reading and spelling.

> What other speech factors are related to articulatory/phonologic disorders?

Other Speech Factors

Several researchers have investigated the relationship between articulatory/phonologic disorders and other speech disorders, namely stuttering and voice disorders. Results have shown a higher than expected simultaneous occurrence of these deviations. Articulatory/phonologic disorders have been shown to occur in 30–40% of children who stutter (Louko, Edwards, & Conture, 1990; Nippold, 1990, 2001; Ratner, 1995). One study even showed the percentage to be 44% in 467 preschool through high school subjects who stutter (Arndt & Healey, 2001). Thus, speech sound disorders seem to occur more frequently in individuals with stuttering (30–40%) as compared with the normal population (2–6%). Paden, Yairi, and Ambrose (1999) compared phonological abilities of persons who recovered from stuttering with those of persons who did not recover. Although both groups showed typical phonological developmental patterns, those who did not recover from stuttering had more delayed phonological development. Interestingly, the phonological complexity of words did not seem to affect which words were stuttered on in a group of 24 children aged 2 to 5 years who were diagnosed with mild and severe stuttering (Throneburg, Yairi, & Paden, 1994).

Articulation/phonological deviations occur in persons with voice disorders more frequently than would be expected. Most students in grades 1 to 12 with voice disorders had concomitant articulatory disorders; articulatory disorder occurred simultaneously in 58% of those with severe voice disorders and in 62% of those with moderate voice disorders (St. Louis, Hansen, Buch, & Oliver, 1992). In the same database, 75% of the students with articulatory disorders had coexisting voice disorders with hoarseness being the most frequent.

Certainly, not every person who has an articulatory/phonologic disorder has a fluency or voice quality impairment, but it is clear that articulatory/phonologic disorders often coexist with stuttering; voice disorders; and morphologic, syntactic, and semantic language disorders. The simultaneous occurrence of these disorders has implications for intervention, making treatment planning and implementation more complex. Four treatment approaches for concomitant stuttering and articulatory/phonologic disorders were identified by Arndt and Healey (2001):

- Blended—treat both disorders simultaneously
- Cyclic—treat each disorder for specific time periods
- Sequential—treat one disorder, then the other
- Concurrent—treat both disorders for equal amounts of time within the context of the lowest phonological and linguistic demands

Survey results showed that 45% of clients with stuttering and phonologic disorders were treated with a blended approach and 21% with a concurrent approach (Arndt & Healey, 2001). These different approaches in terms of allocation of treatment time need to be considered for any combination of concomitant disorders.

SUMMARY

Terminology for speech sound disorders has evolved over the years. Articulatory/phonologic disorders can be defined as speech sounds produced and used at variance with the linguistic community and age-level expectations. Several factors should be considered in making a diagnosis of articulatory/phonologic disorder. Various classification systems are used in describing individual articulatory/phonological impairment. A delay describes an immature phonological system and a disorder describes a deviant system. A phonetic disorder involves the motor system, whereas a phonologic disorder involves the linguistic system. Classically, articulatory/phonologic disorders are classified as dyslalia (rarely used term), dysarthria, and apraxia of speech. Traditionally, speech sound errors are described as omissions, substitutions, distortions, and additions occurring in the initial, medial, and final positions of words. Severity levels of impairment are identified as mild, moderate, severe, and profound.

Many etiological factors potentially affect articulation. However, no general, systematic deficiency of any factor exists that is of sufficient size to have predictive value. No factor is consistently absent. All are found in some cases; all are absent in some cases. Factors that seem to be related to articulatory/phonologic disorders include structural, physiologic, neuromuscular, sensory/perceptual, cognitive, heredity, environmental, psychosocial, personal, linguistic, academic, and other speech disorder factors. One should look for known and potential etiologies, because several factors may be operating to cause an articulatory/phonologic disorder in a particular child or adult. Some factors precipitate the deviancy, whereas others maintain it. The precipitating factors may no longer be operative or may not be treatable. Understanding both the **precipitating causes** and **maintaining causes** is important in planning an intervention program.

REVIEW QUESTIONS

1. What term(s) are currently used to label a speech sound impairment?

2. Delineate the variables that would lead to a diagnosis of articulatory/phonologic disorder.

3. What is the difference between an articulation delay and an articulatory disorder?

4. Differentiate between a phonetically-based speech sound disorder and one that is phonologically based.

5. Describe the classification system proposed by Shriberg and colleagues for child speech disorders.

6. Describe the dysarthrias.

7. What are the characteristics of apraxia of speech (verbal apraxia)? What is oral apraxia? Differentiate between acquired apraxia of speech and childhood apraxia of speech.

8. How are misarticulations often described?

9. Differentiate between organic and nonorganic (functional) etiological factors of articulatory/phonologic disorders.

10. Provide some examples of structural, physiologic, neurological, and sensory/perceptual etiological factors contributing to articulatory/phonologic disorders.

11. What seems to be the relationship between speech sound discrimination ability and articulatory/phonologic disorders?

12. What is the relationship between cognition and articulation/phonological skills? Between linguistic and articulation/phonological skills? Between academic performance and articulation/phonological skills? Between stuttering and articulation/phonological skills? Between voice disorders and articulation/phonological skills?

13. What evidence exists that some articulatory/phonologic disorders may be genetically based?

14. What environmental, psychosocial, and personal factors may be related to articulatory/phonologic disorders?

15. Why might speech-language pathologists look for etiological factors when assessing individuals with articulatory/phonologic disorders?

16. Differentiate between precipitating and maintaining etiological factors.

CHAPTER 6

Assessment of Articulatory/Phonologic Disorders

"A man is hid under his tongue."
—Ali Ibn-Abi-Talib

CHAPTER OBJECTIVES

- Describe the process of screening for articulatory/phonologic disorders.
- Identify the contents of an articulation/phonological assessment battery.
- Describe each component of the assessment battery: articulation/phonological tests, stimulability, connected speech sample, intelligibility, specialized articula-

tion/phonological tests, case history, oral-peripheral exam, hearing sensitivity exam, speech sound discrimination (optional).

- Propose some optional ancillary areas of assessment.
- Discuss the assignment of a severity level to an articulatory/phonologic disorder.
- Describe principles and sequence of the assessment process.

Amajor stage of articulation and phonological management is assessment and diagnosis; that is, gathering and synthesizing the information about a problem and defining the problem. Diagnosis involves assigning an individual to a particular category within a classification system based on attributes, characteristics, or behaviors (Witt, Elliott, Kramer, & Gresham, 1994). It "includes a thorough understanding of the client's problem and not merely the application of a label" (Haynes & Pindzola, 2004, p. 2). The purposes of an initial evaluation are to (a) determine the reality of the problem, (b) determine the etiology(ies), and (c) provide a clinical focus as to potential treatment approaches (Haynes & Pindzola, 2004). After a thorough differential case history is collected, a careful assessment should be completed as a basis for diagnosis and for planning appropriate and effective treatment. This process is perhaps the single most important aspect of clinical management, and it is an ongoing process. If a client is misdiagnosed, then the subsequent plan of treatment may be inappropriate to meet the specific needs of the client.

Conducting a diagnostic workup is a complex undertaking. Not only must appropriate tests be selected, but also information should be obtained beyond the standardized test results. To obtain relevant, important information, the diagnostician must possess an armamentarium that includes good observational skills. Often, the informal assessment information is as important as the formal, standardized test results. Through observation, the astute examiner obtains significant information about the client's speech sound system, motivation, approach to a problem, interests, perseverance, cosmetic characteristics present when talking, and other important idiosyncrasies. The two observational skills—looking and listening—coupled with the cognitive functions of assimilating, analyzing, and interpreting, provide the diagnostician with the necessary tools for making an accurate diagnosis and a reasonable statement about prognosis.

An ample amount of time must be taken to conduct a thorough evaluation. Assessment or evaluation does not need to be limited to a set time frame as is often the case in clinical settings, but rather it should be based on the needs of individual clients. Realistically, there are time restrictions for assessment so that the clinician needs to select tests and diagnostic procedures carefully, selecting procedures that will yield appropriate information efficiently (Khan, 2002). The more relevant information that can be obtained about a client and the better understanding the clinician has of a client and the client's problem, the greater the chance of outlining an appropriate, specific, and effective treatment plan, which is an essential goal of the diagnostic workup. There are situations in which sufficient diagnostic information is unobtainable in specified assessment sessions and evaluation continues into the beginning of treatment. In this case, the clinician conducts trial or diagnostic treatment to learn more about the client so that appropriate treatment strategies can be formulated and implemented as treatment is carried out. Thus, assessment is ongoing. Clinicians monitor clients' progress over time to modify the course of treatment as needed and to decide when to terminate intervention.

> What are two characteristics of individuals with articulatory/phonologic disorders that might complicate the diagnosis?

PRELIMINARY CONSIDERATIONS

Requisites for conducting an accurate assessment are knowledge and awareness of the general characteristics of persons with articulation/phonological deviances. Although there are a great many behavioral differences, a number of likenesses are present among persons with these speech disorders. Furthermore, not all of the characteristics may have been clearly implicated, yet familiarity with those characteristics that are more commonly associated with deviant articulation and phonology, as well as with typical speech sound development, should assist the diagnostician in testing appropriate areas and focusing on the specific problem. The typical course of speech sound development and factors related to articulatory/phonologic disorders are described in Chapters 3 and 5, respectively.

A characteristic common in articulation/phonological testing is variability in speech sound production or inconsistency of test results. Variability in test results can be attributed to variability in the client, diagnostician, diagnostic test, and the interaction between the client and the diagnostician (Shriberg, 1982; Winitz, 1969). A phoneme misarticulated at one time, in one context, or in one emotional state may be correctly articulated at another time or in another phonetic context (Oller, 1973). Because of this variability, the client's articulation and phonological performance should be assessed in several contexts, including connected speech. Connected speech, however, is not the sole answer to obtaining a valid and representative speech sample. As with communication samples of isolated words, connected speech samples may not always be spontaneous; the contexts may be too simple, too complex, or too stereotyped; the contexts may sample only familiar words and an insufficient number of phonemic contexts and positions; or the procedure may be too time-consuming. Nevertheless, determining the contexts in which a typically misarticulated sound is produced correctly or in which a phonological process is suppressed assists the clinician in identifying a starting point for intervention (Ingram, 1989; McDonald, 1964b; Van Riper & Erickson, 1996; Weston & Irwin, 1971). Given the presence of variable speech sound production and inconsistent test results, the diagnostician has an even greater challenge in selecting a treatment approach and speech sound targets.

Another characteristic common to articulation and phonological problems is that of multiple causes (Haynes & Pindzola, 2004; Powers, 1971; Shriberg, 1982). Sometimes, there may be an obvious reason for the speech disorder and, consequently, the diagnostician fails to consider other possibilities. The effective diagnostician is not content with having found one cause for the problem. Instead, a thorough assessment should be conducted to identify multiple causes or causal patterns, if possible. For example, a client who was born with a cleft palate may not undergo the diagnostic scrutiny in areas unrelated to cleft palate, such as use of phonological deviations, because the presence of the cleft may have obscured the importance of these and other causes. Dichotomizing etiology into organic and nonorganic categories should be avoided because it tends to narrow the approach to assessment. Furthermore, the diagnostician may become preoccupied with deciding into which category to place the disorder and overlook the possibility of its having both organic and nonorganic etiologies. It is not uncommon for etiologies to be impossible to ascertain. With clients for whom the etiology has been determined, causes often are multiple. Remember that speech sound production is not always normal when all conditions for its development appear to be favorable, and vice versa, thus complicating the process of making a differential diagnosis in terms of etiology.

An aspect that varies considerably among persons with articulatory/phonologic disorders is client level of awareness. Some clients seem to be keenly aware and sensitive to their deviant speech, while others seem to be unaware of, or at least unconcerned about, their speech differences. Several factors can influence the level of awareness, but it is the responsibility of the clinician to ascertain how aware clients are of their speech. This information can be helpful in determining the client's motivation and thereby provide some useful information about prognosis. If the level of awareness is relatively low, then the clinician may want to increase the emphasis on self-monitoring skills to achieve eventual **carryover**. If the level of awareness is high, then the client may be well motivated to correct the problem, which suggests a favorable prognosis, or the client may be overly sensitive to the problem, which suggests a less positive prognosis.

What is the purpose of screening for articulatory/phonologic disorders?
What three types of instruments are available for screening articulation/phonology?

SCREENING PROCEDURES

Sometimes, before administering a full assessment, a speech screening is done. The purpose of screening is to identify those who may have an articulatory/phonologic disorder, but not to describe it nor make a diagnosis. The amount of time spent with each individual is just long enough to determine whether speech and language are probably deviant, generally no more than 10 minutes per person. A full assessment is the usual recommendation for individuals who do not pass the screening.

Screening most often occurs in preschool or school settings. Screening of preschool and school populations typically includes all of the domains of communication, including articulation/phonology, language, voice, fluency, and hearing. Under IDEA (1997) regulations, individual students are not to be singled out for screening; rather, an entire group of students with specific characteristics, such as all members of certain grade levels, are screened. The same screening items and

procedures are to be applied to all students in a particular category. Permission from parents is not required for screening, but informing them ahead of time is appropriate. Following IDEA guidelines, a multidisciplinary team that includes the classroom teacher, parents/caregivers, and other specialists must recommend the student for assessment and the parent/caregiver must consent to the assessment before the clinician proceeds.

Screening instruments are either informal or formal. Informal procedures are those designed by individual speech-language pathologists and include items such as saying one's name and address, counting, naming colors, describing pictures, and repeating sentences that contain frequently occurring misarticulations, such as "Sit in the swing sister" and "Charles purchased a brand new watch." Older individuals might be instructed to read a passage containing most of the English speech sounds. (See Fig. 6.1 for two examples.) From the informal screening, most experienced clinicians can make predictive judgments based on normative data about speech sound acquisition, such as the pattern of the students' misarticulations. Do they follow the developmental hierarchy, but at a delayed age level? If so, is the delay a major one or is maturation likely to correct the delay? Are the misarticulations unusual? What is the individual's intelligibility level? Is there an ethnic, cultural, or community explanation for the different articulation/phonological patterns that might indicate no speech deficiency? The answers to these questions give the clinician a basis for making a sound subjective judgment concerning whether or not to recommend further assessment.

Formal screening tools for articulation/phonology, such as published instruments, are of three types (Table 6.1). First, there are several general speech and language screening instruments available to speech-language pathologists for screening preschool and early elementary school-aged children, including the *Fluharty Preschool Speech and Language Screening Test, Second Edition* (Fluharty-2; Fluharty, 2000); the *Joliet 3-Minute Preschool Speech and Language Screen* (Kinzler, 1992); the *Joliet 3-Minute Speech and Language Screen, Revised* (Kinzler & Johnson, 1993); the *Preschool Language Scale-4* (PLS-4) *Screening Test Kit* (Zimmerman, Steiner, & Pond, 2005); the *Riley Articulation and Language Test,* Revised (Riley, 1966); the *Slosson Articulation Language Test with Phonology* (SALT-P) (Tade & Slosson, 1986); and the *Speech-Ease Screening Inventory* (K–1) (Speech-Ease, 1985). These instruments include a section for assessing articulation production skills; most have been standardized with

---

Grandfather Passage: You wish to know all about my grandfather. Well, he is nearly 93 years old, yet he still thinks as swiftly as ever. He dresses himself in an old black frock coat, usually with several buttons missing. A long beard clings to his chin, giving those who observe him a pronounced feeling of the utmost respect. When he speaks, his voice is just a bit cracked and it quivers a bit. Twice each day, he plays skillfully and with zest upon a small organ. Except in winter when the snow or ice prevents, he slowly takes a short walk in the open air each day. We have often urged him to walk more and smoke less, but he always answers, "Banana oil." Grandfather likes to be modern in his language.

Rainbow Passage: When the sunlight strikes raindrops in the air, the two act like a prism and form a rainbow. The rainbow is a division of white light into many beautiful colors. These take the shape of a long round arch, with its path high above, and its two ends apparently beyond the horizon. There is, according to legend, a boiling pot of gold at one end. People look, but no one ever finds it. When a man looks for something beyond his reach, his friends say he is looking for the pot of gold at the end of the rainbow.

FIGURE 6.1   Reading passages containing most of the English phonemes to be used for screening the speech production of adolescents and adults.

guidelines for setting the criteria for passing the screening. Second, some screening tools have been developed specifically for articulation/phonology, including the *Phonological Screening Assessment* (Stevens & Isles, 2001), the *Quick Screen of* *Phonology* (Bankson & Bernthal, 1990b), and the *Rules Phonological Screening Test* (Webb & Duckett, 1990). Finally, others are a part of, or a subtest of, a more extensive test (Fisher & Logemann, 1971; Hodson, 2004; Templin & Darley,

TABLE 6.1

Formal Screening Tools for Articulatory/Phonologic Disorders

Type of Screening Tool	Test	Age Levels
General speech/language screening instruments	*Fluharty Preschool Speech and Language Screening Test, Second Edition*, 2000	3–7 years
	Joliet 3-Minute Preschool Speech and Language Screen, 1992	2.5–4.5 years
	Joliet 3-Minute Speech and Language Screen, Revised Edition, 1993	Kindergarten, 2nd grade, 5th grade
	Preschool Language Scale-4 (PLS-4) *Screening Test Kit*, 2005	3–7 years
	Riley Articulation and Language Test, Revised Edition, 1966	Kindergarten, 1st grade, 2nd grade
	Slosson Articulation Language Test with Phonology (SALT-P), 1986	3–5:11
	Speech-Ease Screening Inventory (K–1), 1985	Kindergarten, 1st grade
Specific articulation/ phonological screening instruments	*Phonological Screening Assessment*, 2001	Child–Adult
	Quick Screen of Phonology, 1990b	3–7:11
	Rules Phonological Screening Test, 1990	2–8 years
Subtest of articulation/ phonological test	Screening Form of *Fisher-Logemann Test of Articulation Competence*, 1971	Preschool–Adult
	HAAP-3 Preschool Phonological Screening, 2004	Preschool, Elementary
	Screening Test—Templin-Darley Tests of Articulation, 1969	3–8 years

1969). These instruments provide guidelines in the form of cutoff scores regarding whether a more complete assessment is recommended.

> What components comprise a comprehensive articulation/phonological assessment battery?

ASSESSMENT BATTERY FOR ARTICULATORY/ PHONOLOGIC DISORDERS

Accurate assessment of articulation/phonology involves eliciting various types of speech samples including formal articulation/phonological testing, assessment of stimulability of misarticulated sounds, assessment of articulation/phonology production and intelligibility from spontaneous speech samples in and out of context, and other special tests and observations. Ancillary analyses are also important in the assessment of individuals with articulatory/ phonologic disorders. Such analyses include collecting case history information, assessment of speech structures and functions, auditory sensitivity, and possibly assessment of speech sound discrimination skills. The assessment of speech structures often includes diadochokinetic tasks, which are ways to sample speech rate. Results of a speech rate task, such as rapid naming, rapidly saying "buttercup" 10 times, or the traditional "put-tuh-kuh," may provide useful information relative to later development of literacy skills (Hodson, Scherz, & Strattman, 2002). A flowchart of assessment battery components for articulation/phonological evaluation appears in Figure 6.2. Additionally, to get a total picture of the client's communication abilities, assessment often includes screening or testing the areas of language, voice, fluency, prosody, and phonological awareness.

Four steps are involved in speech sound evaluation procedures:

- Obtaining the speech sample
- Tape recording the client's responses (optional)
- Transcribing the sample
- Scoring and analyzing the sample

The sample to be collected can be in the form of single words, phrases, sentences, and conversation. Additionally, the words, phrases, and sentences can be elicited spontaneously or imitatively. As might be expected, there are advantages and disadvantages for each type of sample. Newman & Creaghead (1989) pointed out that the "optimal

sample should (a) reflect the child's production in actual communicative situations, (b) reveal both inconsistencies and consistent patterns, and (c) contain the full set of English phonemes. Ideally the sample should include conversational speech" (p. 89). The primary disadvantage of single words, phrases, and sentences, particularly when elicited through imitation, is that the sound productions may not truly reflect the child's productions of these same sounds in spontaneous speech; thus, the sample may not be an accurate representation of the child's phonological system, and consequently, the conclusions of the analysis may be inaccurate. This seems to be particularly true for clients who have experience in articulation/phonological treatment. Nonetheless, research findings support a positive correlation between speech sound productions obtained from naming pictures and from spontaneous speaking situations, although differences between these two types of measures are noted for some clients (Bernthal & Bankson, 2004). Few differences have been noted in overall phonological profiles when comparing connected speech and sentence completion tasks with single-word production tasks (Khan & Lewis, 2002). From their review of the literature, Khan and Lewis noted that "the frequency of process usage was greater in connected speech, but the relative importance of any single process overall remained fairly constant" (p. 8). The assets of single-word samples (usually picture naming) are that the phonemic inventory and context can be controlled so that the client's phonetic skills can be noted, the child's speech is more intelligible to the examiner because the intended words are known, the sampling procedure is quicker, and the sample is elicited in a more objective, standardized manner.

Conversational speech can be elicited in a variety of ways, such as by using toys and pictures, talking about the client's interests, retelling a story, and observing the client and parent interacting verbally. The primary difficulties with spontaneous speech samples are that the sample may not tap a complete phonemic inventory, the phonemic contexts are random and uncontrolled, the sample may be unintelligible to the diagnostician, and the procedure can be quite time-consuming. The all-encompassing advantage is that, theoretically, the sample is a more valid representation of the client's speech production and thus of the phonological system. The technique of retelling a story should help alleviate the problems associated with spontaneous speech samples because the examiner can exert more control over the phonemes and phonemic contexts tapped. At least the opportunity exists for such control. From our viewpoint, a sample for

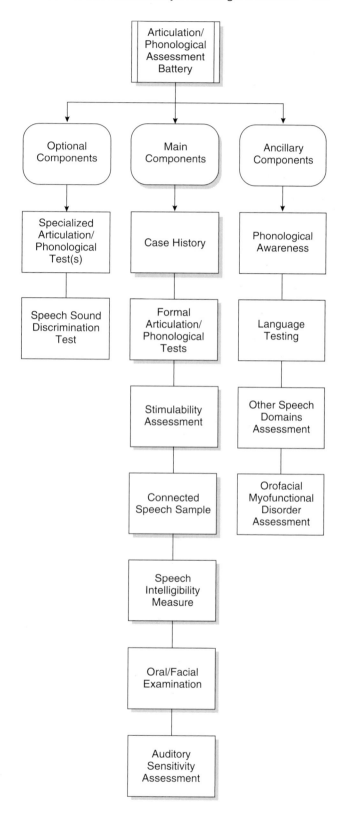

FIGURE 6.2 Components of an assessment battery for articulatory/phonologic disorders.

articulation/phonological analysis should include specified single-word or sentence productions and spontaneous productions.

The speech sample needs to be transcribed online (live), such that the diagnostician makes notes about the productions and transcribes them as accurately as possible while the client is speaking. Additionally, the client's productions can be recorded on audiotape or videotape and listened to or watched later so that the final transcription of the sample will be more reliable and accurate. The examiner then can compare the live transcription with the perception of the sound productions from the tape recording. It is important that the transcription be precise and accurate so that a valid articulation/phonological analysis can be done. The last step in articulation/phonological testing is to analyze the sample.

> Describe traditional articulation tests, combined articulation/phonological tests, and phonological tests.

Articulation/Phonological Tests

Assessment of the client's speech sound production system should include formal articulation/phonological tests. There are three types of formal tests, most of which are standardized:

- Traditional articulation tests
- Combined articulation and phonological tests
- Phonological tests

Most of these tests are normed for children up to 8 or 9 years of age. This does not preclude administering them to older individuals; the norms cannot be applied to their performance on the test, but they can be compared with adult speech in their linguistic community.

Formal Traditional Articulation Tests

Generally, formal traditional articulation tests sample speech sound production in isolated words that typically are elicited by pictures without a model from the examiner. Some tests also provide written word lists or written sentences for individuals who prefer to read; hence, in the latter case, speech sounds are elicited in words produced in the context of sentences. Often, the test items are sequenced in a developmental order of phoneme acquisition. Typically, all American English singleton consonants (except possibly /ʒ/) and selected consonant blends (usually /s/, /r/, and /l/ blends) are tested; sometimes, vowels and diphthongs are also tested. In most tests, the singleton

consonant sounds are sampled in the initial, medial, and final positions of words, although some sample consonants only in the initial (releasing) and final (arresting) positions; blends are usually sampled in the initial position. Test results provide information about types of misarticulations (omissions, substitutions, distortions, and additions) and the word positions in which the errors occur. Sometimes, the manner of or the place of production of the misarticulated consonants is also specified. Further, most tests provide norm-based guidelines to be used for interpreting results.

Each test manual provides instructions on how to administer the test. Generally, for the picture tests, the client is shown the picture stimuli and is asked to name it; or the client is given a question or statement to elicit the target word. The clinician can give cues to help the testee identify the word. However, it is preferable not to spend an excessive amount of time attempting to elicit the target word. Rather, if the client does not say the word with one or two cues, the clinician provides a delayed model in which the clinician says the word followed by a comment (such as "It's a *house*; now, you say it"). Finally, if the client still does not utter the target word, the clinician provides a direct (nondelayed) model (such as "Say *house*"). The goal is for the client to utter the word spontaneously. However, some clients may need to be provided with several indirect models, while others may require all direct models possibly (a) because they do not have the vocabulary necessary to identify the words, (b) because of being reluctant to talk because of their speech problems, (c) because of being shy, or (d) because of innumerable other reasons. Sometimes, the clinician does not "hear" how the client produced a sound being tested. In this case, it is preferable for the clinician to "take the blame" rather than just asking the client to repeat the word. Because of past experiences with listeners who do not understand, the client may be reluctant to repeat when the clinician asks "What?" Instead, the clinician might say, "You said the right word; I just wasn't fast enough to write it down. Please say it again."

The test should be transcribed online (live) rather than attempting to transcribe it from a tape recording. Tape recording the administration of articulation tests is recommended to verify the online transcriptions later. There are three ways to record (transcribe) responses:

- Correct/incorrect method in which the targeted sound is scored as either produced correctly or incorrectly
- Types of errors, including omissions, substitutions, distortions, additions
- Whole-word phonetic transcription

Whole-word transcription is used mostly for phonological process analysis. In traditional articulation tests, only the targeted sounds are transcribed. Most tests use the following system:

- Use the phonetic symbol of the substituted sound for a substitution.
- Use a dash (-) for an omission.
- Use the phonetic symbols for the target sound and for the added sound for an addition (such as transcribing /bəl/ for /bl/).
- Use an X, D, allophonic transcription, or a number (1,2,3) that signifies the severity for a distortion.
- Use NR (no response) for sounds not elicited.
- Leave blank or use a checkmark (√) for a correctly produced sound.

We prefer leaving the column blank for correctly produced sounds so that the diagnostician can readily visualize the client's performance on the test. Those who prefer a checkmark do so to know that this item was tested. In some test manuals, the instructions specify ± scoring merely indicating that a sound was produced correctly or incorrectly. We recommend that the diagnostician use a more detailed scoring system to indicate the type of error rather than only indicating that a sound was in error. Descriptions of the types of errors provide valuable information for planning treatment.

Several tests are available, each having unique characteristics. Certain tests are useful for various aspects of assessment, but the diagnostician will make selections for each testing situation. These selections will be based partly on client characteristics, test characteristics, and availability. Tables 6.2 and 6.3 provide information about several articulation tests. These particular tests are norm-referenced, and they primarily sample articulation skills in single-word utterances.

Although similar, each test has some unique characteristics. The *Arizona Articulation Proficiency Scale, Third Revision* (AAPS-3; Fudala, 2000) was standardized on more than 5,500 children and teens. The unique feature of the AAPS is that it provides a total articulation score based on a weighted phonemic value according to frequency of occurrence of consonants and vowels. Guidelines show how to interpret the score in terms of speech intelligibility. Additionally, the test provides guidelines for severity levels and indicates the age levels at which the normative sample had 90% mastery of each tested phoneme and cluster.

The *Goldman-Fristoe Test of Articulation, Second Edition* (G-FTA-2; Goldman & Fristoe, 2000) was standardized on 2,350 individuals. It provides

a systematic means of assessing an individual's articulation of consonant sounds in words and in context by using a story retell task using pictures. It also includes a stimulability assessment of each misarticulated phoneme in syllables, words, and phrases. Thus, it provides information for three types of speech samples: (a) sounds in words, (b) sounds in sentences, and (c) stimulability. The testee's responses can be analyzed for phonological processes and phonetic inventory with the *Khan-Lewis Phonological Analysis, Second Edition* (KLPA-2; Khan & Lewis, 2002). A companion software program (ASSIST) helps score, calculate, and compare normative data for the G-FTA-2. The software program also assists in writing diagnostic reports including a recommendation section.

The *Photo Articulation Test, Third Edition* (PAT-3; Lippke, Dickey, Selmar, & Soder, 1997) was standardized on 800 subjects. It consists of 72 small, colored photographs with the last three pictures testing connected speech. It also provides a supplementary word list to sample the testees' ability to imitate the sounds in other words. The use of photographs makes it particularly appropriate for older clients, in addition to younger clients.

The *Templin-Darley Tests of Articulation* (Templin & Darley, 1969) was standardized on 480 children aged 3 to 8 years. It includes the Diagnostic Test (picture and sentence forms), Screening Test, and Iowa Pressure Articulation Test. The last subtest assesses the adequacy of the velopharyngeal mechanism by sampling the pressure consonants. The Diagnostic Test is designed to obtain a detailed sample of the client's articulation. The Screening Test includes 50 items. If the clinician desires to analyze groupings of sound elements, overlays can be used to look separately at initial and final consonant singletons, vowels, diphthongs, /r/ and /ɚ/ clusters, /l/ clusters, /s/ clusters, other clusters (such as /ŋk/, /mp/), Iowa Pressure Articulation Test, and the screening test.

The *Weiss Comprehensive Articulation Test* (WCAT; Weiss, 1980) was standardized on 4,000 children. It incorporates several methods for quantifying articulation abilities, such as articulation score, articulation age, intelligibility score, auditory-visual stimulability score, and number of misarticulations. Different methods of quantification are recommended for clients of different ages. Interpretations are provided for each category. The test also includes guidelines for testing areas related to articulation in an attempt to help determine etiology, need for treatment, prognosis, and baseline from which to measure and report

text continues on page 133

TABLE 6.2

Characteristics of a Sample of Standardized Traditional Articulation Tests

	Arizona Articulation Proficiency Scale, Third Revision (Arizona-3)	Goldman-Fristoe Test of Articulation-2 (G-FTA-2)	Photo Articulation Test, Third Edition (PAT-3)	Templin-Darley Tests of Articulation (TDTA)	Weiss Comprehensive Articulation Test (WCAT)
Author(s), publication date	Fudala, 2000	Goldman & Fristoe, 2000	Lippke, Dickey, Selmar, & Soder, 1997	Templin & Darley, 1969	Weiss, 1980
Age levels	1.5–18 years, can be used with older clients	2–21 years	3:0–8:11	3–8 years	3–adult
Subtests and/or forms	Articulation Test Word Reading Articulation Test Language Screening Continuous Speech Language Sample	Sounds-in-Words Sounds-in-Sentences Stimulability	Articulation Test	Diagnostic Test (Picture & Word Forms) Screening Test Iowa Pressure Articulation Test	Picture response forms; Sentence response forms
Sample types	Single words, spontaneous speech	Single words, connected speech, stimulability in syllables, words, and sentences	Single words, spontaneous speech	Single words, sentences, stimulability in isolation, syllable, and word	Single words, simple sentences, storytelling
Stimuli	42 line-drawn picture cards and additional verbal prompts, list of words, optional picture cards for spontaneous speech	Picture plates and verbal prompts	72 color photographs, 9 to a page or 1 per card	141 colored line-drawn pictures	Color pictures, sentence card story pictures
Number of sounds tested	24 singleton consonants, 8 blends, 20 vowels and diphthongs	23 consonants, 16 clusters	24 consonants, 9 blends, 18 vowels/ diphthongs	24 consonants, 56 blends, 11 vowels, 6 diphthongs, 19 /ɚ/s	26 consonants, 22 clusters, 12 vowels, 7 diphthongs
Consonant word positions*	IF	IMF	IMF	IF	IMF
Scores	Total score (1–100 that expresses successful speech production) based on frequency of occurrence value (.5–6.0) intelligibility descriptions, severity designations, percentiles, standard scores	Standard scores, percentiles, test-age equivalents for males and females for Sounds-in-Words subtest	Percentiles, standard scores, and age equivalents	Mean scores and standard deviations	Articulation scores, age-equivalents, number of misarticulated phonemes, intelligibility scores, and stimulability scores
Administration time	3 minutes	5–15 minutes for Sounds in-Words subtest	20 minutes	Not Reported	20 minutes

(continued)

TABLE 6.2 Continued

Characteristics of a Sample of Standardized Traditional Articulation Tests

	Arizona Articulation Proficiency Scale, Third Revision (Arizona-3)	*Goldman-Fristoe Test of Articulation-2 (G-FTA-2)*	*Photo Articulation Test, Third Edition (PAT-3)*	*Templin-Darley Tests of Articulation (TDTA)*	*Weiss Comprehensive Articulation Test (WCAT)*
Standardization sample	5,500+ children and teens representative of the US ethnicity, region, and parental education, gender specific norms for 1:6–3:11	2,350 examinees stratified to match US census data on gender, race/ethnicity, region, and SES	800 subjects from 23 states	480 children	4,000 children
Validity	High correlations with clinical evaluations of articulation problems; high concurrent validity correlations; moderately high relationship with cognitive ability	Adequate content and construct validity	Adequate content and construct validity; .85 correlation with TOLD-P: 3	Not reported	Adequate content and construct validity
Reliability	Internal consistency ranged from .78–.96; test–retest reliability ranged from .96–.98, high intra-rater and inter-rater reliability	Internal consistency ranged .85–.98; test–retest reliability ranged from 79 to 100 % (Median of 98%); inter-rater agreement ranged 70–100% (median of 90+%)	Internal consistency, test–retest, and inter-scorer reliability coefficients approximate .80 at most ages with many in the .90s	Test–retest reliability of Screening Test ranged from .93–.99; correlates >.94 with 176-item test	Test–retest reliability is .90 to .96
Other features	Word reading list for older examinees, language screening task, spontaneous speech task Total score to reflect frequency of occurrence of error sounds (100 minus frequency of occurrence value of misarticulated sounds)	Color-coded response form for word position Samples single word, spontaneous, and imitated productions Response form allows for easy comparison of three types of samples Allows for observation of all vowels and diphthongs Story retelling task allows for informal screening of expressive language	Groups sounds by ages at which 90% of the sample correctly articulated them	Overlays and normed scores for consonant singletons, vowels, diphthongs, /r/ and /ɚ/ clusters, /l/ and /!/ clusters, /s/ clusters, miscellaneous clusters, pressure articulation test, and screening test	Reveals type of misarticulation patterns Provides articulation age, intelligibility, articulation, and stimulability scores

Note: I = initial position, M = medial position, F = final position

TABLE 6.3

Characteristics of a Sample of Standardized Articulation and Phonological Tests Assessing both Articulation of Phonemes and Phonological Deviations Usage

	Bankson-Bernthal Test of Phonology (BBTOP)	Clinical Assessment of Articulation and Phonology (CAAP)	Computerized Articulation and Phonology Evaluation System (CAPES)	Smit-Hand Articulation and Phonology Evaluation (SHAPE)	Structured Photographic Articulation Tests II (SPAT-D II)
Author(s), publication date	Bankson & Bernthal, 1990	Secord & Donohue, 2002	Masterson & Bernhardt, 2001	Smit & Hand, 1997	Dawson & Tattersall, 2001
Age levels	3–9 years	2:6–8:11 years:months	2 years–adult Age comparisons based on Iowa-Nebraska norms (3–9 years)	3–9 years	3–9 years
Subtests	Word Inventory Consonant Inventory Phonological Process Inventory	Articulation Inventory Phonological Checklist	Phonemic Profile Individualized Phonological Evaluation	Articulation Inventory Phonetic Inventory Syllable and Word Shape Inventory Phonological Processes	Articulation Inventory Consonant Inventory Word Shapes Phonological Processes
Sample types	Single words	Single words (1-, 3-, 4-syllable, cluster) Sentences	Single words Connected speech	Single words	Single word production Optional connected speech sample Stimulability
Stimuli	80 color pictures	Pictures	Colored photographs, carrier phrases	80 color photographs grouped by semantic category, verbal cue sentences	48 color photographs featuring Dudsberry (dog), verbal prompts, photographic illustrated story
Number of sounds tested	22 consonants, 15 clusters, 10 phonological processes	23 consonants, 8 clusters, 9 multisyllabic words, 10 phonological processes	23 consonants, 12 clusters, vowels and diphthongs	23 consonants, including IF singletons, 27 2- and 3-element clusters, and 4 words to assess unstressed syllable productions	23 consonants, 10 blends, 14 vowels, 7 phonological processes
Consonant word positions*	IF	IF	IMF	IF	IMF

	Test 1	Test 2	Test 3	Test 4	Test 5
Scores	Percentiles and standardized scores, scaled score (0–5) based upon frequency of occurrence of misarticulatory or phonology processes	Percentiles, standard scores, age equivalents, critical difference score, percentage of occurrence of phonological processes	Percentages, indication of below age level performance	Percentiles & z-scores, normative sample information regarding use of phonological processes and each phoneme and cluster by gender	Standard scores, percentiles, test-age equivalents for females and males
Administration time	15–20 minutes	15–20 minutes	Not reported	20–30 minutes	10–15 minutes
Standardization sample	1,000+ children	1,707 children in 35 states closely representing US population and 4 Canadian provinces	Based on Iowa/Nebraska data (Smit et al., 1990)	2,000+ children (997 children from Iowa and Nebraska and 1,094 nationwide closely representative of national ethnic and gender characteristics) from various socioeconomic levels, geographical areas, and urban/rural residences	2,285 children from 5 US geographical areas
Validity	Good content and construct validity	Good content and discriminate validity; concurrent validity ranging from .62–.88 with BBTOP	Not reported	Good content, construct, and predictive validity	Good content and construct validity; Correlation of .97 with G-FTA-2
Reliability	Internal reliability coefficients ranging from .92 to .98; test-retest from .74 to .85, inter-rater from .93 to .99	Test-retest reliability of .975; inter-rater reliability of .99	Not reported	Inter-rater reliability of .98	Test-retest reliability range of .85–1.0; mean inter-judge reliability of .98; internal consistency ranged from .77 to .95
Unique features	Yields whole word accuracy score. Multiple exemplars for each sound/sound position and phonological processes. Lists common responses for each target	Yields a critical difference score, five foam stimuli figures, checklist for scoring phonological processes	Dialect filters for African American English and Spanish-influenced English. Provides treatment suggestions. Can record productions for later review. Personalized letter to parents. Generates a wide variety of reports	Multiple exemplars of frequently used phonemes and clusters. Checklist transcription (i.e., response form includes likely substitutions and narrow transcription descriptors). Provides information on age of acquisition of consonants, presence or absence of phonological processes, and	Provides analysis of errors according to syllabic function and manner of articulation, consonant inventory, percentage of consonant correct, word shapes, sample vowel repertoire. No whole word transcription necessary

(continued)

TABLE 6.3 Continued

Characteristics of a Sample of Standardized Articulatory/Phonologic Tests Assessing both Articulation of Phonemes and Phonological Deviations Usage

Bankson-Bernthal Test of Phonology (BBTOP)	Clinical Assessment of Articulation and Phonology (CAAP)	Computerized Articulation and Phonology Evaluation System (CAPES)	Smit-Hand Articulation and Phonology Evaluation (SHAPE)	Structured Photographic Articulation Tests II (SPAT-D II)
		Administered and scored by computer program Yields a wide variety of independent and relational analyses	criterion scores indicating possible speech disorders Generates an independent analysis (phonetic inventory and list of syllable structures) and a relational analysis (phoneme-by-phoneme comparison with adult system and a list of phonological processes used)	Tables and explanation of dialectical variations Color-coded response form word position

*Note: I = initial position, M = medial position, F = final position progress. The last 10 pictures assess not only consonant blends, but also contextual speech. In addition to the picture test, the WCAT has a 38 semi-nonsensical sentence test for adults and other clients who can read.

Standardized Combined Articulation/Phonological Tests

Some tests assess both individual phoneme misarticulations, as just described, and phonological deviations or processes (Table 6.3). These tests have the advantage of being able to do a phonetic analysis and phonological deviation analysis from the same speech sample; however, it takes more time to complete the analysis than in traditional articulation tests.

The *Bankson-Bernthal Test of Phonology* (BBTOP; Bankson & Bernthal, 1990a) was standardized on more than 1,000 children. Its three standardized subsections are: (a) Word Inventory that indicates the percentage of test items in which all consonants are correctly articulated, (b) Consonant Inventory that specifies the production accuracy of the consonants in initial and final position of words, and (c) Phonological Process Inventory that specifies the number of times each of 10 phonological processes are used. Each singleton consonant and consonant cluster is sampled several times. The response sheet lists common production errors of the test items, categorizing them into phonological process usage. The test also uses scale scores (ranging from 0 to 4) to characterize the amount of difficulty the testee has with each initial and final consonant depending on the frequency of occurrence of the sound and the number of times it is misarticulated on the test. Scale scores are also used to indicate the level of usage of each phonological process. It yields percentiles and standard scores for each of the three subtests.

The *Clinical Assessment of Articulation and Phonology* (CAAP; Secord & Donohue, 2002) was standardized on 1,707 children. It uses colored drawings to elicit singleton consonants, consonant clusters, and phonological processes in one- to four-syllable words. It also assesses articulation of words in sentences of varying lengths and complexity in older children (5 years and older). Five foam three-dimensional figures and a "warm-up" story designed to increase attention can be used for younger children. It requires little to no whole-word transcription, utilizing a checklist for transcribing the testee's productions. An error difference score can be calculated that reflects a comparison between performance on the single word inventory and the sentence inventory. It generates percentiles, standard scores, and age equivalents

for the consonant inventory and sentence production. It also generates the percentage of occurrence of 10 phonological processes based on 10 to 20 words for each process.

The *Computerized Articulation and Phonology Evaluation System* (CAPES; Masterson & Bernhardt, 2001) uses the age norms developed by Smit et al. (1990). As the name implies, a computer program analyzes the assessment. The stimuli are photographs of 46 words with various word lengths, structures, and stress patterns in the single-word task that are displayed on the computer screen. Words from other articulation tests and words from a connected speech sample can also be analyzed using the CAPES. The testee names the items, the computer audio records the responses (which can be played back later), and the clinician transcribes the client's words directly into the computer as the test is being administered. The results of this profile are used by the computer program to display 10 to 115 additional words for the Individualized Phonological Evaluation, which is a deeper analysis; the words selected are based on the client's performance on the 46-word profile. The CAPES also provides video clips that can be used to elicit narratives. Transcription of the responses incorporate the English IPA and stress markers. On the computer screen, the tester chooses among predicted word productions or transcribes the client's productions using the IPA. The types of analyses that can be done are quite extensive and include independent and relational analyses. Word length, word shape, and consonant and vowel productions (segment-by-segment, phonetic features, nonlinear features, and phonological processes) can be analyzed. The analysis can be performed with a dialect filter for African American English or Spanish-influenced English. The computer program generates reports that can be edited and provides treatment recommendations.

The *Smit-Hand Articulation and Phonology Evaluation* (SHAPE; Smit & Hand, 1997) was standardized on more than 2,000 children. It uses colored photographs to sample singleton consonants and consonant clusters. It generates both an independent analysis (phonetic inventory and a list of syllable structures) and a relational analysis (phoneme-by-phoneme comparison with adult system and a list of phonological processes) of the testee's speech sound system. A checklist is used to transcribe clients' utterances, so the examiner does not need to transcribe the client's productions. The checklist yields percentiles and z-scores for the client's performance on the test. The manual provides normative information about the usage of each phonological process analyzed and each consonant sound and consonant cluster elicited on the test. The use of photographs makes it appropriate for older clients as well as for the younger ones.

The *Structured Photographic Articulation Test II* (SPAT-D II; Dawson & Tattersall, 2001) was standardized on 2,270 children. It uses 40 colored photographs featuring Dudsberry (a dog) to elicit the consonant sounds. Normative information is available for consonant singletons and blends at the word level. As an option, the consonant singletons can be elicited in connected speech using a story, the results of which can be compared to the single-word measure. Other optional assessments include stimulability, vowel production, and production of consonants in complex phonetic contexts, such as /s/, /r/, and /l/ blends in final position. The response form provides for analysis of the single-word productions by manner of production, consonant inventory, percentage of consonants correct, word shapes, and frequency of occurrence of nine phonological processes. The manual provides guidelines for the phonological processes analysis, although there are no normative data for them. It yields standard scores, percentiles, and test-age equivalents for the consonant inventory.

Phonological Tests

In addition to these tests, which can be used for analyzing the client's productions phonologically and for assessing articulation traditionally, formal tests for assessing the use of phonological deviations have been devised (Hodson, 2003, 2004; Ingram, 1981; Khan & Lewis, 2002; Oller & Delgado, 1990; Shriberg & Kwiatkowski, 1980; Shriberg, 1986; Weiner, 1979). Clinicians often report that analyzing phonological deviations on many of these tests is time-consuming when done by hand, but they are recommended to be used with clients whose speech is highly unintelligible. These phonological tests provide a basis for developing more efficacious intervention programs for selected clients by providing a clearer and more precise understanding of the client's underlying phonological system. Phonological tests generally provide the following information: types of phonological deviations used, frequency of their occurrence, percentage of occurrence when considering the number of opportunities, and phonetic inventory, which is a listing of the phonemes that were produced at least once during the sample and of those that were never produced.

Some formal phonology tests have been selected for discussion. These tests and those described in the earlier section represent various sampling techniques, as well as several selected phonological deviations and types of analysis.

Some are computer-based. All of the tests reviewed identify, under various labels, syllable omission, cluster reduction, final consonant omission, velar fronting, stridency deviation (including stopping and deaffrication), and liquid deviation (including gliding and vocalization). Some also identify voicing errors, palatal sound deviations, and affricate sound deviations, while others identify nondevelopmental errors, such as initial consonant omission and backing, as well as other miscellaneous patterns (Table 6.4).

The *Hodson Assessment of Phonological Patterns, Third Edition* (HAPP-3; Hodson, 2004) test was designed to assess children with highly unintelligible speech. Words are spontaneously produced by the child who identifies objects (with the exception of two pictures) rather than the more typical picture stimuli. Three-dimensional objects are used because young children typically find objects more interesting than pictures. Also, objects are more likely to yield a valid representation of children's actual phonological pattern usage because, while manipulating objects, they tend not to produce patterns that have not yet been generalized into conversational speech (Hodson, 2004). In addition to the full HAPP-3 that elicits 50 words, there are two screening protocols: the 12-word Preschool Phonological Screening and the 12-word Multisyllabic Word Screening. The words are elicited and transcribed live and tape recorded for later verification of the transcription. Transcription of the child's responses is done by noting deviations from the adult standard production; the phonemic transcription of the standard consonants is provided on the response form with blank spaces for examiners to write in vowel and diphthong phonetic symbols for the sounds typically used in their linguistic community. The deviations (processes) identified include the major phonological deviations of omissions (including syllables, sound sequences, and singletons) and class deficiencies (including sonorants and obstruents) as well as miscellaneous error patterns composed of glottal stop replacement, phonemic substitutions (such as stopping, backing, and gliding), assimilations (harmony), voicing alterations, epenthesis, and articulation place shifts (such as frontal lisp and lateral lisp). Frequency counts are made and totaled for all major deviations to yield the total occurrences of major phonological deviations (TOMPD) score. Severity levels are assigned based on the TOMPD. The percentage of occurrence for each of the 11 major deviations is also calculated. Hodson and Paden (1991) suggested that the basic processes that occur in 40% or more of the opportunities for occurrence should be targeted for intervention. Additionally, a phonetic

TABLE 6.4

Phonological Deviations Sampled by Standardized Tests of Articulation/Phonology

Hodson Assessment of Phonological Patterns (HAPP-3), 2004/Hodson Computerized Analysis of Phonological Patterns (HCAPP), 2003	Bankson-Bernthal Test of Phonology (BBTOP), 1990	Clinical Assessment of Articulation and Phonology (CAAP), 2002	Khan-Lewis Phonological Analysis 2 (KLPA-2), 2002	Smit-Hand Articulation and Phonology Evaluation (SHAPE), 1997	Structured Photographic Articulation Tests II (SPAT-D II), 2001
Syllable omission	Weak syllable deletion	Syllable reduction	Syllable reduction	Weak syllable deletion	Syllable reduction
Consonant sequence omission (cluster reduction) (with stridents and without stridents)	Cluster simplification	Cluster reduction	Cluster simplification	Cluster reduction—/s/ Clusters; Cluster reduction - Clusters without /s/	Cluster reduction
Postvocalic singleton omission	Final consonant deletion	Final consonant deletion	Deletion of final consonants	Final consonant deletion	Final consonant deletion
Strident deficiency (anterior and palatal)	Stopping	Stopping	Stopping of fricatives and affricates	Stopping of initial fricative and affricate singles	Stridency deletion; Stopping
Velar obstruent deficiency	Fronting	Fronting (velar and palatal)	Velar Fronting	Fronting of initial velar singles	Velar fronting
Prevocal liquid deficiency (/l,r/)	Gliding	Gliding	Liquid simplification	Gliding of initial liquids	Gliding of liquids
	Vocalization	Vocalization		Vocalization of final and postvocalic liquids	
	Assimilation	Prevocalic voicing	Initial voicing	Voicing of initial voiceless obstruents	
		Postvocalic devoicing	Final devoicing		
			Palatal fronting		Palatal fronting
	Depalatalization		Deaffrication	Depalatalization of final singles	
	Deaffrication				
Prevocalic singleton omission					Initial consonant deletion
Intervocalic singleton omission					
Nasal deficiency					
Glide deficiency					
Backing					

inventory for consonants, consonant sequences, and vowels is derived for identifying missing sounds that are stimulable. The HAPP-3 was standardized on 886 children representative of the national school-age population. The consonant category deficiencies sum is converted to a percentile rank, its corresponding standard deviation, and an ability score (or standard score).

The *Hodson Computerized Analysis of Phonological Patterns* (HCAPP; Hodson, 2003) is a computer software program that was developed to analyze the major phonological deviations appearing on the HAPP-3. This simple program compares the client's phoneme-by-phoneme productions to the adult standard production. The program works on IBM-compatible and Macintosh computers. The computer analysis yields the percentage of occurrence of each of the 11 major phonological deviations described by Hodson (2004), including the severity rating of the client's phonological system and a goal statement specifying potential target patterns. Analysis by the HCAPP is considerably faster than analysis by hand of the HAPP-3, but the computer program does not identify substitutions and other strategy patterns.

The *Khan–Lewis Phonological Analysis, Second Edition* (KLPA-2; Khan & Lewis, 2002) is a norm-referenced test of phonological process usage designed to accompany the G-FTA-2. Word production on that test is analyzed for phonological processes. The norms are based on the G-FTA-2 data for 2,350 persons. The entire word as produced by the testee is transcribed. The diagnostician then compares it to the standard adult production to identify phonological processes used by the client. The Sound Change Book provides sound matrices for the initial, medial, and final position of consonants to assist the clinician in identifying the phonological processes used by the client. The 10 phonological processes analyzed are divided into three categories:

- Reduction processes (includes omissions and substitution errors)
- Place and manner processes
- Voicing processes

It should be noted here that reduction process category typically refers to omissions, but in the Khan–Lewis system, it also includes some substitution processes. Optionally, the clinician can note the presence of 34 other phonological processes (identified in the Sound Change Book) and vowel alterations for qualitative analysis (not included in the normative data). The phonological processes are placed in the order of "how severely they affect intelligibility" (Khan & Lewis, 2002, p. 9). In addition to the normed standard scores, percentiles, and test-age equivalents, there are procedures for determining frequency of occurrence of the 10 normed phonological processes and for conducting a phonemic inventory for the testee that displays the sounds by positions produced correctly; sounds by positions produced, but incorrectly; and consonant clusters used by word position. As with the G-FTA-2, there is a companion software program (ASSIST) that helps score, calculate, and compare normative data for the KLPA-2 as well as assists in writing diagnostic reports with a recommendation section.

Criterion-Referenced Articulation/Phonological Tests

All of the articulation/phonological tests just described and appearing in Tables 6.2, 6.3, and 6.4 are norm-referenced, but there are some criterion-referenced test instruments available that can provide valuable information for planning treatment.

The *Test of Articulation in Context* (TAC; Lanphere, 1998) is designed to assess the ability to produce speech sounds in connected speech. It uses four color-illustrated picture boards of familiar scenes to elicit spontaneous speech from preschool through elementary school-aged children. Cues are provided for the clinician to use when a specific stimulus is not elicited spontaneously. Consonants are assessed as singletons in the initial, medial, and final positions as well as in /s/, /r/, and /l/ clusters. The testee can also be evaluated on a severity and intelligibility rating scale that utilizes the variables of sound production, stimulability, speech mechanism, intelligibility, and adverse effect on educational performance for scaling. Determination of whether or not an individual needs intervention is done by looking at the articulation performance in relationship to the developmental scale of articulation acquisition and the severity and intelligibility rating scale. The TAC was developed through field-testing of more than 200 children across the country.

The purpose of the *Fisher-Logemann Test of Articulation Competence* (F-LTOAC; Fisher & Logemann, 1971) is to provide a distinctive feature analysis of the client's phonological system. The age range is from 3 years through adulthood. The distinctive features of consonants analyzed are voicing, place of articulation, and manner of articulation. Analysis of vowels includes the distinctive features of tongue height, place of articulation, degree of tension, and lip rounding. Analysis is by phoneme according to syllabic function: prevocalic, intervocal, and postvocalic. Test materials are colored picture stimuli that test consonants, consonant blends, vowels and diphthongs. This test includes a short form for screening and a sentence form for older clients.

The *Spanish Articulation Measures, Revised Edition* (SAM; Mattes, 1995) is:

. . . an informal criterion-referenced assessment instrument designed to provide information about performance in Spanish . . . . SAM is used primarily to provide descriptive information . . . and is really a collection of informal, descriptive assessment measures and observational tools and is not designed to give the child a "score." (L. Mattes, personal communication, September 4, 2002)

Tasks include picture naming, imitation of verbal stimuli, and spontaneous speech production. The SAM evaluates production of 18 consonants in initial, medial, and final positions and /s/, /r/, and /l/ blends in single words. There is a section for probing, in more in-depth fashion, spontaneous production of some sounds and a section for word repetition probes of individual consonants and blends. It can be used to identify the presence of seven phonological processes. SAM yields the measures of spontaneous word production, word repetition articulation screening, and sound stimulability in syllables and articulation in conversational speech.

> How do speech-language pathologists test stimulability of sounds that are misarticulated by the client?

Assessment of Stimulability

The assessment of stimulability provides information about the client's articulation abilities and is used for determining prognosis and for planning treatment (Miccio, 2002; Powell & Miccio, 1996). Testing of stimulability requires the client to imitate the clinician producing the phonemes that were misarticulated during articulation testing. It demonstrates the client's ability to produce a sound in a highly supportive condition (Bain, 1994). Some formal articulation and phonological tests include sections for stimulability testing; however, if it is not included in the tests given, stimulability should be informally tested because it provides valuable information. Imitations may be of the phoneme in isolation, in syllables, in words, and/or in sentences. A suggested procedure is to elicit three repetitions in isolation and

three in words containing each phoneme that is misarticulated. Then, the percentage of correctly imitated productions can be calculated for each sound and a total or composite percentage calculated for all of the error sounds. In this way, a stimulability score is recorded for each sound, and an overall stimulability score is recorded for all misarticulated sounds. Even though each repetition is scored either right or wrong, the diagnostician can also note whether the client showed any improvement during subsequent repetitions or imitations (e.g., t/s substitution followed by a frontally distorted /s/). Improvement might be indicative of a more favorable prognosis.

A more expansive procedure for testing stimulability is recommended by Miccio (2002). In a complete probe, each sound that is missing from a client's phonemic repertoire is probed for stimulability in 10 trials, in isolation and in three word positions for three vowel contexts (/i/, /u/, /ɑ/). Alternatively, in consideration of time, the stimulability of missing sounds is done in isolation and only one vowel context (/ɑ/). A form that can be used to record the client's responses appears in Figure 6.3.

Ability of young children to imitate phonemes correctly has been used to suggest favorable probability for spontaneously outgrowing the misarticulations (Carter & Buck, 1958; Farquhar, 1961; Kisatsky, 1967; Powell, Elbert, & Dinnsen, 1991; Powell & Miccio, 1996; Sommers, Leiss, Delp et al., 1967). Conversely, sounds that are not stimulable "are least likely to change without direct treatment" (Miccio, 2002, p. 225). Additionally, stimulability scores have been used in selecting target sounds for treatment and in determining at what level to begin treatment, such as isolation, **nonsense syllables**, words. Low stimulability scores indicate unfavorable prognosis, but high stimulability scores do not necessarily indicate favorable prognosis (Pollack & Rees, 1972). A client may achieve a high stimulability score, yet progress in treatment may not be rapid. This may be related to the concept that high stimulability scores reflect good phonetic skills (motoric skills) but not necessarily phonological competence (cognitive skills) (Turton & Clark, 1971). Ease of production may also be an important variable here. The client who easily produces misarticulated sounds may show faster progress in treatment than the one who displays effort or has difficulty when imitating sounds. Generally, the higher the stimulability score, the more favorable the prognosis for improvement, more rapid rate of improvement, or even spontaneous correction of misarticulations.

Sound	Isolation	#__i	i__i	i__#	#__ɑ	ɑ__ɑ	ɑ__#	u__#	u__u	#__u	% Correct
b											
w											
tʃ											
k											
s											
h											
r											
d											
f											
θ											
l											
ʃ											
v											
z											
ð											
m											
p											
n											
g											
j											
dʒ											
t											

Note: # = utterance boundary; __ = sound

Test stimulabillity for misarticulated sounds. Write client's response in the appropriate box. Calculate the percent of correct responses out of 10 trials (i.e., 1 trial in isolation and 9 trials in the prevocalic, intervocalic, and postvocalic in the context of three vowels (i, ɑ, u).

FIGURE 6.3 Form for stimulability probe. (From Miccio, A. W. (2002). Clinical problem solving: Assessment of phonological disorders. *American Journal Speech-Language Pathology, 11,* 221–229. Copyright 2000 by American Speech–Language–Hearing Association. Adapted with permission.)

What does the speech-language clinician look for in a connected speech sample?

Connected Speech Assessment

Because the ultimate goal of articulation/phonological treatment is correct speech sound production in spontaneous speech, collecting a connected speech sample is important so that the diagnostician can note correct and incorrect sound productions and speech sound patterns in a more "natural" speaking context. The sample is used for analyzing expressive articulation/phonology in connected speech. Engaging the client in casual talking; discussing favorite hobbies, sports, games, pets, movies, and television programs; retelling stories; answering questions; playing with toys; role playing; and describing pictures and objects are ways of obtaining contextual speech samples. A client who is taciturn or otherwise reluctant to say much might be more talkative in the presence of a sibling, friend, or parent. The client's spontaneous speech during this procedure should also be tape recorded for later analysis. Obtaining 20 or more utterances, or a minimum of 100 words, is effective for eventual analysis. From a speech sample, the clinician notes which speech sounds are misarticulated as well as types of errors, which sounds are produced correctly, the consistency of the production of speech sounds, and which phonological deviations are used. The speech sound production during the spontaneous speech sample should be compared to the speech sounds produced in the formal, single-word articulation/phonological test to get a clearer picture of the client's speech production system. This same connected speech sample can be used for determining the level of intelligibility as well.

Sometimes, connected speech samples are problematic. Some clients will be reticent to provide such a sample, especially when interacting with an adult they barely know. Also, it can be difficult, if not impossible, to transcribe the speech of individuals who are highly unintelligible. In this case, the clinician does not know the intended words and thus, has difficulty doing a relational analysis of the speech sample. Nonetheless, it is good clinical practice to attempt to elicit a connected speech sample. At the very least, the clinician will be able to observe the prosodic patterns of the client's speech and obtain data to complete an independent speech analysis that includes the client's phonemic repertoire, speech sound patterns, and syllable structures.

The clinician will also probably be able to understand a few words.

What factors contribute to speech intelligibility?
What are some ways to assess speech intelligibility?

Assessment of Intelligibility

The understandability of oral speech is one of the most important factors, if not the most important factor, in the evaluation of articulation and phonology. Speech intelligibility has been characterized as the single most practical measurement of oral communication competence (Metz, Samar, Schiavetti, Sitler, & Whitehead, 1985). The degree of unintelligibility is perhaps the most important single pragmatic indicator of articulation/phonological severity and should be routinely assessed. However, attaining an accurate, reliable, and valid measurement of intelligibility is problematic because of the numerous factors that affect it:

- Articulation/phonological characteristics (e.g., number of speech sounds in error, consistency of misarticulations, frequency of occurrence of error sounds, speech sound error types, and phonological deviations used)
- Suprasegmental factors (e.g., prosodic features such as pitch inflection, open and closed juncture, pauses, speaking rate, and stress)
- Voice characteristics (e.g., voice quality, loudness level, and oral/nasal resonation)
- Fluency
- Linguistic features (e.g., syntax; mean length of utterance; morphology; morphophonemics; semantics; pragmatic features such as communication intent, message content, and social environment)
- Contextual features (e.g., known or unknown topic to the listener, listener's listening skills, type of stimulus material, and the nature of the transmission, such as face-to-face, audio only, audio/video, noise level of the environment) (Bernthal & Bankson, 2004; Boothroyd, 1985; Connolly, 1986; Cullinan, Brown, & Blalock, 1986; Gordon-Brannan, 1994; Grunwell, 1987; Kent, 1996; Kent, Kent, Weismer et al., 1990; Kent, Miolo, & Bloedel, 1992, 1994; Metz, Schiavetti, Samar, & Sitler, 1990; Shriberg & Kwiatkowski, 1982c; Vihman & Greenlee, 1987; Weiss, 1982; Weston & Shriberg, 1992; Yorkston & Beukelman, 1981).

By rating the degree of adequacy or inadequacy of each factor, the diagnostician can determine which factors are contributing most to unintelligible speech.

An important question is: In what type of speech sample should intelligibility be measured: words, sentences, or conversational speech? If the clinician wants to determine overall intelligibility in everyday communication situations, longer utterances (spontaneous speech or sentences) seem more appropriate because connected or contextual speech more closely resembles natural speaking situations. Also, both suprasegmental and segmental factors are available to the listener, factors that affect intelligibility in everyday communication settings. On the other hand, if the objective is to ascertain how phonemic components contribute to untintelligibility, assessment in words is probably more appropriate and efficient (Kent et al., 1992). Sometimes, persons who are unintelligible are unable or unwilling to produce a spontaneous speech sample for various reasons, such as self-consciousness. Also, measurement of intelligibility in spontaneous speech may not be sensitive enough to indicate short-term changes.

The measurement of speech intelligibility has been approached in a number of ways (Gordon-Brannan, 1994):

- Open-set word identification is a procedure in which the percentage of words correctly identified in a speech sample, often a connected speech sample or reading sample, is calculated
- Closed-set word (multiple–choice format) identification is the percentage of words correctly identified from a word list
- Rating scales in which listeners judge, on a predetermined rating scale, how well they understand a speaker's utterances produced in a speech sample (e.g., word list, paragraph reading, or spontaneous speech sample)
- Estimation from articulation/phonological testing

Scores generated from various ways of measuring intelligibility are highly correlated, although the exact scores (e.g., percentages) vary among listeners and from measure to measure (Bern, 1999; Cave, 1999; Clarke, 1997; Dukart, 1996; Gordon-Brannan, 1993; Gordon-Brannan & Hodson, 2000; Mowe, 1997; Sugarman, 1994). Based on percentage of words understood on a closed-set intelligibility test, Monsen (1981) described five levels of intelligibility. A speaker is judged to be essentially intelligible when the percentage of words understood is greater that 70% and difficult to understand with intelligibility ranging from 60 to 70%. How-ever, when the percentage is less than 60%, the speaker is essentially unintelligible to the listener. Perhaps, these competency levels apply to other types of intelligibility measures, although further research is needed to clarify the relationship between intelligibility percentages and listener perceptions.

Some formal assessment instruments are available to measure intelligibility (Weiss, 1982; Wilcox & Morris, 1999; Yorkston & Beukelman, 1981; Yorkston, Beukelman, & Traynor, 1984). The *Assessment of Intelligibility of Dysarthric Speech* (Yorkston & Beukelman, 1981) and the computerized version (Yorkston, Beukelman, & Traynor 1984) are tools designed for quantifying intelligibility of adolescents and adults with dysarthric speech in single words and sentences. Clients either read the stimuli (either single words or sentences of increasing length) or repeat the stimuli after the examiner. The client's utterances are tape recorded for later presentation to a judge who identifies the single words or sentences in an open-set format. Alternatively, single words can be selected from a list of phonetically similar words. Norms are provided for various intelligibility and communication efficiency (speaking rate) measures for persons with various levels of expressive speech functioning.

The *Children's Speech Intelligibility Measure* (Wilcox & Morris, 1999) is a closed-set word identification procedure designed "to provide clinicians with an objective measure of single-word intelligibility of children ages 3:0–10:11 whose speech is considered unintelligible" (p. 1). The client repeats 50 words modeled by the clinician. Only the client's productions are tape recorded. Later, a judge who is not familiar with the client's speech listens to the tape recording and, from a list of 12 phonetically similar words, selects the word he or she thinks the client said. The test yields a percentage of intelligibility score based on the number of words correctly identified by the judge.

The *Weiss Intelligibility Test* (Weiss, 1982) was designed "to quantify intelligibility of isolated words, contextual speech, and overall intelligibility of children and adolescents" (p. 5). Black and white pictures are used to elicit spontaneous production of 25 single words and a 200-word connected speech sample. The client's productions are tape recorded for later **orthographic transcription** and analysis. The judge (who can be the examiner) may either orthographically transcribe (traditional spelling as opposed to phonemic transcription) using a dash (-) to indicate an unknown word or use a score sheet with numbered boxes representing individual words to indicate the words definitely understood (√) or words not understood (left blank). The percentage of intelligibility is an average of the percent of single words understood and the percent of words understood in a spontaneous speech sample. An additional optional assessment procedure is to indicate the degree of impact of 22 factors, such as articulation and mean length of response, on intelligibility of the person being assessed.

Oftentimes, rather than administering a formal test, speech intelligibility is informally assessed by eliciting a spontaneous speech sample (as just described) and evaluating it for speech intelligibility. This is believed to be good clinical practice because a spontaneous speech sample is considered the most valid representation of a client's intelligibility because it is similar to natural communication situations (Kwiatkowski & Shriberg, 1992). Currently, many speech-language clinicians make impressionistic estimates of intelligibility by listening to a connected speech sample; however, this procedure may not be accurate and reliable. Calculating the actual percentage of words understood in a speech sample is probably a more accurate and valid measurement of intelligibility (Kent, Miolo, & Bloedel, 1994; Kwiatkowski & Shriberg, 1992). Unfortunately, this is a time-consuming procedure and, therefore, is not often done by practicing clinicians (Bacon, 1995; Wilcox & Morris, 1999).

Following is a feasible way to assess intelligibility of a speech sample that is not done by estimation. Randomly select 200 consecutive words from the client's audiotape or audio-visual tape recorded contextual speech sample, calculate the percentage of words understood, and compare it with normative data (Table 6.5). This recorded sample should be played back by the diagnostician, or someone unfamiliar with the client's speech system, who listens to the sample and identifies the number of words understood and not understood using the check/minus notation system (/ = words understood, - = words/syllables not understood). Figure 6.4 illustrates a form that can be used for this procedure. The number of unintelligible words is counted and subtracted from 200 then divided by two. The answer is the intelligibility percentage score for that client. If the client's speech is so unintelligible that words cannot be differentiated from syllables (whether "uh-uh" is one two-syllable word or two one-syllable words), the number of syllables should be counted and the percentage of intelligibility calculated based on this system. Another option is to calculate the percentage of intelligible utterances in a 50-, 100-word, or 200+- word speech sample and calculate the percentage of words understood. Of course, the percentage of words understood can be calculated from an orthographic transcription, but this analysis procedure is more time consuming (Bacon, 1995).

An alternative approach is to apply a five-, seven-, or nine-point interval rating scale for assessing intelligibility. An example of a five-point rating scale is one developed by the National Technical Institute for the Deaf, or NTID (Johnson, 1975). The scale includes descriptors for each point as shown in Table 6.6. An example of a seven-point rating scale with descriptors for the endpoints is illustrated in Figure 6.5. Other terms that have been used for describing the endpoints of rating scales for intelligibility include *completely not understandable* to *completely understandable* and *no abnormality* to *totally unintelligible* (Enderby, 1983; Platt, Andrews, Young, & Quinn, 1980; Schiavetti, 1992).

If the audiotaped sample is assessed by someone other than the diagnostician who obtained the speech sample, the score may be slightly lower than the client's actual level of understandability because of the absence of visual clues. Clinically, it is probably acceptable for the clinician who tested the client to listen to the sample for the purpose of assessing intelligibility if this it the first or second time the client and clinician have interacted. But for subsequent analysis, it is preferable for a person who is not familiar with the client's speech patterns to be the listener because of the accommodation effect (i.e., the clinician being able to understand more because of familiarity with the client's speech patterns). The importance of intelligibility testing is not merely to derive a score, but also to identify which variables are interfering with intelligibility.

An important adjunct to the diagnostician determining intelligibility is having the caregiver assess intelligibility as well. Ideally, caregivers orthographically transcribe a spontaneous speech sample from an audio or audio/visual tape recording of their child. The percentage of words understood by the caregiver would be calculated from the transcript. Alternatively, caregivers could be asked to estimate the percentage of their children's utterances that they understand in known and in unknown contexts. Additionally, they could be asked to estimate the percentage of understandability of the client by grandparents, siblings, teachers, friends, or strangers.

In summary, it is recommended that speech intelligibility be determined by the diagnostician from a spontaneous speech sample, if feasible, with a notation as to whether the measure is in a known or unknown context. For the initial assessment, the listener can be the speech-language clinician or a person who is not familiar with the client's speech patterns. The intelligibility measure from this sample can be in the form of: (a) the percentage of

TABLE 6.5

Development of Intelligibility with Age

Age in Months	Percent of Intelligible Speech
18	25%
24	50%
30	64%
36	80%
42	92%
48	100%

words understood derived from an orthographic transcription, (b) the percentage of words understood derived from the check/minus method of notation (Fig. 6.4), or (c) in the form of a rating on a rating scale (Fig. 6.5, Table 6.6). In highly unintel-

ligible individuals, this measure could be supplemented with a single-word intelligibility measure in which the intended word is known so that the clinician has information about how speech sound production contributes to unintelligibility in the client being assessed. Finally, a measure of intelligibility as judged by caregivers should be obtained.

Identify three purposes of specialized tests.

Specialized Articulation/ Phonological Tests

Assessing Consistency of Misarticulations/phonologic Deviations

Knowing the consistency of articulation can be of value in making a statement about etiology, prognosis, and treatment (where and how to begin). An analysis of consistency usually includes a com-

Directions: For each word you understand, place a checkmark (✔) in a square representing that word. For each word (or syllable if you don't know the word boundaries), place a minus (-) in the square representing that word.

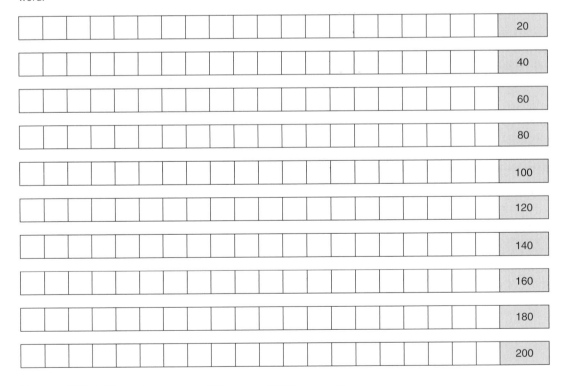

Number of Words Understood _____ ÷ 200 = _____ X 100 = _____%

FIGURE 6.4 Form used to track client's connected speech samples using the check/minus method for measuring the percentage of words understood.

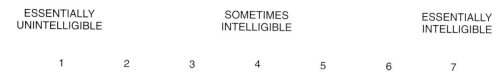

FIGURE 6.5   Seven-point interval rating scale for intelligibility of speech.

parison between articulation of isolated words from articulation/phonological tests and contextual speech. However, for some clients, it is helpful for treatment planning to assess consistency/inconsistency more extensively. Inconsistent phoneme production can be suggestive of apraxia of speech.

Some criterion-referenced tests are designed to evaluate misarticulated sounds in several phonetic contexts. The earliest one developed is *A Deep Test of Articulation* (Deep Test; McDonald, 1964a), which samples articulation in many different phonetic contexts; hence, the "deep" testing. The Deep Test assesses consonant production in the releasing position following all consonants and vowels/diphthongs and in the arresting position preceding all speech sounds, testing each phoneme in approximately 60 different contexts. In this manner, the test helps to identify phonetic contexts in which a misarticulated phoneme is correctly articulated (that in facilitative phonemic contexts). The test stimuli in-

clude pictures of words containing 25 consonants and 10 vowels/diphthongs in arresting and releasing positions. The format of the Deep Test is unique in that the testee is to produce two words without pausing as if it is one word (such as *watch-fish* to test /tʃ/ in the arresting position when followed by /f/). Thus, two pictures are presented simultaneously until a specific phoneme is sampled in about 60 different contexts and the percentage of correct responses is calculated for each one. There is also a sentence form appropriate for testees who can read in which each consonant sound is tested in the releasing and arresting positions in approximately 60 contexts. Results from the Deep Test are helpful in planning treatment for clients who produce only one or a few sounds in error.

The *Articulation Consistency Probe* (Tattersall & Dawson, 1997) is a criterion-referenced test designed to evaluate the consistency of production of consonants and consonant blends in words and connected speech. It provides probes for 20 consonant sounds as well as /s/, /l/, and /r/ blends. It is to be used to supplement traditional articulation tests and helps to determine which contexts are facilitative for misarticulated speech sounds.

The *Contextual Test of Articulation* (CTA; Aase, Hovre, Krause, Schelfhout, Smith, Carpenter, 2000) was designed "to help speech-language pathologists identify phonetic contexts that facilitate young children's correct productions (i.e., facilitative contexts) of previously identified phonemes produced in error" (p. 3). The CTA is to be administered as a follow-up to the administration of a formal articulation test to provide additional information about a client's articulation production of error sounds in several other words. It tests four frequently misarticulated consonant singletons (/s/, /l/, /k/, /r/) in prevocalic positions followed by seven vowels/diphthongs and in postvocalic positions preceded by five vowels/diphthongs; /ɝ/ as a nucleus in a syllable preceded by nasal/glide, fricative/affricate, and plosive sounds; and prevocalic /s/ + nasal, /s/ + liquid, /s/ + stop, stop + liquid, and postvocalic nasal + stop clusters. The stimuli are large colored pictures with three prompts (two devised to elicit the target spontaneously and one to elicit the target as a delayed imitation) provided for

TABLE 6.6

Descriptions of Ratings on the NTID Speech Intelligibility Scale

Intelligibility Rating	Description
1	Speech cannot be understood.
2	Speech is very difficult to understand with only isolated words or phrases intelligible.
3	Speech is difficult to understand; however, the gist of the content can be understood. Two- to three-word utterances are intelligible.
4	Speech is intelligible with the exception of a few words or phrases.
5	Speech is completely intelligible.

From Johnson, D. D. (1975). Communication characteristics of NTID students. *Journal of the Academy of Rehabilitative Audiology, 81,* 17–32. Copyright John Willy and Sons Ltd. Reprinted with permission.

each word when needed. A context is considered facilitative if the sound being assessed is produced in all trials of that context. The CTA was field tested throughout its development.

The *Secord Contextual Articulation Tests* (S-CAT; Secord & Shine, 1997) is the most extensive contextual test reviewed here, although, except for the story component, it uses written and imitative stimuli rather than pictures. It has two components that are designed to assess speech sounds in various phonetic and phonological contexts, to assess articulation production across different levels (prevocalic and postvocalic words, consonant clusters, sentences, and connected speech), and to plan intervention by providing words listed by contexts. It allows clinicians to pretest speech sound production, assess individual speech sounds indepth, identify facilitative contexts, measure progress during treatment, and posttest performance. One of the components of the S-CAT, the *Contextual Probes of Articulation Competence* (CPAC; Secord & Shine, 1997), is an instrument that probes 23 consonants, /ɝ, ɚ/, 12 vowels, 4 diphthongs, and 16 phonological processes in various contexts for each sound/phonologic process. The probes for the individual phonemes are written words that can be read or imitated by the client; the stimuli are single words containing singleton phonemes, consonant clusters (two words or compound words containing consonant clusters), and sentences. For the phonological processes, the probes are written single-words and sentences. A second component of the S-CAT, the *Storytelling Probes of Articulation Competence* (SPAC), is an instrument that probes the production of 23 consonants, /ɚ/ and /ɝ/, and vowels and diphthongs in connected speech through storytelling. Stimulus materials include 25 children's stories with accompanying colored pictures used for story retelling and 25 adolescent-adult stories to be read by the clients. Each story contains 10 to 20+ exemplars of the target sound in various word contexts and syllable functions.

Consistency of speech sound production can be approached in another way—by noting whether the speaker produces a word differently or in the same way during subsequent trials of the same word. A 25-word test of consistency was devised by Dodd (1995) that yields an index of consistency. The examiner asks the client to name pictures of 25 words three times, with each trial being separated by another activity (Fig. 6.6). Production of a word is considered inconsistent when one or more sounds

---

Children are asked to name pictures of the following 25 words three times, each trial being separated by another activity. Imitated data should be avoided by giving semantic cues or, if necessary, teaching the item's name and reassessing its pronunciation later.

dinosaur	witch	vacuum cleaner
slippery slide	tongue	rain
shark	chips	parrot
Bert	girl	bridge
thank you	teeth	kangaroo
jump	scissors	helicopter
birthday cake	zebra	ladybird
fish	umbrella	
elephant	five	

Note:

1. Variable production of 10 or more words on two of the three trials warrants classification as inconsistent disorder. Consonants and vowels should be included. If not all words can be spontaneously elicited, then a percent score can be derived (e.g., 6/23 = 26%). A score of more than 40% would indicate a diagnosis of inconsistent disorder.

2. Variable phonetic distortions of fricatives, affricates, and /r/ should not be counted as inconsistent.

FIGURE 6.6 Stimulus words and collection procedures used in the Index of Consistency. (From Dodd, B. (1995). *The differential diagnosis and treatment of children with speech disorder.* London: Whurr Publishers. Copyright John Willy and Sons Ltd. Reprinted with permission.)

(vowels and consonants) is produced differently, except for distortions of fricatives, affricates, and /r/ on two of three trials. An example of inconsistency provided by Dodd is: *teeth* → /tif/, /tis/, /tit/. A score of 40%+ indicates a diagnosis of inconsistency.

Childhood Apraxia of Speech Tests

Sometimes, diagnosticians suspect that a child who is unintelligible has childhood apraxia of speech (CAS) when that child also demonstrates speech characteristics such as inconsistent misarticulations, unusual misarticulations, sound sequencing errors, and atypical prosody (Table 5.2). In this case, the clinician can further explore the client's speech by administering an assessment tool for CAS. None of the instruments presented next are for the purpose of diagnosing CAS; rather, they provide information leading to such a diagnosis as well as information helpful in planning treatment for the client with CAS.

The *Screening Test for Developmental Apraxia of Speech, Second Edition* (STDAS-2; Blakeley, 2001) was developed to screen for the presence of developmental apraxia of speech (DAS) in children aged 4:0–12:ll. A prescreening task (comparison of receptive and language abilities) is to be completed before administering the STDAS. If the client passes the criteria for the prescreening task (10th or higher percentile in receptive language, 6 months or greater discrepancy between receptive and expressive language age equivalents), three subtests are administered, including prosody, verbal sequencing, and articulation. STDAS-2 was standardized on children with DAS and children with normal speech development. It yields likelihood levels that the person tested has developmental apraxia of speech. Blakeley suggested that when a child falls into the *Very Likely* category, trial treatment utilizing strategies for DAS should be implemented or additional speech and neurological testing should be done.

The *Kaufman Speech Praxis Test for Children* (Kaufman, 1995) was designed to identify the level of breakdown in a child's ability to speak. It can be used as an initial diagnostic tool as well as a measurement of progress. Test items are organized from simple to complex motor-speech movements using meaningful words whenever possible. It is norm-referenced, providing standard scores and percentile rankings for the ages of 2:0–5:11 and a severity rating scale.

The *Verbal Motor Production Assessment for Children* (VMPAC; Hayden & Square, 1999) was designed to identify children who have motor problems that negatively affect normal speech motor control. The areas assessed are global motor control, focal oromotor control, sequencing, connected speech and language control, and speech characteristics with the test items arranged from basic to complex skills. It is standardized and yields percentiles for children aged 3 to 12 years. A treatment approach that complements the VMPAC is the Prompts for Restructuring Oral Muscular Phonologic Targets (PROMPT).

The *Apraxia Profile* (Hickman, 1997) is a criterion-referenced assessment designed to identify and describe apraxic characteristics present in children and to determine the point in the coarticulation process at which a child's specific skills break down. Its purpose is to evaluate articulation movements and movement sequences verbally and nonverbally in children aged 3 to 13 years. It can also be used to chart a child's progress and to share information with parents, teachers, and other professionals. Two profile forms exist—one for preschoolers; the other for school-aged students.

The *Verbal Dyspraxia Profile* (Jelm, 2002) is a resource that provides checklists for automatic and imitative oral-motor movements for the jaw, lips/cheeks, and tongue. The Verbal Dyspraxia: Clinical Picture Checklist assists in the diagnosis of children who may demonstrate CAS. The checklists are descriptive statements that the clinician observes or has noted from other sources, including tests and case history.

> Identify four types of information that can be gleaned from a case history.

Case History

A first step in carrying out a differential diagnosis is to obtain a pertinent case history of the client and the problem (Appendix D). Two common ways of obtaining case history information are: (a) interviews and (b) written questionnaires. Sometimes, both procedures are used for a client. An advantage of the questionnaire is that the person filling out the form has time to reflect on the information requested (Tyler & Tolbert, 2002). Often, the questionnaire calls attention to important factors that can be followed up with a telephone interview and/or a live interview. Using a questionnaire and/or telephone interview can save time in the assessment session and provide helpful information for the diagnostician in planning for the assessment. The advantages of the interview are that it allows the diagnostician to: (a) evaluate and follow up with comments immediately for important clues about the client; (b) clarify answers that are vague, incomplete, or of doubtful accuracy; (c) relieve the parents/caregivers of some anxiety or guilt feelings about past experiences; (d) establish a friendly, professional relationship; and (e) pursue the pertinent behavior of the client. Other ways of obtaining historical data include autobiography, observation, and review of various medical, educational, and other clinical records. Ideally, this type of information, when available, should be obtained and studied before the interview. This information can make the interview much more productive, efficient, and focused.

A case history should provide information about the client, the development and nature of the communication problem, the possible causes of the problem, and the effects of the problem on the client. Areas to explore include relevant educational, cognitive, medical, dental, familial, and psychosocial history and current status as well as personality characteristics of the client. An accurate case history provides information about predisposing, precipitating, and perpetuating etiological factors that often enables the diagnostician to formulate hypotheses regarding the etiologies and to suggest tests and other diagnostic tools for use during the diagnostic intake. In essence, a differential history should provide insights into: (a) the kind of person the client is; (b) the effect the communication problem has on the client; (c) the reasons for the client's problem; and (d) the ways in which the client can best be helped. These determinations, by and large, preclude inaccurate interpretations of the historical data. Errors in interpretation or inaccurate data reported by the informant naturally affect the significance of background information; thus, the diagnostician must be aware of these possibilities and remember that the information provided reflects the perceptions of the informant. Sometimes, discrepancies in information provided by the interviewee occur and should be pursued. This enables a clearer understanding of the problem (Haynes & Pindzola, 2004).

Interviews

Obtaining a case history by interview involves more than merely asking questions and recording responses. It is a dynamic process of purposeful interaction between an interviewer and an informant. A diagnostic interview then "is a directed conversation, carried out for specific purposes such as fact finding, informing, or altering attitudes and opinions" (Haynes & Pindzola, 2004, p. 31). Efforts should be directed toward "the creation of mutual respect and team effort in the understanding and solution of the communication problem" (Haynes

& Pindzola, p. 31). Additionally, history-taking is a continuous process of evaluating historical data and clinical impressions as well as of formulating hypotheses and a diagnosis using all of the information obtained.

In history-taking, at least five requisites are to be met: (a) obtainment of the necessary information about the past status; (b) determination of the present status of the client and the problem; (c) formation of some idea about the future status of the client and the problem, including prognosis; (d) ascertainment of the etiology of the problem; and (e) determination of the age of onset of the disorder and its course of development. When the client is a child, observe the client briefly before beginning the interview. Impressions gleaned during this initial observation can be helpful in guiding the interview as well as in the subsequent diagnostic workup of the client.

Although simplified in this discussion, gathering historical data is not a simple matter. It presupposes considerable clinical and normative knowledge, an individualistic approach, ability to ask and answer pertinent questions, careful listening, sensitivity, objectivity, confidence, curiosity, insightfulness, trustworthiness, and an ability to establish rapport, interpret significant information as it surfaces during the interview, and use it for further questioning. Gathering background information is a science and an art. It is an ongoing process, not a one-time entity, that includes a purposeful exchange of information (Haynes & Pindzola, 2004; Nation & Aram, 1977). Additionally, diagnosticians should always be cognizant of why they ask for specific information and what it may contribute toward understanding the client. Interviewing techniques should be designed to encourage comments, conversation, and questions from the client, parents, or others involved. Much information can be gained from this kind of client participation. Awareness of the rationale at all times helps to avoid unnecessary questions.

In addition to interviewing the client, another effective way of obtaining historical information is to interview the person or persons most familiar and knowledgeable about the client. Appendix E provides guidelines for effective interviewing. Interviewing persons other than the client is a helpful way of obtaining the necessary information about the client, but because information from such sources is based on past observation, caution must be exercised in categorically accepting all of the information as fact. Moreover, objectivity may not always be possible from an informant because of a relationship with the client that may have caused a bias of some kind. Also, the extent and accuracy of the information obtained may have been influenced by interviewee–interviewer factors such as rapport, cooperation, confidence, trust, memory, and recall of the informant. In the final analysis, the diagnostician must determine whether sufficient, relevant, representative, accurate, and reliable information was obtained and whether the informant's responses may have been inadvertently influenced by the diagnostician. Given these requirements and cautions, the interview can still be one of the best ways of obtaining a complete impression of the client and of possibly explaining the reasons for the articulation/phonological problem.

> Describe what the speech-language pathologist examines in an oral-peripheral examination.

Oral-Facial Examination

Inextricably related to assessment of articulation is assessment of the peripheral oral-facial structures. No speech diagnostic workup is complete without having done one. Assessment of the oral-facial structures includes the structure and function of the speech mechanism. As discussed in Chapter 3, some clients may manifest structural and/or functional differences that affect speech, including marked dental malocclusion, cleft palate, and insufficient velopharyngeal movement; however, one should remember that a broad range of variability exists from individual to individual, and individuals can make adjustments to compensate for structural and functional deviations. Structural assessment should include the face, mouth, pharynx, and nasal passages. Assessment of function includes the movable structures comprising the speech mechanism: lips, tongue, mandible, soft palate, and pharyngeal muscles. These structures should be assessed during speech and nonspeech functions, which is accomplished by asking the client to perform some activity while the diagnostician observes and takes notes. Generally, the "range of motion, strength, rate of movement, and accuracy of hitting the speech target" is assessed (Buckendorf & Gordon, 2002, p. 89).

Usually, the assessment of an individual should not begin with an oral examination. Probing inside the mouth can be intimidating and uncomfortable to children and adults. It is helpful for the clinician to use a friendly, conversational tone while doing the examination to relax the client. It is also helpful for examiners to explain to the client what they are doing and why. Using a tongue depressor, flashlight, rubber or latex gloves, stopwatch, and possibly a small dental mirror and gauze is helpful for conducting the examination. Universal precautions should be followed. An appropriate seating arrangement is to sit next to the client during the oral examination. The oral-peripheral examination should not conclude until the following have been observed and evaluated: (a) face; (b) lips; (c) teeth; (d) tongue; (e) palate; and (f) velopharyngeal mechanism. Sometimes, observing all of these structures is not possible during the initial visit.

Assessment of Speech Structures

Assessment of the speech structures and function are addressed separately here, but often in an oral exam, these two areas of examination are commingled. The face and head should be examined for any unusual features of the hair, skin, eyes, nose, and chin. These features may include deviations in coloration, texture, size, symmetry, scarring, tissue excess, or tissue deficiency. Deviations in these structures may only be indirectly related to articulation, if at all, but they may be very helpful in the total assessment or in detecting other possible problems or syndromes that the client may have. Early detection and referral to appropriate disciplines are good preventive procedures.

The speech structures should be assessed by carefully observing the client at rest and during speech and vegetative functions. The diagnostician must possess an adequate frame of reference regarding normality of these structures and functions, so that, in comparison, deviations can be readily detected and analyzed. The diagnostician should note any deviations of the teeth, alveolar ridge, tongue, height and width of the hard palate, dental arch alignment, depth and width of the pharynx, and conditions of the tonsils. Whenever significant deviations are noted, examination by a physician or dentist may be indicated. Obviously, not all of the structures are of equal importance insofar as articulation is concerned, but for the clinician to make a differential diagnosis, they should all be observed with a flashlight and tongue depressor.

Nasal cavity clearance is primarily important to nasal resonance (usually hyponasality) and to production of the three nasal consonants. Inadequate clearance may be related to a deviated nasal septum, hypertrophied turbinates, growths, adenoids, or upper respiratory problems causing mucosal swelling or excessive mucus. Nasal cavity clearance can be assessed by having the client breathe and blow through the nose while alternately occluding one naris then the other. Any obstruction in airflow can readily be detected.

Irregularities pertaining to the teeth and dental arches are observed by looking inside the mouth. Intra-oral inspection with the assistance of a flashlight and tongue depressor can provide information about the occlusal relationship and teeth alignment. Determining the significance of dental irregularities is difficult to do. Using a rating scale, such as the one proposed by Darley and Spriestersbach (1978) and presented in Appendix D, may assist in determining their significance. Besides dental arch alignment and teeth alignment, the diagnostician may observe other aspects of the teeth such as dental caries, oral hygiene, size of teeth, discoloration, and any other unusual dental characteristics.

The alveolar ridge and hard palate are involved in many speech sounds in the English language. Fortunately, except for a gross deviation of these structures, they usually do not interfere with articulation. An unusually rough or prominent alveolar ridge may distort the quality of sibilant sounds or be related to a tongue thrust. A markedly narrow (sometimes related to past or present finger- or thumbsucking) or low palatal vault can crowd the tongue and cause distortions of front consonants, but these structures usually are inconsequential as etiological factors in articulation disorders unless traumatic damage has resulted in cleft of the palate or alveolar ridge.

Two other structures that could affect speech, mainly regarding resonance (but also concerning production of the nasal and pressure consonants), are the tonsils and adenoids. Occasionally, their removal results in irreversible hypernasality and weak production of pressure consonants. If they are enlarged, they can obstruct oral airflow and restrict velar movement. The diagnostician should look inside the mouth and observe the tonsils while the client is at rest and while phonating /ɑ/. If the tonsils are of such size that they nearly contact each other at the midline of the oral cavity during rest,

then they probably are too large and may be interfering with speech. Coloration is important from a medical standpoint. A bright red color indicating inflammation or a grayish color suggesting abscess is cause for referral to a physician. Adenoids cannot be visualized without external equipment. If the adenoids are hypertrophied, a marked degree of hyponasality may be present. Enlarged adenoids have been associated with middle ear infections. Normal atrophy of the tonsils and adenoids generally occurs with maturation, so that by around 16 years of age, most children will have experienced a disappearance of their tonsils and adenoids.

Unfortunately, structural assessments are rather subjective. No clear definition exists of what constitutes adequate nasal cavity clearance beyond unrestricted airflow, acceptable dental occlusion for speech, relatively smooth alveolar ridge, or nonrestricting hard palate. Nevertheless, judgments have to be made and usually they are based on the clinician's past experiences. Sometimes, it is helpful to place judgments of each structure on a continuum of severity from 1 (insignificant) to 4 (very significant). It is helpful for student clinicians or beginning clinicians to examine as many persons as possible who have no known structural abnormality so they can better recognize *normal* structures versus atypical structures.

Assessment of Functions of Speech Mechanism

Functional assessments are likewise subjective. Factors such as rate of movement, range of motion, precision, strength, and timing of the movable speech structures should be assessed through visual inspection, also with the assistance of a flashlight and tongue depressor or other instruments. A nasal listening tube and intra-oral dental mirror are also useful (Fig. 6.7). These functions should similarly

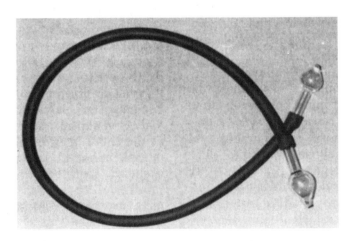

FIGURE 6.7 Nasal listening tube for assessing velopharyngeal closure regarding airflow, resonance, and articulation of pressure consonants.

be assigned a numeric value regarding the relative importance of the deviation (scale of 1 to 4). The movable structures are the mandible, lips, tongue, fauces, pharynx, soft palate, uvula, and cheeks.

The lower jaw or mandible is important to articulation in terms of providing adequate intra-oral clearance and modification for articulation and resonance. If the lower jaw does not or cannot open widely enough, speech can be impaired. Adequacy of mandibular movement should be assessed during speech and nonspeech activities. Asymmetry, restriction, and slow movement should be noted. Excessive overjet, receding jaw (distocclusion), or other malocclusions might affect articulation. Sometimes, the tongue and lips can compensate for mandibular problems; however, compensatory abilities are individualistic. Function can be assessed by having the client open and close the jaw in rapid succession and lateralize the jaw. Temporomandibular joint (TMJ) problems may restrict mandibular movement. These joint problems should be referred to an oral surgeon.

The lips are the most mobile of the facial structures. The symmetry of the lips should be noted during rest, smiling, and movement during speech and nonspeech functions. Function is assessed by having the client open and close the lips, pucker the lips, retract the lips, and lateralize the lips. Also, lip movement is observed and assessed while client says "oo-ee-oo-ee" in rapid succession.

The most important structure of the speech mechanism is the tongue. This mobile, multifunctioning articulator usually has great compensatory ability. It is involved in articulation and resonance for most phonemes. Rate, range, precision, and timing of its movements should be assessed.

Rate of tongue movement is assessed by administering a test of oral diadochokinesis. The client is asked to repeat syllables such as /pʌ/, /tʌ/, and /kʌ/ individually, and /pʌtʌkʌ/ in rapid succession. Each activity should be practiced once, then produced while the diagnostician tape records, counts, and times the repetitions. The amount of time to produce the required number of repetitions is then compared to available norms. The client is instructed to repeat the nonsense syllables as rapidly as possible until told to stop. If the repetitions are so fast that each one cannot be counted accurately, then they should be tape recorded and played back at a slower speed to facilitate counting. However, if the repetitions are that fast, it is doubtful that rate is impaired in that client.

Range of tongue movement is assessed more subjectively by having the client engage in various oral gymnastics: protruding and retracting the tongue, elevating and lowering it, grooving it,

lateralizing it outside the mouth, and lateralizing it inside the mouth by pushing out the cheeks. Each activity should be attempted at least twice. These gross lingual movements provide some information about tongue dexterity, but they do not necessarily correlate with fine lingual adjustments required for consonant production. Oral gymnastic activities could reveal the existence of an ankylosed tongue or neuromuscular involvement. The important determination to make is whether the range of lingual movements is adequate for speech or is adequately stimulable for the eventual acquisition of normal speech.

Timing of tongue movement is closely related to precision. If the tongue shows faulty timing, then it will not arrive within that acceptable positional range in time, causing distorted articulation. Faulty timing could also relate to leaving a target position too late, which would consequently affect contiguous sounds. For normal articulation to occur, the tongue and the other articulators must function in a synchronous manner. Asynergistic movement (faulty timing and coordination) of the tongue in relation to the other articulators must be scrutinized by the diagnostician through inspection and other approaches, such as radiography, when possible. Because of its subtleness, a timing problem may not always be detected.

Precision of tongue movements is important to articulation. The diagnostician should note "overshooting" or "undershooting" of the tongue or a "searching" pattern in trying to locate the correct placement for a sound. Replication of tongue position for speech and nonspeech movements can provide information about the efficiency of kinesthetic-proprioceptive feedback. Judging the precision of articulation physiology is not only very subjective, but very difficult, and requires considerable experience. Looking for imprecise tongue movements during contextual speech and listening for slurring and other types of oral inaccuracies are the two most effective techniques available to the diagnostician. Lack of lingual precision may be associated with central or peripheral nervous system involvement, moderate mental retardation, or heightened emotional states and may relate to vegetative problems or functions.

Additional aspects of the tongue that should be noted include tongue size and other structural deviations, such as deviated lingual raphe (midline depression); fissured tongue; asymmetric tongue posture or size; abnormal tongue position or carriage at rest or during speech; unusual coloration; scarring; tremors; or fibrillations (especially when the tongue is protruded and the eyes are closed); and poor tongue sensitivity.

The pillars of fauces may provide insight into velopharyngeal physiology. They form the archway between the oral and pharyngeal cavities, moving toward the midline of the back part of the mouth and backward during phonation and swallowing. They are involved in velopharyngeal closure. The rate, range, precision, and timing of pillar movement can only be subjectively assessed through intra-oral inspection as the client phonates (as when saying "ah") or pants.

Muscles of the pharynx, particularly of the lateral and back walls, can do much to modify the size and configuration of the pharynx. Because this structure is primarily concerned with velopharyngeal closure, it is most directly related to resonance and production of pressure consonants. In viewing the pharynx, the diagnostician should note height, width, depth, amount of lateral and back wall movement, and of course timing of this movement in relation to velar movement and onset of speech production. For example, if the lateral walls begin to move later than the soft palate or after the onset of speech, speech could be affected.

As with the pharynx, the soft palate or velum is mainly concerned with closure of the velopharyngeal mechanism and production of the velars. As such, it is related to the production and resonation of essentially all phonemes. The diagnostician will want to note the extent, rate, and timing of velar movement during phonation. Look for any deviation to one side or the other of the soft palate. Note whether there is localized contraction during phonation, such as a noticeable depression in the center of the soft palate. Also, look for scarring, discoloration, clefts, and fistulas. Does the soft palate become tense for production of /k/ and /g/? Is its range of motion more or less than that of the average soft palate, compared with observations of others? Does it seem to be long enough? These and other questions should be asked when determining the adequacy or inadequacy of the soft palate. The information is obtained through intra-oral inspection. Make certain that the jaws are parted no more than one inch, the tongue is not protruded, and the head is not tilted backward to avoid restriction of velar movement and distortion of the structural relationships of the oral structures.

The importance of the pharynx and velum functioning in concert should be emphasized. Together, these two structures provide the circle of muscles necessary to effect the sphincteric closure of the velopharyngeal port. Although determination of adequacy or inadequacy of this mechanism is readily possible, the diagnostician cannot always be certain about the reasons. For example, if the client has hypernasality or weak production of pressure consonants, which structure is defective? Are both structures functioning inadequately? Conversely, if one part of the velopharyngeal mechanism is not functioning adequately, how can a particular client still have normal resonance and articulation? Although difficult, an attempt should be made to determine cause and effect so that the most appropriate treatment procedures can be instigated. Although the degree of resonance and articulation distortion may not be indicative of the degree of inadequacy of this mechanism, quantification of the perceived nasality and articulation distortion should be routinely practiced (0 = normal nasality of speech distortion to +3 = severe hypernasality or speech distortion).

The uvula is insignificant to articulation per se. However, it can provide helpful information about other aspects of the velopharyngeal mechanism. For example, deviation of the uvula might indicate neuromuscular or structural involvement. Presence of a bifid uvula could suggest the possibility of a submucosal cleft, and the absence of a uvula might be a microform that is of importance to genetics, even though it does not contribute to velopharyngeal closure.

Two techniques that can be effectively used in a clinical setting are the alar flutter test and the nasal listening tube (Fig. 6.7). The alar flutter consists of compressing and releasing the alar cartilages of the client while producing high vowels in isolation, words, and sentences. It is important that none of these phonemic contexts contain the nasal sounds. If there is a positive flutter (perceptible change in resonance between compressed and released nares), then the mechanism may be functioning inadequately. By placing one end of the listening tube to the client's nose and the other end to the diagnostician's ear, perceptible changes in resonance and nasal airflow can be noted, again during production of pressure consonants in various phonemic contexts, but excluding the nasal sounds. By using these two simple techniques, the diagnostician can obtain inferential information about velopharyngeal physiology.

Cheeks tend to serve only an indirect function. Their primary function is to provide lateral walls for reinforcing the lateral dental arches of the oral cavity for sustaining intra-oral breath pressure and resonance. Only rarely are they directly involved in articulation. An example would be buccal speech of a person with a total glossectomy or with a laryngectomy. Looking for deviations in muscle tonus, asymmetry, scarring, discoloration, and unusual contraction should be part of the diagnostic workup, even though deviations may be more medically significant than communicatively significant. A diagnostic summary of the different aspects of structures and functions of the speech mechanism appears in Table 6.7.

Some formal oral peripheral examination protocols are available. The *Oral Speech Mechanism Screening Examination, Third Edition* (OSMSE-3; St. Louis & Ruscello, 2000) provides a protocol for examining oral structures and functions of individuals aged 5 to 78 years. The exam includes a section for diadochokinetic tasks and provides normative data, including screening cutoff scores. The *Test of Oral Structures and Functions* (Vitali, 1986) is a standardized test of oral structures and was developed for individuals from 7 years of age through adulthood. The manual provides information about expected subtest performance for various disorders such as dysarthria, apraxia, and functional disorders. The *Dworkin-Culatta Oral Mechanism and Treatment System* (D-Come-T; Dworkin & Culatta, 1996) consists of a less than 10-minute screening test and a follow-up deep test to evaluate at-risk systems further. The manual provides treatment suggestions and information leading to differential diagnosis and interpretation.

> How should auditory sensitivity be assessed in a client with an articulatory/phonologic disorder?

Auditory Abilities

Auditory abilities are important to articulation and should be assessed routinely. As noted in Chapter 5, auditory sensory problems are significant etiological factors for articulatory/phonologic disorders. Without auditory sensitivity or the ability to hear, typical speech sound production is compromised. At a minimum, a hearing screening should be administered that can be done by a speech-language pathologist. The 1996 ASHA guidelines (ASHA Panel on Audiologic Assessment, 1997) specify screening for the frequencies of 1,000, 2,000, and 4,000 Hz at 20 dB HL (25 dB HL for adults). If the client fails the screening, he or she should be referred to an audiologist for a full audiological assessment. A typical battery for assessing auditory sensitivity often includes pure tone testing with an audiometer to determine thresholds, impedance testing of the eardrum and middle ear structures to measure impedance and transmittance of sound vibrations, speech reception threshold to determine the intensity level required to perceive speech, and speech sound discrimination. Such an assessment battery should be conducted by an audiologist.

> How can speech sound discrimination abilities be assessed?

Speech Sound Discrimination Assessment

Auditory discrimination (the ability to discriminate between different auditory stimuli) is optional in an articulation/phonological assessment and can be assessed in several different ways using various informal procedures and formal tests. Stimuli may include phonemes, words, sentences, nonsense syllables, environmental noises, and rhythmic patterns. For concerns about articulation and phonology, **speech sound discrimination** (the ability to differentiate between different speech sounds) may be assessed. There are several ways for speech-language pathologists to test speech sound discrimination; these are different than the ways in which audiologists test for it. As shown in Table 6.8, speech sound discrimination tasks can be divided into four categories:

- Make a judgment about two externally-produced sounds (produced by the examiner)—clients indicate whether two stimuli are exactly the same or different.
- Make a judgment about an external sound as compared to the client's internal criterion—clients indicate whether or not the stimulus produced by the examiner is correct.
- Make a judgment about an external sound and one produced by the client—clients indicate whether or not the stimulus they produce is the same as that produced by the examiner.
- Make a judgment about a sound produced by the client relative to the client's internal criteria—clients indicate whether or not their own production is correct.

The last two tasks are really subgoals in some articulation treatment approaches so that clients learn to monitor their own speech. There are no formal tests available to measure the client's ability to perform these two tasks, but clinicians often incorporate these tasks into their treatment with clients.

Some formal tests of speech sound discrimination are available to the speech-language pathologist. The *Wepman's Discrimination Test, Second Edition* (Wepman & Reynolds, 1987) and the Short *Test of Sound Discrimination* (Templin, 1943)

TABLE 6.7

Assessment of Speech Structures and Functions

Structure	Features and Function
Head and face	Size and symmetry
	Texture of hair
	Scars
	Grimaces
	Control of facial expression
	Coloration
	Distance between eyes
	Drooping of eyelids
	Intranasal clearance—passageway and nares
	Deviated septum
	Size of mouth
	Nasal "squinting" during production of pressure consonants
Lips	Size and shape
	Symmetry—during rest, smile, and movement
	Mobility—occlude, pucker, retract, lateralize
	Strength
	Rapid repetition of lip movements (e.g., "oo-ee-oo-ee")
Teeth	Size
	Occlusion
	Number—excessive or deficient
	Spacing
	Coloration
	Hygiene
	Caries
	Prostheses
Tongue	Size
	Shape
	Symmetry
	Mobility and strength
	1. Rate—repeating /pʌ/, /tʌ/, /kʌ/, /pʌtʌkʌ/, etc. in rapid succession
	2. Range—grooving, pointing, protruding, lateralizing and pushing against the cheeks, and elevating the tongue
	3. Timing—assuming correctly timed target positions during contextual speech
	4. Precision—repeating tongue tip and /r/ sound positions accurately
	Coloration
	Tremors or fasciculation
	Attachment of frenulum
	Sensation—perception-tactile threshold sensitivity, tactile localization, 2-point discrimination, oral stereognosis, and kinesthesis
	Tongue thrust
Mandible	Size in relation to upper jaw and tongue
	Symmetry of shape and movement
	Mobility—rate and range of opening and closing in rapid succession
	Position in relation to upper jaw—overjet or receding

(continued)

TABLE 6.7 (Continued)

Assessment of Speech Structures and Functions

Maxilla and hard palate	Size—length and width
	Height
	Scars
	Occlusion (whether or not malocclusion is present, list the type)
	Coloration
	Cleft
	Fistula
	Configuration of alveolar bone
	Configuration of palate
Velopharyngeal mechanism	Size of soft palate
	Mobility of soft palate and degree of movement
	Mobility of lateral pharyngeal walls and degree of movement
	Mobility of posterior pharyngeal wall and degree of movement
	Symmetry of movement
	Synchrony of timing of movement
	Coloration
	Scars
	Cleft
	Fistula
	Adequacy of closure
	Movement of posterior pillars in direction of pharynx
	Size and condition of tonsils and adenoids, if present
	Uvula—bifid
	Deviation in movement of uvula
	Type of gag reflex
Breathing	Rate
	Rhythm
	Pattern—clavicular or diaphragmatic or thorasic
	Phonation sustained steadily for 10 seconds

require the client to judge whether two stimuli (words and nonsense syllables, respectively) are the same or different (Appendix F). The *Goldman-Fristoe-Woodcock Test of Auditory Discrimination* (Goldman, Fristoe, & Woodcock, 1976) uses picture identification to indicate the client's ability to differentiate among four phonemically similar words. The *Washington Speech Sound Discrimination Test* (Prather, Miner, Addicott, & Sunderland, 1971) requires the client to judge whether or not the word said by the examiner was correctly produced.

Speech sound discrimination can be informally assessed by having the client say "same" or "different," "yes" or "no," or "right" or "wrong" when given two sounds, syllables, or words; by identifying a picture of the correct stimulus; or by repeating a word (as when tested by an audiologist). The stimuli for discrimination on formal tests include various sounds rather than focusing on those that the client misarticulates. However, it seems logical that the discrimination tasks should include the phonemes that are misarticulated by the client and an analysis thereof. For example, if a child substitutes /t/ for /s/, phonemes may be presented in pairs, such as /se/ and /te/ or /bæt/ and /bæs/ and the differences between them analyzed. The *Farquhar–Bankson In-Depth Auditory Discrimination Test* (Appendix G) assesses varying levels

TABLE 6.8

Types of Speech Sound Discrimination Tasks

Task	Task Description	Examples
Make a judgment about two externally-produced sounds	Clients indicate whether two stimuli are exactly the same or different	Clinician: "Are these two words the same or different: cot, cod?" Client: "Different" Clinician: "Are these the same: /ot/, /ot/?" Client: "Yes."
Make a judgment about an external sound as compared to the client's internal criterion	Clients indicate whether the stimulus produced by the examiner is correct	Clinician: Points to a picture of a house. "Is this word said correctly: /haʊt/?" Client: "No"
Make a judgment about an external sound and one produced by the client	Clients indicate whether the stimulus produced by the client is the same as that produced by the examiner	Clinician: "Say see" Client: "/ti/" Clinician: "Did you say the word exactly as I did?" Client: "No."
Make a judgment about a sound produced by the client relative to the client's internal criterion	Clients indicate whether their own production is correct	Client: Names a picture of a sun. "/tʌn/" Clinician: "Did you say that word correctly?" Client: "No."

of auditory discrimination abilities for individual sounds and is a useful tool for the diagnostician (Bernthal & Bankson, 1981). Discrimination of correctly articulated sounds may be irrelevant and unnecessary, except perhaps for gross discrimination training of right and wrong productions and tuning in, improving overall listening and self-monitoring skills. Also, it is possibly more helpful to evaluate speech sound discrimination abilities regarding self-discrimination, rather than discrimination of someone else's utterances. It may be better for carryover when clients can produce the phonemes correctly and incorrectly in these tasks and decide instantaneously whether the production is correct or incorrect or better than previous production. When tested, problems in speech sound discrimination should be noted for future consideration in specifying the etiologies and treatment approach.

> What ancillary areas might the speech-language pathologist assess in a client with an articulatory/phonologic disorder? Why might these areas be assessed?

ANCILLARY ASSESSMENTS

Oral Sensation-Perception

Although it is seldom assessed, oral sensation-perception of the tongue, lips, and even soft palate can influence the functioning of these structures. Five dimensions of sensation-perception that can be assessed are: (a) tactile sensitivity, (b) tactile localization, (c) oral stereognosis, (d) kinesthesis, and (e) two-point discrimination. Tactile sensitivity is assessed by gently stroking the tongue at different locations with a wisp of cotton and asking the client whether or not the tongue was touched. Tactile localization is assessed similarly, except that the client is asked to point to the exact location of each stimulus. For both activities, several stimuli should be presented. Oral stereognosis is assessed by placing geometric shapes inside the mouth and asking the client to identify the stimulus shape from multiple choices. Kinesthesis is grossly appraised by having the client replicate elevated tongue tip and tongue protruded positions. Kinesthetic feedback is assumed to be adequate when the replications do not vary more than 2 or 3 mm. Two-point discrimination is assessed by placing a two-point object (spaced 2 mm apart), such as dial caliper, on various locations of the tongue. Then, by alternating between a two-point object and a one-point object and asking the client whether one or two points were felt, the diagnostician can make a determination about the adequacy or inadequacy of two-point discrimination. The test manual of the W-CAT is helpful for additional descriptions of how to assess these areas.

Orofacial Myofunctional Disorder

Orofacial myofunctional disorder that includes tongue thrust may occasionally be present to interfere with the production of the sibilants and other dental and alveolar sounds. Orofacial muscle imbalance can be grossly assessed by having the client swallow solids and noting, by parting the lips while swallowing, whether the tongue is thrusting against or between the front or side teeth. It should also be noted whether the masseter muscles contract during swallowing of solids by placing the index fingers near the angle of the mandible, whether there is any associated malocclusion when the teeth are in approximation, whether there is excessive use of the lips in chewing and swallowing, and whether the lip has strength and to what degree. This should be done three times, and the derived scores averaged. If these characteristics, plus deficient articulation, are unfavorable, the client may have a detrimental tongue thrust.

Phonological Awareness

As indicated in Chapter 5, research findings have shown an association between phonologic disorders and deficient phonological awareness skills (Bird & Bishop, 1992; Bird, Bishop, & Freeman, 1995; Hodson, 1994, 1997; Larrivee & Catts, 1999; Stackhouse, 1997; Webster & Plante, 1992). Because these skills are related to articulation/phonological skills, the diagnostician may decide to assess this area. Tests for phonological awareness contain items that require skills such as rhyming, sound blending, syllable blending, sentence segmentation, syllable segmentation, phoneme segmentation, and sound manipulation. Phonological awareness assessment instruments include the *Comprehensive Tests of Phonological Processing* (CTOPP; Wagner, Torgesen, & Rashotte, 1999) normed for individuals aged 5:0 to 24:11, *Phonological Abilities Test* (Muter, Hulme, & Snowling, 1997) for ages 4 to 7 years, the Phonological Awareness Test (Robertson & Salter, 1997) for students aged 5 to 9 along with a companion computer program for scoring the test, the *Phonological Awareness and Reading Profile-*

Intermediate (Salter & Robertson, 2001) for ages 8 to 14, and the *Test of Phonological Awareness* (TOPA; Torgesen & Bryant, 1994) for kindergartners and first graders. The *Phonemic-Awareness Skills Screening* (PASS; Crumrine & Lonegan, 2000) and the *Pre-Literacy Skills Screening* (PLSS; Crumrine & Lonegan, 1999) are available screening tests. It should be noted that significant findings in this or any other area do not suggest cause and effect, merely a relationship. Some speech-language pathologists are now incorporating work on phonological awareness skills in young clients with phonological disorders for the purpose of boosting literacy skills as well as articulation/phonological skills.

Language

Receptive and expressive language abilities should routinely be screened in persons with articulation/phonological problems because it has been shown that 40% to as many as 80% of children with speech sound impairments have concomitant expressive language problems (e.g., Fey et al., 1994; Shriberg & Austin, 1998; Shriberg & Kwiatkowski, 1994; Tyler & Watterson, 1991), and 10–40% have concomitant receptive language problems (Shriberg & Kwiatkowski, 1994). Although variably defined, language includes the domains of syntax, morphology, semantics, phonology, and pragmatics.

Other Speech Domains

Voice, fluency, and prosody should be screened. As noted in Chapter 5, articulatory/phonologic disorders have been shown to occur in 30–40% of children who stutter, and voice disorders have been shown to accompany articulatory/phonologic disorders in some children. Deviations in voice, fluency, and prosody also can adversely affect intelligibility. Informally assessing these speech domains from the speech samples collected during the assessment sessions is recommended.

SEVERITY LEVEL

Assigning a severity level of mild, moderate, severe, and possibly profound involves consideration of several factors. As stated earlier, severity of articulatory/phonologic disorders varies from mild to severe and from barely perceptible to the trained ear to completely unintelligible. The diagnostician can use norms from a standardized articulation/phonological test as a starting point (Table 5.3). Generally, the norms are based upon the number of misarticulations on the test, the age of the person, and sometimes the type of error and the frequency of occurrence of the sounds misarticulated by the client. From there, the clinician considers other factors that are known to affect the severity level to determine whether the severity level should be shifted upward or downward. Some of these factors include: the number of misarticulations in connected speech, the consistency of misarticulations, the types of errors (typical or atypical; omissions, substitutions, distortions), level of intelligibility, stimulability of the misarticulated sounds, the normalcy of suprasegmental features (rate, intensity, stress, and rhythm), and the age of the person (Davis & Bedore, 2000; Perkins, 1977; Powers, 1971).

Another approach is to calculate the Percentage of Consonants Correct, Revised Edition (PCC-R) metric (Shriberg et al., 1997; Shriberg & Kwiatkowski, 1982c). It "is recommended as the most appropriate metric for comparisons involving speakers of diverse ages and of diverse speech status" (Shriberg et al., 1997, p. 720). If vowels and diphthongs are also a concern, the Percentage of Phonemes Correct (PPC-R) can be used. Usually, the PCC-R is more reflective of an individual's speech competence because vowels and diphthongs are seldom an issue. It is calculated on words elicited in a 5- to 10-minute conversational speech sample. The PCC-R is calculated on intelligible words because the analysis is done on the percentage of *intended* consonants that are produced correctly. Omissions and substitutions of consonants are considered misarticulations; whereas, distortions are not counted as errors, but are considered correct productions. Severity levels fall into four categories based on PCC-R scores:

- Mild ($>85\%$)
- Mild to Moderate (65–85%)
- Moderate (50–65%)
- Severe ($<50\%$)

The Articulation Severity Index (ASI; Rochester Hearing and Speech Center, 2000) is a "multidimensional view of a child's speech production" (p. 1). The impetus for developing this instrument was to attain agreement among clinicians because clinicians vary in terms of assigning severity levels. The ASI can be applied to single-word, as well as conversational speech information and is designed to integrate quantitative data with qualitative data. The factors included in the ASI are (p. 2):

- Age
- Number of phoneme errors
- Frequency and type of selected phonological processes
- Intelligibility in conversation
- Oral motor skills
- Stimulability
- Suprasegmental patterns

This information is gathered from a single-word articulation test (number of omissions, distortions, and substitutions of nondevelopmental prevocalic and postvocalic consonants and blends), occurrence of immature phonological patterns (cluster reduction, final consonant deletion, stopping, backing to velars, initial consonant deletion), intelligibility rating of conversational speech (50+ words in known context and 50+ words in unknown context), stimulability of misarticulated speech sounds (that are at or below age level), oral peripheral exam and oral motor skills, suprasegmental features, and age. The total number of points is converted into a severity level rating, including:

- Within normal limits
- Within normal limits to mild (borderline)
- Mild
- Mild to moderate
- Moderate
- Moderate to severe
- Severe

> What is an appropriate sequence of assessment procedures when evaluating a client with a speech sound disorder?

BASIC PRINCIPLES AND SEQUENCE OF ASSESSMENT

The assessment stage of management presupposes that the referral process has proceeded through appropriate administrative channels, received parental approval and endorsement, and met state and federal regulations. Given these requirements, the remaining tasks facing the diagnostician are outlined in Table 6.9. Each basic step should be carefully carried out so that no piece of the diagnostic puzzle is inadvertently omitted, thereby resulting in a possible misdiagnosis. The clinician may choose to follow the sequence as listed, or vary from this order, depending on the specific situation.

> What factors affect a clinical philosophy of assessment? What are three clinical models of assessment and treatment?

Have a Clinical Philosophy

The diagnostician might consider formulating a clinical philosophy, which should incorporate sound behavioral and scientific theory yet be suffi-

TABLE 6.9

Principles and Sequence of Assessment

Steps Involved Before, During, and After the Assessment

Have a clinical philosophy
Plan for the assessment
    Review the background
    Observe the client
    Select appropriate tests and procedures
    Be prepared to modify assessment plan
    Prepare the test room
Conduct the assessment
    Get the client
    Establish rapport and motivation
    Explain the test procedures and instructions
    Administer the assessment instruments/procedures
    Supplement the test data
    Praise the client's performance
    Document and tape record the responses
    Move smoothly from one task to another
    Remove test materials when completed
    Allow for fatigue
    Pleasantly end the session
Process information obtained from the assessment
    Score tests
    Analyze results
    Interpret results
    Draw conclusions
    Determine treatment, if needed
    Make recommendations
Disseminate results, conclusions, and recommendations
    Discuss findings with client and/or significant others
    Write and disseminate the clinical report

ciently open to modification over the years. The philosophy should permeate the clinician's personality, background, knowledge, and worksite. Additionally, the clinical philosophy should include the concepts of thoroughness, treatment orientation, positiveness, and professionalism for dealing with the heterogeneity that exists within persons who have articulatory/phonologic disorders. The approach to diagnosis and treatment varies from clinician to clinician. Speech-language clinicians choose their own style of service delivery from

three clinical models as described by Tomblin (2002, pp. 14–16):

- Medical model—emphasis on "categorization of problems and identification of causes" that lead to the treatment plan
- Behavioral model—emphasis is in "characterizing the client's performance in tasks that are viewed as important for educational or social success" with treatment based on intervention strategies that result in improved communication
- Systems model—equal emphasis is "on the environment and the client and assumes the problem lies in the mismatch of interaction between them" with treatment focused on facilitative contexts and interactions

The model used by the clinician varies with the type of setting and the client as well as with the speech-language pathologist's clinical philosophy. Usually, clinicians use a combination of these three approaches in their particular work settings.

Procedural Guidelines

Several procedural guidelines suggested by Darley and Spriestersbach (1978) might well be a part of basic, sound clinical philosophy. They remind the diagnostician to keep the purpose clearly in mind. Always be aware of the rationale for doing what you are doing. The purpose of conducting an articulation/phonological assessment is to obtain accurate, reliable information about the client's articulation and phonology. They caution against working too fast. Working efficiently is positive, but working too fast can confuse the client and curtail the amount of speech behavior that might otherwise have been elicited. Another important point is to keep the client motivated. Keeping the client on task is the ideal goal, but sometimes that is not possible. By using an appropriate pace and ample positive reinforcement, as well as being genuinely interested in the client's performance, the clinician will more likely maintain the client's interest and motivation. They also suggest using a straightforward approach. Be direct and request specifically and clearly what you want the client to do. Vague or nonspecific commands encourage vague responses and confusion. Remember to answer questions. The clinician who answers the client's questions more likely will maintain interest and cooperation than the clinician who ignores questions, although not all questions need to be answered. Similarly, ask for repetition. Repetitions may need to be requested from the client whose intelligibility is moderately impaired. The extent to which the client is asked to repeat varies according to the client's reaction to those requests and the degree of frustration manifested. Darley and Spriestersbach (1978) also remind us that the test is merely a tool. Do not become so "test-bound" that you overlook significant information. A test is only one means to an end and is only as good as the tester. There are other ways of obtaining information, and there is other information besides test results. Lastly, the client, not the test, must be central. Do not lose sight of the most important dimension in the diagnostic workup—the client. You are attempting to obtain information from that person about that person. If the test becomes an obstruction, discard it, at least temporarily. It is important to establish good rapport with the client.

Possess Clinical Knowledge and Experience

Closely related to having a clinical philosophy is having the necessary clinical knowledge and experience to do the job. It would be inconceivable for a clinician to possess high standards of professionalism and professional ethics and, at the same time, lack the basic knowledge and experience to deal effectively with persons who have articulation/phonological problems. All clinicians have an ethical responsibility to know about articulatory/phonologic disorders before attempting to deal with them. Anything less than that is unacceptable.

From what sources does a speech-language pathologist obtain important background information about the client?

Preplanning

Review the Background

All pertinent background information should be reviewed before seeing the client, if possible. A questionnaire completed by the client or a person knowledgeable about the client is helpful. Background information comes from several sources in addition to the case history. These include verbal or written information from the referral source, medical reports, and clinical reports from other agencies. Information gathered from the client's case history and other sources can be invaluable in formulating a diagnosis, ascertaining the etiology, and developing a plan of treatment.

Observe the Client

Observation, when feasible, is an important step in the diagnostic sequence, especially in a systemic model of service provision. It can provide representative information about the client, especially when the observation occurs in a natural or comfortable environment such as in the home, with another sibling, or in a play situation. Even observation in a clinic or school setting can be more representative than a formal clinician–child interaction in an unfamiliar room. Observation may be passive or active. In passive observation, the clinician observes the client from an adjacent room; whereas in active observation, the clinician is in the same room with the client simultaneously interacting and observing. Not only should the obtained observational data be carefully documented, but it should also be compared with the data obtained through testing, always noting similarities, discrepancies, patterns, and idiosyncrasies. Whenever possible, it is helpful when observation precedes the planning of the testing and test selection.

What are some criteria used in selecting assessment instruments to be used in an evaluation?

Plan the Diagnostic Workup

The next step should be planning the testing procedure. To reiterate, this step includes a review of the historical and observational information so that appropriate testing instruments and procedures are selected. An outline of the activities, materials, and instruments to be used in assessment is helpful. If the client has special or unusual needs or problems, these should be included in the overall plan. The clinician plans the order in which the instruments are going to be administered. Often, the assessment begins with an interview of the client and/or person knowledgeable about the client. Generally, an effective strategy is to first administer tests/instruments that require no verbal responses or only one-word responses followed by tasks requiring more extensive verbalizations. The oral-peripheral exam might be administered last because some clients are initially uncomfortable with the diagnostician using a tongue blade and wearing gloves. Of course, the sequence depends on characteristics of individual clients. Careful and thorough planning at the outset can save time and avoid problems in the future.

Each published test has some unique characteristics, as mentioned earlier. Some articulation/phonological tests take longer to administer; some are more comprehensive; some have one picture per page; some use photographs; some test consonants and consonant clusters only; some are phoneme oriented; some identify phonological deviations; and some are norm-referenced. Diligence must be exercised in selecting evaluation instruments so that the assessment tools will fit the particular client and elicit a representative speech sample. When selecting a test, the clinician considers factors such as the type of sample obtained, stimulus materials possessed, type of information yielded, including standardization factors (such as reliability and validity), length of test, age levels for which it is appropriate, manipulability of materials, attractiveness, availability, and familiarity. The test should fit the particular client. For example, if the client is a child who is referred because of unintelligibility, a standardized test that assesses phonological deviations might be most appropriate; whereas, for an adolescent referred for a lisp, a phonemic-oriented test that can be read and/or a test that assesses production of the stridents in various contexts might be selected. For the child with a visual acuity deficit, a test that contains large, individual pictures per page is a reasonable consideration. For the client who has an orthopedic problem, a test that does not require manipulation of objects would be a logical choice. If the client has a special problem, such as cleft palate or apraxia of speech, further considerations will need to be given to test selection. A child whose speech pattern appears to display considerable variability should be given a test that samples the same phonemes in several different contexts. These are a few examples for underscoring the importance of perusing various test manuals, administering or being familiar with various tests, reviewing background information about the client, and gathering information about the client before deciding on the tests to use.

Be Ready to Modify the Assessment Plan

The size of the clinician's repertoire of methodology is important. Generally, the capable clinician can perform diagnostic workups by using a modicum of different methods and techniques, but occasionally there will be a client who has special needs that are not compatible with the diagnostician's plan. Perhaps the clinician may find a need to administer a different standardized test, such as one that has larger pictures or fewer items; add an assessment tool, such as a phonological test, test of consistency, or a CAS test; ask a parent or sibling to elicit the speech sample; or use only informal, nonstandardized procedures. Other modifications may need to be made as well.

Prepare the Test Room

Besides planning what to do and how to do it, the diagnostician should make certain that the test room is conducive to test-taking. The room should have appropriate lighting and be free from distractions. An outlet should be available for tape recording, and the room should be quiet. Include an appropriately sized table and two chairs or more whenever parents, spouses, siblings, or others will be present in the room during the testing. The chairs should either be arranged in juxtaposition or across from one another. When doing an oral examination, position yourself next to the client rather than observe intra-oral details from across the table. For the more active clients, position the table between them and yourself, preferably with the table positioned diagonally toward the corner of the room to confine the clients. Finally, place the materials used for assessment so that they are readily accessible, but not distracting to the client. A cabinet or shelf works well. Another option is to place unused materials outside the door to minimize distractions.

> What are the procedures used in conducting the diagnostic session?

Conducting the Assessment

Get the Client

The manner in which you approach the client (adult or child), what you say, and how you ambulate to the test room can be very important. Most children will join you when you say, "Let's go play some games" and extend your hand, but some will turn the other way. During these times, you will need to use various techniques. Pleading, begging, bribing, disguising, clowning, and dragging have been tried. Having the mother carry the child to the test room is another technique that has worked in some instances. There will be times when the client's cooperation will not be obtained. Various approaches have been tried, but being friendly, sincere, pleasant, and firm is usually the most effective.

In many instances with children and adolescents, it is appropriate to invite the parents and siblings into the room where the testing is conducted. Some clinicians prefer for the parent and even siblings to be in the room during testing (Tyler & Tolbert, 2002). This is especially appropriate when using a systems model of assessment. Advantages of having parents in the room are that they can provide helpful information about strategies for working with the child, can interpret the child's utterances, and can supplement information provided earlier in the interview. On the other hand, parents often will "help" their child to respond correctly. Usually, this can be alleviated by asking them not to help the child answer the test items because the test instructions must be followed precisely.

Establish Rapport and Motivation

Some of the same strategies used for inviting the client to join you initially can subsequently be used in establishing rapport and motivation. In the case of adults, a friendly, straightforward approach is usually effective. In the case of younger clients, the clinician must convince the child that the activities will be enjoyable, but this has to happen in a rather subtle manner. Be positive, friendly, interested in the child, and perhaps provide the child with some toys at the beginning of the test session. Casual conversation in an atmosphere of play has helped to establish rapport with some children. Occasionally, providing tangible rewards may be advisable. Looking at pictures is generally enjoyable for most younger clients, and because this is a major part of articulation and phonological tests, clients are usually interested. Periodically providing positive reinforcement for the child's good attending behavior and responses can help to maintain motivation and participation. Minimizing frustration and not spending excessive amounts of time on one activity will also assist in maintaining rapport and motivation. The clinician should conduct the diagnostic workup in a spirit of enjoyment. Furthermore, a child who is enjoying the activities will generally provide better (and more) speech samples than the child who is not enjoying the activities. A moderately fast pace of administration of the formal tests is often helpful in keeping the client interested and responsive.

Establishing rapport takes time. Some children and adults "warm up" faster than others, and some never seem to become overly cooperative. The degree or quality of rapport for a diagnostic workup may never equal that for ongoing treatment. That is one reason for implementing the concept of *diagnostic treatment*, because as rapport continues to improve over time, more valuable and valid information about the client tends to be elicited. Remember that a child can be enticed, but not coerced to perform a task. To entice the child, the diagnostician must know the kind of person the child is and adjust the approaches and procedures to fit that particular child's personality and preferences. Each child is unique and will respond in different ways, some of which will be quite unexpected. An individualistic approach routinely should be used.

Explain the Test Procedures and Instructions

Before administering the articulation/phonological test battery, the clinician should briefly explain the assessment procedures by using simple, concise language and a positive approach. The extent of the explanation will vary with the age of the client. Older clients often understand and respond better than do younger clients. A brief explanation can help to allay anxieties if it is not overdone. Because the test instructions must be given verbatim to ensure validity, reading from the test manual is permissible. If, for some reason, the client cannot take a test in the prescribed manner, this departure from standardization protocol should be noted and perhaps a different test or a different technique should be used.

Administer the Assessment Tools

Often, the diagnostic process begins with an interview of the client or someone knowledgeable about the client to collect case history information or to supplement case history information obtained from a questionnaire or other source. Of course, this procedure can be done at another time during the diagnostic session.

The clinician is now ready to administer the tests. Generally, for children, it is recommended that testing begin with a test or procedure that does not require a verbal response, such as a receptive language test, or with a single-word response format, such as articulation/phonological tests. These types of tasks are probably less threatening to a child who has communication problems. From there, the clinician moves to the hearing screening, connected speech sample, stimulability assessment, and oral-peripheral examination in whatever order seems appropriate for the client. The tests should be administered efficiently, while the clinician documents the client's responses. At the same time, the responses can be audio or video tape recorded for later analysis and verification of the online transcription and notes. The diagnostician should positively reinforce while testing. Generally, reinforce test-taking behaviors and not correct responses to maintain the validity of the results.

One of the primary purposes of an articulation/phonological assessment is to obtain a representative speech sample through the use of standardized tests, criterion-referenced tests, and/or informal evaluation procedures. The operative word is *representative*. As mentioned earlier, in addition to a formal single-word or sentence articulation/phonological test, the diagnostician should assess the stimulability of the sounds misarticulated. The clinician should elicit an informal contextual speech sample that will be used to measure speech intelligibility and also will be compared to the client's performance on the formal test. It is good practice to ask the parent or other reporter about whether the client's performance on these assessments is typical of the client's speech. If after trying several of these additional techniques, the clinician judges that a representative sample may not have been obtained, this impression should be mentioned in the written report and further assessment should be done at a later date.

The rest of the assessment battery is then administered, including the oral-peripheral examination and the hearing screening or full audiological assessment. The clinician may opt to administer specialized tests, such as a speech sound discrimination test, word intelligibility test, contextual tests, and tests for childhood apraxia of speech.

The administration of standardized tests and recording of client performance should follow test manual instructions. If they are not, the results are considered invalid. Even though the instructions among different tests may be similar, the clinician should be knowledgeable about each test's idiosyncrasies before administering the test exactly as indicated in the test manual. The selected test should be administered efficiently so that the client's interest is maintained, yet not too fast so that the client can keep up. If a client is unable to supply the target word spontaneously, followed by a delayed direct model, within a few seconds from when the stimulus was presented, the clinician should provide a direct model rather than wait longer for the client to say the word spontaneously. Sometimes, it becomes obvious during the testing that a direct model will be required for all the items on a formal articulation/phonological test because of the client's reticence to respond. Using good listening and looking skills can help the clinician make accurate test administration decisions. Language used in talking with young clients can be important. In addition to using words that are meaningful to the client, the clinician should phrase commands appropriately. Rather than asking young children if they would like to look at some pictures, tell them that they are going to look at some pictures. Use commands rather than questions.

Audio or video tape recording of the assessment can ensure accuracy of the data collection process. The clinician may not always be able to listen to the client's speech and write the responses without omitting some information; therefore, a tape-recorded session can be helpful in protecting against these errors of omission.

In conclusion, do not assume that (a) the client's production of a specific phoneme during assessment by a formal articulation test is a true reflection of all other productions of that phoneme; (b) the speech performance is reflective of all other speaking situations; (c) the responses on single-word tests reflect those responses that would probably occur in contextual speech; and (d) all standardized tests will provide a representative speech sample. Conclusions such as these could significantly distort the accuracy of the client's level of speech functioning.

Supplement the Test Data

A particular client may demonstrate a type of communication behavior that requires assessment beyond that provided by a standardized test. For example, if a client produced /f/ by approximating the lower teeth with the upper lip, the clinician may ask the client to repeat several other words containing /f/ to see whether this somewhat unusual articulation pattern exists in other contexts. Similarly, if a client has an alar squint when producing certain pressure consonants, the clinician would ascertain whether the squint is present among other pressure consonants as well. It is also helpful for treatment planning to try various sound elicitation techniques to determine a workable approach. Obtain as much supplemental information as necessary to reach a valid conclusion.

Praise the Client's Performance

Let clients know that their performance is appropriate. This technique is invaluable for maintaining rapport and interest. Praise can take the form of a supportive word, a smile, a gentle pat on the shoulder, applause, and even an enthusiastic cheer or a "high five." Well-intentioned and well-timed praise usually results in obtaining a child's cooperation and eliciting desired client responses.

Document and Tape Record the Responses

Significant speech information may come forth at a fast pace during the diagnostic workup. Therefore, an efficient method of taking notes is recommended. Some diagnosticians may need to develop an abbreviated note-taking system and supplement it with a tape recording. The purpose is to record all of the speech data so that a thorough and accurate analysis can be made later because omitting or forgetting any information can present problems.

Move Smoothly from One Task to Another

Smooth transitions in assessment are important. The diagnostician must move from one task or test to another in an organized manner to avoid losing the client. If the client becomes confused or fails to realize the response requirements of a new task, the obtained results may be inappropriate and invalid. Let the client know that, when a new test will be administered, a different response is expected. Move briskly but smoothly and systematically from one task to another so that the client can easily follow the assessment sequence.

Remove Test Materials When Completed

The diagnostician should never leave a previously administered test on the table when administering another test or different activity. Too many materials can be distracting and confusing to the client and to the diagnostician. Besides, the client may have difficulty adjusting to a new test when the one just completed is still present. Confusion has been observed among clinicians who failed to remove previously administered materials.

Allow for Fatigue

A formal testing situation can be fatiguing to everyone involved. Attempting to perform one's best can be exhausting. Testing may require a break or recess to avoid fatiguing in the client. The diagnostician needs to remember that the testing environment should be one in which optimum results are obtained. If fatigue or inattentiveness occurs, terminate the testing and take a walk, get a drink of water, or play a fun game. If after this break, the testing still cannot be resumed, schedule another appointment to complete the testing. The appointment may be scheduled later that same day for those clients who may have come from a long distance for the appointment. The diagnostician needs to remember that individuals with neurological etiology tend to fatigue more quickly than others.

Pleasantly End the Session

Two important stages in the assessment sequence are the beginning and the end. Every clinician should expend considerable effort to get the session off to a good start and to end it on a pleasant note. First impressions are important, so be sure to impress the client favorably. Because the clinician probably is setting the atmosphere for later clinical intervention, the impression made can carry over to later interactions with the client. Giving a prize at the end of the diagnostic workup has proven to be effective for younger clients.

> **What does analyzing the diagnostic workup results involve?**

Process Information Obtained from Assessment

After testing has been completed, the test data need to be analyzed and interpreted. Table 6.10 lists the posttesting sequence, some of which has already been mentioned in the discussion of specific principles of assessment. Administering and scoring the assessment battery are the first steps in the assessment process. Analysis and interpretation allows the clinician to answer questions such as:

- Does an articulatory or phonologic disorder exist?
- If a problem does exist, what is the nature of the problem?
- What are the possible compounding or potentially related factors?
- Is treatment appropriate?
- Which treatment approaches are appropriate?
- Where should treatment begin?
- What is the prognosis for improvement?

Scoring

Scoring is the first task. It should be carried out by carefully and accurately following the instructions provided in the test manual and double-checking all of the scores for possible errors. Simple mistakes can cause complex problems. Clinicians are urged to score and analyze the test results as soon as possible after the testing is completed. The greater the elapsed time after the testing, the greater the likelihood that some information may

---

TABLE 6.10

Sequence of Posttesting Tasks

Step	Task
First	Scoring
Second	Analyzing
Third	Interpreting
Fourth	Concluding (Making a Diagnosis)
Fifth	Predicting (Determining a Prognosis)
Sixth	Recommending
Seventh	Reporting

be forgotten, misplaced, or misinterpreted. Ideally, the scoring will occur on the same day that the tests were given.

Analyzing

Analyses should be done immediately after the results have been obtained for the same reasons mentioned in the preceding section. Analyzing the scores requires the use of the clinician's clinical aptitude, knowledge, and experience. This stage requires the nonjudgmental organization of the facts (Nation & Aram, 1977). It requires skill in scoring, objectifying, comparing with norms, and organizing the data in terms of possible solutions with consideration for what supports those solutions, what does not support the hypothesized problem, and what is still missing and know what it all means.

Comparing the data with norms provides a method of analysis. This approach allows the diagnostician to determine how a specific client is doing in comparison with the typically developing person of that age. Comparison with norms eventually aids in the decision of whether the client has normal, accelerated, or delayed articulation/phonological development.

The diagnostician must decide what data are available and how helpful they are in interpreting specific aspects of the client's articulation and phonology. The data analysis may include information about pertinent sound features such as those listed in Table 6.11. Concerning the types of misarticulations, the diagnostician should analyze them in terms of whether they are typical or atypical. For example, a w/r substitution is typical, but a k/r substitution is not. Determining the positions in which the misarticulations occur most often can also provide valuable information for treating the client. If a client shows an orderly developmental delay in acquiring phonemes rather than a nondevelopmental sequence, an articulation delay rather than an articulation disorder may exist. Another analysis might consider the phonemes that are misarticulated more commonly, the more or less frequently occurring phonemes in the English language. Such a determination would surely have implications regarding the degree of unintelligibility of a client's speech. Cosmetic analysis is important. If a person looks conspicuous even while sounding intelligible or articulate, then that person may have a speech problem. Assessment of consistent and inconsistent misarticulations is also important. Placing the misarticulations into sound classes such as sibilants or plosives will facilitate later clinical management. Likewise, if distinctive features of phonemic groups can be categorized, this can provide considerable assistance to the

TABLE 6.11

Factors or Parameters to be Analyzed from Various Speech Samples Collected

Speech Sound Features

Typical and atypical misarticulations

Typical or atypical order of development

Delayed or disordered development

More or less frequently occurring phonemes in error

Word position of misarticulations

Consistent or inconsistent misarticulations

Phonemic categories produced correctly and incorrectly

Distinctive feature analysis

Phonological deviations used

Cosmetic peculiarities of speech sound production

Comparisons of single words with contextual speech

Syllabic and word structures produced

Stimulability of phonemes misarticulated

Intelligibility analysis

clinician who is contemplating treatment strategies. If phonological deviations can be identified as possibly being delayed in their suppression, then this finding can set the stage for a thorough phonological analysis. Does the client have speech difficulties mainly with vowels or mainly with consonants? How stimulable are the misarticulated phonemes? If intelligibility is less than 100%, what speech, language, and contextual factors account for it? Analyses should also quantify baseline scores or levels. Similar to looking for consistent and inconsistent speech, the diagnostician should compare the similarities and differences in the client's speech between productions of single words and contextual speech. Finally, look for physical signs of struggling behavior or atypical use of the articulators. This analysis can help to specify the presence of a possible motor speech problem. If the diagnostician can think of any other reasonable analyses to make, this should be done.

Interpreting

Another important step in the posttesting procedures is interpretation. This problem-solving task is critical to making appropriate recommendations and planning effective treatment. Misinterpretation can be detrimental. The clinical results must be carefully interpreted to explain such aspects as formulating a diagnosis, stating a diagnosis, assigning a severity level, suggesting possible etiologies, offering a prognosis, and formulating a treatment plan or possibly a need for more data. Decisions must be made not only as to whether or not an articulatory/phonologic disorder is present, but also regarding its severity and type. The diagnostician must know what all the obtained data mean and how to interpret them to the client and family. Interpretation includes (a) identifying types of errors; (b) discovering location of errors in context; (c) discerning patterns of misarticulation, if present; (d) scrutinizing variability of performance; and (e) determining causes (Emerick & Hatten, 1986). In a sense, this stage really pulls it all together. It synthesizes and interprets all of the data and impressions obtained from each of the assessment steps. Furthermore, it places all of the pertinent information in its proper perspective regarding other aspects of the client such as personality, attitude, ability, motivation, needs, and concerns. In other words, all of these speech data are only one part of the whole person, a perspective that should never be forgotten.

To summarize, the interpretation step is one of deciding what all of the data mean, what is significant and what is not, which findings require immediate or preferred attention, and which findings can be dealt with at a later time. Interpretation is the sine qua non of diagnosis, and as such, it taxes the diagnostician's cognitive aptitude and clinical and analytic skills in deciding what is relevant and what is not.

Concluding

Reaching conclusions should present no problems once the interpretations have been made. At this time, the diagnostician reviews all data, analyses, and interpretations, and decides what statements, if any, can be made. The major decision typically is one of deciding whether or not the client has a speech problem. Basically, this is making a diagnosis. Assuming this decision is made, the next step of making recommendations logically follows.

Determine Whether Treatment Is Needed

Another part of the diagnostic procedure is to decide whether treatment is indicated, whether additional information should be obtained, or whether treatment should be deferred. Sometimes, treatment and additional information are needed. Sometimes, referral (such as for medical or dental treatment) is necessary, even though speech treatment is not contemplated or before treatment is begun. At this time in the diagnostic workup, the clinician's effectiveness can be enhanced by understanding norms and ethics and being familiar with the factors associated with the client's stimulability, motivation, age, etiology, and familial and psychosocial issues. Case selection is not easy. The clinician must have a clinical impression that the client can benefit from treatment and that the client wants (or can be persuaded to want) to improve speech. If there is any doubt about case selection or about the best way to alleviate the problem, the speech-language pathologist should seek the counsel of other professionals. State and federal regulations have helped the clinician to determine what constitutes a speech impairment in the schools. The final determination as to whether or not treatment is needed is not solely the clinician's decision. The client, caregivers, significant others, and/or the diagnostic team jointly make the determination.

Make Recommendations

One recommendation may have already been made, such as to treat or not to treat the individual's speech. Additionally, the diagnostician may need to make other recommendations such as health, allied health, educational, and psychological examinations or treatment. If speech treatment is recommended, specific recommendations will need to be made concerning the preferred treatment approaches, including where to begin, how to proceed, how many sessions per week, how long the sessions will be, and whether the better setting is group or individual. These recommendations should be made orally and in writing. All recommendations should be clearly stated. A statement about the prognosis should be included in the recommendations. A prognostic statement should include: "(1) a goal statement, (2) a judgment of success, and (3) the prognostic variables that lead to the prognosis" (Peña-Brooks & Hegde, 2000, p. 320). An example is: "The prognosis for producing velars, liquids, and stridents is good based on stimulability and family support." Prognostic variables include severity, nature of the disorder, causal factors, chronological age, motivation, capability, stimulability, inconsistency, associated behaviors, treatment history, and family support (Miccio, 2002; Peña-Brooks & Hegde, 2000). Prognostic factors as described by Peña-Brooks & Hegde appear in Table 6.12.

What methods are used in disseminating the results of the diagnostic workup?

TABLE 6.12

Client-Centered Prognostic Variables

Variable	Underlying Assumption
Severity	The more severe the disorder is, the poorer the prognosis. The less severe the disorder, the better the prognosis.
Chronological age	The younger the client is at the time of treatment, the better the prognosis. It may be easier to remediate articulation or phonological errors in a young child than an adolescent or adult.
Motivation	The less motivated the person is, the poorer the prognosis for improvement. The client who is highly motivated is more apt to have an "attitude" of learning. Such a client will likely follow through with assignments, treatment suggestions, and so forth. This variable is most significant with older elementary school children, adolescents, and adults. Young children may be much more motivated by external factors manipulated by the clinician.
Stimulability	The more stimulable the client is for an improved or correct production of the target sounds, the better the prognosis. A client with low stimulability may not do as well in treatment. However, this logical conclusion has not been strongly supported. Some children with poor stimulability do very well in treatment and vice versa.
Inconsistency	Inconsistency in sound production errors is often considered a positive prognostic variable. When errors can be produced correctly at least some of the time, they may be more amenable to correction once treatment is initiated.
Associated behaviors	Any behavior that may interfere with the client's progress in treatment is believed to have a negative impact on prognosis. A child with a limited attention span or poor cooperation, for example, may not learn as quickly as a child who is willing and ready to learn.
Treatment history	A child with a history of limited progress or poor maintenance of previously learned behaviors may have a poorer prognosis than a child absent of such history. Not every child comes with a history of speech-language pathology services. Thus, this variable may not apply to all clients.
Family support	The stronger the support extended by the client's family is, the better the prognosis for improvement. Research has continually documented that when the client's family takes an active role in treatment, the likelihood is higher that the client will maintain the skills learned in the clinical environment.
*Causal factors	Certain organic etiologies indicate poorer prognosis. Some perpetuating etiologies cannot be eliminated and thus will negatively impact treatment outcomes (such as dysarthrias, verbal apraxia, and total glossectomy). Precipitating causes that can be alleviated indicate a better prognosis.

*Variable added.

From Peña-Brooks, A., & Hegde, M. N. (2000). *Assessment & treatment of articulation and phonological disorders in children.* Austin, TX: Pro-Ed, Adapted with permission.

Disseminating Diagnostic Results, Conclusions, and Recommendations

After the conclusions have been reached, the diagnostician must formulate some recommendations if possible. There may be times when some recommendations have to be deferred because additional information is needed; however, suggesting that additional information is needed is in effect a recommendation. Sometimes, specific recommendations may not be possible because the gathered data are conflicting or contradictory. In this instance, the recommendation for further observation or more articulation testing may be in order, searching for additional trends or patterns. Never make a recommendation that is not scientifically or clinically justified and supported. Exercise caution in making recommendations and always have a rationale for each recommendation. When in doubt, seek the counsel of other professionals and consider more testing until your doubt can be eliminated.

Reporting

Reporting should be done orally and in writing. During the oral reporting, the clinician should make certain that the information is imparted clearly. Also, the clinician should allow the listener to seek clarification and to ask questions about anything that was previously reported. State your findings succinctly and emphasize your statement of the problem and of the treatment needs. Let the client or parents or caregivers know that a written report will follow that will reiterate what has been mentioned orally. If the recommendation is made to seek additional testing or examinations, then provide a list of names and addresses of where the client may receive assistance. This last step in the posttesting sequence is the important culmination step and the reason for having gone through all of the other steps in the diagnostic workup. Complete it tactfully.

Discuss the Findings

Orally sharing the interpreted speech data with parents, teachers, and others after the speech data have been collected, analyzed, and interpreted is one of the last steps in the diagnostic workup. The discussion should be friendly, objective, relaxing, concise, and intelligible. The clinician should avoid the use of esoteric labels and words that might best be described as professional jargon. The purpose of this step is to communicate concisely and effectively what was found and what is to be recommended. The clients and/or their parents or caregivers want to know whether a problem exists, the nature of the problem, the cause of it, the approach to alleviating it, and what are the chances of success (Tyler & Tolbert, 2002). Be careful not to overwhelm the client with excessive amounts of information. Ask for and answer any questions the clients or their representatives may have before terminating the discussion. Follow this oral presentation with a written report.

Write and Disseminate the Diagnostic Report

The final step in the diagnostic sequence is writing and distributing the diagnostic report. All too often this step is taken lightly, curtailed, hurried, or not done in a timely manner. Remember that the report is a written reflection of the diagnostician's competence and a document that may have to withstand a test of litigation at some time in the future. A well-written, carefully stated, well-documented clinical report is one that contains germane information and conveys the type of professional image that exemplifies the qualities of clinical excellence. With the caregiver's or client's consent, such a report should be distributed to the appropriate persons and agencies concerned about the client's welfare. This might include the referring persons or agency, family, physician, school, clinic, public health nurse, medical specialist, and parents.

SUMMARY

Assessment of articulation and phonology involves gathering and synthesizing information that leads to a diagnosis and recommendation for a treatment approach. The purposes of an initial assessment are to define the communication problem, ascertain the etiology if possible, and provide a clinical focus. Sometimes, a quick speech screening is initially done to identify clients who likely have a communication problem. An assessment battery is administered to individuals who potentially have an articulatory/phonologic disorder. Components of an assessment battery typically include a formal articulation or phonological test, stimulability testing, a connected speech sample, intelligibility measure, case history, hearing screening/assessment, oral-facial examination, specialized articulation/phonological tests, and a speech sound discrimination test (optional). It is important to gather several speech samples to obtain a representation of the client's articulation/phonological abilities. Ancillary assessments include oral sensation-perception, oral-facial myofunctional disability assessment, and phonological awareness. To get a complete picture of the client, the assessment should include the areas of language, voice, and fluency. Assigning a severity level and making a prognostic statement are a part of the process of diagnosing an articulatory/phonologic disorder.

Assessment is a challenging task. It requires a philosophy and understanding of basic principles of behavioral management; familiarity with articulation and phonological tests; knowledge of general characteristics and pertinent history of the client; understanding of formal and informal testing procedures; cognizance of assessing competencies and related structures; and ability to score, analyze, and interpret the collected data and organize them in an accurate, meaningful manner. Assessment requires the diagnostician to have established a frame of reference and standards with which to compare the anatomic, physiological, acoustic, and linguistic correlates of articulation and phonology. Implicit in all of these requirements are well-developed visual and auditory observation skills by the diagnostician, skills that nevertheless might need to render a tentative diagnosis while extending the diagnostic process beyond the initial workup and into the treatment process.

REVIEW QUESTIONS

1. What are the purposes of assessing articulatory/phonologic disorders?

2. Characterize the outcome of a screening of articulatory/phonologic disorders.

3. Differentiate between informal and formal screening procedures. What are three types of formal screening instruments?

4. What components are included in an assessment battery for articulatory/phonologic disorders?

5. What are the advantages of a formal articulation or phonological test? Of a connected speech sample?

6. Describe a traditional articulation test.

7. What information is generally obtained from a phonological deviation analysis?

8. How is stimulability of misarticulated sounds assessed? Why is it important to do?

9. What information is gleaned from a connected speech sample?

10. What are various methods of measuring intelligibility?

11. What are types of specialized articulation/phonological tests? Why might they be administered?

12. What are some approaches to gathering case history information? What types of information are gathered in a case history?

13. How can the case history help in diagnosing a communication problem?

14. Describe an oral-facial examination. What is the significance of an impaired speech mechanism?

15. Describe three clinical models: (a) medical, (b) behavioral, (c) systems.

16. How does a clinician assign a severity level?

17. What factors are considered in determining a prognosis?

18. What is involved in a planning assessment session?

19. What are procedures used in conducting the assessment session?

20. What steps are involved after the assessment battery has been administered?

CHAPTER 7

Transition from Assessment to Intervention of Articulatory/ Phonologic Disorders

"Words learned by rote, a parrot may rehearse."
—William Cowper

CHAPTER OBJECTIVES

- Specify the factors that are considered when determining the need for articulation/phonological treatment.
- Describe the relationship of articulation/ phonological treatment to language treatment as well as to treatment of other communication disorders.
- Describe intervention approaches for dealing with the co-occurence of articulatory/phonologic disorders and other communication disorders.
- Discuss the selection of an intervention approach for individual clients with articulatory/phonologic disorders.
- Present guidelines for implementing articulation/phonological intervention.
- Describe the general phases of articulation/phonological treatment.

After the diagnostic assessment is completed, the speech-language pathologist, in consultation with the client and others, such as parents, spouse, multidiscipline team, and teachers, needs to make several decisions regarding whether or not to intervene, what treatment approach to use, where to begin treatment, and so forth. During the assessment process, the clinician not only gathers information regarding the client's speech and language skills and related factors, but also formulates hypotheses regarding future intervention for the client. Some of the questions to answer when transitioning from assessment to intervention include:

- Is the client's communication system, including the articulation/phonological component, within the normal range of the client's linguistic community and age level?
- Is the client in need of an articulation/ phonological intervention program?

- Does the client have other concomitant communication disorders? If so, what approach will be used to deal with the multiple communication problems?
- Should a phonetic, phonological, or combination treatment approach be implemented for the articulatory/phonologic disorder?
- What are the terminal articulation/phonological objectives for the client?
- What are the initial targets of the treatment program?
- What steps should be carried out throughout the intervention?
- What specific sound elicitation techniques, stimulus materials, and clinical activities are to be used?

After analyzing the diagnostic information and consulting with the client and significant others, the speech-language clinician will plan the treatment, answering all or most of these questions. Of course, if the plan turns out to be ineffective for the client, the clinician will revise the plan and continue the treatment process until, hopefully, the objectives are accomplished by the client.

> What factors influence the communication patterns that fall within the range of normal limits?

RANGE OF COMMUNICATION PATTERNS WITHIN NORMAL LIMITS

Before discussing the need for articulation and phonological treatment, it must be emphasized that there is a wide range of communication patterns, including articulation, that falls within the normal limits of acceptability. As addressed in Chapter 4, not every speech difference is a speech disorder. Identifiable standards of language usage exist to which the oral communication of individuals can be compared. In the United States, there are three major dialectical regions—Eastern, Southern, and General American. Distinctive articulation patterns are used by members of each dialect, such as dropping vocalic /r/ by Eastern speakers and using diphthongs instead of vowels by Southern speakers. Differences also exist among speakers within the three regions related to subregional dialectical, ethnic, cultural, and socioeconomic groups. For example, the substitution of /θ/ for /f/ is generally acceptable in the African American language-speaking community. The substitution of /r/ for /l/ by English-speaking Japanese or of /j/ for /dʒ/ by speakers of Swedish origin are not considered articulatory disorders, but normal linguistic community differences.

Factors other than dialect influence judgment of normalcy of communication patterns. Sometimes, differences are accepted by some occupational communities, but not by others. Additionally, different situations for the same speaker may influence the phonological patterns used. An African American speaker might use mainstream American English when talking with a teacher, but use Black English when talking with peers. A college professor will probably use quite precise enunciation in giving a formal lecture and less precise articulation when talking at home with family members. The age of the speaker also influences whether a misarticulation is within normal limits; for example, it is acceptable for a 4-year-old child to substitute /w/

for /r/, but not for an adult speaker. Generally, typical dialectical, occupational, situational, and age differences in speech sound patterns are acceptable and thus are considered normal. A speech-language pathologist needs to be knowledgeable about expected speech patterns for individual clients relative to their linguistic community to provide appropriate service.

> What factors are considered when determining the need for articulation/phonological treatment in an individual client?

NEED FOR TREATMENT

Not every person who misarticulates is in need of articulation/phonological treatment. Analyzing the results of the assessment battery is important, but the decision for implementing intervention involves more than looking at standardized test scores. Clients who perform below the second percentile or more than 2 standard deviations below the mean on standardized articulation/phonological tests usually should be given high consideration for enrollment in a treatment program. In many school districts, the cutoff for inclusion in a speech-language pathology program is at the seventh percentile or 1.5 standard deviations below the mean.

Beyond test performance, the need for treatment is related to social, occupational, cultural, and ethnic aspects of the individual's environment. Thus, evaluation criteria for the adequacy of communication skills are based on social acceptability in the client's linguistic community. This principle is supported by Perkins (1978) who specified that two criteria for determining the extent to which misarticulations are a problem relate to cultural speech standards and vocational goals. When dealing with children, one must assume that the child needs a language system that is useful in many expanding and changing environments, and a system or systems to be used at home, away from home, with the same social group, and with others. Along these same lines, the probable or desired lifestyle or occupation of a person should be considered when determining need for treatment because articulation deficits may become a barrier to social and professional opportunities (Byrne & Shervanian, 1977; Van Riper & Erickson, 1996). To illustrate this point, several law students sought treatment for their /r/ misarticulations or lisping in a university clinic (where one of the authors of this text worked) as a requisite to continuing their pursuit of a law career. As reported in Chapter 1, several studies have shown that even a person with a so-called minor articulatory disorder is perceived negatively by some listeners.

Another factor in determining need for articulation/phonological treatment is the attitude of peers, family, and important others in the person's environment (Andrews, 1996; Andrews & Andrews, 2000; Johnson et al., 1967; Perkins, 1978; Van Riper & Erickson, 1996). How satisfied are individual speakers with their speech? How do parents and teachers view a child's speech? How do people in the environment evaluate a person's speech? Attitudes of speakers range from acknowledgment of the speech problem to rejection and insistence that the problem does not exist to intense concern or preoccupation with it. Important persons in the individual's environment sometimes react to articulation errors by rewarding them and sometimes by penalizing them. Such reactions must be considered in determining need for treatment.

The preceding discussion leads to two questions that must be considered when determining need for treatment. Is an articulation deviancy a problem if the client, family, teacher, or other important persons do not perceive it as one even though the speech-language pathologist does? Speech-language pathologists must be acutely aware of imposing their values on their clients. The misarticulations can be described in relation to normative data and other criteria and may be considered deficient, but if the primary persons in the client's environment do not see a need for treatment, then treatment probably should be deferred. Conversely, is there a problem when the client, family, teacher, or others perceive it as such, but the speech-language pathologist does not assess it to be a disorder? In this case, the clinician may choose to provide services or refer the client elsewhere. Before IDEA, one of the authors once enrolled a kindergarten boy in a public school speech program for misarticulation of /r/ because of student and parental concern. In this instance, the attitudes of the parent and child were the overriding consideration. However, if clinicians judge that they cannot help the client, ethically, treatment should not be implemented.

A third factor in determining need for treatment is the nature of the articulation/phonological deficiency itself; that is, the causes, severity, and effects on communication. Certainly, an important criterion for determining the extent of the problem is the intelligibility of the speaker. Additionally, the frequency with which articulation errors occur, the type of misarticulations (such as distortion,

substitution, omission, and addition), the phonological deviations used, and stimulability for correct production are important considerations. Relative to stimulability, considerable evidence exists that nonstimulable sounds are least likely to be acquired without intervention, and conversely, stimulable sounds are more likely to develop naturally through maturation (Miccio, Elbert, & Forrest, 1999; Powell, Elbert, & Dinnsen, 1991; Rvachew, Rafaat, & Martin, 1999). The consistency with which individual phonemes are misartiuclated is also a factor. One study showed that inconsistent sound substitutions/distortions produced by preschool children with phonological and language disorders was related to greater improvement in the percentage of correct consonants (PCC) after treatment as compared to children whose sound substitutions/distortions were less variable (Tyler, Lewis, & Welch, 2003). In other words, children who were inconsistent in their errors were shown to benefit most from intervention even though not all misarticulated sounds were targeted. Inconsistency accounted for 31% of the variance, meaning that there are other variables that account for improvement as a result of treatment. Finally, another important consideration is whether or not the misarticulations constitute typical or atypical patterns (Leonard, 1973). Examples of atypical productions include lateral lisps, omission of initial consonants, and substitution of glides for fricatives or stops for liquids (Table 3.2). Logically, atypical misarticulations are less likely to correct themselves spontaneously. The more unintelligible the person's speech is and the more conspicuous the speech is, the more severe the articulatory/phonologic disorder is and the greater the need for formal intervention. More frequently occurring errors, more consistency in misarticulated sounds, more frequently occurring phonological deviations, higher usage of atypical misarticulations, and poorer stimulability of misarticulated sounds are also related to a more severe disorder.

Age is also a critical factor in determining need for treatment, as explained in Chapter 3. Although some errors may normally persist until age 7 or 8, articulation/phonological treatment should not always be deferred until then. Postponing may, in fact, disable a child in the educational system, family, or community that rewards good oral communication skills and may result in embarrassment, isolation, and frustration for the child. In other words, developmental age levels of particular phonemes must be considered in determining need for intervention, along with other factors.

A final determining factor pertains to etiology of the disorder. One reason for differentiating between functional and organic causes is to acquire some idea about the seriousness of the communication problem and its possible prognosis. When serious organic causes exist, a client should usually be considered for treatment, regardless of chronologic age or developmental norms, provided, of course, the clinician thinks that intervention will be helpful.

Describe the relationship between treatment for articulatory/phonologic disorders and treatment for language disorders.

TREATMENT CONSIDERATIONS

Relationship Between Articulation/Phonological Treatment and Language Treatment

A discussion of articulation/phonological treatment in relation to language in general is important because articulation and phonology are actually an integral part of the total language system. As discussed in Chapter 6, language is comprised of five integral subsystems: semantics, syntax, phonology, morphology, and pragmatics. The way speech sounds are used is part of the language subsystem known as phonology; therefore, when articulation errors occur, the individual is using a sound system that is at variance with the adult system. Recent linguistic literature has led to a view of articulation as an integral part of the whole language system and of looking for patterns of misarticulations rather than considering each error separately. Articulation/phonological treatment, then, may be considered one dimension of language treatment, but it is confined to the phonemes of language. Thus, it is often differentiated from language treatment involving the other four language subsystems, namely semantics, syntax, morphology, and pragmatics. Articulation/phonological treatment is not to be confused with treatment of morphological errors, such as incorrect use of plurals, past tense verbs, or possessive nouns, nor is it involved with syntactic errors, such as incorrect noun-verb agreement. Different treatment approaches are needed for these types of errors. For example, articulation/phonological treatment should not be implemented for correction of /s/ and /z/ omissions if these omissions occur only in plural nouns or singular verbs or possessive nouns. Articulation/ phonological treatment also is not designed for teaching word meaning; a semantic language treatment approach is suggested.

The preceding statements do not mean that semantics, syntax, morphology, and pragmatics are not involved in articulation/phonological treatment, because the various subsystems of language cannot be completely separated as being mutually exclusive. When teaching correct articulation patterns, the phonemes are taught in the context of correct word forms, syntactic structures (phrases and sentences), word meaning, and appropriate relationships between words and expressions. Therefore, other areas of language may be learned incidentally, although they would not be the focus of the treatment program.

What is the relationship between articulation/phonological treatment and treatment for other communication disorders?

Relationship of Articulation/Phonological Treatment to Other Aspects of Communication

Just as articulation is intrinsically related to language, it is also an important component of communication. Communication has been defined as "any exchange of meaning between a sender and a receiver" (Gilham & Bedore, 2000, p. 27). It involves encoding, transmitting, and decoding messages and takes many forms, including speaking, listening, reading, writing, and using gestures and other forms of nonverbal communication. The speech and hearing communication process is one of the primary modes of communication among human beings. Because it involves at least two people—a speaker and a listener—oral communication is a complex interaction. The information-giver selects and produces symbols to convey an idea, and the receiver perceives and interprets the symbols and responds accordingly.

Communication processes include the five subsystems of language, speech, paralinguistics, nonlinguistics, and **metalinguistics** (Owens, 2002). Paralinguistics refers to the suprasegmentals; that is, intonation, stress, rate, and timing. Nonlinguistic components include gestures, body posture, facial expression, eye contact, head and body movement, and physical distance between the speakers or proxemics. Metalinguistic cues "can signal the status of communication based on our intuitions about the acceptability of utterances. . . . The focus is on what is transmitted but also how this is accomplished" (Owens, p. 31). Oral communication also involves hearing, and cognition (awareness, perception, conceptualization, differentiation, and thought, which enables comprehension, interpretation, and symbol usage). Interpersonal relations are another component of communication. How a speaker's message is interpreted by the listener depends on the previously named factors and probably others. The speaker's articulation skills influence the accuracy with which a message is understood. Certainly, articulation contributes greatly to the intelligibility of a speaker's message; that is, how much of the message is understood. Consequently, a person with an articulatory/phonologic disorder may have a communication handicap. The severity of the communication disability of a person with an articulatory/phonologic disorder is related to the degree of unintelligibility, number of misarticulated sounds and phonological deviations, specific sounds that are misarticulated, type of misarticulation or phonological deviation, consistency of error sounds, and personal and social speech standards and attitudes. When treatment of an articulatory/phonologic disorder improves articulation skills, communication with others will be enhanced.

During articulation/phonological treatment, other aspects of communication cannot be ignored because articulation of sounds does not occur in isolation but rather overlaps with the other parameters of speech production. For example, appropriate speaking rate, correct pronunciation of words, appropriate inflectional patterns, appropriate loudness levels, fluency, and other intelligibility factors should be a part of the practice material. Correct speech sound patterns must be incorporated into everyday communication situations under the guidance of the speech-language pathologist.

> What diagnostic categories are factors in selecting a treatment approach?

Diagnostic Considerations

Some diagnostic categories may determine the treatment approach selected by the speech-language pathologist. One such differentiation is phonetic versus phonological errors. A phonetic error is one in which there is a seeming inability to produce such a sound motorically. This is likely to happen in dysarthrias, apraxias, facial and oral structural anomalies, physiological deficits, and hearing loss. Phonological errors are those in which the individual can motorically produce the correct sounds, but has not mastered the sound system of the language; that is, the phonological or cognitive rules. These errors may also be present in auditory perceptual deficits and in many so-called "functional" disorders cases. It is difficult to state generalities about causes of phonetic and phonological errors because each client must be evaluated on an individual basis and because individual clients often display both phonetic and phonological errors. Certain treatment approaches seem best suited for phonetic errors, whereas others are more helpful for phonological errors, as will be pointed out in Chapters 8 and 9.

A second diagnostic differentiation relates to delayed versus deviant articulation. Delayed articulation refers to following the normal sequence of development, but at a slower rate. The system used is less mature than the adult system. Examples of normal misarticulations are w/r, θ/s, b/v, and f/θ. Children in this category who are 7 years or younger with normal intelligence and without other deficits may acquire normal articulation without intervention, although not always. Cases of deviant articulation are those in which a normal pattern of development is not followed; that is, the misarticulations are different from those of children in the normal process of articulation development. Examples are omissions of initial consonants, gliding of fricatives, and lateralized sibilants. Individuals who show such disordered speech sound patterns usually will not spontaneously correct their errors. Leonard (1973) urged that individuals with deviant articulation patterns be given priority for treatment over persons with delayed articulation. Whether the client has delayed or disordered phonology, treatment is indicated when he or she is 4 years or older and is unintelligible.

Third, the speech-language pathologist needs to differentiate childhood apraxia of speech from dysarthria, language disorder, and functional articulatory disorders, which are formidable tasks indeed (Tables 7.1 and 7.2). In childhood apraxia of speech, articulation treatment can be an arduous process requiring an inordinate amount of treatment time (Caruso & Strand, 1999; Yorkston et al., 1999; Yoss & Darley, 1974). "Even with intense stimulation by the clinician the children experience persistent difficulty repeating phonemes and words" (Chappell, 1973, p. 362). Traditional articulation treatment does not seem to be effective with children who have dyspraxia. To plan effective treatment, it is critical to diagnose childhood apraxia of speech differentially.

TABLE 7.1

Comparison of Apraxia of Speech with Dysarthria

Apraxia of Speech	Dysarthria
Absence of significant paresis, paralysis, ataxia, incoordination of the speech muscles; therefore, client has little difficulty with involuntary oral motor acts such as chewing, swallowing, sucking, and licking	Presence of paresis, paralysis, ataxia, incoordination, involuntary movements; speech behavior and vegetative functions of chewing, swallowing, sucking, and licking reflect types and severity of neurological disease or damage
Inconsistency in articulation performance and difficulty in predicting errors	Speech errors are relatively consistent and predictable
Difficulty with speech initiation, selection of phonemes, and sequencing phonemes	Little difficulty with speech initiation, selection or phonemes, and sequencing phonemes
Most common types of articulation errors are substitutions and repetitions; occasional metathetic errors	Articulation errors are primarily distortions
Increased speaking rate results in improved articulation	Increased speaking rate results in deterioration of intelligibility
More accurate speech production in spontaneous speech, poorer in reading and in imitative activities	Speech production accuracy does not vary appreciably in spontaneous speech, reading, and imitative activities
Discrepancy between voluntary, purposeful, and spontaneous reflexive performance; the former is much more difficult	Accuracy of articulation does not vary appreciably with the situation
Rate, rhythm, and stress (prosody) of speech adversely affected by repetitions, hesitations, and groping for correct articulation positions	Slow, labored speaking rate is present with evidence of strain and tension, especially for difficult consonant clusters; often difficulty with breath control results in inappropriate phrasing, and inappropriate silent intervals
Articulation performance poorer as words increase in length and complexity	Articulation performance is less affected by word length
Result of motor programming deficiency	Result of motor execution deficiency
Oral nonverbal apraxia often present	Absent oral nonverbal apraxia

SELECTION OF AN INTERVENTION APPROACH

After making the diagnosis of articulatory/phonologic disorder and after determining a need for articulation/phonological treatment, the speech-language pathologist must select a treatment approach and design an intervention program for each individual client.

Describe four approaches for treating the concurrence of articulatory/phonologic disorders and one or more other communication disorders.

Multiple Communication Disorders

Oftentimes, clients will present with articulatory/phonologic disorders concomitant with one or more other speech and/or language disorders. In this case, the clinician must decide how to deal with the various communication disorders. Will two or more communication problems be addressed simultaneously, concurrently, cyclically, or sequentially?

Concurrence of Phonological and Language Disorders

Some limited research has looked at the earlier question as it relates to expressive language, but the results have been inconclusive. These studies

TABLE 7.2

Case History Information Contrasted for Developmental Speech Delay and Childhood Apraxia of Speech

Interview Topic	Developmental Speech Delay*	Childhood Apraxia of Speech**
Medical history	Frequent history of otitis media, including the need for pressure-equalizing tubes	May coexist with particular genetic syndromes (e.g., Down, fragile X) History of neurological disease or damage more common
Developmental history	Relatively infrequent reporting of feeding problems Relatively normal milestones regarding quantity of speech	Feeding problems Little vocal play or babbling Little imitation in infancy Delayed language onset One-time use of word token reported
Family history	One or more family members with a history of the same speech disorder	Suspected childhood apraxia of speech in family member Other communication disorders, including written communication disorders in family history
Communication skills	Increased risk for receptive language problems Greatly increased risk for expressive language problems	Frequent concurrent language problems, especially involving expressive language
Psychosocial skills	Relatively frequent concerns about effectiveness of parental behavior management and for parental concerns regarding child's ability to gain acceptance from peers Very common concerns about the child's increased sensitivity (e.g., feelings easily hurt)	Behavioral disorders because of frustration Temper tantrums, inflexibility, excessive motor activity, and withdrawal also noted
Motor skills: fine and gross, excluding oromotor	Few concerns about gross or fine motor skills	Gross/fine motor incoordination not uncommon
Oromotor skills	Few concerns about oromotor skills	Observed abnormalities in movement patterns observed during feeding Observed abnormalities in movement patterns observed during imitative play with sounds or facial expressions
Current medical status	Few neurological concerns Current concerns regarding middle ear disease not uncommon	Soft neurological signs frequently noted
Other observations	Generally good or at least acceptable progress in speech treatment	Slow progress in treatment

*Data from Shriberg & Kwiatkowski (1994).
**Data from Blakeley (1983), Hall, Jordan, and Robin (1993), Hodge and Hancock (1994), Rapin and Allen (1981), and Shriberg et al. (1997).
From Strand E. A., & McCauley R. J. (1999). Assessment procedures for treatment planning in children with phonologic and motor speech disorders. In A. J. Caruso & E. A. Strand (Eds). *Clinical Management of motor speech disorders in children* (pp. 73–107). New York: Thieme. Reprinted with permission.

explored the effects of language treatment on the phonological production skills of children who have phonological and language disorders. Some studies demonstrated that speech sound production skills improved in children who received language intervention (Hoffman, Norris, & Monjure, 1990; Matheny & Panagos, 1978; Tyler, Lewis, Haskill, & Tolbert, 2002; Wilcox & Morris, 1995) while other studies did not show such improvement (Fey et al., 1994; Tyler & Sandoval, 2004). Similarly, some research has shown that morphological skills improved in children who received phonological intervention (Bopp, 1995; Matheny & Panagos, 1978; Tyler & Sandoval, 1993; Tyler & Watterson, 1991), while others did not show language gains (Duder, Camarata, Camarata, Koegel, & Koegel, 1998). As might be expected, children in the Matheny and Panagos (1978) study showed the most gains in the domain targeted (such as articulation or language); that is, children receiving articulation treatment improved more in speech sound production and those receiving language treatment improved more in language skills. Phonological and language treatments were administered cyclically in the Tyler et al. (2002) study with one half of the subjects receiving phonological intervention first, followed by morphosyntactic treatment, with the other half receiving the interventions in the reverse order. Both groups improved significantly in speech sound production and morphosyntactical skills after 24 weeks of treatment. Interestingly, the phonological skills of the children improved after receiving 12 weeks of either phonological or language in-

tervention, and they improved even more after receiving an additional 12 weeks of either type of intervention. On the other hand, the morphosyntactical production of children receiving the phonological treatment did not improve significantly until after receiving the language treatment.

In consideration of the equivocal results of the various studies of children with concomitant articulatory/phonologic and language disorders, what approaches seem to be the most effective? The choices are simultaneous or blended, concurrent, cyclic, and sequential (Table 7.3). If the goal is to facilitate improvement in both domains, the cyclic and concurrent approaches seem to be called for. In the cyclic approach, each disorder is treated for specific time periods, alternating between the two disordered areas. In the concurrent approach, both disorders are treated for equal amounts of time in the same session. A potential problem for a blended (i.e., simultaneous) approach in which both disorders are treated simultaneously is that the linguistic system may be overly burdened with phonological and morphological/syntactical demands being placed on the client at the same time. Alternatively, the sequential approach in which one disorder is treated before the other one would be appropriate if one of the two domains—phonology or language—has a higher priority. For example, a clinician may choose to administer phonological intervention first in a child who is unintelligible rather than focusing on morphology and syntax first because one's inability to be understood is significantly more devastating than the misuse of morphemes and word arrangement.

TABLE 7.3

Treatment Strategies for Clients with a Phonologic Disorder Concomitant with a Language, Fluency, or Voice Impairment

Treatment Strategy	Description
Simultaneous (Blended)	Incorporate goals for language, voice, or fluency while targeting articulation/phonological objectives; both disorders are targeted at the same time.
Concurrent	Equal amounts of treatment for two disorders in the same session. In the case of concomitant phonologic and fluency disorders, avoid providing feedback for articulation errors.
Cyclic	Alternating treatment for each disorder for a specified time period. For example, target articulation/phonology objectives for one session and fluency targets during the next session.
Sequential	Treat one disorder until all targets are met for that disorder then follow with treatment for the other disorder.

Concurrence of Articulatory/Phonologic and Other Speech Disorders

Articulatory/phonologic disorders can also occur concomitantly with stuttering and voice disorders. Again, the simultaneous or blended, concurrent, cyclic, and sequential approaches are options in these cases. For concurrent stuttering/phonologic disorders, a survey of clinicians showed that the blended (simultaneous) approach is the treatment of choice in 45% of the cases, and 21% are treated concurrently (Arndt & Healey, 2001). In the blended and concurrent approaches, neither disorder goes untreated.

No matter which intervention strategy is employed with a concomitant stuttering problem, prudent treatment targets speech sounds in a relaxed, nondemanding environment. The client is encouraged to produce the target sounds with loose articulation contacts, perhaps with a relaxed, slightly breathy voice to reduce tense speech production. The clinician should always model the targets and speak in the same manner to demonstrate that speech can be easy. Usually, fast drill work or timed responses are not used with these clients because such techniques may place undue pressure on them. Sometimes, it is helpful to teach clients progressive relaxation to relax the speech structures. Occasionally, a young client who does not normally stutter begins using dysfluencies while receiving articulation/phonological treatment in or out of the clinic. In these cases, the recommendation is to provide a relaxed speaking environment in as many speaking situations as possible, including the clinic, home, and school. Parents, teachers, and clinicians need to work together to monitor the client's fluency and to react in a manner that facilitates fluency. The clinician's role is to guide parents in using effective communication strategies to increase fluency.

A review of the professional literature demonstrated that treatment of clients with concomitant articulatory/phonologic and voice/resonance disorders has not been the focus of research studies. The same four treatment approaches (Table 7.3) are applicable for these cases as well. For clients with hyperfunctional voice problems, modeling and instructing the client to use soft articulation contacts and soft or breathy, relaxed glottal attacks while producing the targets in clinic and when speaking is helpful. For clients with hypernasality, precise articulation and optimal oral resonance and oral cavity opening often help to camouflage the excessive nasal resonance and nasal air flow.

> When is it appropriate to select a phonetic treatment approach? When is a phonological treatment approach appropriate?

Articulation/Phonological Treatment Approaches

When articulation/phonological treatment is implemented, the first decision is to determine whether a phonetic or phonological treatment approach should be implemented. Phonetic approaches focus on individual speech sound targets, whereas phonological approaches focus on speech sound patterns. Generally speaking, phonetic approaches are most appropriate when the disorder is characterized as a motor or phonetic problem. This is often the case with a structural, physiological, neuromuscular, or sensory etiology. Phonetic approaches are also indicated when a client is intelligible, uses only a few misarticulated sounds, or distorts speech sounds. Specific phonetic treatment approaches are described in Chapter 8. Phonological approaches, on the other hand, are appropriate when the speech sound disorder is characterized as a phonological or linguistic problem. Traditionally, these disorders have been labeled *functional* or nonorganic. Phonological approaches are indicated for clients who are unintelligible and who have multiple misarticulated sounds. However, phonological approaches generally are not indicated for older clients (8 years and older) who have childhood apraxia of speech. Specific phonological treatment approaches are described in Chapter 9.

Consideration of Phonetic Treatment Approaches

When a phonetic approach is used, the following questions need to be addressed:

- How many sounds will be taught at a time?
- Which sound or sounds will be taught first?
- Will specific auditory training or speech perception training be needed?

Traditionally, treatment is begun with work on one or two phonemes if they are cognates of one another; for example, /s/ and /z/ or /t/ and /d/. When carryover on the first sound is occurring, work can begin on a second one while continuing with the generalization stage of the first. One possible exception to the recommendation of working with only one sound at a time is with adults or older children who may be more motivated and better able to handle three or more sounds at a time. More than one sound may also be treated at a time when the treatment method specifies so; for example, motokinesthetic (Young & Hawk, 1938; Young & Stinchfield-Hawk, 1955), multiple phonemic (Bradley, 1989; McCabe & Bradley, 1975), and the wedge (Sommers & Kane, 1974) methods described in Chapter 8.

Target Phoneme Selection

There are several criteria to aid in selection of target phonemes (Table 7.4). It is advisable to begin with a misarticulated phoneme or phonemes that are relatively easy for clients to produce. Some of the following criteria are related to that guideline, but others are concerned with client desires and the contribution of phonemes to improving communication.

- *Phoneme that is the earliest to develop.* Phonemes appearing earliest in speech developmental norms are often presumed to be the easiest to produce, but this is not the case for some clients. Using this criterion means applying the normative approach to target selection.
- *Phoneme that is later developing.* In contrast to the preceding guideline, a nontraditional concept is to target later developing phonemes when initiating articulation/phonological treatment. The rationale for this approach is that targeting later developing sounds will result in greater change in the phonological system (Gierut, Morrisette, Hughes, & Rowland, 1996); however, the results of recent studies have not supported this approach (Williams, 2003).
- *Phoneme that is the most stimulable.* Traditionally, clinicians select a speech sound that is stimulable, such as when the client can imitate the clinician's production of the target sound in

isolation, syllables, words, or phrases. The rationale is that if a phoneme can be produced correctly following auditory stimulation, it probably is not difficult for the client to learn and would be a good place to begin because the client will likely be successful. However, occasionally carryover can be very difficult for a phoneme that is quite stimulable. Other potential target phonemes are those that can be elicited with techniques other than auditory/visual stimulation (Chapter 10).

- *Phoneme that is not stimulable.* Contrary to the above guideline, a nontraditional approach is to select a speech sound that is not stimulable (Williams, 2003). The rationale is that stimulable sounds may develop naturally on their own without direct treatment (Miccio et al., 1999; Powell et al., 1991). Other research has not supported this contention (Rvachew et al., 1999; Rvachew & Nowak, 2001).
- *Phoneme that is produced correctly in a key word.* A key word is a word in which the client correctly produces the misarticulated sound in a spontaneous speech sample (Van Riper & Erickson, 1996). Elicitation of the sound then can begin with a key word. Such words should be noted by the diagnostician when obtaining a speech sample or otherwise interacting with the client. There are also published tests designed to reveal words and phonetic contexts in which clients correctly articulate a speech sound that they typically misarticulate. These tests are described in Chapter 6.
- *Phoneme that occurs most frequently in speech.* Certain sounds occur often in the English language, whereas others seldom are used (Table 2.4). The Arizona (Fudala, 2000) bases the total articulation score on the frequency of occurrence of phonemes. The Weiss Comprehensive Articulation Test (W-CAT) (Weiss, 1980) lists the relative frequency of English phonemes. Those that are used more frequently presumably have a higher impact on intelligibility and therefore are more important to communication. Select an error sound that when corrected will most improve intelligibility. For example, correction of /s/, relative frequency of 7.47%, is more critical to intelligibility than /ʃ/, that has a relative frequency of 0.88%.
- *Phoneme that is visible.* The production of some phonemes can be easily seen by watching the speaker's mouth, whereas the production of other phonemes cannot. Examples of the former are bilabials, labiodentals, linguadentals, alveolars, and some palatals. Examples of articulation placements that are not visible are glides, some palatals, velars, and glottals. It is usually

TABLE 7.4

Selection Criteria for Which Phonemes to Target

Criteria for Selecting Phoneme Targets

Earlier developing phoneme

Later developing phoneme

Stimulable phoneme

Nonstimulable phoneme

Phoneme produced correctly in a key word

Frequently occurring phoneme

Visible phoneme (i.e., labials, dentals, alveolars, some palatals)

Consistently misarticulated phoneme

Phoneme client/others desire to target

Phoneme for which client has been criticized or penalized

Phoneme that is omitted or has an atypical substitution

Phoneme least affected by physical limitations

Same phoneme for a group of clients

easier to teach the visible sounds first because visual as well as auditory stimulation is salient, and clients can see in a mirror whether or not they are accurately placing their articulators as they try to imitate the clinician's articulation placement.

- *Phoneme that is most consistently misarticulated.* Generally, those sounds that are most consistently misarticulated are the ones in greatest need of treatment. Error sounds that are inconsistently produced, such as those produced correctly sometimes and incorrectly other times and in other contexts, are more frequently corrected through maturation without intervention. For this reason, the error sound that is most consistently misarticulated should be considered a high priority for selection in treatment. There is some evidence that it is more fruitful to target sounds that are produced with various substitution errors and omissions, including sometimes omitting /k/, other times using a t/k substitution, other times using a d/k substitution, and still others using a p/k substitution, rather than sounds that are consistently misarticulated with the same error (Tyler et al., 2003).

- *Phoneme that the client/significant others most desire to correct.* Sometimes, clients or their significant others have a preference for beginning with a particular phoneme. This may be a sound that occurs in the client's name or address and therefore is used frequently, or it may be an error sound that has brought the most negative reactions. There are many other reasons for such client desires, and the speech-language pathologist should certainly consider them when deciding where to start. Targeting such sounds may be particularly motivating for the client unless the sounds are extremely difficult for the client to produce.

- *Phoneme for which the client has been most criticized or penalized.* Many clients have received negative reactions for misarticulating particular sounds because of the conspicuousness of the errors. A lateral lisp, nasalized production of /s/ and /z/, a w/r substitution, and facial contortions simultaneously accompanying sound production are examples of articulation and associated errors that may be conspicuous to listeners and can result in teasing, frowning, or other undesirable listener reactions. If a client corrects such errors, self-concept and attitudes toward speech should be enhanced.

- *Phoneme that is omitted or has an atypical substitution.* The type of misarticulation is also an important variable in deciding with which

sound to begin. Presumably, speech sounds that are omitted or have unusual substitution patterns compromise intelligibility. Targeting these types of misarticulated sounds will likely increase intelligibility, which is an important goal of articulation/phonological treatment.

- *Phoneme whose production is least affected by physical limitations.* There are many instances in which articulation skills are complicated by organic causal factors. Again, ease of production is important in deciding where to start; therefore, physical complications must be considered. For example, it often is easier for clients with cleft palate to produce nonpressure sounds than pressure sounds. Children whose upper central incisors are missing will probably experience more difficulty with /s/ and /z/ than with /l/, /k/, and /g/.

- *Phoneme that is the same for a group of clients.* In some clinical settings, especially schools, articulation/phonological treatment may be administered to a small group of clients. The selection of a sound that is misarticulated by all members of a group has some advantages in that all would work on the same sound at the same time.

Speech Perception Training

Much has been written about the relationship between speech perception and articulation/phonological skills. Various opinions are held regarding whether or not to include perception training (variously called auditory training, ear training, and speech sound discrimination training) as part of the treatment for articulatory disorders. For example, Van Riper and Erickson (1996) generally recommended auditory training for all "functional" articulation cases; Winitz (1975) advocated it for many clients, but not all; McDonald (1964b) did not recommend it for any; and Rvachew (1994) recommended it for selected clients. The rationale for implementing auditory training is that speech is learned through the ear. A person has to hear a sound several times before all its salient features are perceived. In other words, the client must be able to detect not only the error, but also the correct sound before attempting to produce it. On the other hand, the rationale for not using auditory training is that individuals usually can learn to produce sounds correctly without it. In fact, discrimination between correct and incorrect productions is probably learned during production training when the clinician provides feedback as to the correctness of the sound produced (Williams & McReynolds, 1975). Proceeding directly to production training seems to be more efficient.

Before deciding whether or not to use auditory training, research results should be considered. Studies on the relationship between speech sound discrimination/speech perception and articulation have been conflicting and inconclusive. Individuals with deviant articulation/phonology seem to have poorer speech perception ability. Refer to Chapter 5 for a review of some of these studies.

Some research has been done to determine if discrimination training has any effect on misarticulations and if production training has any effect on discrimination ability. Briefly, traditional auditory discrimination is done by having clients identify the target sound in a variety of contexts, differentiate that sound from other speech sounds in a variety of contexts, and sometimes evaluate their own productions of the target sound in a variety of contexts (i.e., self-discrimination). Some of the earlier studies tended to look at general discrimination training that did not focus on the target sound. Shelton, Johnson, Ruscello, and Arndt (1978) found that there was no difference in articulation skills between preschool children trained by their parents in speech sound discrimination and children who received no such training. Williams and McReynolds (1975) found that discrimination training improved discrimination ability, but not production of sounds. Conversely, production training improved articulation and discrimination skills. They hypothesized that during production training, discrimination training is simultaneously occurring because the client receives feedback on both acoustic and articulation aspects of productions. Also, clients are hearing a model of correct sounds and are comparing their own productions to that model; therefore, production training may be sufficient to train discrimination or perhaps it is training discrimination simultaneously. However, Winitz (1975) contended that discrimination training will improve articulation if the distinctive features of the misarticulated sounds are in the repertoire of the individual and if the training is extensive and carefully carried out.

Later studies looked at the impact of speech perception training that emphasized the misarticulated sound. In a single subject design study, Jamieson and Rvachew (1992) found that speech perception training can facilitate sound production for some children. Rvachew (1994) found that the articulation skills of children with phonologic disorders improved with speech perception training that was directed toward the misarticulated sound and was provided concurrently with speech sound production training for the same sound. Children who received general perceptual training using nontarget sounds showed lesser ability to produce

the target sound than children who received perceptual training to discriminate between correct production of the target sound versus incorrect production in words as well as children who received training to differentiate between the target sound produced correctly versus a maximally contrasted sound. From her results, Rvachew recommended the following:

- Incorporate perceptual training with children who show difficulties with both the perception and production of the targeted sound contrast.
- Provide production training either along with or shortly after the perceptual training. It was noted that children who were most successful were those who received speech perception training for their misarticulated sounds and who also eventually became stimulable for the misarticulated sound in the production part of treatment.
- Use perceptual contrasts using the misarticulated sound, beginning with a maximal opposition contrast; for example, for /s/, begin with /s/ and /m/ and end with minimal contrasts; use with /s/ and /ʃ/, /s/ and laterally distorted /s/).
- Vary the stimulus from "good quality exemplars" to "more ambiguous exemplars" throughout the training using a variety of speakers.
- Perhaps use amplification during the perceptual training.
- Use a computer-driven feedback procedure if possible. This seemed to engage the children during the perception training tasks.

Thus far, the discussion has been about interpersonal speech perception; that is, clients are making judgments about sounds produced externally by other persons. Intrapersonal perception also has been used as a clinical technique. In this case, clients evaluate their own productions. In self-discrimination tasks, clients evaluate their productions of a target phoneme and record each production as correct or incorrect. This strategy, used in conjunction with production training, has been shown to be effective in generalization of the target sound to outside clinic settings (Ingham & Parks, 1989; Koegel, Koegel, & Ingham, 1986; Koegel, Koegel, Van Voy, & Ingham, 1988; Shriberg & Kwiatkowski, 1987). However, these results were not replicated by Gray and Shelton (1992).

Every speech-language pathologist must consider the preceding information in view of the fact that testing self-discrimination is difficult, and then decide whether or not to incorporate specific auditory training in articulation treatment. Spending much time on auditory training with individuals who can already discriminate their misarticulation from the correct sound would not be efficient. Assessment of the client's auditory perceptual ability must be done to determine this, but there are no published tests available to do this (Gray & Shelton, 1992). Rather, speech-language pathologists must rely upon results of criterion-referenced assessment procedures. It is probably more expedient to teach the client to discriminate between the error sound and the correct sound than to teach general discrimination skills. If discrimination work is done, the sounds should be presented in sentences in addition to isolation and individual words. If speech discrimination activities are included, they should be arranged in a hierarchical order of difficulty and should require the client to be an active participant, especially in learning self-monitoring. Incorporate auditory training with production work; that is, clients should be asked to evaluate their own productions during the latter stages of treatment. Whether or not specific auditory training is done and how it is done will be determined by the treatment approach selected, the needs of the client, and the skills of the clinician.

Phonological Treatment Approach Considerations

When a phonological approach is used, the following questions need to be addressed:

- Which phonological methodology will be implemented?
- Which distinctive features or phonological patterns will be targeted?
- Will speech perception training be incorporated?
- Will the client practice the targeted patterns in nonmeaningful material as well as in meaningful contexts?

Four strategies have been used for targeting phonological patterns in contrast to individual speech sounds in the phonetic approaches:

- Cycling
- Distinctive features
- Contrasting pairs
- Nonlinear

In the distinctive features method, *distinctive features*, such as back and strident, are targeted in the context of two or more phonemes, with one phoneme containing the feature to be learned and the other phoneme not containing the feature. When possible, the two phonemes used should contain the same bundle of features except for the feature being targeted. For example, /k/ and /t/, /g/ and /d/, and /n/ and /ŋ/ would be appropriate minimal pairs for teaching the back feature. (Tables 2.7,

2.8, and 2.9 and Appendix B display distinctive feature systems.) In the phonological *cycling* strategy, phonological sound patterns (such as final consonants, stridency, clusters) are targeted through exemplar sounds/contexts (such as final /p/, final /t/) for a specified period of time. Two strategies used in the **contrasting pairs approach** include minimal contrasting pairs and maximal contrasting pairs. In the contrasting pairs strategy, sets of two words are used as exemplars to demonstrate the phonological pattern (such as clusters versus cluster reduction, stridents versus stridency deletion, final consonants versus final consonant deletion) that is to be learned. One word contains the pattern, and the other word does not. In the minimal word pairs strategy, the word pair stimuli are the same except for the pattern to be learned; for example, *meat* and *me* to teach final consonants. In contrast, the maximal word pairs approach uses word pairs with sounds that are maximally contrasting; for example, *thumb* and *gum*. Finally, in the nonlinear phonology approach, the cycling strategy is used; however, the basis for target selection differs from the phonological cycling approach developed by Hodson and Paden (1991), which will be described in Chapter 9.

When is it appropriate to use each of the phonological intervention approaches briefly described above? Limited research helps answer this question. Generally, all of these approaches have been shown to be effective for some clients and for some patterns (e.g., Carver, 1997; Gierut, 1989, 1990a; Royer, 1995; Saben & Ingham, 1991; Tyler, Edwards, & Saxman, 1987; Tyler & Sandoval, 1994). The cycling approach often is effective with preschool children who present with multiple misarticulations, multiple phonological deviations, and unintelligibility. During later stages of treatment with these children, minimal contrasting word pairs is sometimes called for when carryover of the patterns produced in clinical sessions does not occur to conversational speech and to other settings. The contrasting approaches seem to be difficult for most young children to handle and thus are more appropriate for older clients. The nonlinear approach requires a comprehensive analysis that is quite time-consuming. In some cases, such an analysis may be necessary to determine the contexts in which correct speech patterns are not being used.

Target Distinctive Feature/Phonological Pattern Selection

Several criteria exist to aid in selection of distinctive features and phonological patterns. Some of these overlap with phoneme selection criteria that were presented earlier in this chapter.

- *Distinctive features/patterns that are developed earlier.* Distinctive features and phonological patterns that appear earlier presumably are the easiest to produce. By using this criterion, one can apply a normative strategy for target selection.
- *Distinctive features/patterns that are stimulable.* In phonological treatment approaches, the client produces the speech sound patterns to be learned and, in some instances, contrasts the target with patterns the client is already using. Thus, the client needs to be able to produce sounds that are exemplars for the targeted distinctive feature/pattern as well as the contrast patterns. If the client does not produce the exemplars with auditory/visual stimulus, other techniques, such as phonetic placement, motokinesthetic stimulation, and progressive approximation, are used to elicit the exemplar sounds. For clients to be successful in improving phonological production, they need to have the requisite motor skills necessary for articulating speech sounds.
- *Distinctive features/patterns that are not stimulable.* One strategy used in phonological treatment approaches is to select distinctive features or phonological patterns that are not readily stimulable; that is, the client does not imitate them with auditory/visual stimulation only. As mentioned earlier, clients need to learn to produce the sounds and sound contexts to incorporate correct speech sound patterns into their repertoire. The clinician then needs to use other techniques to elicit the speech sounds in various positions and contexts within words, phrases, and sentences. Often, these are the traditional speech sound elicitation techniques used in phonetic approaches.

- *Distinctive features/patterns that most affect intelligibility.* Generally, phonological treatment approaches are used with clients who have multiple misarticulations and who exhibit various degrees of unintelligibility. A practical strategy is to select targets that will result in increased intelligibility as quickly as possible. Some research has been conducted to identify phonological deviations that compromise speech intelligibility (Hodson, 2004; Hodson & Paden, 1981, 1991). These are appropriate initial targets (Table 7.5).
- *Distinctive features/patterns that are not being used consistently.* Generally, all else being equal, the deviant distinctive feature errors and phonological patterns that are used more consistently are the ones in greatest need of treatment. Because acquisition of the adult sound system is a gradual process, those patterns that are sometimes used correctly and sometimes not may be in the process of being acquired naturally. In the phonological cycling program developed by Hodson and Paden (1991), the correct patterns used in less than 60% of the opportunities are to be targeted, while those that are used more than 60% of the time need not be targeted.
- *Sound or distinctive feature that is used in other contexts.* Several individual speech sounds are used in a particular phonological pattern. For example, the stridency pattern consists of the strident sounds used in all three positions of words and in clusters, and the final consonant pattern includes all the consonants except for the glides /w/ and /j/. Sometimes, a client produces a particular sound in one phonological pattern but not in another pattern. An example is a client who produces singleton /t/ in the initial position of words, but not in word final

TABLE 7.5

Phonological Deviations Associated with Unintelligible Speech

Most Frequently Occurring	Frequently Occurring	Less Frequently Occurring
Cluster reduction	Final consonant deletion	Metathesis
Stridency deletion	Velar deviations	Coalescence
Stopping	Backing	Epenthesis
Liquid deviations	Syllable reduction	Reduplication
Assimilation	Prevocalic voicing	Diminutive
	Glottal replacement	

Hodson, B. W., & Paden, E. P. (1981). Phonological processes that characterize unintelligible and intelligible speech in early childhood. *Journal of Speech and Hearing Disorders, 46,* 369–373.

position nor in clusters. In the early stages of treatment for this client, word-final /t/ probably would be a good choice when the pattern of final consonants is being targeted, or initial /st/ or final /ts/ would be appropriate choices when the target pattern is clusters. The strategy of using sounds in individual clients' phonemic inventory to establish unused phonological patterns takes advantage of their motor ability to produce the sounds.

Phonological Approach Treatment Techniques

In some phonological treatment protocols, speech perception tasks are incorporated in meaningful contexts (Blache, 1982; Fokes, 1982). The focus is on the difference between two patterns or the salience of the target pattern, rather than on the salience of the individual phonemes as is the case in the phonetic approaches. In many of the contrasting pairs methods, one of the steps is for the client to differentiate between the clinician's production of the two stimuli in the pair. For example, when working on final consonant deletion, the client may be asked to point to the picture of *bow* then to the picture of *boat*. Later, the client engages in production of the two pairs of stimuli, often at the word level. The idea is that, through the listening task, the client learns that the use or nonuse of the target pattern makes a difference in the meaning of the word. Auditory input is incorporated in a different way in the cycling approach. At the beginning and end of every session, the client listens with amplification to the clinician producing a few words illustrating the target pattern for the day (Hodson & Paden, 1991). This procedure is also part of the homework done daily outside the clinical session.

In most of the phonological approaches, clients produce the contrasts between the target pattern and the deviant pattern. In the distinctive feature approach, clients produce a sound that has the targeted feature as well as a sound that does not have the feature in several contexts, moving from isolation through sentences and connected speech (Costello & Onstine, 1976; McReynolds & Bennett, 1972). In the contrasting pairs approach, clients produce the contrasting patterns in meaningful contexts, words, and sentences (Blache, 1982; Fokes, 1982; Tyler et al., 1987). In the phonological cycling and nonlinear phonology approaches, production of contrasting patterns is used as needed in the later stages of treatment (Hodson & Paden, 1991).

One of the differences between most phonological treatment protocols and the phonetic treatment protocols is that only meaningful stimuli are used. With the exception of the distinctive feature approach, clients produce real words rather than isolated sounds and nonsense syllables and words. Even in the distinctive features approach, meaning is attached to the sounds produced by connecting the isolated sound and nonsense syllables with its written symbol or graphic representation of the unique features of the sound. Thus, the focus of the speech production practice in the phonological approaches is on the linguistic components of the speech sound system rather than on the motor components. Of course, the motor components cannot be ignored in clients who have difficulty producing the sounds needed to produce the target features and phonological patterns. In this case, clinicians teach the clients the motor skills they need to produce the sound pattern being targeted.

> What are some guidelines to follow when providing articulation/phonological treatment?

GENERAL GUIDELINES OF ARTICULATION/ PHONOLOGICAL INTERVENTION

Some general guidelines to follow in administering articulation/phonological treatment have evolved over the years (Table 7.6). These guidelines are not adhered to by all speech-language pathologists, but they are general principles that provide a good base for the treatment of articulatory/phonologic disorders.

Be a Humanist, Artist, and Scientist

To be an effective and efficient clinician, one must be a scientist, humanist, and artist. The assessment and treatment processes can be likened to scientific experiments. The clinician develops hypotheses about the client's ability to improve articulation/ phonology, devises a treatment plan, carries out the plan perhaps with modification, and analyzes the results. Thus, the speech-language pathologist functions as a scientist. Additionally, competent clinicians have knowledge about anatomy and physiology of the typical speech and language system, typical speech and language development, etiologies of disabilities, and they apply this knowledge to their work with clients. Because the treatment process involves two or more people,

TABLE 7.6

Guidelines for Implementation of Articulation/Phonological Treatment

Treatment Guidelines

1. Be a humanist, artist, and scientist.
2. Have available a large repertoire of treatment approaches.
3. Use individualized approaches.
4. Eliminate or minimize the effect of maintaining causative factors.
5. Write behavioral objectives.
6. Specify treatment procedures.
7. Use logically sequenced steps in the treatment plan.
8. Begin treatment at the client's skill level.
9. Expect less-than-perfect articulation from some clients.
10. Have available a large repertoire of specific techniques.
11. Elicit sounds in the simplest way.
12. Teach the distinction between the error and standard production.
13. Use a minimum of motivational devices.
14. Teach several sounds at a time (if feasible).
15. Provide many opportunities for client practice of target(s).
16. Ensure the client is an active participant.
17. Involve parents, siblings, teachers, and spouses when possible.
18. Continuously assess the articulation/phonological problem and progress.
19. Include work on transfer and maintenance.
20. Conduct treatment follow-up.

the clinician needs to be a humanist, establishing a relationship that will facilitate changes in the client's speech. Generally, this is spoken of as *rapport building*, which means to develop an understanding, accepting, and warm relationship. Because what is known about disordered articulation is incomplete and imprecise and because no two persons or problems are alike, clinicians must be artists by being creative in dealing with individual clients. Such creativity should be based on scientific information and certainly will be influenced by the clinician's educational background, participation in continuing education activities, consultation with colleagues, and analysis of past experience. Perhaps someday researchers will identify, with greater certainty, the treatment pro-

cedures that are most effective with different types of clients; however, until that time the speech-language pathologist must make creative use of clinical impressions, reasoning, judgments, and intuition to strengthen those treatment procedures that have been most productive in the past.

Have Available a Large Repertoire of Treatment Approaches

The competent speech-language pathologist should have a large repertoire of treatment approaches as well as specific techniques to use for sound elicitation and for transferring target sounds to different contexts. An individualistic approach to diagnosis and treatment is strongly recommended. Certainly, competent clinicians will not be limited to two or three approaches and will continue expanding their repertoire through reading professional literature; consulting with other clinicians; creating and experimenting; and attending classes, short courses, and seminars.

Use Individualized Approaches

Historically, clinicians have not used different treatment approaches for different clients. There is a great temptation to continue using the approach that has worked in the past for many clients and is most comfortable for the clinician. However, current pressures to be more efficacious and accountable with treatment present the challenge of improving our intervention. At the same time, older approaches are being refined and new approaches are being developed that provide clinicians with options so they can select treatment approaches and techniques that will be more efficient and effective in remediating a specific articulatory/phonologic disorder.

The same treatment approach should not be used with every client. This guideline is predicated on a thorough, accurate assessment of the client in which the speech-language pathologist becomes familiar with the individual and with the exact nature of the patterns of articulation and misarticulations and related factors, including those that are maintaining the problem. During the assessment process, the speech-language pathologist should be alert to any indication of a positive response to a particular learning procedure. Such responses are hints at potentially effective treatment approaches for particular clients. For some clients, it may not be essential to go through the entire treatment sequence if probing shows that they already have the skills for certain steps of the program; perhaps only certain steps need to be emphasized. This is one way of individualizing articulation/phonological treatment approaches for particular clients. Different clinical approaches may be better suited to different clients. The assessment procedures should differentiate among various clinical groups such as those displaying deviant articulation patterns versus delayed articulation, phonetic errors versus phonological errors, and organic versus nonorganic etiologies. Such information has implications for selecting an appropriate intervention approach. Also, a period of trial treatment is often helpful in finding an effective approach.

Eliminate or Minimize the Effect of the Maintaining Causative Factors

The principle of eliminating or minimizing effects of maintaining causes is contingent on a thorough evaluation of the client. In adhering to this guideline, the maintaining causes are of primary concern. Those that precipitated the disorder, but are no longer operative are usually not critical. Of course, there are instances in which the precipitating and maintaining causes are not fully determined, but it may not always be essential to do so. Many times, the articulatory/phonologic disorder may be the result of multiple causative factors or may be of unknown etiology. In the latter instance, articulation/phonological treatment will be truly symptomatic treatment as is much of behavioral and medical treatment.

Before planning a treatment program, the speech-language pathologist should investigate the changes that can be made to eliminate, minimize, or compensate for the maintaining causes. If a physical problem significantly contributes to the disorder, correction to the extent possible should be made such as repairing the cleft palate, clipping the lingual frenulum, improving the hearing, or providing orthodontic treatment. The degree of improvement to be expected from correcting facial and oral cavity structural anomalies is uncertain and must be considered on an individual basis. Certainly, such changes will not automatically guarantee correct articulation. In some cases, such as in partial glossectomy and cerebral palsy, individuals must be taught compensatory movements. Depending on one's professional background, place of employment, philosophy, and the age of the client, the speech-language pathologist may choose to correct tongue thrust swallow before or while initiating formal articulation treatment for a frontal lisp. Unfavorable parental, sibling, or teacher attitudes and interactions with the client may be alleviated through counseling while the

client is in the treatment program. These are only a few examples of eliminating or minimizing causes before or during articulation treatment. Each case must be considered individually and handled accordingly. The clinician should never be reluctant to change a planned treatment program when the client is not responding as expected or when new information indicates that a different approach might be more effective.

Write Behavioral Objectives

One of the most important contributions that operant philosophy has made is in writing specific behavioral goals and objectives. These goals and objectives enable the clinician to observe and measure progress in treatment and allow for replication of results (Hegde, 1998; Roth & Worthington, 2001). If objectives are not observable and measurable or if they are written with vague wording, they are not useful for determining whether the intervention is effective, how the intervention is progressing, whether (and when) the goal has been achieved, or when treatment should be terminated. From a practical viewpoint, specific goals are needed for individualized family service plans (IFSPs) in many preschool settings, for individualized educational plans (IEPs) in public school settings, and for third-party payers. Therefore, it is important for every clinician to become proficient in writing clear, concise, quantifiable objectives that delineate what the client is supposed to do, under what conditions it is to be done, and how well the task is to be accomplished (criterion level).

Specify Treatment Procedures

A corollary to writing behavioral objectives is the guideline for specifying procedures. Again, this allows for accountability and replication of treatment results (Hegde, 1998). Procedures include the specific treatment approach being implemented, types of stimulus materials, and the steps to be followed in going from where the client starts to where the client achieves the objectives. Sometimes, the type of reinforcement to be used, the consequences of incorrect responses, and the reinforcement schedule are also specified. A sample IEP with behaviorally stated objectives is included as Appendix H.

Use Logically Sequenced Steps in the Treatment Plan

Often, an intervention plan in which the course of treatment occurs in logically sequenced steps is efficient and effective in the achievement of the speech objectives. Most treatment approaches are described in steps leading to the goal of improved habitual speech sound production in context. The intervention facilitates success by building on what the client can do and introducing new skills gradually while providing positive reinforcement and pleasant, meaningful experiences for the client. A stepwise treatment plan does not eliminate a humanistic component or some other modifications because the clinical sessions involve interaction between two or more people. The clinician can be, and in most cases should be, warm, that is "human," in carrying out the behavioral program.

Here are some requirements of a programmed behavioral treatment plan to remember when developing a plan of intervention (Collins & Cunningham, 1976):

- Make sure the client has the necessary prerequisite behaviors before initiating the program. Examples of behaviors include: demonstrating the concepts of *same* and *different*, maintaining eye contact, and attending to and following instructions of the clinician.
- Write the objectives in behavioral terms. State objectives so that they are observable and measurable. An objective should specify exactly what the client is to do, under what circumstances, and how well.
- Specify small, logically sequenced steps that eventually lead to a final objective. A criterion level should be set for each step. Do not move on to the next step until the current one is completed. If the current step seems unachievable, add a branching or intermediate step to the program.
- Specify the type of positive reinforcement and schedule for providing reinforcement for correct responses. Types of reinforcement include food, drink, tokens, social, e.g., "good," smile, pat on the hand, and points earned for a prize or activity. A clinician may choose to ignore or punish incorrect responses by saying "no" or "that's not right," taking away a token, or giving a black mark. This is a way of providing feedback to the client.

Begin at the Appropriate Level

Begin at the articulation level of the client so that eventually, new speech sound patterns replace incorrect ones. The clinician should begin with what the client can already do easily or at a level slightly beyond what the client can do and gradually move toward developing new speech skills. If a client has multiple articulation errors, it usually is advisable to begin remediation with a sound or sound pattern that can most easily be produced correctly, is likely to result in early success for the client, and creates a positive client attitude toward the clinical process. Later, clients will probably be more amenable to producing the more difficult phonemes or patterns. Easily produced sounds include those that are most stimulable, visible, and earlier developing. For some clients, production of the error sound in nonmeaningful material, such as sounds in isolation, nonsense syllables, and nonsense words, tends to be easier than production in meaningful material because the client has habitually used misarticulations in meaningful contexts but not in unfamiliar contexts. Therefore, it is suggested that the error sound be produced first in nonmeaningful material and later in meaningful contexts (Bernthal & Bankson, 2004; Gerber, 1977; Johnson et al., 1967; Winitz, 1969, 1975). Contrarily, practice in nonmeaningful contexts may not be useful for a phonologic disorder (Hodson & Paden, 1991).

The clinician does not have to start the treatment program at the beginning stage if the client is beyond that level. Different clients can enter the treatment program at different levels. Not all clients function on the same level insofar as speech sound production is concerned. Some clients may be at the isolation level, and some may be at the sentence level. Because it is of utmost importance to start where the client is, the clinician must determine the level for each individual and begin treatment at that level. An example of a hierarchy of treatment levels appears in Table 7.7. A particular client may enter treatment at any of these levels—once again emphasizing the importance of using an individualistic philosophy in treatment.

Expect Less Than Perfect Articulation from Some Clients

The guideline for accepting less than perfect speech sound production from some clients applies to organic and nonorganic cases. If an organic deficit, such as may result from cleft palate, cerebral palsy, dysarthria, apraxia, and mental retardation, is not correctable, the speech-language pathologist must formulate treatment objectives that are within the client's potential. This does not mean that such goals cannot be changed during the treatment process because the client may perform better or poorer than expected. Nevertheless, the goals must be realistic in terms of the physical, mental, and emotional capabilities of the client. The clinician's responsibility to assist the client and family in acknowledging, accepting, and adjusting to the speech limitations.

TABLE 7.7

Example of a Hierarchy of Treatment Levels

Level*	Step	Goal
I		Perceptual training
	1	Identification of target sound in isolation, words, sentences, and connected speech
	2	Discrimination between target sound and other speech sounds
	3	Discrimination between correctly and incorrectly produced target phonemes
	4	Discrimination of own productions of target
II		Establishment of phonemes
	1	Target phoneme produced in isolation
	2	Target phoneme produced in nonsense syllables
	3	Target phoneme produced in words
	4	Target phoneme produced in phrases and sentences
	5	Target phoneme produced in monologue and dialogue
III		Transfer of phonemes
	1	Transfer to various phonemic contexts
	2	Transfer to various physical environments
IV		Maintenance of target phonemes
	1	Production in all phonemic contexts
	2	Continual production over a period of 3 to 6 months

*Training in self-monitoring should continue throughout the entire treatment process.

In instances of nonorganic cases, the client also may not achieve perfect articulation even though the necessary physical and mental capacities seem to be present. There may be unknown physiological or psychoemotional limitations, or the client may not have the need or desire to achieve the goal set by the clinician. In this instance, the speech-language pathologist should use all feasible techniques for attaining the terminal objective of correct articulation, but should not become frustrated or feel dejected because of failure to achieve the present goal. Not every person in the clinician's potential caseload will be able to achieve perfect or even acceptable articulation.

Have Available a Large Repertoire of Specific Techniques

It is necessary to have several general treatment approaches, such as those that are described in Chapters 8 and 9. A speech-language pathologist must also have a number of different techniques for eliciting sounds in isolation and for putting sounds into nonsense syllables and words (Chapter 10). For example, a certain technique for eliciting correct /s/ from persons with a lateral lisp will not work for all who have a lateral lisp; therefore, the clinician must be ready with an armamentarium of techniques for the face-to-face situation with the client. The same is true for eliciting /r/, /l/, /f/, and, as a matter of fact, for all sounds. Go into the clinic room with at least 4 to 8 different techniques for eliciting the target. Similarly, a client does not often automatically produce sounds correctly in nonsense syllables or words even when production is correct in isolation. The clinician must be prepared with several techniques for accomplishing this task. Thus, an effective speech-language clinician will use various articulation/phonological treatment approaches and specific techniques with various clients.

Elicit Sounds in the Simplest Way

When teaching a client to produce a particular phoneme, the clinician should use few and simple directions. The easiest way is to instruct the client to imitate the clinician's model. If this procedure is not successful after a few trials and if the phoneme is a visible one, a technique such as having the client look in the mirror and imitate the clinician's oral movements should be tried.

The clinician's provision of **motokinesthetic stimulations** is effective in many instances (Appendix I). These stimulations involve the clinician moving the client's tongue, lips, and jaw on the outside of the face. Other fairly simple procedures involve manipulating the client's tongue with a tongue blade; moving the articulators from a sound the client can produce to the target sound; showing pictures illustrating placement of the articulators; and, with a tongue depressor, touching the points of two articulators that should contact one another when the sound is produced. Providing verbal directions for placement of the articulators may be effective if the instructions are not too complex. Unfortunately, such directions are often unclear, lengthy, and confusing. The rationale for this guideline of eliciting sounds simply is that the correct motor movements must eventually become automatic. But if the elicitation procedure is too complex, the automatization process will be more difficult, if not impossible. A person who had received articulation treatment for an /r/ distortion reported that after 30 years, it was still necessary to consciously place the articulators for /r/ because of having been taught to produce the sound through complex directions.

Teach the Distinction between the Error and the Standard Production

There are a couple of treatment methods that focus on the distinction between the error and standard productions: (a) speech sound discrimination and (b) production of contrastive pairs, often word pairs. Speech sound discrimination refers to the client distinguishing between the target sound or sound pattern and other sounds or patterns. One speech perception technique is for the client to identify the target sound when produced by the clinician in various levels of production, such as with isolated sounds, syllables, words, sentences, connected speech. Another technique is for the client to discriminate between sounds produced correctly and incorrectly by the clinician at various levels. A third technique is to have clients identify when their own productions are correct and incorrect; that is, to self-discriminate.

The contrasting pairs technique involves the client producing two sounds or speech sound patterns in various levels of production (syllables, words, sentences), one of which is the target

sound/pattern and the other that is not the target. Often, the two sounds/patterns are minimally contrastive. For example, clients who substitute /k/ for /t/ would produce contrasting word pairs such as *key* and *tea*. Clients who omit final consonants would produce contrasting words such as *bow* and *boat* and *sew* and *soap*. Sometimes, the client is asked to differentiate between the two pairs when produced by the clinician (Blache, 1982; Fokes, 1982; Weiner, 1981). Not all clients need to learn to differentiate between the correct and incorrect productions, but it appears to be helpful for achieving carryover for some.

Use a Minimum of Motivational Devices

At one time, speech-language pathologists spent a great deal of time devising games and other motivational devices to make speech fun. Unfortunately, this sometimes resulted in inefficiency as the number of responses per unit time was minimal and often the game became more important than the speech. It now seems unnecessary to use so many of these devices to motivate clients to learn. This does not mean that clinical sessions should be drudgery; they should still be enjoyable, but not solely through the use of games. After all, the basic objective is using accurate articulation, which should not be obscured by just playing games; however, it is easier to "play" with a child than to "work" with a child, so this attitude of "play" might be preserved in treatment sessions that stress meaningful interaction. Effective reinforcement can be used to maintain the desire to improve phonological skills, and hopefully, the client will become intrinsically motivated to work on speech. It is helpful to explain the sequential steps so that the client understands the need for the drill work or practice of the targets. There are ways of illustrating the sequence to even young children (Fig. 7.1). Having the client record daily progress on a chart also involves the person in the treatment program and provides a way of following their self-progress. As one clinician once said, the ultimate goal is "speech for speech's sake" rather than "games for speech's sake." "Motivation should be harnessed to good speech, not irrelevant to it" (Powers, 1971).

Teach Several Sounds at a Time

In some instances, it is advisable to target one sound at a time. However, most children and adults are capable of learning several sounds at once (Van Riper & Erickson, 1996). Capability should be determined by stimulability testing and the client's age

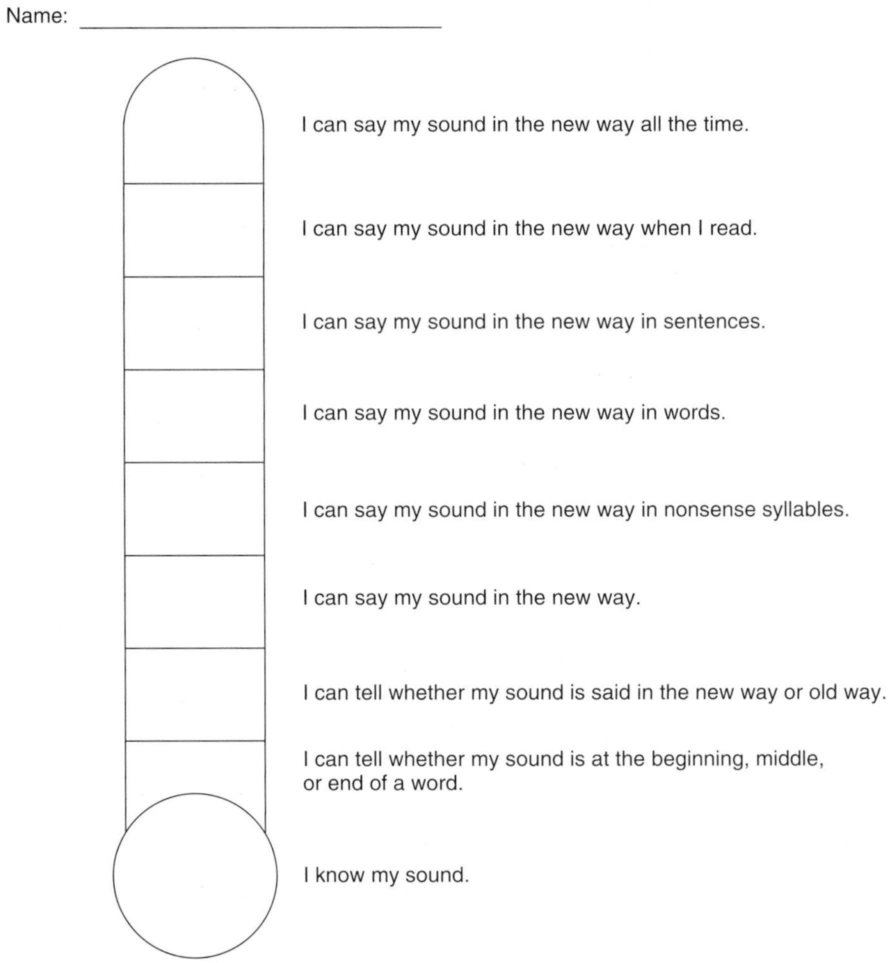

Name: _____

I can say my sound in the new way all the time.

I can say my sound in the new way when I read.

I can say my sound in the new way in sentences.

I can say my sound in the new way in words.

I can say my sound in the new way in nonsense syllables.

I can say my sound in the new way.

I can tell whether my sound is said in the new way or old way.

I can tell whether my sound is at the beginning, middle, or end of a word.

I know my sound.

FIGURE 7.1 Speech gauge.

level and cognitive abilities, and, in some cases, after a few weeks of trial or diagnostic treatment. Reasons for working on several sounds simultaneously include (a) expediting the rate of progress; (b) improving intelligibility more rapidly; (c) maintaining motivation; (d) reducing the chances for overgeneralization; and (e) financial or economic purposes—the faster the progress, the less the cost to the taxpayer or to whomever is responsible. It has been mentioned already that both phonemes of cognates may not always need to receive individual attention; for example, working on /s/ may not always require working on /z/ because there tends to be generalization across cognates. Besides cognates, the clinician may elect to work on entire sound classes (such as all of the stops) or on a major feature that is lacking, such as sibilancy. Using a phonological approach, one can target the reduction of a phonological process such as final consonant deletion or stopping in which several sounds are worked on at

the same time. In this manner, the intervention process becomes more efficient.

Provide Many Opportunities for Client Practice of the Targets

The purpose of a clinical session is to provide maximum opportunity (repetition) for speech practice. Clinical activities should be planned ahead of time, and the materials should be organized and ready for use so that clinical time is not devoted to deciding what to do and to gathering materials. If equipment is used, it should be in working order and checked before the session. Clinical activities should be simple to explain, to understand, and to use; otherwise, valuable time will be spent answering questions and giving further explanations. Fairly rapid presentation of stimuli and provision of reinforcement results in eliciting more responses. It also keeps the client alert and attentive to the task, providing little opportunity to engage in off-task behavior. Providing reinforcement that consumes the least amount of time should be the goal. For example, coloring a picture or working a puzzle can be quite time consuming, whereas stamping a stamper or giving a "high five" is not. Setting time limits for reinforcement activities can alleviate the time problem. These are but a few suggestions for helping the client practice articulation/phonological skills as often as possible during the session. After all, the goal is meaningful repetition.

Keep Clients Actively Participating

With the possible exception of very young children or of persons with extremely limited intellectual capacity, the client must be actively involved in the treatment process for it to be successful (Andrews & Andrews, 2000; Hodson & Paden, 1991). The clinician must know how the client perceives the problem. There should be a cooperative interaction between the client and the speech-language pathologist so that the former is active and informed, aware of the nature of the speech problem, the steps involved in the learning process, and the progress being made. Active participation can be aided by presenting stimuli at a fairly rapid pace, by varying the rhythm or flow of the sessions, and by making the treatment sessions interesting and pleasant. The clinician needs to present the material and provide reinforcement enthusiastically rather than in an uninteresting, routine manner. Such attitudes may be transferred to the client. With young children and some older children, this probably means using participatory activities rather than straight drill work or confining the treatment activities to table work.

The tasks the client is to perform should not be too difficult nor too easy (Hodson & Paden, 1991). The overall correct responding percentage should probably be somewhere in the range of 80 to 95%. The client can be made aware of the progress rate through such techniques as counting the number of correct and incorrect responses, charting the percentage of correct responses, and checking off treatment steps as they are accomplished. The clinician can require the client to self-evaluate responses rather than to rely on the clinician's judgments. Evaluation of responses by the client may be more effective than assessment by the clinician (Gerber, 1977; Koegel et al., 1986; Koegel et al., 1988; Scarry & Scarry-Larkin, 1996). Many clinicians concur with the notion that self-evaluation is much more effective than clinician evaluation because self-evaluation encourages the client to assume the onus of responsibility

while making conscious decisions rather than semi-reflexive responses; thereby achieving carryover more quickly. Group sessions may also encourage active involvement for some children. The clinician should manipulate the clinical sessions to include the client actively in the treatment process.

Involve Parents, Siblings, Teachers, and Spouses

As indicated in Chapter 5, inappropriate attitudes and reactions of important persons toward the client's speech may contribute to articulatory/phonologic disorders. Therefore, involving these people in the treatment process becomes an important part of the management of the client's communication problem. Additionally, this will likely aid in the carryover process. The clinician should inform these persons about the nature of the disorder and frequently work together to develop strategies and guidelines as to what they can do to aid in the remediation process. Every effort should be made to guide them to be supportive and encouraging of the client's efforts and to be constructive in their interest and activity. The counseling can be done on an occasional basis or can be quite intensive, depending on the individual case. The amount of involvement of other persons in the treatment varies with such factors as severity of the problem, stage of treatment, quality of the client–person relationship, and motivation of the interested person. In many cases, parents or others can become very much a part of the treatment program by observing the clinician at work with the child or by working with the child alongside the clinician. Often, there is a tendency to keep parents away from the treatment, but the opposite should be the case as often as appropriate (Andrews & Andrews, 2000; Lillywhite, 1948). The speech-language pathologist and family can frequently work together effectively as co-clinicians.

Assess the Articulation/ Phonological Problem and Progress Continuously

Assessment of the client's articulation should extend throughout the treatment process, allowing for appraisal of the client's progress (Hegde, 1998; Shelton, 1978). One way of doing this is to probe the client's speech sound production in untreated words, varying phonetic contexts, and in higher levels of speech sound production. It is also useful to listen to the client speak in connected speech and observe the client's production of the target sounds or patterns. This ongoing assessment provides a basis for changing the treatment procedures when progress is not commensurate with clinician expectations or when client responses indicate that a different approach would be more effective. The speech-language pathologist needs to be flexible and to modify methods when necessary. This does not mean that treatment should be changed at the whim of the clinician, but occasionally plans do need to be changed when indicated by ongoing reevaluation of the client.

Include Work on Transfer and Maintenance

Transfer or **generalization** refers to applying the newly learned behavior in situations different from those in which it was learned. **Maintenance** refers to the continuing application of the learned behavior. These two processes are commonly called *carryover* (discussed in detail in Chapter 10). In articulation/phonological programming, carryover refers to using the correct sound or pattern in other settings with other people for the rest of the client's life. After correct sound production is acquired, carryover must occur for the treatment program to be considered successful.

Because generalization often does not occur automatically, special attention during treatment must be directed to the process of generalization or carryover. Activities for encouraging generalization to untreated words and to nonclinical settings should begin as soon as or even before the client has completed the establishment phase of treatment. In fact, generalization of the correct phoneme may occur earlier because the sound can generalize or transfer to different positions or contexts within words, to different words and utterances, to other sounds that have similar distinctive features, and to other speaking situations or environments quite early in treatment. Activities for facilitating generalization include periodic probing of the target sound in various phonemic contexts and physical environments, practicing the sound in many different environments, developing a core vocabulary that contains the target phoneme, reducing the frequency of reinforcement, involving various helpers, and eliciting many repetitions in the treatment setting. Additional ideas are included in Chapters 8, 9, and 10. To reemphasize, generalization should be taught because it does not always occur spontaneously.

Conduct Treatment Follow-Up

Prudence suggests follow-up on clients to determine whether or not they have maintained the correct production of speech sounds and patterns in spontaneous speech. "Follow-up is a procedure designed to assess response maintenance in the natural environment and across time" (Hegde, 1998, p. 284). If feasible, when a client seems to have achieved the objectives, suspend treatment for 3 to 6 months without dismissing the client from the caseload (Hedge). Then, schedule a follow-up session to do a conversational probe, ideally in a nonclinical setting with people not associated with the intervention. If the client is not using the correct speech sounds and patterns consistently, arrange for what Hegde calls *booster treatment*; that is, see the client for one or more sessions as a refresher. These booster treatment sessions should then again be followed up with another conversational probe in 3 to 6 months. Another procedure for follow-up is to consult the parents, teacher, spouse, or other appropriate individuals to receive input from them regarding whether or not the client has achieved carryover.

> What are the general stages of articulation/phonological treatment?

GENERAL PHASES OF ARTICULATION/ PHONOLOGICAL TREATMENT

Even though there are different treatment approaches, some general stages exist (Table 7.8).

Elimination or Minimization of Causative Factors

Elimination or minimization of etiological factors is applicable to those clients in whom changes can be made to allow for articulation skills to develop

TABLE 7.8

General Phases of Articulation/ Phonological Treatment

Phases	Description
1	Elimination or minimization of causative factors
2	Auditory perceptual training
3	Acquisition
4	Transfer or generalization to connected speech
5	Maintenance or habituation

more readily. This step usually precedes clinical intervention, but it may also be done concurrently. Examples include fitting a client who has velopharyngeal insufficiency with an obturator or performing palatopharyngeal surgery, fitting a client who is hearing impaired with a hearing aid, waiting for the permanent upper frontal incisors to fully erupt before targeting certain alveolar speech sounds, and discouraging older siblings to speak for the client.

Auditory Perception Training

Speech sound discrimination is not a part of all treatment approaches, but when specific speech perception training is done, it may precede production training. Speech perception may also occur concurrently with treatment, which is recommended by Rvachew (1994) who has researched this area for a number of years.

Acquisition

During the acquisition stage of treatment, the client learns to produce the sounds/patterns correctly in various contexts. Treatment may begin with production of the phoneme in isolation and proceed to nonsense syllables, words, phrases, sentences, and conversation. In some treatment approaches, the client works on production of words, phrases, sentences, connected speech only in meaningful contexts. This stage is generally conducted in the clinical setting. The client should achieve automatic, rather than deliberate, production at each level before moving to the next higher level, unless a cycling approach is being implemented.

Transfer or Generalization to Connected Speech

After production is strengthened, transfer should occur. This stage involves the client using the sound in connected speech within the clinical setting, outside the clinical setting, with the clinician, and with others. Here, the client transfers correct articulation to everyday speaking situations.

Maintenance or Habituation

Maintenance is the last stage of treatment in which the client habitually uses correct speech sound patterns in all situations over a long period of time. Whether or not the treatment program is successful depends on retention or automatization of the re-

sponses learned in the clinical setting. The clinician should periodically recheck the client's speech to ensure that the new behaviors are retained and that carryover has occurred. If articulation skills do not become automatic, they will tend to revert back to earlier error patterns.

These stages are not mutually exclusive; they are overlapping. How each stage is accomplished varies with the particular treatment approach used and the individual clients and clinicians involved.

SUMMARY

Articulation and phonology are subsystems of language and occur concurrently with the use of other language systems. Thus, articulation and phonological treatment includes all categories of language. They also are part of the communication process that contributes greatly to the intelligibility of a message. There is a wide range of articulation and phonological patterns that are within the normal limits of acceptability depending on the dialect, the speaking situation, and the age of the individual. Not every person who has misarticulations or phonological deviations needs treatment. Need is dependent on the social, cultural, ethnic, and occupational environment of the individual, client and family attitudes toward the speech problem, nature of the speech deficiency, client's age, and etiology of the problem.

Sometimes, clients have concomitant communication disorders along with the articulatory/phonologic disorder. In those situations, treatment for the various disorders can be implemented simultaneously, concurrently, cyclically, or sequentially. Treatment should be carefully planned so that special consideration is given to the diagnostic categories of phonological versus phonetic errors, delayed versus deviant articulation, and organic versus nonorganic causes. After the speech-language pathologist (in consultation with the client, family members, and others) decides to initiate articulation/phonological intervention, a treatment plan is devised. The clinician selects a treatment approach that may be a phonetic approach, a phonological approach, or a combination of the two approaches. Before implementing a treatment plan, however, the speech-language pathologist has other decisions to make such as which sounds, features, or patterns to target, whether or not to incorporate speech perception training into the treatment program, whether or not to use contrastive pairs practice, and whether or not to use nonmeaningful stimuli in addition to meaningful speech in the intervention. There are some general guidelines to be followed in treatment that help to plan for each client on an individual basis. Five general stages of treatment include: (a) elimination or minimization of causative factors; (b) auditory perception training; (c) acquisition or production; (d) transfer or generalization; and (e) maintenance or **habituation**. Methods of providing treatment are discussed in Chapters 8 and 9.

REVIEW QUESTIONS

1. What are some questions speech-language pathologists must answer when transitioning from assessment to articulation/phonological intervention?

2. Identify factors that determine whether or not misarticulations/phonological deviations need treatment.

3. Describe four ways to provide treatment to clients with multiple communication disorders. Which approaches are appropriate for the coexistence of phonologic and language disorders? For the coexistence of phonologic and stuttering disorders? For the coexistence of phonologic and voice disorders?

4. Briefly contrast phonetic and phonological intervention approaches.

5. What types of cases call for a phonetic treatment approach? What types call for a phonological treatment approach?

6. What criteria are to be used in selecting target phonemes? In selecting target distinctive features and phonological patterns?

7. What do research findings suggest about the use of speech perception training in articulation/phonological treatment programs?

8. Identify and characterize four phonological treatment methods.

9. Explain and give a rationale for the statement, "The clinician must be a humanist, artist, and scientist."

10. What are some guidelines for providing efficacious articulation/phonological treatment?

11. What are the general stages of articulation/phonological intervention? Briefly describe each stage.

CHAPTER 8

Phonetic Treatment Approaches

"Nothing is more useful than to speak clearly."

—Phaedrus

CHAPTER OBJECTIVES

- Describe the general characteristics of phonetic treatment approaches.
- Identify the types of articulatory/phonologic disorders that are most suitably treated with phonetic treatment approaches.

- Characterize each of the various phonetic treatment approaches.
- Provide a rationale for each phonetic treatment approach presented.
- Identify the advantages and limitations of each phonetic treatment approach.

Various approaches for articulation/phonological treatment have been used over the years, beginning with the phonetic placement approach of the 1920s and continuing to those currently being developed for phonological deviations. All of the approaches imply the existence of a treatment sequence: planning, establishment or learning of the sound, transfer or generalization, and maintenance or stabilization. Although these common elements exist, different rationales and philosophies relative to the nature and causes of articulatory/phonologic disorders have influenced specific procedures and techniques that have been devised for each treatment approach.

Phonetic (motor) approaches for treating articulatory/phonologic disorders are described in this chapter. Generally, these approaches focus on the mechanics of producing the speech sounds, and the methods vary among the approaches. The approaches are categorized according to their underlying premises and historical significance. Considerable overlap exists in the procedures used for the phonetic approaches described here. Some incorporate sound discrimination training; others do not. Some begin production at the isolation level, others at the syllable level, and still others at the word level. Some include practice of the target speech sounds in meaningful and nonmeaningful contexts. Many incorporate a self-evaluation or a self-monitoring component. The clinical techniques vary, but the goal for all approaches is for the client to produce the target sounds correctly in spontaneous speech as quickly as possible.

This chapter presents several phonetic treatment approaches that have been used by speech-language pathologists over the years (Table 8.1). Some of these are of historical significance. Descriptions of these approaches include the developer's rationale; goals and procedures used; and additional comments relative to the types of clients for whom the approach is most appropriate, the advantages and limitations of the approach, and how the approach is used today. As might be expected, some clinicians prefer to implement certain approaches, even though other approaches might be more effective for some clients than others. In reality, clinicians often use

TABLE 8.1

Types of Phonetic Treatment Approaches for Articulatory/Phonologic Disorders

Type of TX Approach	Specific Approach	Brief Description
Articulator placement/movement	Phonetic placement	Instruction in specific placement of the articulators to produce speech sounds
	Palatometric instrument	Use of a pseudopalate to provide visual feedback
Traditional	Stimulus	Auditory training and production practice of target sound in progressively increasing levels of linguistic complexity
	Wedge	Target two or more speech sounds at a time using sounds that have dissimilar phonetic features
	Multiple phonemic	Target production of all error sounds at a time with each progressing at its own rate
Tactile-kinesthetic	Motokinesthetic	Manipulation by the clinician of the articulators externally on the face and neck to guide the articulation mechanism in speech sound production
	PROMPT	Use of multidimensional tactile prompts to guide the articulation mechanism in producing speech sounds
Phonetic context	Sensory-motor	Bisyllable and trisyllable drill for multisensory awareness of speech sound patterns and production of error sound in facilitating phonetic contexts that gradually are expanded
	Paired-stimuli	Use key words paired with words in which the target sound is produced incorrectly at the word, sentence, and conversational levels
Stimulability	Integral stimulation	Imitation of clinician's multisensory models in stimulable sounds
	Stimulability enhancement	Production of consonants in isolation or CV to increase number of stimulable sounds
Behavior modification	Programmed instruction	Specification of stimuli, client responses, and consequences (reinforcement, punishment, and/or differential reinforcement) in small sequential steps
Other	Heterogeneous group	Incorporation of all types of communication problems in a group setting, targeting sounds from whole to part to whole
	Nonsense material	Simultaneous auditory training and speech production. Sounds targeted in nonmeaningful material at all levels before meaningful material

components of the various approaches, even incorporating procedures from phonological approaches (Chapter 9) into phonetic treatments and vice versa.

What primary feature characterizes articulator placement/movement treatment approaches?

ARTICULATOR PLACEMENT/MOVEMENT TREATMENT APPROACHES

Two approaches are categorized here as articulator placement/movement treatment approaches: (a) phonetic placement and (b) palatometric instrumental system. Phonetic placement techniques were developed in the 1920s, and the palatometric instrumental system is a more recent approach that incorporates technology to show clients where to place and how to move their articulators to produce speech sounds.

> Describe the phonetic placement treatment approach, including its advantages and limitations. How has the approach been modified for use today?

Phonetic Placement Approach

Perhaps the first articulation treatment approach was the **phonetic placement approach** developed by Scripture (1923) and Scripture and Jackson (1927). In this method, the client is given general speech exercises and is instructed to perform specific placements of the articulators to produce specific speech sounds.

Rationale

According to Scripture (1923), to move the speech structures correctly, a person must feel the movements and hear the sounds while producing them. An individual with an articulation deviancy must develop the ability to place the articulators in whatever position necessary for speech purposes and, consequently, have complete control over them. The client then must attend to and consciously position the articulation structures, in addition to controlling articulation movements. An implicit assumption of this approach is that each sound is always produced in the same way using the same placement. Thus, the role of the clinician is to teach the client "to carefully correct his faults" (Scripture, 1923, p. 123). Tongue exercises are recommended especially for generally indistinct speech, while breathing and relaxation exercises are recommended for those persons who appear tense. Exercises for the tongue and lip and procedures for strengthening the velar musculature are to be used with "organic" disorders, but other clinicians today suggest more direct velopharyngeal exercises for improving velopharyngeal physiology. Scripture (1923) emphasized that correction of articulation deficits is important to a person's social and mental development and well-being; thus, an individual with articulation deviances should receive training in articulation skills.

Goals and Procedures

The implicit goal of the phonetic placement approach is correct articulation of all speech sounds. Production of the sound begins in isolation and progresses through syllables, words, sentences,

and prepared dialogue. General relaxation, breathing, tongue, and lip exercises are performed by the client. Various techniques and devices are used to demonstrate to the client where to place the articulators and how to direct the breath stream:

- Manipulation of articulations or holding articulators in place with tongue blades and sticks
- Manipulation of articulators with clinician's gloved fingers
- Verbal description and instruction
- Breath indicator for mouth and nose, such as a mirror
- Graphic records, such as a spectrogram
- Feeling of breath stream with hand or seeing effects of breath stream on a tissue
- Observation of clinician and client in mirror while producing sounds
- Feeling of laryngeal vibration
- Observation of diagrams, pictures, or drawings of articulators while producing certain sounds
- Observation of palatograms of articulators while producing certain sounds

Over the years, other techniques to demonstrate placement of the articulators have been devised by speech-language pathologists, but the preceding list gives an indication of the procedures that have been used. Recently, Fletcher and associates (Fletcher SG, personal communication, November 14, 2003) developed a palatometer to assist clients in the placement of their articulators for producing speech sounds. When using the phonetic placement approach, the client should understand exactly which tongue, lip, and jaw positions should be assumed before attempting the target sound (Van Riper & Emerick, 1996). When produced correctly, the sound should be strengthened by repeating it immediately many times with no distractions so that the client gets the tactile and proprioceptive sense of how to produce the sound.

Comments

The phonetic placement approach can be used with individuals or groups and with children or adults. Specific instructions and techniques need to be adapted to fit the level and needs of particular clients. Scripture (1923) indicated that the approach can be used with any articulation disorder, and Van Riper and Emerick (1996) suggested that the approach is especially useful for individuals who are hearing impaired and for clients with whom other sound elicitation procedures are unsuccessful.

Advantages of this approach are that it is faster than other methods in eliciting sounds from some clients and that it is useful in teaching compensatory articulation movements. Limitations are that it is a less direct procedure for producing sounds than others, sounds are less stable at first, and the exact articulation placement of a sound varies with the phonemes that precede or follow it (Aase et al., 2000; Johnson et al., 1967; McDonald, 1964b; Powers, 1971; Van Riper & Emerick, 1966). Also, the mechanics of phonetic placement often require so much attention from the client that a sound taught in this way cannot be produced quickly or subconsciously in conversational speech. Furthermore, contextual speech does not consist of discrete tongue, jaw, and lip placements, but rather of dynamic movements that are quite different from tongue placements for isolated sounds.

Today, phonetic placement procedures are frequently used to elicit individual speech sounds in isolation. It is a useful approach especially for clients who are not stimulable for the target sound and for whom other elicitation techniques have not been successful. They are also useful in teaching compensatory articulation placements and movements for clients with structural and neuromotor deficits in the articulation mechanism. They provide valuable clues to clients in their sound production. Clinicians are often inventive in devising effective phonetic placement techniques when working with individual clients.

A second component of the phonetic placement approach outlined by Scripture (1923) is general nonspeech exercises for the speech structures. Some speech-language clinicians have used devices and procedures for strengthening the articulators, controlling the articulators, and controlling respiration in nonspeech functions (Boshart, 1998, 1999; Marshala, 2001; Rosenfeld-Johnson, 2004). Use of these techniques has been called *oral-motor therapy*—a controversial, yet potentially helpful approach when there is a rationale for using them as a precursor to working on speech per se; however, its indiscriminate use is not recommended. To date, minimal research data exists on the effectiveness of oral-motor exercises for improving speech sound production, and the few available studies generally do not support the contention that these exercises lead to improved articulation skills (Davis & Velleman, 2002; Lof, 2002, 2003; Pannbacker & Lass, 2003). Clinicians should be cautious in using oral-motor exercises for the purpose of improving speech sound production and in making claims about their effectiveness until clinical research results demonstrate positive treatment outcomes for articulation skills (Lof, 2003; Pannbacker & Lass, 2003). With the current state of evidence, it seems prudent to work on speech sound skills directly.

> Describe the palatometric instrument treatment approach, including its advantages and limitations.

Palatometric Instrument Approach

In the **palatometric instrument approach**, a palatometer is used to provide visual feedback of how the client produced the target sound. It registers "the place and pattern of linguapalatal contact against the palate, alveolar ridge, and inner margins of the teeth" (Fletcher, 1992, p.198). In the recent computerized version, the client and clinician can view a palatogram of where sounds are formed in the mouth and can compare them with the palatogram of how the client is producing these sounds (http://www.LogoMetrix.org). This is done through a visual display on a split screen on a computer monitor. The visual displays can be static or dynamic; that is, in real time, slow motion, or frozen in time. Through a modeling-imitation paradigm, clients learn to produce speech sounds correctly using the visual displays of palatograms.

Rationale

The intent of the palatometric instrumental system approach is "to link oral sensations directly with spatial and temporal properties of normal speech articulation" (Fletcher, 1992, p. 217). The client learns to perceive articulation postures and gestures accurately and is guided in how to physically execute the required motor skills to articulate the error sounds correctly. The client imitates the visual displays (palatograms) of correct speech models of the target sounds in various phonetic contexts. In this way, clients change their speech motor patterns to produce the target sounds correctly.

Traditionally, speech-language pathologists rely upon their perception to determine the correctness of speech sounds. However, even though two phonetic elements are perceived to be alike and have the same phonological features, they may be produced differently. Although one can predict the acoustic outcome of certain articulation postures and movements and most talkers produce sounds generally in the same way, listener perceptions are only inferences about how the client produced the sounds. On the other hand, because the articulation structures are basically the same from one speaker to another, the same physical placements and movements of the articulators likely will result in standard acoustic outputs. The palatometer helps the client achieve the standard articulator placements and movements that presumably will result in correct speech sound production. It focuses the client's attention on the "physiological details of speech articulation" (Fletcher, 1992, p. 222).

Goals and Procedures

Instrumentation in the palatometric system includes two pieces of equipment in addition to a computer: (a) a pseudopalate placed inside the mouth with 116 sensors and (b) a minicomputer (Fig. 8.1). The pseudopalate picks up the points of tongue contact with the palate and the minicomputer translates the information that is then transferred to the computer monitor (Fig. 8.2). Various types of visual displays can be shown to the client, including static and dynamic patterns, client patterns, clinician patterns, and a split screen showing both the clinician model and client production.

Ideally, the ultimate goal of the palatometric instrumental system approach is "to establish articulatory gestures and movements that are executed easily and accurately by the talker in finely coordinated, rhythmical, connected speech patterns" (Fletcher, 1992, p. 243). The speech articulation patterns should be automatic and result in intelligible speech output. Treatment begins at the subphonetic level; that is, tongue and palate postures and movements for vowels and consonants. Intervention first focuses on vowels, starting with /i/, moving to the back, rounded vowel /u/, then to the other vowels. Diphthongs are targeted next, followed by

the consonants. The anterior stop and sibilant postures function as referents for all of the other consonants.

The client is first acclimated to the palatometric instrumentation. The clinician explains the visual display to the client, indicating that each dot on the computer screen represents the sensor locations on the pseudopalate. When the dots brighten on the screen, it means that part of the palate was touched. Six steps are involved in this approach:

- Focused attention
- Pattern recognition
- Mental imaging
- Response rehearsal
- Systematic practice
- Verification and evaluation

Each of the six steps is followed for each production of contrasting word/nonsense syllable pair. The first step is *focusing the client's attention* on the physiology of producing the target. The clinician produces the target that is translated into a visual display of the palatogram on the computer monitor. The clinician guides the client to perceive, recognize, and extract properties of the modeled articulation skills. The client is to focus on the key articulation features, such as where the tongue tip touches the alveolar ridge in the production of /t/. Explanations should be brief and explicit. According to Fletcher (1992),

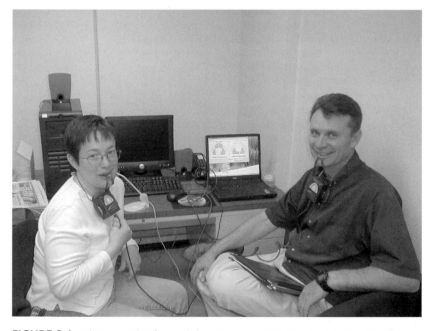

FIGURE 8.1 Photograph of pseudolarynx, minicomputer, and computer monitor in place. (From LogoMetrix (2005). *Helping People Talk*. Glendale, AZ: LogoMetrix. Used with permission.)

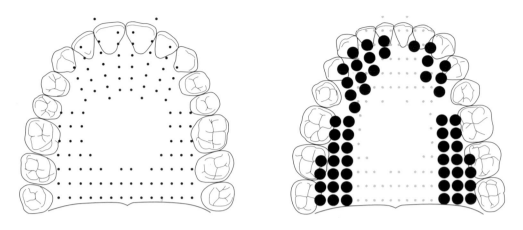

Contacts before and after

FIGURE 8.2   Schematic of pseudolarynx visual display showing sensor points. (From LogoMetrix (2005). *Helping People Talk*. Glendale, AZ: LogoMetrix. Used with permission.)

"overexplaining can cause confusion. For example, simply point to the location where an important part of an essential movement will be taking place and say little more than 'watch here'" (p. 223). The second step, *pattern recognition*, involves the client pointing to the salient articulation pattern on the computer screen. Focusing and pattern recognition are alternated. *Imaging*, the third step, involves instructing clients to form a picture in their minds of what the articulation contact pattern looks like and having them describe the pattern or point to the visual display of the pattern. This is to provide a cognitive link between imagined and actual actions. Next, in *response rehearsal* or mental practice, the client silently rehearses the articulation patterns, without moving the articulators. Most of the rehearsal practice should be in real words or nonsense syllables rather than isolated sounds. However, it is sometimes necessary to practice isolated sounds, especially for younger children, but it should be kept to a minimum. The fifth step is to execute the articulation motor patterns with much *repetition*. Appendix J provides samples of a clinician's instructions for each step. In the last step, *verification*, clients evaluate how closely their production matched the clinician's model by comparing the visual images on a split screen display.

Comments

The palatometric instrumental system is best used with individual clients, rather than groups. Individual pseudopalates are custom made for the client and the clinician and are suitable for use by children and adults. The six-step treatment approach as outlined by Fletcher (1992) can be difficult for preschool children to understand, especially the imaging and rehearsal steps. The approach with the current technology has been used successfully with clients who are hearing impaired (who incidentally have had access to similar instrumentation for several decades) and those who are bilingual (LogoMetrix, 2005). It might be an effective approach for most individuals with articulation disorders, including childhood apraxia of speech. It also could be particularly useful for eliciting speech sounds that are not readily stimulable.

The advantages of the approach is that it provides objective computer-based information about articulation placements and movements, split-screen displays show model and client patterns simultaneously, model patterns can come from either the clinician or computer-stored images, and various types of visual displays assist in analysis of client productions. Limitations include the need to purchase equipment, cost of the equipment, the potential discomfort of the pseudopalate in the mouth, and the inability of a few clients to relate the visual display to actual articulator positions and movements. It may be better suited for older children, adolescents, and adults.

This approach continues to be developed and currently is not widely available to practicing clinicians. Perhaps the six-step program could be simplified to become a modeling-response-feedback paradigm. Such a treatment paradigm may be easier for young children. Further research and clinical use of the instrumentation is needed to determine its usefulness, but it holds promise.

Who is credited with developing the traditional approach to articulation/phonological treatment?

TRADITIONAL TREATMENT APPROACHES

The **stimulus approach**, developed by Van Riper (Van Riper & Erickson, 1996), is considered by most to be the traditional treatment approach for articulatory/phonologic disorders. Over the years, it has formed the basis for subsequent intervention strategies.

Describe the stimulus treatment approach, including the advantages and limitations.

Stimulus Approach

In 1939, Van Riper first formulated what now is generally considered the traditional approach to articulation treatment, often called the *stimulus approach*. The latest published version of this approach appeared in 1996 (Van Riper & Erickson, 1996), which is used here as a bibliographic source. The stimulus approach emphasizes auditory training or speech perception training that precedes and accompanies sound production. After the sound is elicited in isolation, it is produced at various levels, including nonsense syllables, words, phrases, sentences, and spontaneous speech, by the client through auditory-visual stimulation.

Rationale

In the stimulus approach, the basic error in an articulatory disorder consists of a misarticulated sound or sounds, and thus the individual sound in error becomes the focus of treatment (Van Riper & Erickson, 1996). Identification and isolation of an error sound are especially difficult for the client because production of a sound is brief, it varies with the phonetic context, and it involves different sensory modalities in the discrimination process. Characteristics of the sound must be made vivid enough to be mastered. Therefore, auditory perception training is emphasized and sound production begins in isolation rather than in more complex articulation movements involved in syllable, word, and sentence production. If the client can learn to produce the sound in isolation, syllables, and some words, the tools are present for the client

to correctly articulate the error sound in all words in which it occurs (Van Riper & Emerick, 1990).

The treatment process should begin where the client is so that progression through each phase of the recommended program is not necessary; that is, work can begin at any level appropriate to the client's pretreatment skills. The clinician must design a treatment plan, but should be flexible enough to make revisions as new information about the client's skills and progress arises. Further, the approach can be programmed according to operant conditioning principles and methods (Van Riper & Erickson, 1996). As a matter of fact, many articulation programs written by others follow Van Riper and Erickson's principles and techniques.

Goals and Procedures

In the stimulus approach, the goals of articulation intervention for the client are:

- To become aware of characteristics of the standard phoneme
- To recognize characteristics of misarticulations and how they differ from the target sound
- To produce the standard sound at will and to stabilize or strengthen the use of the target sound in isolation, syllables, words, phrases, and sentences
- To use the standard sound in spontaneous speech of all kinds and under all conditions; that is, to achieve carryover

Generally, one sound or one pair of cognates is practiced at a time so as not to confuse the client. Characteristics of sounds that are initially selected for treatment include those that are correct in some phonetic contexts, that require simple coordinations, that are most stimulable, that are earlier developing, that the client is motivated to practice, and that are most helpful in improving intelligibility. The treatment process is illustrated in Figure 8.3. The first two goals of treatment involve auditory training (speech perception training). The first steps deal with *identification of the standard sound* as produced by the clinician. During this phase, the client does not attempt to produce the *new* sound. From the clinician's productions, the client is to locate and isolate the sound and to *discriminate* it from others. In the next steps of treatment, clients listen to themselves; that is, the speech perception training becomes a self-hearing or self-evaluating process. The standard sound is discriminated from its error through scanning the client's own speech and comparing it with the standard phoneme production. Initially, the clinician signals when errors occur. Progressively, the client identifies the error after, during, and before it occurs; that is, progress

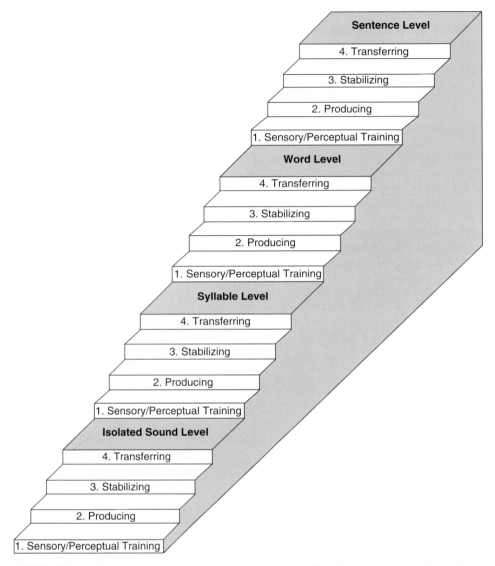

FIGURE 8.3   Design of articulation therapy in the stimulus (traditional) approach. (From Van Riper, C., & Erickson, R. (1996). *Speech correction: An introduction to speech pathology and audiology* (9th ed.). Boston: Allyn & Bacon. Reprinted with permission.)

goes from recalling to perceiving to predicting misarticulations. This procedure is continued throughout the treatment process because it is critical that clients continuously evaluate their own productions.

The third goal of treatment involves *elicitation of the target sound* through the process of varying and correcting the client's attempted productions. This is accomplished at all successive phonetic levels and may begin at whichever level is appropriate for the client's skills. Typically, production begins at the isolation level. Five alternate methods for evoking the sound were specified by Van Riper and Erickson (1996):

- **Progressive approximation**, or **shaping**, which consists of a series of sounds that progressively approximate the target sound until it is produced correctly; that is, a gradual shift from a sound the client can produce to the standard sound
- Auditory stimulation in which the clinician produces the sound several times and instructs the client to imitate
- Phonetic placement in which various procedures are used to teach the client where to place the articulators and how to direct the breath stream
- Modification of other sounds, in which the client makes a sound and then moves the articu-

lators while continuing to produce the first sound
- Key word in which production begins on a word in which the target sound is correctly articulated

The fourth treatment goal is *stabilizing the target sound*. The *new* sound must be strengthened before it will be produced correctly in conversation. Techniques for strengthening include repetition, prolongation, increased intensity, whispering, and simultaneous talking and writing. The sound is then evoked and stabilized in successive phonetic levels from nonsense syllables to nonsense words,

real words, phrases, and sentences. The final step includes *transfer and carryover*. At this point in treatment, the client develops a feedback system, first consciously and later subconsciously, that will scan utterances and automatically identify and correct any errors that occur. Numerous techniques for achieving the objectives for each phase of the auditory stimulus treatment approach can be employed. Some of these techniques include creating key words, slow motion speech, echo speech, unison speech, correcting the clinician's production, and role playing. The design of articulation intervention with the stimulus approach is illustrated in Table 8.2.

TABLE 8.2

Treatment Steps in the Stimulus (Traditional) Approach

Step	Description	Example
Phase I—Auditory training		
Step 1: Identification	Give sound vivid character	/f/ is the *angry cat* sound
Step 2: Isolation	Identify sound in series of phonemes, words, phrases, sentences, reading, conversation	When you hear the /f/ sound, tap the table
Step 3: Stimulation	Bombardment with the target sound	Listen to the story with multiple /f/ words
Step 4: Discrimination		
a. Error detection	Identifies errors in clinician's speech	/pɪʃ/ for /fɪʃ/
b. Error correction	Assists clinician in correcting the error	Help me say *fish* right
Step 5: Self-hearing	Client identifies own errors throughout the production and transfer phases	Did you say *fish* right?
Phase 2—Production		
Step 1: Isolation	Vary and correct sound in isolation	Watch me in the mirror and make the sound just like I do–/f/
Step 2: Stabilization in isolation	Practice the sound in various ways (e.g., softly, quickly, whispered)	Say /f/ every time I ring the bell
Step 3: Nonsense syllable	Vary, correct, and stabilize in CV, VC, CVCV, with all vowels and diphthongs	/fi/, /if/, /ifi/
Step 4: Words	Vary, correct, and stabilize in monosyllabic and multisyllabic words in the initial, final, and medial positions	/fit/ (model, then no model) /lif/ (model, then no model) /kæfe/ (model, then no model) /fit/, /lif/, /kæfe/ (no model)
Step 5: Sentences	Vary, correct, and stabilize in sentences in all positions	The shoe did not fit. A calf is a baby cow. She is laughing. (model, then no model)
Phase 3—Transfer and carryover	Use the sound in spontaneous speech in all situations by enlarging treatment situation (activities, conversational partners, settings, etc.), with the incorporation of self-evaluation and self monitoring	Role playing in clinic session. Speech assignment to use /f/ at the dinner table at home

Comments

The stimulus approach, or variations thereof, is used widely. It is particularly appropriate for clients with only a few errors. Because only one sound or a cognate pair is targeted at a time, variations of this approach in which more than one sound is targeted at a time are probably more efficacious for clients who have several misarticulations. It is useful for cases in which the focus is on precise articulation placement or adapted placements for persons with structural or physical limitations. This approach can be easily adapted for group sessions in addition to individual sessions, and it can be used with children and adults. Advantages include ease and simplicity of use, directness, and absence of distracting or irrelevant cues (Johnson et al., 1967). It provides for repetition of the motor patterns of target sounds. One limitation is that the auditory perception training component is difficult for some clients. Also, focusing on one or two sounds at a time can result in a long treatment process for clients with multiple misarticulations, and overgeneralization (using the target sound as a substitution for other speech sounds) of the target sound often occurs, although this usually abates without intervention.

Today, the stimulus approach is often referred to as the traditional approach and is widely used. Many times, the methodology is modified to omit the auditory training except for the self-evaluation and self-monitoring component. Speech sound production is often implemented as outlined by Van Riper and Erickson (1996); that is, systematic target sound production practice beginning with the lower levels of complexity, including isolation, syllables, and words, and progressing to higher complexity culminating in spontaneous speech. Often, clinicians will work on more than one sound at a time. Many behavioral articulation programs and computer programs incorporate all or part of the stimulus approach. For example, the Speech Assessment and Interactive Learning System (SAILS, 2004) is a computerized program for speech perception training and LocuTour (http://www.LocuTour.com) has developed a series of computerized programs for most of the consonants and consonant clusters that follow the traditional approach procedures, including the auditory training component for each sound.

What distinguishes the wedge treatment approach from other approaches?

Wedge Approach

The **wedge approach** does not include different treatment procedures or techniques (Sommers & Kane, 1974). Rather, it is a system of selectively targeting more than one sound at a time using one of the popular articulation treatment approaches, such as stimulus, integral stimulation, or programmed. The client works on two or more sounds at a time, targeting sounds that have dissimilar phonetic features, such as /k/ and /l/.

Rationale

The wedge approach is based on the assumption that not all error sounds need direct treatment because learning to produce one sound often generalizes to other sounds with similar phonetic features. Therefore, not all phonemes need to be targeted. The sounds selected for treatment have dissimilar phonetic features and thus are *wedges* because they open up the incorrect articulation pattern. The features of the selected sounds often transfer to other error sounds that have the same features, often without direct intervention. In these instances, this approach is more efficacious than targeting all misarticulated sounds one at a time. Working on two or more dissimilar sounds at a time is not confusing to clients, even preschoolers, because the sounds are so different in terms of their distinctive features (Sommers & Kane, 1974).

Goals and Procedures

The goal of the wedge approach is correct production of all misarticulated speech sounds. The client's speech sound system is analyzed thoroughly to determine the error sounds that have similar and dissimilar features. The phonetic features that are considered include voicing, nasality, affrication, duration, and place (some clinicians today would add frication and stridency to this list). Similarities between pairs of sounds are based on the number of distinctive features in common. The clinician selects two or more misarticulated sounds that have phonetically dissimilar features, such as an unvoiced labial fricative /f/, unvoiced velar stop /k/, and voiced alveolar liquid /l/. Transfer often occurs on the nontargeted sound that is similar to the target. If not, the other misarticulated sounds are subsequently targeted.

Comments

The wedge approach can be used with children and adults, as well as with groups and individuals. It is suited to clients who have several misarticulations because more than one sound is targeted at a time and the sounds are strategically selected, providing the opportunity for transfer to occur for other sounds with similar features. The advantages of the approach are that the treatment is more efficient than one-sound-at-a-time strategies, and it capitalizes on transfer patterns so that not all misarticulated sounds need to be directly targeted. Today, many clinicians use this approach with clients who have multiple misarticulations, often following the steps of the stimulus approach without the auditory perception training component.

> Compare and contrast the multiple phonemic approach with the stimulus approach.

Multiple Phonemic Approach

The **multiple phonemic approach** was developed by McCabe and Bradley (1975; Bradley, 1989). In this approach, all misarticulated sounds are treated at the same time. Each sound is produced at the client's proficiency level; that is, isolation, syllables, monosyllabic words, or phrases. Sounds are elicited in isolation with whatever techniques are appropriate for the client. No auditory discrimination training is done. An essential part of the program is that the client works on all misarticulated sounds in every session.

Rationale

The multiple phonemic approach is quite similar to traditional approaches except that several sounds are worked on at the same time (Bradley, 1989; McCabe & Bradley, 1975). The client proceeds at an appropriate pace for each error sound. The rate of progress for each sound varies depending on the difficulty for the individual client. In the first phase of treatment, the client produces all consonants, including those produced correctly, as well as those produced incorrectly. This is done to provide success from the beginning of treatment and to train the client to attend to several phonemes at a time rather than only to those that are misarticulated. In the final stages of treatment, the objective is to articulate whole words correctly instead of only the target sound. The client then is responsible for correct production of several phonemes at once. In phrases, the client must attend to articulation of more than one phoneme, to word sequences, and to semantic aspects of the utterance. According to McCabe and Bradley, when this is accomplished by the client, progress through the remaining steps will be relatively easy.

Throughout treatment, the client's own vocabulary is used rather than words that happen to contain target phonemes but that may not be useful to the client. The client should experience success throughout the treatment process. Each session begins and ends with an activity that the client can achieve. Additionally, if the percentage for correct responses for all tasks falls below 80% during one session, the tasks are modified to allow for a higher success rate. McCabe and Bradley (1975; Bradley, 1989) used a programmed approach and emphasized the necessity for tracking all client responses so that the clinician can determine when to proceed to the next step for each sound, when to modify tasks to accommodate the client's skill level, and when to branch.

Goals and Procedures

The goal is correct production of all speech sounds in spontaneous speech. There are three phases of articulation treatment in the multiple phonemic approach:

- Establishment
- Transfer
- Maintenance

Each phase is composed of steps, each of which has a specific stimulus, client response, reinforcement schedule, and criterion level. The purpose of Phase I, the *establishment phase*, is to achieve correct production of all error sounds in isolation using only visual stimulation; for example, the client is presented the grapheme of a sound printed on a card and asked to say it. If the client initially needs more than visual stimulation to achieve correct production, auditory and tactile stimulation are added. The second step of the establishment phase is considered a holding procedure for sounds that have reached the criterion level in the first step, but for which there is insufficient time to work on in subsequent steps. In this step, each phoneme is produced once in isolation with only visual stimulation. In this way, the client practices all error sounds during each session.

Phase II, *transfer* of sounds into syllables, words, phrases, reading, and conversation, comprises six steps. Step 1 is characterized as a "word probe" or test of the sound in monosyllabic words. If the client does not produce the sound in 6 of 10 words, step 2, practice of the sound in CV and VC syllables and in multisyllables, is implemented. When the client meets the criterion on the word probe, treatment proceeds to step 3, production of the target sound in monosyllabic and multisyllabic words. Words used are selected on the basis of the client's age and vocabulary and include nouns, verbs, adjectives, and other parts of speech. Step 4 consists of practice of the target sound in phrases and sentences. At this stage, the objective may change from correct production of the sound to correct articulation of the whole word. In step 5, the client reads stories or paragraphs. Usually, the objective is correct articulation of whole words rather than only of a specific sound. Error words are practiced after the reading. Last, step 6 involves spontaneous speech with the objective of whole-word accuracy.

The last phase of training, Phase III, is *maintenance* of correct articulation in various speaking situations. In step 1, the client engages in conversational speech in the clinical setting with minimal cues. Step 2 involves maintenance of articulation skills over time without direct intervention. The client is evaluated 3 and 6 months after treatment is terminated.

Each misarticulated phoneme progresses through all three phases at a pace that is appropriate for the client. For example, three sounds may be in Phase I, four sounds in Phase II, and two sounds in Phase III. Thus, all error sounds are worked on at the same time. Table 8.3 outlines the steps of the multiple phonemic approach as presented by Bradley (1989).

Comments

The multiple phonemic approach is deemed most appropriate for clients who have six or more misarticulated sounds (Bradley, 1989). It has been used with children who have repaired cleft palates and other corrected orofacial anomalies as well as with those who have functional articulation problems. The age range has been 5 to 14 years, although it certainly is an approach appropriate for older individuals. The approach seems to be more usable with individuals than with groups because it would be difficult to record client responses for more than one person at a time. The advantage of working on more than one sound at a time is that intelligibility is improved more rapidly. The approach also seems to be more efficient than traditional approaches that focus on one or two sounds at a time. A limitation is that working on several sounds at a time may be confusing to some clients. It may not be necessary to target all sounds in error because of generalization to nontarget sounds that have similar phonetic features.

What feature characterizes tactile-kinesthetic treatment approaches?

TACTILE-KINESTHETIC TREATMENT APPROACHES

Some treatment approaches involve the clinician's external manipulation of the client's articulators. The first such approach, motokinesthetics, was developed in the 1930s. A more recent version of this approach is PROMPT (Prompts for Restructuring Oral Muscular Phonetic Targets), which was devised in the 1980s.

Describe the motokinesthetic treatment approach, including its advantages and limitations.

Motokinesthetic Approach

Motokinesthetic articulation treatment was developed by Young and Hawk (1938) in the 1930s. In this approach, the speech-language pathologist directly manipulates externally parts of the client's speech mechanism (external mouth, jaw, nose, and neck regions), especially the articulators. Later, Vaughn and Clark (1979) expanded on these stimulation techniques. A subsequent derivation is the PROMPT (Chumpelik, 1984; Hayden & Square, 1994).

Rationale

The air current from the lungs is the source of speech production, and this air current is acted on by muscles to produce speech sounds (Young & Stinchfield-Hawk, 1955). The sounds are not produced in isolation, but in a sequence. In typical speakers, the muscles of the speech mechanism produce an easy flow of movements proceeding from one sound to the next. Articulation learning requires coordination of muscular activities used in speech, control of the air current, and facial expression. Individuals who have misarticulations need to learn the feel of articulation movements.

Through the clinician's manipulations and productions of the sounds, the client associates the articulation movements with the auditory input and learns to articulate sounds. The client reproduces the articulation movements through the kinesthetic sense. Presumably, positive kinesthetic and tactile feedback is established by the clinician manipulating the client's articulators.

Goals and Procedures

The stated objectives are to prevent incorrect articulation learning and to aid in the correction of misarticulations (Young & Hawk, 1938). Manipulations by the clinician set the patterns for the location, di-

TABLE 8.3

Treatment Steps for Each Target Sound in Multiple Phonemic Approach

Phase	Step	Description	Target Response	Criterion	Example
I—Establishment	Step 1: Sound in isolation	1. Auditory, visual (grapheme), phonetic placement, etc. stimulus 2. Auditory, visual stimulus 3. Visual stimulus	All consonants in isolation or in CV with a neutral vowel	4/5 in 2 consecutive sessions or 5/5 in 1 session	/kə/, /gə/, /s/, /z/, /f/ /v/
	Step 2: Holding pattern	Visual stimulus (Grapheme)	All consonants in isolation	1/1	/kə/
II—Transfer	Step 1: Word probe	Auditory model	10 monosyllabic words (5 initial position, 5 final position)	60%	cat, comb, can, key, come, back, sock, like, lake, sick
	Step 2: Syllable (if client fails word probe)	1. Open stimulation * 2. 1 Auditory-visual model for 5 responses	25 CV and VC	80% for two consecutive sessions or 90% for one session	/ki/, /kæ/, /kʌ/, /kɑ/, /ku/, /ik/, /æk/, /ʌk/, /uk/, /ɑk/
	Step 3: Word	1. Open * 2. Visual stimulation	25–30 words that are frequently occurring and represent various parts of speech (e.g., nouns, verbs, modifiers, and prepositions)	80% for two consecutive sessions or 90% for one session	cat, come, catch, color, kind, key, cold, take, like, black, back, sock, make, dark, kick
	Step 4: Phrase/sentence	1. Open or visual/auditory * 2. Open or visual/auditory * 3. Open or visual * 4. Open or visual *	1. Target sound 2. Whole word ** 3. Target sound 4. Whole word **	80% for two consecutive sessions or 90% for one session	The shoe is black. The cat is purring. Make me a picture. Is it in back of me? Are you cold?
	Step 5: Reading/story	Visual stimulus	1. Target sound 2. Whole word **	80% for two consecutive sessions or 90% for one session	"Read this page of your book." "Now, you tell me story I just told you."
	Step 6: Conversation	Auditory stimulus	1. Target sound 2. Whole word **	80% for two consecutive sessions or 90% for one session	"Tell me about the TV program you watched last night."
III—Maintenance	Step 1: In-clinic conversation	1. Auditory	Whole word **	90%	"What did you do during the holidays?"
	Step 2: Out-of-clinic conversation	2. Observation	Whole word **	90%	Observe in class room, playground, etc.

*Open = Any type of stimulation needed

**Whole Word = All sounds in the words are to be produced correctly rection, and form of articulation movements; that is, they indicate where the movement is to occur, the direction in which the articulators are to move, and the manner in which the sounds are to be produced. There is a standard stimulation for each sound, and the clinician uses that stimulation each time the sound is produced. Thus, the speech-language pathologist guides the muscular actions that act on the air current. The sounds so stimulated are produced sequentially, without pausing between sounds. No procedures are given for transferring the client from passive to active sound production then on to carryover.

The clinician says the syllables while manipulating the client's articulators, and the client watches the clinicians face; therefore, the client receives kinesthetic, tactile, auditory, and visual stimulations simultaneously. The feeling of movements is learned and becomes associated with the auditory input of the clinician. In other words, after the client feels the movements, the articulation movements can be reproduced through the kinesthetic sense.

The whole client needs to be considered, and manipulation rarely begins during the first meeting with the client (Young & Hawk, 1938). When using this approach, the client is placed in a supine position to facilitate relaxation. The clinician then manipulates the articulators with the "skill of a typist." Sometimes when initially teaching a speech sound, a tongue depressor is used inside the mouth if the standard manipulation is ineffective. The use of the tongue depressor is discontinued as soon as possible. No auditory discrimination training is done, and sounds are not produced in isolation, but rather in syllables, words, phrases, sentences, and paragraphs. Table 8.4 outlines the steps to follow in a motokinesthetic approach, and Appendix I describes the stimulations for each sound.

Comments

The motokinesthetic approach can be used only with individuals, not with groups. It is appropriate for children and adults. Young and Hawk (1938) recommended the approach for the categories of sound substitutions, delayed speech, speechlessness, cleft palate, hard of hearing, deaf, blind, deaf-blind, cerebral palsy, and aphasia and for the development of infant speech. More detailed information about adaptations of the method for various types of clients are provided by Young and Stinchfield-Hawk in their book. The approach is likely to be most effective with neurological and motor deficits, such as cerebral palsy, other dysarthrias, acquired apraxia, and childhood apraxia of speech (Sommers & Kane, 1974).

The most effective way for a speech-language

TABLE 8.4

Treatment Steps in a Motokinesthetic Approach

Step	Description	Example
1	Target sound + /ə/	/pə/
2	Monosyllables	/pɑ/, /pɑp/, /hɑp/, /pi/, pip/, /hip/
3	Repetitive bisyllables	/pɑpɑ/, /pipi/,/pʌpʌ/
4	Multisyllabic words	/pepɚ/, /hæpi/, /pʌpi/, /læptɑp/
5	Phrases and sentences	/pɪk mi ʌp/, /hi wɑnts ə pʌpi/
6	Comparative practice in words and phrases	/pɛt, bɛt, dɛt/, /kep, ket, kem/ /ʃi wɔr ə kep/, /hi rɛd ə pepɚ/

---

pathologist to learn this method is to be taught by another who has skill in using the approach. It would be extremely difficult, if not impossible, to learn to use motokinesthetics by reading the textbook, although Vaughn and Clark (1979) clearly described the stimulations for all phonemes and provided practice materials for clinicians to learn the techniques. This is perhaps the primary limitation of the approach. Another limitation or potential problem is the supine position because some clients may not feel comfortable lying down, and many treatment rooms are not equipped appropriately for it. While it may not be necessary for some clients, a supine position may be facilitative in other cases. The approach, however, can be implemented with a client in a seated position with the clinician and client seated in adjacent chairs facing in opposite directions as shown in Figure 8.4.

Today, clinicians use motokinesthetic stimulations, often modified versions of Hawk and Young's (1938) or invented ones, to elicit individual speech sounds and to aid in speech sound production in syllable, word, phrase, and sentence contexts. Manipulations for individual sounds seem to be particularly useful in eliciting speech sounds and for comparing and contrasting a target sound with a substitute sound when a client is confused about when to use each. A modification of the approach was found to be effective (Bashir, 1980) with childhood apraxia of speech in which clients were taught to use the sound stimulations on themselves. Some clients have used the motokines-

Respondent

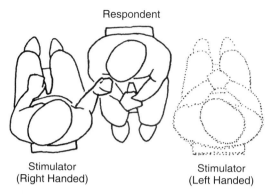

Stimulator
(Right Handed)

Stimulator
(Left Handed)

FIGURE 8.4 Seating of client during extra-oral manipulations when implementing the motokinesthetics treatment approach. (From Vaughn, G., & Clark, R (1979). *Speech facilitation.* Springfield, IL: Charles C. Thomas. Reprinted with permission.)

thetic stimulations on themselves without direct instruction; they have indirectly learned them from the clinician.

> Describe the PROMPT treatment approach, including its advantages and limitations.

PROMPT Treatment Approach

The PROMPT treatment approach was formally devised by Hayden in 1980 (Hayden,1999) and first published in 1984 (Chumpelik, 1984). Its roots are in the motokinesthetic approach (1938). In this approach, multidimensional tactile cues or prompts are provided by the clinician to guide the articulation mechanism in speech production. Each speech sound has a different prompt. "The prompts are given externally using muscles of the face, under the chin, of the structures associated with voicing and nasality, and of the jaw opening" (Chumpelik, p.144). Treatment proceeds through a seven-stage motor-speech hierarchy.

Rationale

PROMPT is based on neurological, anatomical, cognitive-linguistic, and motor theories (Hayden, 1999). Producing speech sounds involves the speech mechanism reaching a phonetic target within a "three-dimensional space-coordinate system" (Chumpelik, 1984, p. 141). The process of reaching these targets is dynamic as the articulators move from one phonetic target to the next, and each target can be reached from various locations. It is hypothesized that the neuromotor control of the speech system occurs through a combination or

closed loop and open loop systems. "In this framework, the higher levels of the motor nervous system may determine the overall timing and movement toward end positions (open-loop), but the programming of details and actual execution are accomplished through lower level pathways and mechanisms (closed-loop)" (Chumpelik, p. 142).

The PROMPT system provides tactile stimulations using touch, pressure, kinesthetic, and proprioceptive cues for the phonetic targets as well as for the *feed-forward* or sequential movement needed to go from one target to the next. It specifies the articulator positions while assisting the client in reaching these positions. The clinician's manipulation provides "a framework for spatial and temporal motor speech programming" (Square-Storer & Hayden, 1989, p. 190). Using the tactile prompts, the clinician has almost complete motor control of the peripheral and some of the proximal articulators. Clients are provided with the number of clues they need with all or most of the prompt components being given during earlier stages of treatment and fewer as treatment progresses until the client produces the targets without external tactile prompts by the clinician. Treatment progresses through a motor-speech hierarchy as shown in Figure 8.5 (Hayden, 1986, as cited in Hayden, 1999). The principle of the system is that the client gains speech motor control over levels of speech movements and each newly acquired skill is integrated with the previous levels.

Goals and Procedures

The goal for the client is to approximate phonemes, independently produce words/phrases, and produce conversational speech, depending upon the client's capabilities. The treatment generally progresses through the stages of the motor-speech hierarchy (Fig. 8.5). Level I focuses on attaining the postural support for speech with a focus on trunk, neck, and head control and the suppression of abnormal oral-motor reflexes. Level II stresses control of phonation, including voicing, so that the duration of speech for /ɑ/, /h/, and /m/ is 2 to 3 seconds. Level III involves movement on a single plane with voicing focused on jaw movement that is limited to vertical movement with the anterior–posterior movement controlled by the clinician. In level IV, additional planes of movement are added with an emphasis on control of lip retraction and rounding and symmetry and coordination of lip movements. There is integration of voicing, jaw, facial contraction, and lip rounding. Level V involves control of tongue height and location and integration of tongue movement with jaw and lip movements. Level VI includes sequenced movement on

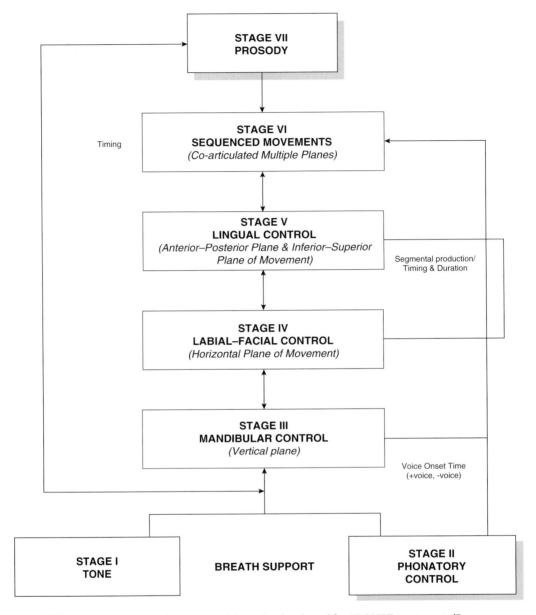

FIGURE 8.5 The motor speech treatment hierarchy developed for PROMPT treatment. (From Hayden, D. (1999).*The P.R.O.M.P.T. System Level 1: Manual.* Santa Fe, NM: PROMPT Institute, Inc. Reprinted with permission.)

multiple planes, encompassing voicing, jaw and facial contraction, tongue control, and timing. Level VII focuses on suprasegmentals, including intonation, stress, juncture, and speech rate in sequenced motor movements.

There are three phases of treatment with motor-speech and interaction and language goals specified for each phase:

• Phase I—Single plane of movement (vertical or horizontal)

• Phase II—Two planes of movement (vertical and horizontal across two syllables)

• Phase III—Three planes of movement (vertical, horizontal, and anterior–posterior)

In Phase I of treatment, levels I, II, and III of the motor-speech hierarchy are addressed; Phase II, level IV; and Phase III, levels V, VI, and VII. Table 8.5 displays the motor-speech goals and objectives for PROMPT intervention. The clinician gradually fades cues throughout each phase

TABLE 8.5

PROMPT Motor-Speech Goals and Objectives

Phase	Motor-Speech Goals	Interaction and Language Goals
I	To develop or refine speech motor control at the *single plane of movement* (vertical or horizontal) *without combining* them within the same syllable	To develop structure and routines that use sounds or syllables for interaction and use of oral communication or word
II	To further develop speech-motor subsystem control on at least two *planes of movement* (vertical and horizontal across two syllables)	To develop a lexicon using the speech-motor movements for the creation of semantic-syntactic relations and *short phrases* that may be used for turn-taking and to support interaction routines
III	To further develop and refine speech-motor subsystem control on *three planes of movement* (vertical, horizontal and anterior–posterior), either partially or wholly within the same word or phrase	To expand linguistic phrase structures and develop more flexibility in interaction

of intervention. The prompts are integrated into a communicative framework throughout the treatment process.

Before speech production, it is important for the client to be in a postural state for maximum readiness for speech movement. The client's body posture should be symmetrical. The clinician's hand is placed behind the client's head to restrict it from moving when the prompts are provided. The angle between the mylohyoid and neck is always 90° or less and the mylohyoid should be relaxed to allow maximum penetration of the mylohyoid tactile cues provided by the clinician.

Prompts provide information about several speech parameters including place of contact, extent of mandibular excursion, resonance and phonation, number of muscles in the contracted state, duration of segments relative to one another, manner of production, and coarticulation. There is a standard prompt specified for each English vowel, diphthong, and consonant. For each sound, tactile cues are provided by the clinician for the place of contact on the mylohyoid muscle (under the chin) and/or facial structures, the jaw position or excursion, the timing (such as fast, hold, quick release), and pressure. Nasal resonance and voicing features are cued by touching the nose and the laryngeal area, respectively. Mandibular excursion refers to the amount of jaw opening needed for each sound. The pressure prompts on the mylohyoid and facial structures provide cues about the number of muscles to be used, the duration of the contraction, and the de-

gree of tension of the muscles. The distinctive features of manner for the consonants—the management of the airstream—is cued through the prompts for position, pressure, and timing. Co-articulation is addressed using the PROMPT system by working at the phrase level with the clinician dynamically using surface prompts to move from one sound to the next. The clinician can prompt each target phoneme in a syllable, word, or phrase guiding the client's articulation movements during production of speech. In connected speech, the clinician modifies the standard prompt to account for co-articulation. For example, the lips may be rounded on the /s/ sound when saying the word *soap*, but retracted when saying the word *seed*. Prompts also vary based on the individual client's disability profile.

There are three levels of prompts:

• Parameter
• Complex
• Surface

Parameter prompts provide the base support and are the large organizing gestures (such as voicing, rounding, retracting). *Complex* prompts are multidimensional and specify as many components as possible. *Surface* prompts are noncomplex cues that signal place, timing, and transition (such as omission of voicing and jaw excursion cues). As treatment progresses, the parameter and complex prompts give way to surface prompts. At the word or phrase level, the clinician does not need to prompt every sound. Perhaps only the initial and final consonants or certain misarticulated sounds need to be cued. Still later, all prompts are faded and the client produces words and phrases without the tactile prompts.

Comments

The PROMPT system can be used with children and adults and with groups and individuals. It is effective in "controlled behavior conditions" and "in unstructured group situations in which language is also a treatment focus" (Chumpelik, 1984, p. 153). It was devised for childhood apraxia of speech and has been used effectively with other motor-speech disorders. It has been used successfully with persons who have phonologic disorders, hearing impairments, aphasia, dysarthria, dyspraxia, autism, head injury, and dysfluency (Jones EM, personal communication, February 20, 2001).

The only feasible way to learn to use the PROMPT system is to go through extensive training and practice, which is probably the primary limitation of the approach. Advantages include the flexibility of the approach to meet the needs of individual clients and the tactile cues provided by the clinician that vary from complex to surface (depending upon the clients needs). It can be applied in structured and unstructured settings. The approach provides for transitioning from isolated sound production to conversational speech. Often, speech sounds and sound sequences can be elicited with the prompts when other elicitation techniques have been ineffective. As with the motokinesthetics approach, clients have been observed using the PROMPT cues on themselves to assist them in producing speech sounds (Marriner N, personal communication, March 8, 2001).

> What feature characterizes phonetic context treatment approaches?

PHONETIC CONTEXT TREATMENT APPROACHES

Some articulation treatment approaches use the strategy of taking advantage of the phenomenon of phonetic context or co-articulation to target speech sound production. This was the idea in Van Riper's (Van Riper & Erickson, 1996) use of key words to elicit target speech sounds. Others have expanded on this technique (McDonald, 1964b; Weston & Irwin, 1971).

Co-articulation refers to the phenomenon in which the articulators simultaneously move in the production of speech sounds that are perceived to occur sequentially. In other words, the articulation

movements of a sound are influenced by sounds that closely precede and follow it. McDonald (1964b) considered this aspect in the sensory-motor approach when he referred to *overlapping movements* and contended that coarticulation must be considered when evaluating and treating articulatory disorders. Co-articulation factors can be used to facilitate production of sounds (Eisenson & Ogilvie, 1977; Schuckers, 1978). For example, to help prevent lip-rounding of /r/, /r/ should be used in combination with an unrounded vowel. To aid in the production of /k/, a back vowel rather than a front vowel should be used. A second application of this phenomenon is to practice the target sound in systematically varied phonetic contexts so that correct production is achieved no matter which sounds precede or follow it (Shelton, 1978). The client needs to learn to co-articulate a wide variety of phonemes.

> Describe the sensory-motor treatment approach, including its advantages and limitations.

Sensory-Motor Approach

The sensory-motor approach was devised by McDonald (1964b). In addition to the strategy of coarticulation, the client becomes aware of tactile and kinesthetic aspects of speech sound patterns. Production begins at the syllable level (as opposed to the isolation level), which is considered the basic unit of speech. Sounds that the client already produces correctly are practiced in the context of bisyllables and trisyllables. After production of each bisyllable, the client describes the movements of the articulators by stating which two articulators touched and in what direction the tongue moved. Stress patterns are varied during this bisyllabic and trisyllabic drill, and the client identifies the stressed syllable. Actual training of a misarticulated phoneme begins in a phonetic context in which it was produced correctly; that is, in a two-word combination in either the releasing or arresting position as determined by the results of *A Deep Test of Articulation* (McDonald, 1964a).

Rationale

The sensory-motor articulation treatment method emphasizes all the sensory and motor processes involved in speech production, because speech results from the interaction of certain sensory and motor processes. These processes evolve from simple to complex skills as a child matures from birth through 8 years of age. The integration of auditory, proprioceptive, and tactile sensations results in the use of precise, intricate articulation movements that normal speakers learn. McDonald (1964b) described the movements of articulation as ballistic and overlapping.

Ballistic movements occur as a result of rapid contraction of a muscle group followed by a short period of no contraction with the involved structure continuing to move because of momentum. The movement is subsequently stopped by contraction of the antagonist muscle group. According to McDonald, all skilled movements, including articulation, are ballistic. Articulation movements also are overlapping; that is, articulation of a particular phoneme is influenced by the sounds that precede and follow it. Stated another way, ". . . when a group of movements typical of an isolated consonant is combined with another consonant or vowel, the result is not the sum of the two movements, but a new group" (Shohara, 1939, as cited in McDonald, 1964b, p. 2). Thus, the exact articulation of any sound depends on its phonetic environment or context; each different context means that a different movement pattern must be used. For example /s/ followed by /t/ is phonetically produced differently than /s/ followed by /k/ in that the tongue position, mouth opening, and such, are not the same. There are three types of overlapping movements:

- Overlapping of different parts of the same structure; for example, in the articulation of *oaks* (/ks/), two different parts of the tongue are used
- Overlapping of different structures adjacent to one another; for example, in the articulation of *spool* (/sp/), the lips and tongue tip are involved
- Overlapping of different structures remote from one another; for example, in the articulation of *something* (/mθ/), the lips, soft palate, and laryngeal muscles are used

From his viewpoint then, McDonald (1964b) defined articulation as a "process consisting of a series of overlapping, ballistic movements which place varying degrees of obstruction in the way of the outgoing air stream and simultaneously modify the size, shape, and coupling of resonating cavities" (p. 87).

These overlapping, skilled articulation movements are superimposed on the syllable, which McDonald (1964b) considered the basic unit of speech, both physiologically and morphologically. A syllable has three components:

- Release, which may be through a consonant or by chest muscles
- Vowel shaping

- Arrest, which may be through a consonant or by chest muscles

Sounds do not occur normally in isolation nor even in the initial, medial, or final positions of words. Instead, sounds are parts of the movement sequences of syllables. Consonants function to release or arrest syllables. Words are not physiological units in running speech, but sequences of syllables. The syllables are produced with differing rates and stress patterns. McDonald identified three types of consonants as they occur in syllables:

- Simple—a single consonant that arrests or releases a syllable, as illustrated by /se/
- Compound—two or more consonants that function as a single consonant, as in /ste/
- Abutting—adjacent consonants with one arresting the first syllable and the other releasing the second syllable, such as /æstɚ/.

McDonald (1964b) criticized more traditional articulation approaches for several reasons. He contended that testing sounds in the initial, medial, and final positions of words is haphazard sampling rather than a representative sample of the client's articulation skills. Sounds should not be taught in isolation because they do not occur naturally in isolation; the syllable is the basic unit of speech. Ear training emphasizes only one sensory channel and uses analysis of another person's production rather than attending to all sensory input channels. Finally, commercially prepared or clinician-prepared materials do not place responsibility for learning on the client and likely do not use the client's own vocabulary. Thus, McDonald devised a treatment approach with a consideration of these factors and of his viewpoint of the articulation process.

Goals and Procedures

The goal of the sensory-motor approach is to increase the number of phonetic contexts in which the target phoneme is produced correctly rather than to teach a *new* sound. This is based on the idea that deficient articulation is not always consistent, some phonemes may never be produced correctly, others are sometimes produced correctly, and still others are always produced correctly in certain contexts. This variability is because articulation develops from simple to complex skills as the sensory and motor processes mature over time.

There are three general goals to be reached in the sensory-motor approach. The first is "to heighten . . . responsiveness to patterns of auditory, proprioceptive, and tactile sensations associated with overlapping ballistic movements of articulation" (McDonald, 1964b, p. 138). In this first phase of treatment, the client *imitates* the clinician's auditory stimuli and *describes tactile and kinesthetic sensations* by indicating which two articulators touched, in which direction the tongue moved, and which syllable was stressed. The stimuli progress from simple to complex movements, using varying stress patterns. On the bisyllabic drills, only correctly articulated consonants, as shown by testing, are used. The stimulus sequence is as follows:

- CVCV (consonant-vowel-consonant-vowel) with the same consonant and vowel and with equal stress; for example, /bibi/
- 'CVCV with the same consonant and vowel and with trochaic stress patterns; for example, /'bibi/
- CV'CV with the same consonant and vowel and with iambic stress patterns; for example, /bi'bi/
- CVCV with different vowels and various stress patterns; for example, /'bibu/, /bɑ'be/
- CVCV with different consonants and various stress patterns; for example, /bi'ki/, /te'me/
- CVCV with different vowels and consonants and various stress patterns; for example, /'biku/, /tɑ'mo/
- CVCVCV with different vowels and consonants and various stress patterns; for example, /pu'toni/, /'mɑwebə/.

Different movement sequences are practiced beginning with larger changes of movement so that diverse parts of the articulators are used, such as with /po ki te/, in which the movement shifts from the front of the mouth at the lips to the back of the tongue and, finally, to the tongue tip. Progressively, smaller articulation movement shifts are used as in /ti se mo/, in which the tongue tip is used twice in succession followed by a front bilabial consonant. At this point in the program, phonemes that were incorrectly produced on the articulation test are presented. The earlier bisyllabic practice and descriptions of various movement sequences may result in correct production of these error phonemes because clients are now more aware of how speech sounds are produced (McDonald). However, if the client continues to misarticulate these error sounds, no attempt is made to teach correct production at this trisyllabic drill stage of treatment. Sounds that continue to be produced incorrectly are dropped from the drill stimuli.

The second general goal is "to reinforce correct articulation of the error sound" (McDonald, 1964b, p. 142). The client is allowed to select the target sound. Additionally, a sound should be selected that can quickly be habituated, is earlier developing, and is not correct in a high percentage of phonetic contexts (but is correct in at least one phonetic

context). The Deep Test (McDonald, 1964a) is administered for the target sound. The phonetic context in which the sound was produced correctly during assessment is the starting point for *production of the error sound*. Procedures for practicing the correct articulation in the phonetic context include slow motion speech, equal stress on both syllables, prolongation, and practice in short sentences.

The third goal is "to facilitate the correct articulation of the sound in systematically varied phonetic contexts" (McDonald, 1964b, p. 146). This phase of treatment begins by changing the vowel following the target sound. The *phonetic context* is then further *modified* in additional word combinations and sentences. At this stage, the client makes a list of words beginning and ending with the target sounds. These words are used in various combinations, stress patterns, and rate patterns. Sentences with these words are constructed and practiced with different stress and rate patterns. Table 8.6 outlines the steps in a sensory-motor approach.

Comments

McDonald (1964b) recommended this approach for children whose articulation errors seem to be the result of arrested or delayed articulation development and for those who correctly articulate the sound in at least one phonetic context. This approach seems to be especially appropriate for clients who have multiple errors; it is a bit tedious for those with only one or two errors. A variation of this method has been recommended for children with childhood apraxia of speech (Rosenbek, Hansen, Baughman, & Lemme, 1974). The approach can be adapted to group treatment, to individual work, and to adults, although it was designed for children. Because clients are to describe the positions of the articulators as well as to specify stress patterns, it is usually not appropriate for children younger than 7 years of age.

Emphasis on varying stress patterns is a positive aspect of the sensory-motor approach because suprasegmentals are an important part of speech production. The early stages of this approach on developing an awareness of the placement and movement of the articulators may assist clients in learning to produce misarticulated sounds without directly targeting them in treatment. Giving the client responsibility for treatment material and using the client's vocabulary may facilitate carryover. Incorporating the concept of overlapping movements in articulation treatment, more commonly referred to as *co-articulation*, may also expedite management. Some limitations of the approach are the tedious nature of the drill, imitation, and description of articulation sequence movements, and

TABLE 8.6

Treatment Steps in the Sensory-Motor Approach

Phase	Step	Description	Example
I		Practice with sounds already produced correctly in varying phonetic contexts	
	Step 1	CVCV with same C and V, equal stress	/toto/ "How did you make that sound? What two parts of your mouth touched?"
	Step 2	CVCV with same C and V, stress on first syllable	/'toto/ "How did you make that sound?"
	Step 3	CVCV with same C and V, stress on second syllable	/to'to/ "How did you make that sound?"
	Step 4	CVCV with same C and different V, varying stress	/'totu/, /ti'te/ "How did you make those sounds?"
	Step 5	CVCV with different C and same V, varying stress	/to'bo/, /'timi/ "How did you make those sounds?"
	Step 6	CVCV with different C and different V, varying stress	/'tomi/, /ta'do/ "How did you make those sounds?"
	Step 7	CVCVCV with different C and different V, varying stress (use some sounds client produced incorrectly)	/'tomiku/, /mako'te/, /du'seni/ "How did you make those sounds?"
II		Practice correct production of error sound in facilitating context	"Say *kitship* slowly. Say '*kitship* is a funny word'"
III		Systematically vary phonetic contexts	
	Step 1	Change vowel following target sound	kitshop, kitsheep
	Step 2	Change other sounds before or after target sound	kidshop, kimsheep
	Step 3	Combine words from lists of words beginning and ending with target sound, varying stress patterns	top ship cup shed dish top wash dog
	Step 4	Sentences	The fish took the bait. My boat should float.

the client is given no feedback about how to change incorrect production attempts.

Today, the sequence of producing bisyllables and trisyllables with varying stress patterns in the initial stages of the approach is often incorporated into treatment with childhood apraxia of speech and acquired apraxia. Some recommend that persons with apraxia begin their articulation work with nonmeaningful syllable production (Strand & Skinder, 1999). Finding facilitative contexts for producing individual speech sounds, particularly /l/, /r/, and the stridents is an effective strategy currently used by clinicians. In this case, the nonsense bisyllable and trisyllable drillwork is omitted from the treatment process.

Paired-Stimuli Approach

The **paired-stimuli approach** was initially devised by Weston and Irwin (1971) who later devised articulation treatment kits (Irwin & Weston, 1971–1975) based on the paired-stimuli method. It is a highly structured approach in which treatment sequentially progresses from words to sentences to conversation. Words in which the target sound is correctly produced are used as a frame of reference and as a starting point for transfer of that sound to other words. The client says a key word followed by a training word; that is, a word in which the target sound was produced incorrectly prior to treatment. Sounds are targeted in initial and final positions and are targeted one phoneme at a time.

Rationale

The basis of the paired stimuli approach is operant conditioning principles (Weston & Irwin, 1971). Weston and Irwin noted that while operant conditioning focuses on symptoms, it has been shown to be effective in modifying behavior in the realm of communication as well as in other areas. The paired stimuli method adheres to the operant paradigm of discriminative stimulus, response, and contingent reinforcer. Using key words as the conduit to correct articulation of the target in other words takes advantage of beginning with what the client can already do.

Goals and Procedures

The goal is correct production of the target sounds in conversational speech. One sound is targeted at a time. There are three stages in the paired-stimuli approach:

- Word level
- Sentence level
- Conversation level

The *word level* stage requires selection of a target sound and key words, words that contain the target sound only once and in which the client correctly produces the target sound in 9 of 10 trials. Four key words are identified, two containing the target phoneme in the initial position and two in the final position. If no word exists in which the target sound is used correctly, they are taught to the client. Then 20 training words, 10 with the target sound in the initial position and 10 in the final position, are selected. A training word is one in which the sound is misarticulated in two of three trials.

Pictures representing a key word with the sound in the initial position and 10 training words are placed on a picture board with the key word in the middle. Criterion for movement to the next step is 80% correct productions of the training words in two consecutive training strings. A training string is the pairing of a key word with each of 10 training words. In the first step of stage 1, the client is instructed to produce the key word followed by the first training word and is reinforced for correct productions. Misarticulations are ignored. This procedure is repeated for each of the successive training words. In the second step of stage 1, the same procedure is repeated for a key word and 10 training words in the final position. In the third step, a third key word is taught that has the target sound in the initial position. The client produces pairs of words, the key word and a training word as a unit, instead of producing the key word and training word separately. The client is reinforced for correct production of both the key word and the training word. In the fourth step, the client produces pairs of words, the fourth key word which has the target sound in the final position, and the training words. The frequency of reinforcement is decreased to reinforcement of two correct response units.

During stage 2, the client says the first key word and the 10 training words in *sentences* in response to the clinician's questions. Reinforcement is decreased to every third correct response. In the second step, the procedure of asking questions is repeated for the second and third key words and their respective 10 training words alternately so that a question is asked about the second key word (final position) followed by a question about the third key word (initial position), and so on, until all 20 training words are produced. In the third step, the first and fourth key words are alternated, again alternating the initial and final positions.

The last stage, *conversation*, involves the clinician and client engaging in conversational activities. If the client misarticulates the target sound, the clinician models the correct production and asks the child to imitate the correct response. As the treatment continues in this stage, the client is sequentially reinforced for four correct productions, then seven, and finally 10, 13, and 15 consecutive productions in consecutive trials. Intervention for the target sound is ended when the client produces it in conversation in 15 consecutive opportunities on two successive treatment days. Table 8.7 outlines the stimulus shift approach.

Comments

The paired stimuli approach was designed for children, but could be used with adults if modified to use written words rather than pictures. It is most appropriately used with individual clients and not with groups. It is most appropriate for clients who have only a few misarticulations because only one sound is targeted at a time. The advantages of the approach are that clients begin treatment with a task that they are able to do, they progress at their own pace, they receive considerable practice on their target sound in successively more complex tasks, and they achieve success. Appropriately trained and credentialed paraprofessionals can carry out some steps of the procedure. The limitations are that only one sound is worked on at a time, so it may not be efficacious for clients with multiple misarticulations. Clinicians may become mechanistic in administering the treatment, and if followed precisely, there is no flexibility in implementing the approach.

Today, the technique of paired stimuli is used by some clinicians with some clients who do produce key words. It is one of the effective ways of eliciting target sounds in clients who are not readily stimulable. Speech-language pathologists tend to be flexible in the techniques they use with individual clients and do not follow a rigid behavioral approach.

> What feature characterizes stimulability treatment approaches?

STIMULABILITY TREATMENT APPROACHES

Some approaches revolve around the phenomenon of stimulability in the treatment process. One of

TABLE 8.7

Treatment Steps in the Paired Stimuli Approach

Step	Description	Criterion	Example
Stage I—Word	Identify 4 key words (2 initial, 2 final) Select 20 training words (10 initial, 20 final)		1. /ʃu/ 2. /hʌʃ/ 3. /ʃo/ 4. /puʃ/ /ʃʌt/, /ʃɑp/, /ʃɚt/, etc. /fɪʃ/, /wɑʃ/, /kæʃ/, etc.
Step 1	Produces key word 1, then training word 1; key word 1, training word 2; key word 1, training word 3; . . . key word 1, training word 10	80% of two consecutive training strings	/ʃu/, /ʃʌt/ /ʃu/, /ʃɑp/ /ʃu/, /ʃɚt/, etc.
Step 2	Produces key word 2, then training word 11; key word 2, training word 12; key word 2, training word 13; . . . key word 2, training word 20	80% of two consecutive training strings	/hʌʃ/, /fɪʃ/ /hʌʃ/, /wɑʃ/ /hʌʃ/, /kæʃ/, etc.
Step 3	Produces key word 3 followed immediately with training word 1, then key word 3 immediately followed with training word 2, . . . to key word 3 with training word 10	80% of two consecutive training strings; both words must be correct	/ʃo/-/ʃʌt/ /ʃo/-/ʃɑp/ /ʃo/-/ʃɚt/, etc.
Step 4	Produces key word 4 followed immediately with training word 11, then key word 4 immediately followed with training word 12, to key word 4 with training word 20	80% of two consecutive training strings; both words must be correct	/puʃ/–/fɪʃ/ /puʃ/–/wɑʃ/ /puʃ/–/kæʃ/, etc.
Step 5: Probe	Conversational sample	80% in 15–20 words	Talk about recent activities
Stage II—Sentence			
Step 1	Produces key word 1 with training word 1 in a sentence, then key word 1 with training word 2 . . . to key word 1 with training word 10	80% of two consecutive training strings; both words must be correct	Clinician: "Is the *shoe shut* up in the closet?" Client: "Yes, the *shoe* is *shut* up in the closet."

(continued)

TABLE 8.7 (Continued)

Treatment Steps in the Paired Stimuli Approach

Step	Description	Criterion	Example
Step 2	Produces key word 2 with training word 11, then key word 3 with training word 1, alternating between key word 2-training word and key word 3-training word in sentences	80% of two consecutive training strings; both words must be correct	Clinician: "Did the whale tell the *fish* to *hush* up?" Client: "Yes, the whale told the *fish* to *hush* up." Clinician: "Did he *shut* the door at the *show*?" Client: "Yes, he *shut* the door at the *show*."
Step 3	Produces key word 1 with target word 1, then key word 4 with target word 11 . . . key word 1 with target word 10, then key word 4 with target word 20	80% of two consecutive training strings; both words must be correct	Clinician: "Did you *shut* the door with *your shoe*? Client: "Yes, I *shut* the door with my *shoe*." Clinician: "Do the *fish push* the pole." Client: "Yes, the *fish push* the pole."
Stage III— Conversation			
Step 1	Converses by answering open-ended questions. Clinician stops conversation when client has 4 correct target sounds or 1 incorrect word.	Correct production of target sound in four words produced spontaneously	"What did you see at the aquarium?"
Step 2	Converses by answering open-ended questions.	Correct production of target sound in seven words produced spontaneously correct	"Tell me about . . . "
Step 3	Engages in conversational speech	Correct production of target sound in 10 words produced spontaneously	"Tell me about . . . "
Step 4	Engages in conversational speech	Correct production of target sound in 13 words produced spontaneously	"Tell me about . . . "
Step 5: Probe	Engages in conversational speech	Correct production of target sound in 15 consecutive words produced spontaneously in two consecutive opportunities	"Tell me about . . . "

the earlier approaches, integral stimulation, prioritized speech sounds for treatment based on their stimulability or ease of elicitation. The most stimulable sounds are targeted initially and as articulation skills improve, the more difficult sounds become more easily stimulated and are subsequently targeted. A later approach, stimulability enhancement, targets nonstimulable sounds all at once in young children to increase their phonetic repertoire early.

> Describe the integral stimulation treatment approach, including its advantages and limitations.

Integral Stimulation Approach

In 1954, Milisen and associates devised and reported on an articulation treatment program called **integral stimulation**. This approach has also been referred to as the most common approach to dealing with speech disorders (Strand & Skinder, 1999). In it, clients use all relevant stimuli, including auditory, visual, and perhaps kinesthetic, to produce speech sounds correctly. Clients imitate the clinician's model by focusing attention on both the auditory stimulus and visual stimulus by listening and watching the clinician's face. Clients then hear, see, and feel their productions. Finally, both the client and clinician evaluate the response. Treatment begins with production rather than with auditory perception training.

Rationale

The basic premise of Milisen et al. (1954) is that deviant articulation results from a disruption in the normal learning process that can be corrected when treatment is appropriate, initiated early enough, and continued long enough. Treatment is based on learning principles appropriate for the skill level of the client. The focus is on producing correct responses rather than on unlearning incorrect responses.

Milisen et al. (1954) enumerated four criteria of a good treatment program:

- Should handle all types of articulation deviances, all age levels, and all environmental and physical limitations
- Should involve methods that are based on learning theory, that are easy to understand and teach, that enable successful performance, and that challenge the client
- Should present material in a whole or complete speech response that enables the client to produce it correctly
- Should not conflict with psychotherapy

According to Milisen (1954), "A speech movement skill cannot be learned until it is produced" (p. 10). Thus, the stimulus complex must elicit correct production. To elicit a correct response, the stimulus must be vivid for the client. Use of all available sensory stimuli aids in obtaining correct responses. Other techniques such as phonetic placement and tongue and lip exercises fractionalize or "break up" the speech process. Use of multiple stimuli is supported by a study that showed visual-auditory stimulation to be more effective than either visual or auditory stimulation alone (Scott & Milisen, 1954). Further, the results of another study showed that large amounts of stimulation resulted in better ability to produce sounds after a time lapse (Romans & Milisen, 1954).

The integral stimulation approach is based on the assumption that clients are most strongly motivated when they can see and hear themselves producing the whole sound correctly. Thus, treatment begins with sounds that are most easily stimulable. Milisen (1954) hypothesized that features learned while producing easily stimulable sounds are transferred to sounds that were not stimulable at first, but later become stimulable because of the success in producing other sounds.

Goals and Procedures

The ultimate goal for the integral stimulation approach is for the client to articulate speech sounds correctly under the most advanced condition of three factors, namely, amount of assistance needed for correct production, complexity of the speech configuration, and audience threat to good speech (Milisen et al., 1954). Sound selection is a key component of the approach. Basically, misarticulated sounds are listed in the order of stimulability and in terms of level of distraction to listeners. Sounds that occur more frequently as well as severity of the misarticulation are considered the most distracting. Sounds produced correctly or better (such as distortion instead of a substitution) after stimulation are considered the most stimulable. Visibility of the sounds, auditory acuity and discrimination abilities, general speech environment (including others in child's environment displaying similar misarticulations), organic conditions, and motivational influences are secondary factors to be considered in sound selection. Only one sound is targeted at a time. Ideally, treatment begins with sounds that are stimulable and distracting to the listener. Nonetheless, the sound initially targeted is stimulable. It progresses to sounds that were initially not stimulable but have become more stimulable because of "transfer of training of common elements from the recently learned sounds" (Milisen, 1954, p. 10). Sounds remaining nonstimulable are stimulated to elicit a change in their production that can be modified into a correct imitation of the target sound. Finally, if any phonemes remain nonstimulable after intensive stimulation, auditory perceptual training procedures are used; or, as a last resort, fractionalizing methods are used.

Once a sound is selected, the clinician uses integral stimulation, which includes: (a) clinician production of the sound such that the client hears, sees, and perhaps feels it; (b) the client's response, which the clinician sees, hears, and feels; and (c) evaluation of the response by the clinician and the client. The clinician uses every device to make the sound heard and seen. All points of articulation should be made as visible as possible to the client.

Throughout the treatment process, the clinician manipulates three variables so that the client is challenged (but does not completely fail):

- Amount of clinician assistance needed
- Complexity of the speech unit
- Listener reaction

Generally, two variables are held constant while the third one is being manipulated. The first variable is the amount of assistance needed for the client to produce the speech unit. In other words, the clinician varies the amount of stimulation and help given to the client depending on how much is needed to elicit a correct response at a particular stage of treatment. A second variable is the complexity of the speech unit. Treatment begins with easier speech units such as an isolated consonant and proceeds to more complex configurations such as nonsense syllables, sentences, and conversation. Also, sounds are usually easier to produce in singletons rather than blends, and memorized material is usually easier than reading material and conversation. The third variable is audience or listener reaction. "Friendly" listeners tend to facilitate more accurate responses, whereas an "unfriendly" audience may cause a client to regress to incorrect speech patterns. At the later stages of treatment, the three variables should be at the most adverse level with the client using correct productions. Milisen et al. (1954) believed that success of articulation treatment frequently is dependent on the amount of success experienced with the first sounds worked on because improved speech positively changes the attitudes of the client and persons in the environment. Success with the first sounds provides a model learning pattern and motivation for the client.

Comments

The integral stimulation approach is adaptable with groups and individuals, and with children and adults. It has been recommended for children with apraxia of speech (Strand & Skinder, 1999), for dysarthria (Rosenbek & LaPointe, 1985), and for acquired apraxia of speech (Rosenbek, 1985; Rosenbek, Lemme, Ahern, Harris & Wertz, 1973). Advantages seem to be the multisensory input that provides multiple clues for sound elicitation, early success because the most stimulable sounds are targeted first, and the focus on movement patterns needed by clients who have motor impairment (Strand & Skinder, 1999).

Today, the integral stimulus approach is used for children with apraxia of speech and acquired apraxia with an emphasis on movement patterns and sound sequences rather than focusing on isolated sounds. It entails repetitive practice. The im-

itation method from multisensory input has been modified to provide clients with phonetic placement information, to use shaping for sound elicitation, and to incorporate rhythm, intonation, and stress into the intervention.

> Describe the stimulability enhancement treatment approach, including its advantages and limitations.

Stimulability Enhancement Treatment Approach

In the **stimulability enhancement approach**, several consonants are targeted in isolation at the same time. The purpose is to increase the size of the phonetic inventory. Each sound is associated with a character, such as an animal or object, and a movement or gesture. The client produces the sounds in playlike activities. This approach was specifically designed for "children with very limited phonetic inventories and for whom most sounds missing from the inventory are nonstimulable" (Miccio & Elbert, 1996, p. 337).

Rationale

Stimulability refers to the speaker's ability to improve production of sounds through imitation of the correct sound production. Stimulability provides evidence that the speech mechanism has structural and functional integrity necessary for speech sound production. However, the opposite is not necessarily true; that is, the lack of stimulability does not mean that there is a structural or functional problem with the speech mechanism (Lof, 1996; Powell & Miccio, 1996). When a sound is not stimulable, the client's motoric, perceptual, or linguistic abilities may be deficient or other factors may negatively affect stimulability, including poor attending or noncompliance. A stimulable sound is likely to be added to the client's phonetic inventory even without direct targeting of that sound in treatment (Miccio, Elbert, & Forrest, 1999; Powell, 2003; Powell, Elbert, & Dinnsen, 1991). On the other hand, a sound that is not stimulable is unlikely to improve without direct intervention. Thus, generally, the prognosis for clients who are stimulable is more favorable than for those who are not stimulable (Powell & Miccio, 1996). Keep in mind, however, that this prediction is not true of all individuals.

Stimulability seems to affect generalization of sounds targeted in treatment (Powell & Miccio, 1996). When sounds that are not stimulable are targeted and become stimulable, they are more likely to generalize. When these nonstimulable sounds become stimulable, the clients phonetic repertoire will increase, which in turn increases the phonetic contrasts that the client can produce and, consequently, increases intelligibility.

Goals and Procedures

The goal of the stimulability enhancement treatment approach is to increase the client's phonetic inventory as quickly and efficiently as possible. Specifically, the objective is to increase the number of stimulable sounds in the client's repertoire. Consonant sounds are targeted in isolation (e.g., /f::/) or consonant-vowel combinations for the stops and glides (e.g., /tʌ/). Each

consonant sound is associated with an animal or object and with a gesture or movement (Table 8.8). At the beginning of every session, each targeted sound is modeled for the client along with a character card and the movement. The client is encouraged to produce the sounds with the clinician, but is not required to do so. Then, the clinician and client engage in developmentally appropriate playlike activities, providing the opportunity for the client to imitate the consonants (e.g., "Go Fish," spinner game). The client and clinician take turns so that the clinician is continuously providing models of the target consonants. The clinician reinforces the client for correct responses with verbal feedback and provides multiple modality (auditory, visual, tactile)

TABLE 8.8

Stimulus Characters Used to Elicit Consonant Production in the Stimulability Enhancement Approach

Consonant		Character	Example of an Associated Gesture
Stops	/p/	Putt-putt pig	Hands move in a skating motion
	/b/	Baby bear	Pantomime rocking a baby
	/t/	Talkie turkey	Nod head from side to side
	/d/	Dirty dog	Dig and frown
	/k/	Coughing cow	Cough with hand at throat
	/g/	Goofy goat	Roll eyes toward ceiling
Fricatives	/f/	Fussy fish	Hand fussily pushes away from body
	/v/	Viney violet	Move arm up as a winding vine
	/θ/	Thinking thumb	Tap thumb on chin
	/s/	Silly snake	Slinkily move finger up arm
	/z/	Zippy zebra	Hastily move finger up arm
	/ʃ/	Shy sheep	Clutch hands together and look down shyly
Affricates	/tʃ/	Cheeky chick	Sassily tap hand on cheek
	/dʒ/	Giant giraffe	Move eyes upward in stair steps
Nasals	/m/	Munchie mouse	Push lips together and rub tummy
	/n/	Naughty newt	Shake head back and forth negatively
Glides	/w/	Wiggly worm	Shiver
	/j/	Yawning yoyo	Yawn with hand tapping mouth
	/h/	Happy hippo	Laugh and shake shoulders
Liquids	/l/	Lazy lion	Stretch arms lazily
	/r/	Rowdy rooster	Crow with head and shoulders held high

From Miccio A. W., Elbert M. Enhancing stimulability: A treatment program. *Journal of Communication Disorders, 29,* 335–352. Reprinted with permission.

instruction when the client incorrectly produces the target. To ensure success for the client, all consonants are included in the clinical activities, including sounds that are produced correctly and/or are stimulable. Thus, the client receives treatment for nonstimulable sounds while stimulable sounds are reinforced and stabilized. The idea is that with success on the stimulable sounds, the client becomes more willing to attempt to produce the nonstimulable sounds that are more difficult.

Probes can be inserted into the treatment sessions to denote progress. Miccio and Elbert (1996) used the procedure of administering one third of the total probe during each session. Probes consist of the consonants produced in nonsense syllables and words in the initial, medial, and final positions using the vowels, /i/, /æ/, and /ɑ/ (Fig. 6.3).

Comment

The stimulability enhancement treatment approach can be used in individual and group sessions. It was designed to be used with young children with very limited phonetic inventories in conjunction with poor stimulability. The advantages of the approach are that it capitalizes on the research findings that generalization occurs for sounds that are stimulable, the play activities are usually motivating for young children, and targeting most consonants at once is efficacious—resulting in increased intelligibility. A limitation may be that some young clients will become confused when working on so many sounds at a time. In practice, clinicians may choose not to probe nonsense syllables and words in every session.

> What elements characterize behavior modification treatment approaches?

BEHAVIOR MODIFICATION TREATMENT APPROACHES

During the 1970s and early 1980s, many speech-language pathologists used programmed instruction articulation treatment programs. Many such programs were published (e.g., Baker & Ryan, 1971; Brown, Timm, & Evans, 1978; Irwin & Weston, 1971–1975).

Programmed Instruction Approach

The **programmed instruction approach** to articulation treatment can be accurately referred to as operant conditioning, **behavior modification**, behavior therapy, or as learning theory because it is based on principles formulated in these areas. It is an approach that can be overlaid onto other approaches; that is, programmed instruction can be applied to other approaches, such as stimulus, sensory-motor, integral stimulation, and enhanced stimulation. Programmed instruction is an approach in which the stimuli and client responses are behaviorally specified before initiation of treatment. Stimuli are arranged in small, sequential steps leading to the desired terminal objective. The client is given immediate feedback about the adequacy of responses in the form of reinforcement for correct responses and sometimes in the form of **punishment** for incorrect responses. Progress is continuously monitored through tracking and recording procedures.

Rationale

In the 1960s and 1970s, there was a rapid increase in the use of behaviorism in which operant conditioning techniques play a major role and from which programmed instruction was developed for articulation intervention. In this approach, treatment is directed toward modifying observable problem behaviors or symptoms rather than toward the underlying causes. A specified behavior is modified through the manipulation of stimuli that both precede (antecedent event) and follow (consequent event) the client's responses. Behavior modification procedures are characterized by specification of behavioral objectives in quantifiable terminology, by precise measurement of behaviors, and by systematic use of reinforcement schedules and programmed instruction.

An important component of programmed instruction is observing, assessing, and recording speech behaviors in an objective way. Appropriate and accurate observation helps the clinician assess the effect of treatment. To assess a behavior objectively, the behavior must be clearly described so that anyone observing would see the same behavior. Subjective estimates of progress merely provide a feel for the effectiveness of treatment, but knowing the exact increase or decrease in the frequency of correct or incorrect responses allows the clinician to evaluate the effectiveness of treatment procedures accurately. A critical component is stating the objectives behaviorally by identifying objectives that can be observed and measured. A behavioral objective describes what the learner will be able to do as a result of a learning experience; thus, the objective specifies what the learner is to do, under what conditions, and how well.

Clinicians present stimuli to elicit a response. The learning principle to which this is related is referred to as the S-R laws, which can be written as $R = f(S)$ under c. This formula refers to the relationship between stimulus events (S) and response events (R) under certain environmental conditions—c (Mowrer, 1988). It is reasoned that when a specified response always varies directly as the stimulus is manipulated, the stimulus causes the response. Thus, one can control the response by manipulating the stimulus that precedes it by controlling the antecedent event. Of course, 100% control never occurs when dealing with human behavior. However, if speech-language pathologists desire to change speech behaviors, the use of the functional relationship between stimuli and responses can result in such a change.

In addition to manipulating antecedent events, behavior is controlled by the consequence that follows a response to increase or decrease the frequency of a specified client response. This process has been called *contingency management*, which seems to be a term analogous to behavior therapy and behavior modification. There are three basic procedures for increasing and decreasing responses by manipulating consequent events (Hegde, 1998; Mowrer, 1988). The first procedure is reinforcement that may be either positive or negative. Positive reinforcement is a pleasant consequence that increases a particular response. If the frequency of a response does not increase, the consequent stimulus is not a positive reinforcer. The effect of positive reinforcement is influenced by the amount of reinforcement, the number of trials reinforced, and the schedule of reinforcement. The reinforcement schedule refers to how often a response is reinforced. Negative reinforcement also increases the frequency of a response, but it does so through escape from or avoidance of an aversive stimulus. Unlike punishment, the unpleasant stimulus may be presented before the response and is removed as a consequence of a desired response (escape) or the client performs the target behavior in order to avoid the presentation of an aversive stimulus.

A second procedure used to control behavior is the use of punishment, in which an aversive stimulus is presented following a response to decrease the frequency of occurrence of the response (Hegde, 1998; Mowrer, 1988). The aversive stimulus or consequence of an incorrect response may be verbal, nonverbal, or mechanical (such as "that's incorrect, try it again," marking an X instead of a +). Time out is a form of punishment in which positive reinforcement is removed. The client may be removed from the environment, may be excluded from activity, or may receive no reinforcement for a brief period. Another form of punishment is response cost, in which a positive reinforcer is removed, such as taking away a token, a good mark, or a penny.

A third procedure of manipulating consequent events is **differential reinforcement**; that is, the combination of positive reinforcement and **extinction** (Hegde, 1998). Extinction is a procedure in which reinforcement is terminated and the behavior is allowed to occur until it disappears. With extinction, the clinician essentially ignores incorrect responses. The combination of extinction (or ignoring incorrect responses) and reinforcement of correct responses results in faster extinction of the undesired behavior, in this case, misarticulations. Thus, the client is simultaneously increasing one behavior and decreasing the other. Such a procedure is used in shaping behavior as in progressive approximation as described by Van Riper and Erickson (1996). Behaviorists sometimes call the procedure response *differentiation*. A certain response is reinforced initially in treatment, but later is not reinforced or is extinguished because the client is now using a behavior that is closer to the terminal behavior. This process of reinforcement and extinction of a certain response continues until only the terminal behavior is reinforced and the approximations are extinguished. Thus, the initial response becomes extinguished while another response is rewarded. A second way in which a combination of positive reinforcement and extinction is used is in discrimination training in which different clinician responses are given to different stimuli (Hegde, 1998). Thus, a response is reinforced in the presence of one stimulus, but not reinforced in the presence of another stimulus. For example /s/ is to be used when a picture of a *sink* is shown, but not when a picture of a *drink* is shown. This also may be what occurs when a client produces /s/ correctly when talking to the clinician, but not when talking to the teacher. The clinician is a discriminative stimulus for /s/, but the teacher is not.

Procedures for acquisition of behaviors have been discussed, but now the subject turns to principles of transferring or generalizing behaviors to other situations. Generalization of learning refers to the process by which the learning of one behavior facilitates learning of another behavior. There are two forms of transfer: (a) stimulus generalization and (b) response generalization (Hegde, 1998; Mowrer, 1988). **Stimulus generalization** occurs when a response is elicited by a stimulus that is not the same as the training stimulus. Types of general stimulus generalization include physical stimuli (such as picture versus actual object), verbal stimuli (such as "Say sun." versus "What is this?"), physical setting (such as clinic room versus playground), and audience (such as speech-language pathologist versus teacher). Because of this process, clinicians do not need to teach a sound in every possible word in which it occurs or in every setting or with every communicative partner; instead, the correct response generalizes to words not taught. The second form of positive transfer is **response generalization**, in which one stimulus elicits several different responses. An example of this in articulation/phonological treatment is when the client participates only in speech sound discrimination training and produces the target sound in words even though production of the target sound was not a part of the treatment. Sometimes, *old learning* interferes with using new responses to old stimuli (such as using the target sound in words that the client misarticulates). In this phenomenon, the learning of a second behavior is seemingly more difficult because of what was previously learned, which results in more time needed to learn the second response. This may be what is happening when attempting to teach new articulation responses. The misarticulation has been learned and, consequently, interferes with the learning of a different, correct response. Use of unfamiliar stimuli in the form of nonsense syllables or nonsense words may facilitate teaching a *new* sound in that the misarticulation has never been used in the nonmeaningful speech unit.

In summary, the behavioral principles and characteristics of programmed instruction include (Costello, 1977):

- **Successive approximations**—Program begins with a response that the learner already has and gradually changes in small, logically sequenced steps to terminate with the target behavior
- Active participation—Learner responds overtly and frequently
- Immediate *knowledge of results*—Immediate feedback is provided to the learner
- Mastery learning and *self-pacing*—Responses given correctly on each step is a prerequisite to moving on to the next step so that clients proceed at their own pace
- Fading *stimulus* support—Models, prompts, and cues are gradually faded so that the stimulus becomes less supportive
- Concept learning through *varied* repetition—Many examples of a rule or principle are presented so that the concept or rule will be learned

Goals and Procedures

The goals of treatment of a programmed instruction approach are often determined by the clinician, although clinicians are urged to include clients, parents, and other significant persons in the decision-making process. Parenthetically, parent input is mandated by IDEA (1997) during the Individualized Education Plan (IEP) process. Whatever the objective, it is to be behaviorally stated in that the behavior to be achieved must be observable and measurable. The objective should specify what the client is to do, under what conditions, and how well. Each program generally has a terminal objective; that is, the goal of the entire program (including subobjectives or transitional objectives) must lead to the terminal objective. The intent of the objective should be specified whenever it is not the same as the behavior that indicates the intent (Meyer, 1998; Mowrer, 1988). Following is such a statement: *To discriminate between /s/ and /θ/ by pointing to a red card when the clinician says /s/ and pointing to a blue card when the clinician says /θ/ in 19 out of 20 trials*. To rephrase this objective as *to point to a red card when the clinician says /s/ and to point to a blue card when the clinician says /θ/ in 19 out of 20 trials* would not accurately reflect the intention of the objective, although it accurately reflects what the client is to do. An example of stated goals, behavior objectives, and procedures is included in Appendix K.

A method for speech-language pathologists to use when writing their own programs follows:

- Identify a target behavior that the client needs to attain; examples are *articulation of /f/* and *discrimination of /s/ from other sounds*.
- Formulate a *terminal objective*.
- Construct a pretest and posttest that assess for the behavior identified in the terminal objective.
- Develop a *task sequence* that delineates the steps of the program.
- Complete a *task analysis* in which prerequisite behaviors for each task are listed.
- Put the *task sequence* into a delivery system that specifies stimuli, client responses, reinforcement schedule, reinforcers, criteria for passage and failure for each step, and a procedure for recording performance and progress (Collins & Cunningham, 1976).

Costello (1977) described the components of a program that are similar to those used by Collins and Cunningham. Each component is to be specified for each step. The function of the stimulus is to elicit a response. It is modified throughout the program from providing very supportive conditions to providing minimal cues. The client response begins with a behavior in the client's repertoire and progresses toward the terminal objective. Effective reinforcement must be determined for each client.

Initially, reinforcement is usually administered for every correct response; however, reinforcement should become more natural and intermittent as the program progresses. Both pass and fail criteria should be specified. Determining whether or not a criterion is met depends on tracking and recording the client's correct and incorrect responses.

Over the years, many articulation programs have been developed and published and thus are readily available for clinician use.

Comment

The programmed approach is used with children and adults. It probably is easier to implement on an individual basis, but it is certainly adaptable to group situations.

This approach has been quite controversial in the field of speech-language pathology, as well as in other fields. Critics contend that humans are free to do as they choose and that their behavior should not be controlled, that it is dehumanizing to reduce behavior to S-R laws, that the approach deals with specific behaviors only and not with the whole person, and that the clinician may develop into a mechanistic and inflexible technician (Mowrer, 1988). Shelton (1978) believed that the client is relatively passive, although others indicate that the client must actively respond. After analyzing several articulation programs, Gerber (1977) concluded that the greatest shortcoming of the approach is reliance on a prewritten approach that restricts flexibility. She believed that, ideally, each clinician should apply principles of programming, but with knowledge, skills, and sensitivity, so that each individual client is optimally served.

There are several advantages of the approach according to Costello (1977). Treatment is effective because terminal behaviors are usually learned thoroughly and quickly at a high rate of success. Procedures can be replicated because they are standardized and often can be used by paraprofessionals. The method is economical because the time required for learning is often brief and applicable to several students. Also, it reduces the time needed for lesson planning and preparation. A good client–clinician relationship is fostered because of the reinforcement. Finally, a clinician gains a better understanding of the communication process and learning principles. An additional advantage is that clients progress at their own pace and use such programs because they facilitate accountability, which is demanded by federal, state, and local agencies. Certainly, most other articulation approaches are adaptable to using programmed instruction principles and procedures.

Today, speech-language pathologists apply many of the learning principles specified by the operant conditioning approach. Behavioral objectives are usually specified, especially by public school clinicians in Individual Family Service Plans (IFSPs) for preschoolers and Individualized Education Programs (IEPs) for school-aged clients and clinicians who receive funding through third-party payers. Data are likewise collected to report progress or lack of progress. The treatment sequence moves from lower levels of complexity to highly complex tasks; daily objectives (subobjectives) go from easier tasks to harder tasks throughout the course of treatment. Clinicians vary the stimuli provided beginning with lots of support to minimal or no support. Feedback is provided to clients usually in the form of positive reinforcement and sometimes also in the form of punishment. Reinforcement schedules are probably not as rigidly applied as specified by behavioral management methodology, but clinicians tend to use rich reinforcement schedules (100% reinforcement) during earlier stages and leaner and intermittent variable schedules in the later stages of intervention. Clinicians tend to use secondary reinforcers, including social and token reinforcers, rather than primary reinforcers, such as food and drink.

> What are other phonetic treatment approaches?

OTHER ARTICULATION TREATMENT APPROACHES

It is not possible to discuss all articulation treatment approaches that have been developed. However, it is useful to comment briefly on a couple of additional approaches (for historical purposes) and additional techniques that may be helpful to clinicians in their work with persons who have articulatory/phonologic disorders.

> Describe the heterogeneous group treatment approach including its advantages and limitations.

Heterogeneous Group Approach

While not used today, the **heterogeneous group approach** is described here for historical purposes. Backus (1957) and Backus and Beasley (1951) devised a method of working with all types of speech deviances in a group setting. Speech skills are taught through developing interpersonal relationships and group interactions. The clients begin with a speech pattern in a context or situation. The pattern is then broken down and finally put back into context. In other words, the sequence of working on speech patterns proceeds from whole to part to whole.

Rationale

Backus and Beasley (1951) developed the group approach because their observations showed that changes in speech behavior depend more on variables of interpersonal relationships between the client and clinician and among groups of clients than on speech drills and ear training. Additional observations revealed that the ability to produce correct speech patterns in structured drill situations does not necessarily create carryover to social situations (Backus, 1957). Backus further noted that persons with different types of speech disorders showed some similar behaviors and that persons with the same disorder displayed basic differences; therefore, the use of speech-disordered labels becomes meaningless. These observations led to the development of a group interactive approach rather than an individual drill-type approach. Speech is therefore viewed as an aspect of the total behavior of an individual rather than merely as a motor skill.

Backus and Beasley (1951) made the following assumptions about learning, which apply to speech development as well as to other areas of human development:

- Learning proceeds from the whole to parts by a process of progressive differentiation.
- Learning involves a process of organization in which the individual must perceive the whole or a patterning of the parts.
- The whole person does the learning.

With a consideration of these assumptions, treatment procedures deal with the functional organization, social skills, and speech patterns, thus going from the whole person (functional organization) to parts (social skills) and finally to subparts (speech patterns). The functional organization of a person is comprised of perceptions of self; perceptions of the environment; basic needs, which include a feeling of belonging and safety; value standards; and techniques for adjusting to the environment. The social skills are adjustive techniques that allow the individual to develop positive interpersonal relationships that facilitate learning.

The clinician's role in the group approach is based on three assumptions of interpersonal theory (Backus, 1957):

- Individuals do their own growing, changing, and learning.
- An individual will grow and learn unless barriers block the growth.
- Critical learning variables are contained in interpersonal relationships.

Treatment is defined as "a particular kind of interpersonal process in which at least one of the participants seeks consciously to keep creating the sort of environment in which the other participant can develop his own potentialities to the greatest extent possible at successive points in time" (Backus, p. 1034). It is not the speech-language pathologist's role to provide psychotherapy, although the two fields interrelate and use some of the same techniques. However, the speech-language pathologist is primarily concerned with speech and language usage and the mechanics of speech production, whereas the psychotherapist deals with other behaviors.

In summary, Backus and Beasley's approach (1951) adheres to four treatment principles that evolved from these viewpoints. The first principle is that group instruction should be the core of management. In this way, various interpersonal situations and real speaking situations can be structured. The value lies in an optimum situation for meeting individual needs. Second, group membership should not be segregated by types of disorders or symptoms. Individual group members are exposed to a range of problems to be solved. The positive aspects of speech are stressed. Third, treatment should provide a corrective "emotional" experience. This is not to be construed as psychotherapy. Instead, speech is used as a means to create significant interpersonal relationships. Last, treatment should be structured in terms of interpersonal relationships involving conversational speech. The interpersonal relationship comprises the whole, the speech behavior is a functional part of the whole, and the subpart is sound production mechanics.

Goals and Procedures

The goal of the speech-language pathologist in the heterogeneous group approach is to help individual clients change behavior in interpersonal relationships to function more adequately in terms of satisfaction and security. Backus and Beasley (1951) explained that speech is one of the behaviors to be changed in order for speech to be used adequately in social situations.

Goals of the individual client are different at different stages of treatment and are different for each person within a group. The goals revolve around changing the functional organization, social skills, and speech patterns of the clients. The first goal, improving the functional organization of individuals, is achieved by developing a positive psychological climate by interacting warmly, being relaxed, developing a group structure in which each client is encouraged to participate and will experience acceptance and success, being permissive, accepting feelings, helping clients succeed, keeping the situation speech-oriented, and setting rational limits. Individual group members contribute to verbal interaction, serve as a model for others, and reinforce others (Sommers & Kane, 1974). Social skills that are to be developed include the ability to follow conventional social patterns, win acceptance and support from others, share attitudes, and develop flexibility in role-taking.

The final goal is speech development. As stated previously, a speech pattern is introduced in context and patterned language is used. All group members respond with the same pattern and evaluate one another while the clinician gives directions to aid in production. The correct aspects of speech production are reinforced, and the incorrect aspects are described as needed improvement for the whole group. No techniques for eliciting individual sounds are provided, but repeated experience with selected sounds is provided by using the same response in various situations. The response is one that is used frequently in real-life situations. Sounds are selected on the bases of ease of learning, needs of the group, and frequency of occurrence, but not on the basis of developmental order. They often begin with /θ/ and /v/ and later add /s/.

Seven types of interpersonal situations provide the means for achieving the objectives:

- Experiences in human relatedness occurring in everyday life, such as greetings, introductions, invitations, asking favors, sharing, and apologizing
- Specialized experiences in analyzing use of speech by enacting everyday situations and discussing them
- Specialized experiences in observing part functions in which speech patterns are observed through the senses and motor patterns and evaluated in terms of the difference between what a person did and what is usually done
- Specialized experiences in using the method of science in behavior by making available tools for observing, evaluating, and solving problems using general semantic principles
- Specialized experiences in communicating about feelings

- Experiences in acquiring specific information (applied in skills), such as telling time, colors, calendar, and arithmetic
- Experiences in developing certain abilities for pleasure, such as sewing, singing, card tricks, and sports

A sample lesson is presented in Appendix L to aid in understanding the group approach.

Comments

The number of clients per group varies, but Backus and Beasley (1951) indicated that 8 to 10 is an effective number. Subgroup sessions can be scheduled to meet individual needs, or the larger group can be divided into smaller groups during regular sessions. The approach can be used with all age levels, including adults, and with all types of speech disorders. Backus (1957) recommended that levels of locomotion ability, age, and interest levels are important considerations in grouping. She further suggested that at least two members of the same gender should be included in a group rather than only one member of a gender. Short-term intensive management, using fairly long sessions, is preferable to shorter sessions meeting over a longer period.

Advantages of the approach are that it tends to provide motivation for success and to facilitate carryover (Sommers & Kane, 1974). Backus (1957) cautioned that a person needs to become thoroughly acquainted with the rationale and procedures she recommended before implementing them. A limitation is that it does not efficiently change incorrect speech patterns. The approach appears to resemble small group, interpersonal communication as much as intervention for oral communication disorders.

Certainly, many clinicians today work with clients in small groups and sometimes in the classroom as in this approach. However, the speech patterns are usually targeted more directly.

> Describe the nonsense material treatment approach, including its advantages and limitations.

Nonsense Material Approach

The **nonsense material approach** to articulation treatment was developed by Gerber (1973). In this method, the client achieves correct articulation of error sounds in nonsense syllables and words used with the characteristics of conversational speech before proceeding to real-word production. In other words, nonmeaningful words are produced automatically, rapidly, and effortlessly with normal stress, juncture, and intonation patterns. Only then does the client produce the error sound in meaningful words.

Rationale

Gerber (1973) developed the nonsense material approach because of the frustration over clients not achieving carryover. She observed, as have many clinicians, that when a newly acquired sound is used in conversational speech, it is deliberately and carefully produced, but when the client's attention changes to the content of the message, misarticulations often recur. Initially, the sound must be produced with careful and deliberate attention because the former articulation response (misarticulation) interferes with the correct response because the person is focusing on the sound rather than on the meaningful word as a whole, or perhaps because of other reasons. Whatever the reason, this deliberate speech production interferes with carryover to spontaneous speech, which is not deliberate.

Gerber (1973) hypothesized that there are two different levels of speech: *deliberate* and *spontaneous*. Table 8.9 compares the characteristics of the two modes of speech. The overriding principle of the nonsense material approach is to bridge the gap between these two levels. The use of nonsense syllables and words with the characteristics of spontaneous speech aids in bridging the gap and facilitating carryover. Sound production occurs effortlessly in sentences and stories with normal prosody before meaningful words are introduced. According to Gerber, after this objective is achieved, the client will likely produce the sound in meaningful material without undue effort and exaggerated articulation. The client, then, is free to focus more attention on content because of the prior practice on nonsense material. The nonsense material is programmed with a consideration of phonetic complexity in that stimuli using easier articulation movements that are introduced before more difficult ones.

Accuracy in evaluating and monitoring the client's own speech is critical, in most instances, for achieving carryover. In Gerber's method, this skill is systematically trained to develop a more effective means of monitoring speech by detecting and correcting misarticulations. Generally, auditory speech perception is stressed, but some clients may need training in visual, tactile, or kinesthetic perception or any combination of these.

Gerber recommended using an approach midway between a *game* approach and operant conditioning. In this way, the client responds at a rapid rate to material designed to arouse interest. Active client participation is required while focusing on the quality of speech production, not on the game. A game approach is not effective because games tend to distract attention away from speech and because the response rate is reduced. Conversely, an operant conditioning approach tends to be uninteresting because of straight drill work. Therefore, a combination of the two approaches is used.

Goals and Procedures

The goal of the nonsense material approach is automatic production of the target sound in sponta-

---

TABLE 8.9

Contrastive Analysis of the Attributes of Spontaneous and Structured Speech

Spontaneous Speech	Structured Speech
Articulatory movements are rapidly overlapping and effortless	Articulatory movements are frequently artificially prolonged and strenuous
Articulation is subordinated in consciousness to the content of the message; therefore, production is relatively automatic	Attention is focused on the mechanics of sound production; therefore, production is deliberate, frequently emitted from a preparatory set
Segmental sounds are modified by natural patterns of stress, juncture, and intonation related to meaning	Stress patterns are frequently distorted through exaggerated production; rhythm and melody are often stilted and artificial

From Gerber, A. (1973). Goal: Carryover an articulation manual and program. Philadelphia, PA: Temple University Press. Reprinted by permission.

neous speech with the criterion specified as "90 to 100 percent correct production of the target sound in a communicative situation wherein the client's attention is focused on the content of the message and not on the deliberate control of the mechanics of speech production" (Gerber, 1973, p. x). No procedures for acquisition of sounds are provided except for /r/; other sources can be consulted for sound-acquisition techniques.

The nonsense material is presented in levels of increasing complexity:

- CV, VCV, and VC syllables
- More complex syllables; for example, CVCV, VCCV, and VCC
- Simple nonsense words; for example, CVC
- Multisyllabic nonsense words; for example, /'kakɪ/
- Phrases comprised of nonsense words; for example, /'kakɪ pʌnəd fæk/
- Conversations in nonsense words
- Using nonsense words in meaningful contexts; for example, "I saw a /sot/"

Each level of nonsense material is programmed to be produced eventually with the characteristics of spontaneous speech; that is, consistently correct with normal juncture, with rapidness, in stressed and unstressed syllables, in varying levels of phonetic complexity, and in natural syntactic structures. After the highest level of nonsense material is produced as though it were conversational speech, real words are introduced. The client's own vocabulary is used and the words are eventually produced in sentences and connected speech. Gerber (1973) provided several techniques for the previously described treatment process, including *sound hopscotch, sound hurdles*, riddles, word-building blocks, *follow the beat, model sentence drills*, and stories. The procedures emphasize speed of production and natural prosody.

Simultaneously with the production training, self-monitoring training is incorporated. This is programmed in the following six steps to be used at each level of production work:

- Evaluate clinician's live speech productions
- Evaluate clinician's taped speech productions
- Evaluate taped samples of clinician and client productions with each producing one sound unit
- Evaluate taped samples of clinician and client productions with each producing three sound units
- Evaluate taped client productions without clinician model

- Evaluate client productions without clinician model before playing back the taped utterances

The client strives to produce the sound consistently and to evaluate productions accurately at increasing levels of speed.

Comments

The nonsense material approach is designed for older children who have passed the stage of articulation development through maturation; that is, children who are 7 or 8 years of age and adolescents. The material can be adapted for adults, although it has not been widely used with adults. Less direct approaches are recommended for children under age 7 years. The approach can be used on an individual or group basis. Gerber indicated that not all clients need to perform all activities at all levels. The advantages of Gerber's approach are that the client develops strong internal motivation, the material is highly organized, and carryover is facilitated (Sommers & Kane, 1974). Limitations include producing the target sound in nonsense phrases and sentences may not be motivating for some clients. The characteristics of spontaneous speech production often can be incorporated in practice of meaningful words, phrases, and sentences without first working on these levels in nonmeaningful words.

Today, many clinicians include practice of target sounds in nonmeaningful syllables and words, although seldom do they go the extreme of producing entire phrases and sentences in nonsense words. The rationale for using nonsense contexts is to develop motor patterns needed for producing the target sound. The sequence suggested for speech sound discrimination seems to be a good one for developing speech perception skills and for teaching self-evaluation and self-monitoring.

SUMMARY

Several widely used phonetic treatment approaches, categorized as articulator placement/movement, traditional, tactile-kinesthetic, phonetic context, stimulability, behavior modification, and others, have been described. These approaches focus on the mechanics of producing individual speech sounds. The specific approaches presented here include phonetic placement, palatometer instrumental system, stimulus (traditional), wedge, multiple phonemic, motokinesthetics, PROMPT, sensory-motor, paired stimuli, integral stimulation, stimulability enhancement, programmed instruction, heterogeneous group, and nonsense material. Certainly, each approach has unique features, but there are also commonalities among them. Some are older classic approaches upon which later procedures and techniques have been developed. Each approach has been effective in treating at least some clients with articulatory/phonologic disorders.

Practicing speech-language pathologists need to be familiar with these approaches to plan and carry out treatment programs for individuals with articulatory/phonologic disorders. Often, it is efficacious to combine elements of the various approaches when working with individual clients. Speech-language pathologists do not necessarily need to use an approach in its entirety to be successful.

REVIEW QUESTIONS

1. In general, what is the focus of phonetic or motor treatment approaches for articulatory/phonologic disorders?

2. What is the primary feature of each of the following groups of treatment approaches?

   a. Articulator/placement
   b. Traditional
   c. Tactile-kinesthetic
   d. Phonetic context
   e. Stimulability
   f. Behavior modification

3. In one or two sentences, characterize the following treatment approaches: (a) phonetic placement, (b) palatometer instrument, (c) stimulus, (d) wedge, (e) multiple phonemic, (f) motokinesthetics, (g) PROMPT, (h) sensory-motor, (i) paired stimuli, (j) integral stimulation, (k) stimulability enhancement, (l) programmed instruction, (m) heterogeneous group, and (n) nonsense material. What is the rationale or basis for each approach?

4. Describe and relate principles to be followed and components that need to be specified in a programmed instruction approach.

5. What are the advantages and limitations for each of the phonetic approaches listed in #3?

6. Which of the phonetic approaches in #3 is/are most suitable for clients with only a few sound errors? For clients with multiple misarticulations? For preschoolers? For school-aged clients? For adults? For clients with childhood apraxia of speech and acquired apraxia? For clients with dysarthria?

7. How is each of the phonetic treatment approaches currently incorporated in treatment provided by speech-language pathologists?

Phonological Treatment Approaches

"A child, when it begins to speak, learns what it is that it knows."

—John Hall Wheelock

CHAPTER OBJECTIVES

- Describe the general characteristics of phonological (linguistic) treatment approaches.

- Identify the types of articulatory/phonologic disorders that are most suitably treated with phonological treatment approaches.

- Characterize each of the following phonological treatment approaches: distinctive features, phonological cycling,

  minimal meaningful contrasting pairs, maximal opposition contrast, Metaphon, nonlinear.

- Provide a rationale for each phonological treatment approach.

- Identify the advantages and limitations of each phonological treatment approach.

- Describe how each approach currently is used or adapted by practicing clinicians.

Over the years, numerous treatment approaches for articulatory/phonologic disorders have been developed by various researchers and clinicians. Many of the more recent approaches have emanated from the psycholinguistic literature (e.g., Bernhardt & Stemberger, 1998; Chomsky & Halle, 1968; Compton, 1970; Ingram, 1989; Jakobson, 1968, 1971; Morehead & Morehead, 1976; Stampe, 1969, 1979). In this book, these approaches are categorized as phonological or linguistic, in contrast to the phonetic approaches described in Chapter 8. While the underlying bases of these approaches are different, there is considerable overlap between the actual clinical procedures used in the two types of treatment approaches. In point of fact, phonetic sound elicitation techniques are often needed during the initial stages when using a phonological treatment approach in order for

clients to learn to produce sounds missing from the speech sound inventories of persons with phonologic disorders, sounds that contain targeted distinctive features and speech sound patterns. These approaches are generally appropriate for clients who have multiple speech sound errors that appear to be systematic and who do not have major limitations to their motor speech mechanism.

Generally, phonological approaches focus on distinctive features and/or phonological patterns of the speech sound system rather than on individual phonemes as is the case for phonetic approaches. The specific intervention strategies and methodologies vary among the specific phonological intervention approaches, although again there is considerable overlap in the procedures used. Some begin treatment with isolated speech sounds, although most begin production in words. Some

TABLE 9.1

Specific Phonological (Linguistic) Treatment Approaches for Articulatory/Phonologic Disorders

Type of Approach	Brief Description
Distinctive feature	Distinctive features of sounds are targeted through the production of contrasting exemplar phonemes, one of which contains the feature and the other not containing the feature
Phonological cycling	Phonological patterns are targeted in words containing exemplar sounds/sound contexts for a specified time period through the production of words
Meaningful minimal contrasting pairs	Phonological patterns are targeted in contrasting word pairs, one of which contains the targeted pattern and the other not containing the pattern
Maximal opposition	Production of contrasting word pairs differing in multiple phonetic features with the goal of increasing the phonetic inventory and complexity level of the phonological system
Metaphon	Targets phonological rule system (phonological processes) through phonological awareness training, communication awareness training, and production of contrasting word pairs
Nonlinear	Various segmental and syllable/word structure levels are targeted through the production of exemplar words for a specified time period

include practice in nonsense syllables and words, but most include production practice only in real words. Some incorporate contrastive production of speech sounds and words, while others focus only on production practice of the targeted sound or syllable/word structure pattern. Finally, some incorporate speech perception training, some use phonological awareness training, and others use only production practice. Table 9.1 provides a list and brief description of the specific phonological treatment approaches presented in this chapter.

The first type of phonological treatment approach that was developed focused on distinctive features of phoneme classes. Later, specific phonological deviations (processes) treatment approaches were developed by Howell and Dean (1994), Hodson and Paden (1991), Fokes (1982), Weiner (1979, 1981), and others. In the phonological deviation intervention strategies, rather than focusing on the production of individual phonemes, the task is to reduce the frequency of occurrence of certain phonological deviations while increasing correct phonological patterns. Basically, two types of phonological deviations treatment programs have been devised:

- Meaningful contrasting pairs (Fokes, 1982; Weiner, 1979, 1981);
- Cycle format that targets deficient phonological patterns (or reduction of phonological deviations) (Hodson, 2004; Hodson & Paden, 1991).

A variant of the contrasts approach was developed by Elbert and Gierut (1986; Gierut, 1989, 1990a, 1990b) in which maximally contrasting

speech sounds are targeted with the later developing phonemes being targeted early in the treatment process. The Metaphon approach was developed in England by Howell and Dean (1994; Dean, Howell, Waters, & Reid, 1995) in the mid-1980s, which begins with phonological awareness activities and proceeds to production of phonological contrasts of target phonological processes. More recently, the nonlinear approach was developed by Bernhardt and Stemberger (2000), in which the client works on speech sound production in various prosodic (suprasegmental elements, such as syllable stress), syllable/word structure, and segmental (such as distinctive features and word position) contexts using a cycling format. Descriptions of each of these approaches include the developer's rationale, goals and procedures used, and additional comments regarding the effectiveness of each, its pluses and minuses, and how the approach is used today.

> Describe the distinctive features treatment approach, including its rationale, advantages, and limitations.

DISTINCTIVE FEATURES APPROACH

The **distinctive features approach** for articulation/phonological treatment was originally developed by McReynolds and Bennet (1972). In this approach, distinctive features (such as voicing, back, and strident) of phonemes are taught, rather than individual phonemes. This is done by the client producing two sounds, one that contains the feature to be taught and the other that does not. The contrasting phonemes are produced in varying levels of complexity, often beginning in isolation followed by nonsense syllables, words, and possibly sentences and conversational speech.

Rationale

The distinctive features approach is based on the premise that distinctive features are the basic elements of sounds; that is, sounds are composed of a bundle of features (McReynolds & Engmann, 1975). They are the elements that distinguish one sound from another. When developing articulation skills, children systematically acquire phonetic features leading to expansion of their phonemic repertoire. As more distinctive features are added, more phonemes are articulated correctly. Distinctive features theorists contend that articulation errors are systematic. Children with articulation errors often use a phonemic rule system that is different from the adult system (Costello, 1975). Misuse or omission of a distinctive feature may result in the misarticulation of several sounds and unintelligibility of some words. The intent of the distinctive features approach is to aid the client in discovering the rules of the adult phonology system (Van Riper & Erickson, 1996). The client learns distinctive features rather than specific sounds. When a feature is acquired, the hypothesis is that it will transfer to other sounds that contain the acquired feature. Thus, more than one sound may be changed by teaching a particular feature without directly teaching all of the sounds containing the feature. If this is true, using a distinctive features approach is more efficient than traditional approaches.

How are distinctive features taught? Distinctive features do not appear in isolation; therefore, they are taught in the context of sounds. Both the presence and absence of a distinctive feature are taught through two or more phonemes that ideally are minimal pairs; that is, the two phonemes contain the same features except that one contains the feature to be taught and the other does not contain the target feature. For example, the contrast pairs of /k/ and /g/ could be used to teach voicing, and /t/ and /s/ could be used to teach stridency. Often, the clinician selects the target sound and its substituted error for the contrast to be taught. Such a procedure enhances the feature contrast the client needs to learn.

As indicated in Chapter 2, various distinctive features systems have been developed and used to analyze and treat articulatory/phonologic disorders. Chomsky and Halle's (1968; Table 2.9) system was used by McReynolds and Engmann (1975) who published an in-depth distinctive features assessment tool, although they indicated that any system can be used. The distinctive features system devised by Singh and Polen (1972) was preferred by Costello and Onstine (1976). A simplified system using phonetic feature terminology familiar to speech-language pathologists (such as vowel, nasal, glide, fricative, and alveolar) was developed by Drexler (1976) (Appendix B). The in-depth feature analysis of a client's articulation/phonological system advocated by Costello and Onstine (1976) and McReynolds and Engmann (1975) were used mostly for research purposes and are rarely used by practicing clinicians because clinical time limitations preclude its use. However, to implement a distinctive features approach, the clinician needs to determine the patterns of feature errors; that is, which features are present, which ones are not, which features are used correctly, and which ones are used incorrectly. In the absence of a specific distinctive features assessment tool, practicing clinicians often analyze data gathered in formal and informal articulation/phonological tests and spontaneous speech samples to describe the distinctive features patterns used by individual clients.

Goals and Procedures

Three different distinctive features treatment protocols are described here. The general goals of the programs are to teach the client how to produce a specified distinctive feature in the context of phonemes and where to use the feature; that is, the client must learn the rules for correct use of a particular distinctive feature. Unlike most of the other phonological approaches, distinctive features treatment programs begin at the isolation level for the contrasting sounds. It is important to produce the contrasting sounds in meaningful contexts. At the isolation and nonsense syllable levels, this can be done by pairing the speech sound production with its orthographic representation (such as /s/ is the letter "s") or with a representative symbol (such as a snake for the /s/ sound). At the word and sentence levels, meaningful contexts are provided by pictures or alternatively by written words for clients who can read.

McReynolds and Engmann's (1975) approach was developed for research purposes. They indicated that the approach may need to be modified for clinical purposes, but the treatment principles are useful nonetheless. From the analysis, the clinician determines the percentage of incorrect usage of the positive (presence of the feature) and negative (absence of the feature) aspects of each of 13 features (vocalic, consonantal, high, back, low, anterior, coronal, round, tense, voice, continuant, nasal, and strident). If a feature error occurs in less than 25% of the trials, it is not necessary to target because the feature is considered established. If a feature is used incorrectly 40 to 50% of the time, it is inconsistently produced probably in one of the following patterns: (a) produced in some phonemes, but not in others; (b) produced in either the releasing or arresting positions; or (c) produced in appropriate and inappropriate contexts. If a feature is incorrect 65% of the time, the feature probably has not been acquired or stabilized. If the percentage of errors for a feature is 80% or above, the feature has not been acquired. Features at the 80% level of error have the highest priority and should be targeted first. Those at the 50 to 60% level of error have the next priority with treatment focusing on the feature in phonemes or word positions where it is omitted. After analyzing the evaluation results, a feature is selected for intervention. Two standard sounds are used for teaching the feature contrast, with one sound containing the feature to be taught and the other sound not containing the target feature.

The client produces both consonants throughout the treatment process; no auditory training is done. A programmed instructional approach is used. Stimuli consist of nonsense pictures and verbal stimuli using the two contrasting consonants and the vowels /ɑ/, /i/, /æ/, and /u/. The responses are initially imitative and progress to spontaneous productions. Reinforcement schedules and criterion levels are specified. Treatment begins with the production of the phoneme containing the feature to be learned, imitatively and spontaneously. Traditional elicitation techniques are used when the client does not imitate the target sound. After the client learns to produce the target feature in a sound, feature contrast training is implemented in which the two sounds are produced in CV syllables with the vowels, imitatively and spontaneously. The two sounds are then produced in VC syllables with the vowels, imitatively and spontaneously. Generalization of the feature to other sounds is tested. If generalization has not occurred, the same treatment protocol is administered again using two other phonemes as a contrasting pair for the same feature. For example, /p/ and /f/ may be used initially to teach stridency. If generalization does not occur to all stridents, /s/ and /t/ could be used as a second contrasting pair for stridency.

A second treatment protocol was devised by Drexler (1976). Although she did not use a distinctive features analysis as thorough as that of McReynolds and Engmann (1975), she expanded on their treatment program. The contrasting phonemes ideally are the same in all features except the one being taught; however, sometimes it is necessary that they vary in two features (such as /ʃ/ and /t/ could be used to teach the fricative even though the two sounds differ not only in fricative feature, but also in the placement features of palatal and alveolar). There are five phases in Drexler's program:

- Initial position, which includes the phonemes in isolation and CV syllables
- Final position in VC syllables
- Words
- Phrases
- Sentences

The first two phases follow McReynolds and Engmann's format. At the word level, minimal word pairs are produced (such as *suit/toot* and *pass/pat* when contrasting /s/ and /t/ for the fricative feature). Sometimes nonsense words, which are assigned a meaning, need to be used at the word level when no two contrasting meaningful words are available. At the phrase and sentence levels, words containing the contrasting phonemes are produced in meaningful, short phrases and sentences. The operative word is *meaningful* such that only one of the two contrasting words is appropriate for the target sentence. For example, rather than using sentences such as *I see a _____* in which either contrasting word (such as _sack_ and _tack_) would fit, it is more effective to use the two sentences of *I put the food in a* sack, and *I pushed in the* tack *with my thumb*. In this case, only one of the two contrasting words fits into each sentence, showing the client that the context indicates when it is appropriate to use the +fricative feature and when it is appropriate to use the -fricative feature.

A third distinctive features treatment format was developed by Costello and Onstine (1976) who advocated a thorough distinctive features analysis. Features are selected for intervention on the following bases:

- Developmental order of feature acquisition
- Complete omission or misuse of the feature
- Number of phonemes affected by the feature

Costello and Onstine also implemented a programmed instruction approach. In contrast to the two protocols described previously, they selected two sounds for training that contain the feature to be taught and one that does not contain the feature.

Examples include using /s/, /ʃ/, and /t/ for teaching stridency and /b/, /d/, and /p/ for teaching voicing. Two sounds with the feature are produced on the assumption that the client can more easily conceptualize the feature than when only one sound is used. The three sounds are each produced by the client in the following sequential levels:

- Isolation
- CV and VC syllables
- Words in releasing and arresting positions
- Phrases in releasing and arresting positions
- Sentences in releasing and arresting positions
- Stories
- Conversation

Table 9.2 illustrates an example of the steps to follow in a distinctive features approach.

Comments

The distinctive features approach has been implemented primarily with children on an individual basis, although group treatment is also possible. It also seems feasible to adapt it for adults. The approach is recommended for phonological deviancies, but not for phonetic deviancies. A distinctive features analysis should be reserved for clients who have four or more sound errors because it is probably not clinically useful to analyze the articulation pattern of those with fewer errors (McReynolds & Engmann,1975).

The approach is often efficient because once a feature is acquired, it tends to generalize to other sounds. Some single-subject studies have shown that such generalization does occur (Costello & Onstine, 1976; McReynolds & Bennett, 1972; Ruder & Bunce, 1981). Overgeneralization usually does not occur. A limitation of the approach is that formal distinctive features analyses are quite time-consuming; however, McReynolds and Engmann (1975) indicated that the time required for analysis must be compared with the hours spent in treatment when such an analysis is not done. Another limitation is that some younger clients become confused when producing contrasting phonemes at the same time. This approach can be used only for substitution errors and not for distortions and omissions.

Today, clinicians generally use informal distinctive features analyses, noting which features are absent or misused in a client's phonetic inventory. Also, phonological deviation analyses like those described in Chapter 5 identify absent phonetic features. The current trend is for clinicians to implement the minimal pair or cycling approaches when choosing a phonological approach rather than a distinctive features approach.

> Describe the phonological cycling treatment approach, including its rationale, advantages, and limitations.

Phonological Cycling

The **phonological cycling approach** was developed by Hodson and Paden (1991). In this approach, deficient phonological patterns are targeted for a specified period of time through production of exemplar words. All major patterns that need remediation are addressed in treatment, one at a time, for a certain period of time. One cycle of treatment consists of production practice of *all* major phonological patterns that need to be targeted. Those patterns that need continued practice after a cycle are targeted again, each for a certain time period in two or more phonemic contexts, constituting another cycle of treatment. The targets become increasingly complex with succeeding cycles. Thus, correct speech sound patterns are allowed to emerge over time.

Rationale

One of the premises of the cycling approach is that misarticulations are systematic; that is, the errors "are based on systematic alterations from the adult model" (Hodson & Paden, 1991, p. 8). The errors are predictable. Thus, assessment and treatment are focused on the broad, underlying characteristics of the client's speech output. These systematic patterns are targeted rather than individual speech sounds. An example is that, instead of addressing each consonant that is omitted in final position as in sound-by-sound approaches, two or three exemplar final consonants are targeted in a cycle. A second premise is that speech sound acquisition is a gradual process. Individual speech sounds and speech sound patterns are acquired over time. Thus, each phonological pattern is targeted for a certain amount of time rather than targeted until a certain criterion level is achieved.

The phonological cycling approach is based on seven underlying concepts and the treatment procedures outlined by Hodson and Paden (1991) take into account each of them.

Phonological acquisition is a gradual process (p. 76). Initially, treatment facilitates a target pattern for a short period of time and moves on to another pattern, allowing clients to internalize the pattern on their own. The first pattern is revisited or recycled at a later point in time during the intervention process. In this way, correct phonological patterns are allowed to emerge gradually.

TABLE 9.2

Steps in a Distinctive Features Treatment Plan

Levels of Sound Production	Steps	Example Target: Stridency
Isolation	1. Imitate target sound	Show picture of letter *s*. "Say /s/"
	2. Produce sound without a model	Show picture of the letter *s*. "What sound is this?"
	3. Imitation: Contrast target sound with its minimal pair sound	Point to picture of the letter *s̩t*. "Say (/s/ or /t/)."
	4. Production: Contrast target sound with its minimal pair sound	Point to picture of the letter *s* or *t* in a random order. "What sound is this?"
Syllables	5. Imitate CV syllables of target sound	Point to picture of letter *s*. "Say (/si/, /sæ/, /sɑ/, /su/)"
	6. Imitate VC syllables with target sound and its minimal pair	Point to picture of the letter *s* or *t*. "Say (/si/, /ti/, /sæ/, /tæ/, /sɑ/, /tɑ/, /su/, /tu/)" in random order.
Words	7. Imitate words with target sound in initial words	Show picture of a *sack*. "Say *sack*."
	8. Produce words with target sound in initial words	Show picture of *sack*. "What is this?"
	9. Imitate words with target sound in initial words and minimal pair words with contrast sound	Show pictures of *sack* and *tack*. "Say *sack*. Say *tack*."
	10. Produce words with target sound in initial words and minimal pair words with contrast sound without a model	Show pictures of *sack* and *tack*. "What is this? And what is this?"
	11–14. Repeat steps 7–10 using target and contrast sounds in final position	Use pictures and words such as *nice* and *night*.
Phrases	15. Imitate phrases with target sound in any position	Show picture of *sack*. "Say *paper sack*." Show picture of *nice*. "Say *nice lady*."
	16. Produce phrases with target sound without a model	Show picture of *sack*. "Describe this picture."
	17. Imitate phrases with target and contrast sounds	Show pictures of *sack* and *tack*. "Say *paper sack*." "Say *little thumbtack*."
	18. Produce phrases with target and contrast sounds without a model	Show pictures of *sack* and *tack*. Point to the *sack*. "Describe this picture. Point to the *tack*. Now, describe this picture."
Sentences	19–22. Repeat steps 15–17 using complete sentences	Use pictures and sentences such as "I filled up the sack. I hit the tack with a hammer."
Stories	23. Retell a story that uses words with the target sound and its minimal pair	"I'm going to tell you a story about _____." "Now you tell me the story."

Children with normal hearing typically acquire the adult sound system primarily by listening (p. 76). Treatment includes auditory bombardment or amplified auditory stimulation at the beginning and end of each session. Auditory stimulation involves the clinician reading a list of words exemplifying the target pattern while the client listens through low-level amplification. According to Hodson and Paden (1991), the amplification improves the client's image of the utterance.

As children acquire new speech patterns, they associate kinesthetic with auditory sensations, en-

abling later self-monitoring (p. 76). Clients need to learn what the speech sounds feel like as well as how they sound. When a misarticulation is used repeatedly, incorrect kinesthetic sensations are reinforced. Thus, it is the goal for clients to produce the speech pattern correctly as close to 100% of the trials during the treatment session so that the clients are hearing and feeling the correct speech pattern rather than an incorrect pattern which will facilitate self-monitoring.

Phonetic environment can facilitate correct sound production (p. 76). Clinicians have observed that children often can more easily produce a certain sound in some words than in other words. The word position of the sound, as well as the phonetic context (the sounds that precede and follow it), affect how easily the client produces a given sound. Consequently, the words used for production practice in treatment are selected carefully. Initially, those words that provide the most facilitating context are used as stimuli. For example, a velar is usually easier to produce in the context of back vowels than front vowels as well as in words that do not contain an alveolar sound. Surprisingly, /s/ is produced correctly more frequently when followed by /t/ and /d/ than as a singleton fricative (Gallagher & Shriner, 1975a, 1975b). This finding is consistent with the observation that /s/ is often produced more easily in the context of a cluster /st/ than in singleton /s/ followed or proceeded by a vowel. As treatment continues, more difficult contexts are used as stimuli.

Children are actively involved in their phonological acquisition (p. 76). "Children are aware of and participate in their own phonological development" (Hodson & Paden, 1991, p. 82). They appear to need to be assisted overtly in discovering the sound system used by the speakers of a language. This is done through production practice of the targeted patterns in treatment.

Children tend to generalize new speech production skills to other targets (p. 77). Children transfer a speech sound characteristic or feature from the sound targeted in treatment to other sounds with the same feature. Therefore, it is not necessary to target every misarticulated sound. In the cycling approach, as is the case with most phonological approaches, only a few phonemic contexts for each targeted pattern are directly addressed in treatment allowing for more efficient treatment.

An optimal "match" facilitates children's learning (p. 77). Optimal learning occurs when there is a match between the objective and the client's ability to meet the objective. In the cycling approach, this is implemented through target selection. The target is one step above the client's current performance level. The target is a task that the client does

not currently do, but has the capability of doing. "An important concomitant is that complexity is increased gradually so that the child is always challenged, but satisfaction and enjoyment can be experienced at each session" (Hodson & Paden, 1991, p. 85).

Goals and Procedures

Suggested goals for the phonological cycling approach are to (a) increase intelligibility to at least 90% in connected speech and (b) reduce the percentage of occurrence of phonological deviations to less than 40% (90% for liquid deviations; Hodson, 2004). When necessary, the misarticulations remaining are addressed with a more traditional phonetic approach. The treatment process really begins with a phonological assessment. The most compatible assessment for this approach is the HAPP-3 (Hodson, 2004), although other phonological assessments can be used for target selection. Clients who fall into the moderate, severe, or profound categories on the HAPP-3 are appropriate candidates for this approach.

After selecting the children who should be seen for intervention, the speech-language pathologist determines the phonological deviations that are to be targeted for remediation and the order in which they will be targeted. Target selection is done for each cycle of treatment. "A cycle is a period of time during which all phonological patterns needing treatment are facilitated in succession. Phonemes with the phonological patterns are used to facilitate emergence of the respective patterns; (i.e., phonemes are a means to an end)" (Hodson, 2004, p. 33). Major phonological deviations present in at least 40% of the possible occurrences are to be targeted except for glide deviation and anterior nonstrident deviation (backing) that should be at 60% or more. Each phonological pattern is targeted in at least two contexts (e.g., final /p/ and final /t/ for final consonants) for approximately 60 minutes per context before going on to the next pattern. Only one pattern is targeted per session especially during the first few cycles. Three or four cycles are usually required for a client who is unintelligible to become intelligible (Hodson, 2004). The length of a cycle varies from 5 to 16 weeks, depending on the number of target patterns and phonemes/contexts as well as the frequency and length of sessions.

The major phonological deviations are those that most adversely impact intelligibility (Hodson & Paden, 1981). All of the major patterns that are deficient are targeted in each cycle of treatment unless a pattern is not stimulable, which is often the case for velars. Nonstimulable patterns are skipped until later cycles when they become stimulable. Within a cycle, the early developing patterns are generally targeted first, followed by the posterior/anterior contrasts, /s/ clusters (for targeting the deficient patterns of cluster reduction and/or strident deviation), and finally the liquids. This sequence may be altered for some clients depending upon an individual's stimulability for sounds/sound contexts within the patterns. We have often found that clients can more easily produce /s/ clusters than posterior obstruents (such as /k/, /g/) and thus target /s/ clusters before velar obstruents. Some children have great difficulty producing velars initially. Table 9.3 displays potential deficient patterns, target patterns, and targets for the initial cycles. The criterion for sound/context selection is ease of production for the client. At least two individual sounds/contexts from a particular pattern are selected for a cycle, and each are presented for a specified period of time. Other more complex sounds/contexts are selected for the same pattern in later cycles. Cycle 1 basically "lays a phonological foundation," while the target patterns seem to be easier for the client to produce during cycles 2 and 3 (Hodson & Paden, 1991, p. 97). Note that consonant sequences (addressing cluster reduction or consonant sequence omission) and stridency (addressing stridency deviation that includes omission of stridents and substitution of a strident by a nonstrident) are targeted together in the initial cycles through the context of /s/ clusters. Because two patterns are targeted simultaneously, at least four /s/ clusters are addressed for 60 to 90 minutes each. Initial /s/ clusters (such as /st/, /sp/, /sm/, and /sn/) are targeted successively either before or after successively focusing on final /s/ clusters (such as /ps/, /ts/, and /ks/). Intermingling initial and final /s/ clusters usually is confusing to clients in the beginning cycles (Hodson, 2004).

Upon completion of each cycle, it is advisable to readminister the HAPP-3 to determine the major phonological deviations that need to be recycled. Syllableness and final consonants often resolve after cycle 1 of treatment. Target sounds/contexts for cycle 2 and subsequent cycles usually should be a little more difficult for the client than the cycle 1 targets. Appropriate targets include combining two cycle 1 targets in a 60-minute period; for example, targeting /sp/ and /st/ together in one session or initial /k/ and initial /g/ when each of these targets were worked on individually during cycle 1. Other strategies for later cycles are to target other exemplars of the desired pattern, the same sound in a different word position, /r/ clusters, /l/ clusters, three-element clusters (including /spl/, /str/), and contrasting word pairs (including *key* and *tea* for the velar obstruent pattern). Sometimes, in cycle 2,

initial /r/ and initial /l/ are retargeted in the same context for stabilization if a client did not produce them in words easily during cycle 1. The objective for /r/ in the initial cycles is to suppress gliding of /r/ rather than striving for completely correct /r/ production. In later cycles, velar obstruents could be targeted in words that include alveolar consonants, but such words should be avoided in earlier cycles because of the strong potential for alveolar assimilation to occur. Another strategy to use during the third or fourth cycle is to incorporate "It's a _____" phrases for working on stridency and/or consonant sequences with one 60-minute time period spent on "It's a *nonstrident word*" followed by 60 minutes of "It's a */s/ cluster word.*"

After the basic phonological deviations are suppressed, other targets might need to be addressed, such as palatals (/j, j clusters, ɚ, ʃ, tʃ, dʒ/), voicing contrasts, vowel contrasts, singleton stridents (/f, s/), and other consonant clusters (/kw, tw, sw, bj, hj, fj, kj/, and final /st/) (Hodson & Paden, 1991). In the cycling approach, inappropriate targets for clients with unintelligible speech include final voiced stops (/b/, /d/, /g/), unstressed (weak) syllables, dental fricatives (/θ/, /ð/), velar nasal (/ŋ/), and final /l/ (Hodson & Paden, 1991). The rationale for not addressing final voiced stops is that clients often add a schwa when attempting to produce final voiced obstruents resulting in epenthesis. Also, devoicing commonly occurs in the speech of young children as they develop their speech, and adults also devoice some final consonants (Hodson & Paden, 1991). Both children and adults tend to omit unstressed syllables in multisyllabic words (e.g., /prɑbəbli/ → /prɑbli/), to substitute final /n/ for /ŋ/, and not produce final /l/ with an elevated tongue tip. Incorrect production of /θ, ð/ does not seem to affect intelligibility appreciably. Appendix M displays assessment results, cycle 1 projection, and cycle 2 projection for a child with a severe phonologic disorder.

Appropriate selection of words for production practice during treatment sessions is critical. During the earlier cycles, words that have facilitative phonetic contexts should be used. In the event that a client uses velar fronting, a typical deviant pattern, use words that do not contain anterior consonants, especially alveolars. Select words such as *cow* and *cook* rather than *cane* and *kite*. Whenever a client has velar deviations, target /s/ clusters that do not contain velars; that is, work on /st/ (both sounds have the same phonetic placement) or /sp/ instead of /sk/ or /ks/. On the other hand, if the client backs, select /sk/ or /ks/ as targets because the client easily produces /k/. Similarly, if a client has /l/ deficiency, do not target /sl/ before the client produces /l/ easily.

TABLE 9.3

Potential Target Patterns/Phonemes for Initial Phonological Cycles

Deficiencies (If Consistent)	Targets (If Stimulable)
Early Developing Patterns	
Syllable deletion	Spondaic words (i.e., equal-stress compound words)
	2-syllable spondaic words
	3-syllable spondaic words
Initial consonant deletion	Word-initial
	Anterior nasals /m, n/
	Anterior stops /b, d, p, t/
	Labial glide /w/
Final consonant deletion or glottal replacement	Word-final
	Voiceless stops /p, t, k/
	Anterior nasals /m, n/
Nasal deviation	Anterior nasals /m, n/
	Word-initial
	Word-final
Glide deviation	Labial glide /w/
Lack of CVC structure	CVC words with same consonant (e.g., "toot")
Posterior/Anterior Contrasts	
Velar deviation (fronting)	Word-final /k/
	Word-initial /g, k/
	Word-initial /h/
Anterior nonstrident deviation (backing)	Word-final /t/
	Word-initial /d, t/
/s/-Clusters	
Cluster reduction/Stridency deletion	/s/ clusters
	Word-initial /sp, st, sm, sn, sk, sw/
	Word-final /ts, ps, ks/
Liquids	
Liquid /l/ deviation	Suppress gliding
Liquid /r/ deviation	Word-initial /l/
	Word-initial nonglided /r/

Source: Hodson, B. W., Gordon-Brannan, M. (1992). *Phonological assessment and remediation: Expediting intelligibility gains.* Conference sponsored by Portland Center for Hearing and Speech, Beaverton, OR.

When working on /s/ clusters in a cycle, select at least one target to be in the final position (such as /ts/ or /ps/) that facilitates use of stridency at the end of words, and as a bonus, works on plurals. Note that it is not appropriate to target final /s/ clusters such as /st/ or /sp/ as these are more difficult for children to produce. Often, production of /r/ (or a distorted /r/ that is a nonglide) is facilitated in context with back vowels. The nonfacilitative phonetic contexts should be reserved for later cycles after the client has been successful producing the desired patterns in facilitative contexts.

The components of a phonological cycling lesson include:

- *Review of the words used in the previous session.* When the same pattern is targeted in the current session, these words can also be included along with the new ones in some of the activities. When the current session is targeting a different pattern, the previous session's words are not incorporated.
- *Amplified auditory stimulation.* Auditory stimulation entails the client listening through earphones to the clinician read, once or twice, a list of 12 to 15 words containing the current session's target sound/context. The clinician reads the words conversationally without emphasizing the target through an amplifier set at a low level of amplification. The list contains the potential production-practice words plus other words representing the pattern that may be more complex words. The client is not to repeat the words during this portion of the session.
- *Selection of production-practice stimuli.* Two to five words that the client can produce are selected from a potential list of words that can be elicited through pictures or objects. It is often helpful to use the microphone-amplifier-earphone apparatus while the client is attempting to say the potential word stimuli. The client makes 5″ X 8″ cards displaying the words to be selected by drawing pictures, pasting pictures on the cards, or coloring the picture cards. This makes the cards personal for individual clients. The words are written on the front of the cards so that others can identify the pictures, and there is an added bonus of including a literacy component.
- *Experiential-play production practice.* In this step, clients practice the target pattern multiple times in a few words. The children's interest is maintained by using several different activities in which the same words are practiced throughout the session. At the beginning of the production practice step, the 2 to 5 selected words are elicited using whatever cues (including modeling, tactile cues, visual cues, auditory cues, etc.) are necessary for correct production of the pattern. Note that the operative word is *pattern*. The client is reinforced when the correct pattern is used even though an incorrect sound may be used. For example, a client is reinforced for using a final consonant when the target is final consonants even though the incorrect final consonant was used (e.g., /bot/ instead of /bon/).

Also, a lingually distorted /s/ that has the strident component would be reinforced because the target pattern is stridency. In these cases, the client is praised for producing the correct pattern, but the clinician then attempts to elicit the correct sound production (e.g., "Good, you put a sound at the end. Now watch me and say boat."). With children who are working on bisyllables, the goal is for the client to produce two distinct syllables, even when they are only vowels. Throughout the practice, the goal is for the client to be 100% correct in using the targeted pattern; thus, the clinician provides as many cues as necessary to achieve a high level of achievement. Producing incorrect patterns, which need to be corrected by the clinician, provides an inaccurate kinesthetic image. Modeling and cues are gradually decreased throughout the session as the client's ability to produce the correct patterns improves. Words from other sessions focusing on the same pattern can be incorporated in the current session activities which does expand the number of practice words. For children who can read, a few minutes of oral reading at a reading level lower than their reading ability is included in each session.

- *Probing to select next session targets.* Near the end of the session, the target phoneme/context is selected for the next 60-minute period of the cycle. The clinician instructs the client to imitate models of appropriate targets. The target that is most stimulable or is the easiest to elicit is selected. For example, when the next session is to target /s/ clusters, the clinician may attempt to elicit /st/, /sm/, and /sp/ to determine which one is easiest for the client. Another example is to determine whether it is easier for the client to produce a velar or an /s/ cluster when moving to later developing patterns within a cycle.
- *Repetition of amplified auditory stimulation.*
- *Home program.* The production practice cards for the current pattern are sent home or to school with the client. The home program involves someone reading the auditory stimulation word list to the client and the client saying the production practice words displayed on the cards to someone once a day. This entails about 2 minutes daily. The home program can be done by a parent, educational assistant, sibling, older student, and so on in the home, classroom, or another appropriate place. Table 9.4 shows a sample lesson.

Incorporation of phonological awareness activities is recommended during clinical sessions for most clients (Hodson, 2004).

TABLE 9.4

Sample Phonological Cycling Lesson Plan

Lesson Plan Components	Examples
	Prior Lesson's Target: Three-syllable spondees for targeting syllables
	Target: final /p/ for targeting final consonants
Review	Client names word cards from previous session: *baseball bat, cowboy hat, hot dog bun, ice cream cone*
Amplified auditory stimulation	Clinician reads list to client with amplification. Client listens:
	mop, stop, hop, up, envelope, potato chip, pop, skip, soap, gallop, sleep, ketchup, wipe, tulip, help, pipe
Selection of production practice words	With amplification, client imitates clinician saying potential production practice words. Selects words in which final /p/ is stimulable. Child draws (pastes, colors) pictures on 5″ × 8″ cards. Client imitates words several times: *up, pop, mop, hop, pipe*
Production practice activities	Picture cards made in prior step are used in various activities.
	Clinician provides a model and/or other stimuli as needed for the client to use correct production (final consonant) as close to 100% accuracy as possible.
	Client names pictures as they are "caught" during fishing activity.
	Client names pictures as they are hit with a bean bag.
	Client names pictures as they are found during a treasure hunt.
	Client names pictures when the music stops during musical chairs.
Probe for next target	Client imitates clinician saying words with the next potential target for final consonants: /t/, /m/
	eat, boat, hat, Mom, time, home
	Note: Done after final /p/ has been targeted for 60–90 minutes
Amplified auditory stimulation	Repeat amplified auditory stimulation step
Homework	Instructs child/parent/teacher's assistant/older sibling to do the following once a day:
	1. Read the listening (amplified auditory stimulation) list to client
	2. Listen to client name the word cards for the final consonant pattern

A **focused auditory input** cycle is an alternative technique to use with clients who have been unwilling or are unable to produce any target at the beginning of treatment. This is particularly appropriate for children below the 3-year level of functioning. In this strategy, major phonological patterns are stimulated, but the client is not required to say anything. Rather, the clinician provides the stimuli for the target pattern in activities, and the client interacts with the clinician in the activities. Each phoneme within a pattern is the focus for about 30 minutes. Auditory stimulation with slight amplification (if possible) is incorporated in the session. Parents or others read the stimulation word list to the client daily.

Comments

The phonological cycling approach has been implemented primarily with children who are unintelligible. Group treatment as well as individual treatment is appropriate. It is generally recommended for phonological deviancies, but not for phonetic errors. It has been used effectively with children who have cognitive deficits by doubling the amount of time spent on each target (Hodson BW, personal communication, Fall, 1990). It has also been used with children who have hearing impairments (Gordon-Brannan, Hodson, & Wynn, 1992). This approach should be reserved for multiple articulation errors because the focus is on speech sound patterns rather than individual speech sounds.

An advantage of the cycling approach is that it is often efficacious because not all sounds in a pattern need to be addressed in treatment; that is, the correct target pattern often spontaneously transfers to other sounds within the pattern. It has been shown to be particularly effective with clients whose speech is unintelligible (Hodson & Paden, 1983). One limitation of the approach may be that a phonological processes analysis is quite time-consuming, but is offset by the efficient intervention results. Several single subject and case study research has shown the phonological cycling approach and modifications of the approach to be effective (Carver, 1997; Gordon-Brannan et al., 1992; Hodson, 1994; Hodson, Chin, Redmond, & Simpson, 1983; Hodson & Paden, 1981; Kemper, 1996; Ozanich, 1997; Rheault, 2002; Royer, 1995; Tyler, Edwards, & Saxman, 1987). Overgeneralization tends not to occur. Unlike the distinctive features approach, the phonological cycling approach can address omissions as well as substitutions. It is not appropriate for distortions that really are phonetic errors rather than phonological errors.

Today, clinicians are beginning to perform phonological analyses to use as a basis for selecting phonological deviations in treatment. Increasingly, the newer articulation/phonological tests include both a phonological deviation analysis along with traditional sound-by-sound analysis. These tests are becoming more user-friendly, and some can be done with computer analysis software that decreases the amount of time needed to analyze clients' speech. Clinicians use phonological cycles approach with children, particularly young children, who have multiple articulation errors and who have no apparent organic problem that contributes to the articulatory/phonologic disorder.

> Describe the meaningful minimal contrasting pairs treatment approach, its rationale, advantages, and limitations.

MEANINGFUL MINIMAL CONTRASTING PAIRS APPROACH

In the meaningful minimal contrasting pairs approach, phonological processes or deviations are targeted to be suppressed. In other words, the objective is to decrease the frequency of occur-

rence of the incorrect phonological deviations and to increase the occurrence of the correct speech sound pattern. This is accomplished by the client producing pairs of words, one word containing the desired pattern and the other word containing an opposite pattern. It is thus demonstrated to the client in which meaningful words the targeted pattern is to occur and in which words it does not occur.

Rationale

The meaningful minimal contrasting pairs approach originally emanated from the natural phonology theory which posits that children acquiring a phonological system begin with a set of innate and universal processes and learn to suppress those that do not occur in their home language. The approach is based on the premise that sound errors are the result of faulty learning of phonological rules; therefore, the client needs to learn and apply the linguistic rules for phonology to use correct phonemic patterns. The assumption is that the client is using early-developing rules or inappropriate rules, and the task of treatment is to eliminate inappropriate rules or processes, such as final consonant deletion or velar fronting.

A second premise of this approach is that treatment of one or a few phonological processes will result in correction of several phonemes at once. For example, elimination of the deviation of stopping may affect all fricatives. Similarly to the distinctive features approach, intervention is more efficient than the more traditional approaches which focus on individual phonemes. Because the approach has been developed to deal with phonological rather than phonetic disorders, intervention usually begins at the meaningful word level. Seldom does the clinician focus on speech sound production in isolation or nonsense syllables.

How are the appropriate phonological rules taught? Inappropriate phonological patterns are targeted to be reduced or eliminated which is quite different from approaches in which the client is taught to use a particular sound or feature correctly. A common strategy is to compare and contrast two words, one that uses the targeted pattern and one that does not. For example, contrasting word pairs such as *bow/bone* and *me/meet* could be used for final consonant deletion; *cake/take* and *game/dame* for velar fronting, and finally, *feet/fleet* and *soon/spoon* for cluster reduction. These contrasts demonstrate to the client that meaning is affected when the incorrect pattern is used.

Goals and Procedures

The objective of the meaningful minimal pairs approach is to decrease the occurrence of inappropriate phonological processes while increasing appropriate phonological patterns. The client is not required to use correct articulation per se, but to use the appropriate pattern, although it is preferred that the client does produce the correct sound. The first step is to select the phonological processes to be targeted. Assessment results, including formal articulation/phonological test performance and analysis of spontaneous speech samples, are used for this purpose. Several bases can be used for selecting the deviations to be targeted along with the sequential ordering of the targets. Factors to be considered include normative data information, percentage of occurrence of phonological deviations, developmental order, and probable influence on intelligibility (Khan & Lewis, 2002). One approach to target selection is to begin with the earlier-developing basic deviations as proposed by Hodson and Paden (1991) followed by the later-developing basic deviations, and finally proceed to the secondary deviations. Another strategy is to pick three phonological processes for targeting at the same time, one from each of the categories of syllable structure, harmony or assimilation, and feature contrast or substitution (Weiner, 1979). Table 9.5 presents the treatment order recommended by Weiner for phonological processes in each of three categories. We have found that the voicing deviations (such as prevocalic voicing and final consonant devoicing) do not need to be addressed initially in treatment because they usually do not affect in-

telligibility and often are suppressed (corrected) without direct intervention (Hodson & Paden, 1991; Howell & Dean, 1994). Also, targeting weak syllable deletion is not recommended because adult speakers often delete unstressed syllables in their speech (Hodson & Paden, 1991). However, addressing syllable deletion is recommended when the client seldom uses multisyllables.

Various treatment protocols have been developed to use meaningful contrasts for target phonological patterns. They all use pictures of words representing minimal pairs, one that is an exemplar of the targeted pattern and the other that is not. A procedure for contrasting phonemic patterns using pictures of word pairs was outlined by Fokes (1982). Initially, the client discriminates between the clinician's productions of 8 to 10 word pairs. The client then produces the words. The responses are scored on the basis of whether or not the specific contrast was correct rather than whether the sound was correctly articulated. The words are then used in sentences and stories. One or more phonological patterns are targeted during each session.

A similar intervention protocol using contrasting word pairs was described by Blache (1982):

- *Discussion of words*—Determine whether client understands the words used in the treatment activity by pointing to the picture stimuli representing the words
- *Receptive testing and training*—Determine whether client perceives the phonological feature separating the two words; that is, client points to the correct picture when the clinician says one of the two words

TABLE 9.5

Order of Phonological Process Targets in Each of Three Categories of Phonological Processes Recommended by Weiner (1979)

Order of Targets	Phonological Processes Categories		
	Syllable Structure	*Harmony*	*Feature Contrast*
Target 1	Deletion of final	Prevocalic voicing	Stopping
Target 2	Glottal replacement	Final consonant devoicing	Affrication
Target 3	Weak syllable deletion	Velar assimilation	Gliding of fricatives
Target 4	Cluster reduction	Labial assimilation	Fronting
Target 5		Alveolar assimilation	Denasalization
Target 6			Gliding of liquids
Target 7			Vocalization

- *Production training*—Client becomes the "teacher" and says one of the two words; clinician points to the word the client actually produced
- *Carryover*—Engage in activities to produce the words in phrases, sentences, and conversation in the clinic and outside the clinic

A third variation is illustrated by the following instructions to the client: "We are going to play a game. The object of the game is to get me to pick up all five pictures of the _____. Every time you say _____, I will pick one up. When I have all five, you may paste a star on your paper" (Weiner, 1981). The pictures represent minimal pairs. If the client uses incorrect productions on two consecutive trials, the clinician gives instructions to correct the errors. Table 9.6 presents a sample lesson plan using the meaningful minimal contrasts strategy.

Comments

The meaningful minimal contrasting pairs approach has been implemented primarily with children, although it seems feasible to use with adults. Group management is also possible with the approach. It is recommended for phonological deviancies, but not for phonetic deviancies. This approach should be reserved for multiple articulation errors because it is probably not useful to analyze the phonological patterns of those with fewer errors.

An advantage of this approach is that it is often efficacious because once the target pattern is learned (that is, the deviant pattern is suppressed), it generalizes to other affected sounds and word structures. Results of treatment have shown the minimal contrasting pairs approach to be effective (Blache, 1982; Blache, Parsons, & Humphreys, 1981; Fokes, 1982; Kemper, 1996; Royer, 1995; Tyler et al., 1987). Overgeneralization usually does not occur probably because the client contrasts two correct speech sound patterns. Unlike the distinctive features approach, the contrasting pairs approach can address omissions as well as substitutions. It is not appropriate for distortions which really are phonetic errors rather than phonological errors. A limitation of the approach is that many formal phonological analyses are quite time-consuming; however, the time required for analysis must be compared with the

TABLE 9.6

Sample Minimal Pairs Lesson Plan

Steps	Examples
Stimulus: Pictures of 5–8 minimal opposition word pairs (five copies of each word)	Target: Final Consonants
1. Establish meaning of words	Client and clinician discuss the meaning of the pictures: *pie-pipe, me-meat, bow-boat, be-bean, hoe-home*
2. Receptive testing and training	Lay out five pictures of *pie* and *pipe*. "Pick up *pie/pipe*." Continue until the client picks up all 10 cards correctly. Follow the same procedure for the other word pairs.
3. Production training	Present two stacks (five cards each) of *pie* and *pipe*. "Now, you be the teacher and tell me which cards to pick up." Continue until the client correctly names each word pair five times, assisting the client as needed in producing the words by putting on a final consonant. Follow the same procedure for the other word pairs.
	"I have pie and pipe. Which card would you like?" Clinician provides feedback and assists in production as needed. Child must acquire all 12 cards.
4. Carryover activities	Play "Go Fish" with two of each minimal pair words.
	Play "Treasure Hunt" using the cards as the treasure. Client says "I see/found a _____."
	Tell a story using the 10 cards. Client retells the story.

hours spent in treatment when such an analysis is not done. Another limitation is that some younger clients and persons who are cognitively challenged become confused when producing contrasting patterns at the same time.

Clinicians are beginning to perform phonological analyses as a basis for selecting phonological deviations to address in treatment, and the newer articulation/phonological tests tend to include a phonological deviation analysis along with traditional sound-by-sound analysis. Clinicians use the minimal contrasting pairs approach with children who have multiple articulation errors and who have no apparent organic problem that contributes to the articulatory/phonologic disorder. Production of contrasting word pairs is done in later stages of the cycling approach when necessary.

> Describe the maximal opposition treatment approach, including its theoretical basis, advantages, and limitations.

MAXIMAL OPPOSITION APPROACH

The **maximal opposition approach**, also known as maximal pairs contrast approach, was developed as an alternative approach to the minimal opposition strategy just described (Elbert & Gierut, 1986). In this approach, two phonemes that are different in the multiple phonetic features of voice, place, and manner are contrasted. In other words, the sound pair contrasts differ by as many distinctive features as possible (Gierut, 1990a). Examples include contrasting /m/, a voiced bilabial sonorant, with /k/, a voiceless velar obstruent; and contrasting /b/, a voiced bilabial stop, with /s/, a voiceless alveolar fricative. Thus, rather than targeting a particular speech sound feature or pattern, individual clients presumably select the specific features that they identify as relevant to sound production (Gierut, 1989). In this approach, clients produce contrasting word pairs with one of the words containing a sound that is not in the client's repertoire and the other word containing a sound the client already produces correctly.

Rationale

According to Gierut (1989), the maximal opposition approach is supported by developmental psycholinguistic literature. "Young normally developing children initially seem to attempt and to maintain maximal distinctions and contrasts among sounds and sound classes" (Gierut, p. 10). The development of sound contrasts progresses from major oppositions to finer distinctions; for example, initially distinguishing between oral and nasal sound production and between obstruent and sonorant sounds, and later adding voicing, place, and manner distinctions. Thus, when developing their speech, children initially focus on the wide differences between sounds rather than on the smaller differences. The maximal opposition approach gives them an opportunity to contrast phonemes that are widely different. An additional basis for the approach is that young children are active and creative when acquiring the phonological system (Elbert & Gierut, 1986; Gierut, 1989). They are individualistic and unique in the type of sounds and contrasts they add to their phonological systems and seem to experiment with and revise their phonological system as they are learning it. Finally, generalization seems to be facilitated by loosely structured intervention that does not limit the range of correct responses. Thus, a maximal opposition approach is based on the following characteristics (Gierut, p.10):

- Emphasizes phonemic contrasts along a more grossly differentiated range of features
- Allows a child considerable flexibility in identification of relevant feature contrasts
- Encourages broad generalization of those features identified as relevant

In maximal oppositions, the client has many more unique distinctions to discover than in minimal oppositions, and the contrast is easier to identify from other sound pairs that are minimally contrasting.

Another rationale for the maximal opposition approach is the concept of marked and unmarked sounds as described in Chapter 3. Marked sounds are those that are more difficult to learn, occur later in development, and occur less frequently in the languages of the world. According to implicational linguistic theory, the presence of marked (difficult) sounds in an individual's speech sound inventory implies that the unmarked (easy) sounds are also present in the inventory, but not vice versa. The hypothesis for treatment then is that when clients learn to produce marked sounds, the unmarked sounds will also be learned. The contention is that when a client learns to produce the marked sounds, both marked and unmarked sounds are learned; however, when the client only learns to produce unmarked sounds, the marked sounds will not necessarily be learned (Gierut, 1989, 1990a, 1990b).

Goals and Procedures

The goals of the maximal opposition approach are to increase the phonetic inventory and the complexity level of the phonological system (Fig. 3.6). In the simplest, level A, children produce nasals, glides, and labial and alveolar stops. In level B, the contrast between voiced and voiceless stops is added, and in some cases, /k/ and /g/ are added, giving a contrast between anterior and posterior. Level C phonemic inventories include fricatives and/or affricates. In level D, a liquid consonant, either /r/ or /l/, is added. Finally, the most complex, level E, includes either the inclusion of both /s/ and /θ/ giving a stridency contrast in the fricatives, or the inclusion of both /l/ and /r/ giving a lateral contrast in liquids. (Gierut, 1990b).

Prior to treatment, a phonological assessment of the client's speech sound system is done using a combination of a spontaneous speech sample and elicitation of all consonants in the initial, intervocalic, and final positions in a variety of exemplars. The analysis includes descriptions of a client's phonetic inventories; phonemic inventory (the sounds that are used contrastingly); distribution of sounds; phonological rules and positional, inventory, and sequence constraints; and underlying representations of morphemes (Geirut, 1990a). From the analysis, maximally contrasting sounds are selected for intervention. In the case of inventory constraints (the sound does not appear in the child's phonetic inventory), one of the contrasting sounds is a sound that is absent from the child's phonetic inventory and the other one is present in the child's inventory. In the case of positional constraints, one of the contrasting sounds is one that does not appear in the initial, intervocalic, or final position and the other contrasting sound does appear in that position. The two contrasting sounds differ along multiple feature dimensions that can include major class distinctions (such as consonantal, sonorant, syllabic). The sound that is excluded from the client's phonetic or phonemic inventory is referred to as the *target* sound and the contrasting sound that is in the client's inventory is identified as the *comparison* sound.

The intervention is a behavioral programmed approach (Gierut, 1989, 1990a). Treatment consists of two phases: (a) imitation and (b) spontaneous. Five to eight word pairs for each contrasting sound pairs are used as stimuli. An option is to produce contrastingly the target sound with two or three comparison sounds that are already in the client's speech sound inventory (Elbert & Gierut, 1986). During imitation, the clinician models a word pair and the client imitates it. A third option

is to contrast two sounds that do not appear in the client's phonetic inventory (Gierut, 1992). This phase continues until a preset criterion level is reached (75 to 90% correct production of both sounds over two consecutive sessions). No speech sound discrimination or perceptual work is incorporated. During the spontaneous phase, the client names the picture pairs without a clinician model. This phase is continued until the preset criterion is reached (90% over two or three consecutive sessions). The word pairs are produced at the single word level. Treatment activities include:

- *Drill*—Client names the word pair stimuli
- *Sorting*—Client names pictures and puts them in their respective sound piles
- *Matching*—An array of pictures presented from which the client selects one, names it, and finds its matching pair, then names it
- *Informal storytelling*

Ideally, the word pairs used in treatment are minimal pairs; that is, "two words which differ in meaning when only one sound is changed" (Crystal, 1985, p. 195). To achieve this, the stimuli can be real words (Elbert & Gierut, 1986; Gierut, 1989) or nonsense words that have been assigned lexical meaning (Gierut, 1990a). Nonsense words that are consistent with English phonotactics can be introduced in the context of stories and illustrated with pictures. The pictures are used in the production activities of the contrasting word pairs. It is sometimes difficult to identify suitable minimal pairs. An alternative is to use *near minimal pairs;* that is, words that differ by more than one sound with the vowel preceding or following the target being the same vowel (Elbert & Gierut, 1986). Examples include *cheek-meat, goat-phone, shine-bite* when contrasting /tʃ/ with /m/, /g/ with /f/, and /ʃ/ with /b/, respectively. Table 9.7 illustrates the treatment steps in a maximal opposition approach.

Comments

The maximal opposition approach has been implemented primarily with children and in individual treatment sessions, although it also seems applicable for adults and with groups. It was developed to teach phonemic distinctions. First, the client learns to produce the target sound motorically then conceptualizes it through spontaneous production of the target in contrast with a comparison sound or sounds. This approach probably should be reserved for multiple articulation errors, perhaps six or more, because it is probably not useful to analyze the phonological patterns of those with fewer errors.

TABLE 9.7

Sample Maximal Opposition Lesson Plan

Steps	Examples Maximal Opposition Pair: /m/ and /k/
Phase 1: Imitation	
A. Client imitates clinician's productions of 5–8 maximal opposition word pairs in initial position	Show pictures of words, one at a time. "Say _____:" *might-kite, May-Kay, mop-cop, miss-kiss, man-can*
B. Client imitates clinician's productions of 5–8 maximal opposition word pairs in final position	Show pictures of words, one at a time. "Say _____:" *comb-coke, Tom-talk, buck-bum, limb-lick, beam-beak*
Phase 2: Spontaneous	
A. Drill—Client says the words	Show pictures of words, one at a time. "What is this?"
B. Sorting—Client says both words of a pair and puts each into its own sound pile of cards	Give client a pair of words. "Name the cards and put each one in its own sound pile."
C. Matching—Client says one word of a pair, finds its contrasting word, and names it.	Lay the /m/ cards (representing the contrasting words) on the table. Hand a /s/ card to the client. "What is this?" "Find its match and name it."
D. Informal storytelling	Present some of the picture cards to the client. "Tell me a story using these cards."

Note: One can do the initial and final positions together or separately, depending on the client's abilities.

An advantage of this approach is that it may be efficient because once the client has learned to produce the target sound in contrast to the comparison sound, other sounds that were omitted may be added to the client's phonetic and/or phonemic inventory. Some single subject research has shown evidence of its effectiveness, especially with children who have a moderate phonologic disorder (levels B, C, and D) (Gierut, 1989, 1990a, 1992; Tyler & Figurski, 1994). Overgeneralization usually does not occur probably because the client practices the correct speech sound patterns. Unlike the distinctive features approach, the contrasting pairs approach addresses omissions or excluded phonemes. The maximal opposition approach only targets speech sounds that are either entirely missing from a client's phonetic inventory or that are excluded from certain word positions; other types of phonological deviation patterns, such as assimilations, are not addressed with this approach. A minimal opposition approach is recommended as a follow-up of the maximal opposition treatment. As with all phonological approaches, the approach is not appropriate for distortions. A limitation of the approach is that the phonological analysis recommended for assessment can be quite time-consuming. Another limitation is that some younger clients become confused when producing contrasting words.

The maximal opposition approach has been investigated primarily in single subject studies (Gierut, 1989, 1990a) and seems not to be used extensively by practicing clinicians. This approach certainly is a departure from the typical learning framework in which learning progresses from easy to difficult rather than from difficult to easy as is advocated in the maximal opposition approach. Further research on using this approach with a variety of clients, including those with more severe phonologic disorders (such as at levels A and B), is needed to determine the effectiveness of such an approach.

> Describe the Metaphon treatment approach, including its theoretical basis, advantages, and limitations.

METAPHON APPROACH

The **Metaphon treatment approach** originated in the mid-1980s and has been further developed by Howell and Dean to facilitate change in the simplification rules or phonological processes used by children with phonologic disorders (Dean et al., 1995; Howell & Dean, 1994). It is a metalinguistic approach to phonological/articulation treatment designed to enhance "knowledge of the phonological and communicative aspects of language, set within a therapeutic environment which maximises learning opportunities" (Howell & Dean, 1994, p. *vii*). In this approach, clients first develop an awareness of the properties or features of sounds, the contrasts between speech sounds, relationship of sound contrasts to meaning, and the way in which sounds can be manipulated to improve their ability to be understood. Clients subsequently produce the sound contrasts needed to convey meaning.

Rationale

The Metaphon treatment approach evolved from two principles, namely: (a) some children with disordered speech have problems acquiring adult phonological patterns and should be working on the contrastive function of speech sounds rather than with articulation of individual speech sounds and (b) children in treatment should take an active and informed role. It was Dean and Howell's (1994; Dean et al., 1995) contention that current treatment approaches do not take into account the nature of such phonologic disorders and the way children learn; instead intervention for speech sound disorders tends to incorporate discrimination and production of specific phonemes and is an unexplained, adult-led activity that does not always motivate the child to take an active role in the process.

Children with phonologic disorders are differentiated from those who have phonetic disorders by Howell & Dean (1994). Children with phonologic disorders are described as those who consistently use patterns of pronunciation that are different from adult speakers; that is, they have their own phonological rules that contrast sounds and combine sounds into meaningful utterances. Some probably also have a phonetic component because many have restricted phonetic inventories. Individuals have a unique combination of rule usage; they may use developmental phonological rules, atypical rules, or a combination of rules. A phonologic disorder arises from "a difficulty with learning and applying the phonological rules of adult language rather than from a difficulty with articulatory production. . .phonological disorder is essentially a phonemic/organizational problem rather than a phonetic/production difficulty" (Howell & Dean, 1994, p. 7). Therefore, treatment is focused on

helping children with phonologic disorders eliminate the simplification phonological rules and adopt the adult phonological rules. Having children simply imitate contrastive pairs "will be of limited value because. . .these children are not fully aware of the nature of their communication failure. . .they have little knowledge of the precise nature of their difficulty" (Howell & Dean, p. 59).

Metalinguistics refers to thinking about and reflecting on the nature and functions of language. One component is phonological awareness or **metaphonology** defined as "the ability to pay attention to and reflect upon the phonological structure of the language" (Howell and Dean, 1994, p. 65). According to Howell and Dean, language acquisition theories and some research results support the hypothesis that there is a role for some aspects of linguistic awareness in phonological development. Also, some research has shown that some children with phonologic disorders have poor metalinguistic skills, and that phonological awareness skill can be developed through intervention. Therefore, in the first phase of Metaphon treatment, clients learn that sounds have certain combinations of features that differentiate them from other sounds, that some of the features also occur in other sounds, and that these sounds can be grouped according to features. Metacommunication, that is, "knowledge that successful communication depends upon the person who is speaking being understood by those who are listening" (Howell & Dean, 1994, p. 65), is another important concept. In Phase 2 of Metaphon intervention, clients become aware of communication breakdown and are encouraged to make repairs which are facilitated by applying their knowledge of the phonological system which they learned earlier.

Goals and Procedures

The goal of the Metaphon approach is to attain a phonological developmental level commensurate with children of the same age and psycholinguistic ability (Howell & Dean, 1994). The aim is for clients to acquire and apply the adult phonological rules in their speech production.

The first step is to conduct a linguistic analysis of the phonologic disorder that involves a phonological process analysis. A process is a rule type defined as "a rule which can be applied to varying extents across a class of sounds or different word positions" (Howell & Dean, 1994, p. 25). Although other phonological assessment tools can be used, the Metaphon Resource Pack (MPR; Dean, Howell, Hill, & Waters, 1990) was developed as a companion to Metaphon intervention. It assesses 13 simplification phonological processes as shown in Table 9.8. The diagnostician should also determine the other patterns that are used by individual clients, because children with phonologic disorders

TABLE 9.8

Simplifying Phonological Processes Assessed by the Metaphon Resource Pack

Process	Approximate Age of Suppression
Systemic	
Velar fronting	3.00 to 3.06
Palatoalveolar fronting	4.00 to 4.06
Stopping of fricatives	
/f/	2.6 to 3.00
/v/	3.00 to 3.06
/θ/	2.06 to 3.00 → fronting to '[s] type'
/ð/	3.06 to 4.00 → fronting to [d] or [v]
/s/	2.06 to 3.00
/z/	3.00 to 3.06
/ʃ/	2.06 to 3.00 → fronting to '[s] type'
Stopping of affricates	3.06 to 4.00 → fronting to [ts; dz]
Backing of alveolar stops	(atypical process)
Syllable final devoicing	3.00 to 3.06
Syllable initial voicing	2.06 to 3.00
Liquid glide simplification	4.06 →
Dental fronting	4.06 →
Structural	
Initial consonant deletion	(atypical process)
Final consonant deletion	3.00 to 3.03
Initial cluster reduction/deletion	3.06 to 4.00
Final cluster reduction/deletion	(not available)

Notes:

Approximate age of suppression = Age at which these processes have ceased to be used, or are used inconsistently, by most children of this age

Atypical process = Process that is not recorded in normal acquisition data

Not available = Process reported in normal acquisition but where no age of suppression is given

From Howell, J., & Dean, E. (1994). *Treating phonological disorders in children* (2nd ed.). London: Whurr Publishers Ltd. Reprinted with permission.

often use unique or idiosyncratic patterns. The MRP consists of the following components:

- *Screening procedure*—Single word sample that provides an overview of the phonological processes used by the client
- *Process-specific probes*—Set of stimuli for each of the 13 phonological processes and administered as needed to provide more in-depth information about an individual client's speech
- *Monitoring procedure*—Assesses the extent and pattern of change throughout the treatment process

Additionally, a phonetic analysis is to be done on the data sample that includes a spontaneous speech sample as well as the single word sample. The assessment consists of the phonetic inventory, phonetic distribution, cluster usage, syllable type usage, and imitation ability of sounds missing from the inventory. A vowel analysis is done when needed. From the analysis, specific targets and the order of addressing the targets is determined with a consideration of factors such as chronological age, variability of process usage (e.g., used in one word position, but not in another position), potential effect on intelligibility, and availability of speech sounds (e.g., produced in data sample, stimulability). Generally, phonological processes that occur in 50% or more of the available opportunities should be targeted.

The Metaphon treatment approach has two phases of treatment: (a) developing phonological awareness and (b) developing phonological and communicative awareness. The goal of the first phase is to develop awareness of the properties of sounds and their interrelationships in a motivational setting. The clinician and child explore "the properties of sounds; how sounds differ from each other due, for example, to place and manner distinctions; and the importance, for meaning, of maintaining those distinctions" (Howell & Dean, 1994, p. 87). For systemic phonological processes (substitution of one sound for another), the following steps comprise Phase 1:

- *Concept level*—Use the vocabulary (e.g., *long-short, front-back, noisy-whisper*) that will later be used to describe sound properties at the non-sound level
- *Sound level*—Transfer the concept level vocabulary to describe nonspeech sounds
- *Phoneme level*—Engage in activities involving manipulation of speech sounds in which the listener (client and clinician both function as listeners) describes speech sounds, often using visual representations

- *Word level*—Introduce minimal word pairs differing in the contrast being targeted. Child makes a judgment about the sound property used to produce the word (e.g., *long* for fricatives or *short* for stops; *noisy* for voiced sounds or *whisper* for unvoiced sounds). Words containing different sounds demonstrating the target contrasting features are incorporated in the activities (e.g., *tea-key* and *dough-go*).

For structural phonological processes (the syllable or word structure is changed), a different sequence of steps is followed:

- *Concept level*—Illustrate the vocabulary, to be used later, at the nonspeech level (e.g., hitting notes on a xylophone representing number of speech sounds; trains with/without engines for CV/V structures; trains with two engines for clusters)
- *Syllable level*—Describe syllables that represent the targeted contrast in nonsense and/or real words using the vocabulary established at the concept level
- *Word level*—Introduce minimal word pairs differing in the contrast being targeted. Child makes a judgment about the structure used to produce the word (e.g., two horses pulling a cart for clusters or one horse pulling a cart for singletons; head, body, tail for CVC and head, body for CV or final consonant deletion). Words containing different sounds demonstrating the target

contrasting features are incorporated in the activities.

The focus of Phase 2 of treatment is to convey the intended message. The three goals of Phase 2 are to transfer the metaphonological knowledge to communication situations, build up communication awareness, and develop phonological awareness so that the client alters or repairs output to convey meaning. The core clinical activity involves the client recognizing and producing distinctions between minimal pair words (two words differing in one of the sound properties targeted in Phase 1, e.g., /ti/-/ki/). The stimuli are 6 to 9 pictures of each word of a targeted minimal pair. The pictures are placed face down in a pile on the table except for one pair of words that are placed face up and are the "answer cards." The speaker picks up one picture and says what it is. The listener points to one of the answer cards and may also say the word. The pictures are then compared to see whether they match. Clinician feedback relates to the success of the communication rather than on the client's production of the word. Possible scenarios appear in Table 9.9. After the client distinguishes between minimal pairs at the word level, treatment proceeds to sentences. The sentences used are identical except for the minimal pair words (for example, "Draw a picture of a _____ on the chalkboard," "Put the picture of _____ in the box."). Table 9.10 illustrates the treatment steps in the Metaphon approach.

TABLE 9.9

Clinician's Feedback to Client's Responses During Phase 2 of Metaphon Treatment

Client's Role	Client's Response	Clinician's Feedback	Client's Reply
Listener	Points to correct referent	Reinforce knowledge (e.g., "That's right. How did you know to point to that one?")	Describe the sound (e.g., "Because you said the long sound.")
Speaker	Says the correct referent	Reinforce utterance (e.g., "Right, you said the long sound. I bet you know other long sounds.")	Identify other sounds in the same class (e.g., "Yes, /ʃ/ and /z/ are also long sounds.")
Listener	Points to incorrect referent	Provide feedback (e.g., "I think I said the long sound, not the short sound. Listen to the two words—see/tea. Which one is the long sound?")	Points to correct referent
Speaker	Says the incorrect referent	Provide feedback (e.g., "I heard the short sound. Should it have been the long sound?")	"Yes, it's _____."

Chapter 9 • Phonological Treatment Approaches 249

TABLE 9.10

Treatment Steps in Metaphon Approach

Phase	Step	Description	Example Target: Suppress stopping fricatives
Phase 1		Developing phonological awareness	
	Concept level	Use the vocabulary that will later be used to describe sound properties at the nonsound level	Activities using the terms *long* and *short:* Match up long and short pairs of socks Put long items in one pile and short items in another pile
	Sound level	Use the concept level vocabulary to describe nonspeech sounds	Activities with nonspeech sounds to demonstrate *long* and *short* sounds: Blowing a whistle Singing "la" Musical instruments Noise making toys
	Phoneme level	Describe speech sounds in which the listener, often using visual representations in conjunction with the descriptor words	Clinician and client take turns producing fricatives and stops. Represent fricatives with a long sock and stops with a short sock. Listener identifies the sound heard as being a *long* sound or *short* sound.
	Word level	Introduce minimal word pairs differing in the contrast being targeted using words containing different sounds demonstrating the target contrasting features. Client makes a judgment about the sound property used to produce the word.	Client is the listener. Client makes judgments as to whether the sound in theword said by the clinician is *long* or *short*: "Does this word have a long or short sound? See . . . tea . . . shoe . . . dog . . . pie . . . zoo" "Does this word go in the long pile of cards or the short pile? Sun . . . shirt . . . tie . . . fork . . . boat"
Phase 2		Developing phonological and communicative awareness	
	Word level	Recognizes and produces distinctions between minimal pair words	Core Activity: Place a pile of eight pictures of *sew* and eight pictures of *toe* face down on the table and one picture of each (answer cards) face up. Take turns as speaker and listener. Speaker picks up a picture from the pile and names it without the listener seeing it. Listener points to the correct answer card and may also say the word. Clinician provides feedback of client's responses. Use other minimal pairs.
	Sentence level	Recognizes and produces distinctions between minimal pair words in sentences	Take turns as speaker and listener. "Put the picture of _____ in the box." see/tea fan/pan feet/Pete vest/best shack/tack sack/tack Place the picture cards on the floor. "Stand on the _____."

Comments

The Metaphon approach is explicitly appropriate for linguistically-based phonologic disorders and not for phonetic disorders. It was developed for use with children, but with a change in vocabulary, could potentially be used with older clients. It seems to be inappropriate for children younger than 3.5 years of age. Using the approach in group treatment seems feasible, although it has been described in individual treatment settings. This approach should be reserved for multiple articulation errors because the focus is on speech sound patterns rather than individual speech sounds.

An advantage of this approach is that the recommended analysis, MRP, was developed to meet practicing clinicians' need for analysis instruments and procedures that are not time-consuming allowing appropriate treatment targets to be selected in a time-efficient manner. The Metaphon approach directly targets metaphonological skills so that clients develop an understanding of how sound production relates to communication and communication breakdown. Some research results have shown the approach to be effective (Dean et al., 1995; Howell & Dean, 1994). It seems logical that it is particularly effective with clients who have minimal restrictions on their speech motor skills; those who have phonetic constraints, that is some speech motor skill limitations, may require explicit phonetic (i.e., traditional) training in addition to or instead of a metalinguistic-based approach. Overgeneralization tends not to occur because virtually no attention is placed on the mechanics of speech sound production. A potential limitation is that some children may not be motivated to work on phonological awareness activities. Others may not have the cognitive abilities needed to develop phonological awareness or to translate metaphonological skills to speech sound production in a real communication situation. It may be confusing for some younger children to produce word pairs using different sounds.

The Metaphon approach does not seem to be used widely in the United States. Since it was developed in England, many practicing clinicians in the U.S. may be unaware of it. However, many speech-language pathologists do address various phonological awareness skills in their treatment of children with speech and language disorders.

> Describe the nonlinear treatment approach, including its theoretical basis, advantages, and limitations.

NONLINEAR APPROACH

The **nonlinear approach** was developed by Bernhardt and Stemberger (2000) as a clinical application of the nonlinear phonology acquisition theory. It is based on the concept of hierarchical arrangement of varying levels of speech sounds (Fig. 3.1). From a thorough phonological scan analysis, four types of treatment goals are selected based on two major dichotomies: "(a) syllable and word structure versus segments and features and (b) 'new stuff' versus 'old stuff' in new combinations or places" (Bernhardt & Stemberger, p. 51). The four types of goals include:

- *Goal Type 1*—New syllable and word structures
- *Goal Type 2*—New individual features and segments
- *Goal Type 3*—New simultaneous combinations of "old" features
- *Goal Type 4*—New places for old segments

A phonological cycling approach (Hodson & Paden, 1991) is recommended for addressing the treatment objectives. The difference between the phonological cycling and nonlinear approaches is the selection of targets. Individual targets are selected, one for each goal type.

Rationale

The nonlinear theory of phonological acquisition posits that there are separate levels or tiers of representation for the prosodic and segmental units (phonemes) that are organized hierarchically (Figs. 3.1 and 3.2). Each tier or level is autonomous. Thus, each level is analyzed and separate intervention targets are selected for the various levels. Three levels of syllable/word structure are considered: (a) word, (b) syllable, and (c) skeletal (CV) tiers. Even though the tiers are separate, there is interaction among them such that there may be restrictions or constraints on features in certain syllable positions. For example, certain phonemes may not be used in some syllable positions or only some syllable shapes are used for words. Therefore, these interactions are also analyzed and treatment targets are selected to address these restrictions.

During development of the phoneme level, certain sounds are underspecified or are the defaults. In other words, as children develop their speech, only certain speech sounds are used initially, and they are considered the defaults. For example, the front stops /t/ and /d/ appear early in development and are considered the defaults (underspecified phonemes). Later developing speech sounds are the nondefaults or are specified. In treatment, some targets are set to decrease the use of defaults; that is, to teach the client to produce the later-developing nondefault sounds. The same principle applies to syllable/word shapes. Some syllable/word shapes are defaults (e.g., CV), while other shapes are nondefaults or specified (e.g., CCVC) and goals are developed to increase the use of the nondefault syllable/word shapes. In summary, the rationale for the nonlinear approach is that an individual's phonological system has several levels and these levels interact. Certain phonemes and syllable/word shapes are defaults while others are nondefaults and thus are not used by some individuals. The various levels of the client's phonological system are analyzed and treatment goals are developed for the various levels.

Another concept involved in the approach is that there are two factors to consider when developing treatment goals: (a) syllable/word structure versus segments and phonetic features, and (b) *new* versus *old* features. When targeting a phoneme that is omitted from the client's inventory, it should first be targeted in a word shape that is already in the client's repertoire. When targeting a new syllable/word shape, the new word shape should be targeted in the context of phonemes already in the client's inventory. In other words, only one new element is added at a time.

Goals and Procedures

The goal of the nonlinear phonological approach is use all levels of the phonological system as adult speakers of the language. Specific treatment objectives are selected on the basis of a nonlinear scan analysis that includes a: a) segmental or phonemic analysis and (b) syllable and word structure analysis (Bernhardt & Stemberger, 2000). Such an analysis is key to developing treatment objectives. The scan analysis does not require counting of errors; rather it is a description of the client's phonological system as well as a comparison of it to adult speakers of the language.

The syllable and word structure analysis includes an inventory of word length in syllables, stress patterns of syllables, and CV word shapes. The analysis further includes a comparison of the client's productions with the adult targets for word length, stress patterns, and word shapes. A comparison is made between the client's productions of spontaneous versus imitated utterances and of single word versus phrases.

The phonemic analysis is done for both consonants and vowels. The consonant analysis includes a phonetic inventory by word position as well as a comparison to the adult targets. The analysis also includes a listing of the substitution and omission patterns for manner, voicing, and place features. Further, the segmental analysis explores word position and sequence constraints. It is to be noted when a sound is omitted from one or two word positions while occurring in other word positions and when certain sequences of sounds do not occur. The sequence analysis is done for consonant clusters as well as for consonants separated by a vowel. Generally, assimilations are an example of sequence constraints. Consonant assimilation, coalescence, CV assimilation, epenthesis, metathesis, and migration are included in the phonemic sequence analysis. Vowels are often not a problem because they typically are acquired early. When they are a problem, a vowel analysis is done. A vowel inventory is completed as well as a notation of matches with adult targets. An analysis of vowel features includes looking at the production of the features of tense-nontense, back-coronal/dorsal, high-low, and round.

The scan analysis leads to formulating four types of objectives that are addressed using a cycling approach (Bernhardt & Stemberger, 2000). Table 9.11 illustrates the goal types. Goal type 1 focuses on syllable/word structure that can involve word length in syllables (e.g., use two-syllable words), stress patterns (e.g., use weak–strong stress pattern as in *balloon*), and word shapes (e.g., use CVC). Goal type 2 addresses individual sound features (e.g., continuancy, lateral). Goal type 3 focuses on sound features that are not used in specific feature combinations (e.g., voiced obstruents, coronal continuants). Goal type 4 focuses on sounds in certain word positions and sequences (e.g., final voiceless obstruent, velar-labial sequence with an intervening vowel). Usually, the words selected for type 1 and 4 goals should contain sounds already in the client's inventory. Similarly, the words used for goal types 2 and 3 should be word shapes and stress patterns that the client already uses. Also, sequence constraints should be avoided when initially targeting new word shapes or sound features. Four objectives are selected, one for each goal type. These four targets are worked on in cycles as described by Hodson and Paden (1991). With each successive cycle, additional targets that represent the four goal types increase in complexity.

Comments

The nonlinear approach has been used primarily with children who have disordered phonological systems. Using the approach in group treatment seems feasible, although it has been described in

TABLE 9.11

Goals in a Nonlinear Phonological Intervention Plan

Phonological Level	Syllable and Word Structure	Segments and Features
Totally New Stuff	*Type 1*	*Type 2*
	(Phrases) Word lengths Stress patterns Word shapes	Individual features (and related segments)
Old Stuff in New Places or in New Combinations	*Type 4*	*Type 3*
	1. New word positions for old segments 2. New sequences of segments	New combinations of old features

From Bernhardt B., Stemberger J. P. (2000) Workbook in nonlinear phonology for clinical application. Austin, TX: Pro-Ed. Reprinted with permission.

individual treatment settings. It is generally recommended for phonological deviancies, but not for phonetic errors. This approach should be reserved for multiple articulation errors because the focus is on speech sound patterns rather than individual speech sounds.

An advantage of this approach is that goals are developed for individual clients after a thorough analysis of their sound systems, including the syllable, word, and phrase structure in addition to the individual phonemes. It focuses on both what the client can and cannot do. The approach addresses speech sound production in the context of syllable and word structure, stress patterns, phonemic sequences as well as individual speech sound features. Some research results have shown it to be an effective approach (Bernhardt, 1990, 1992). One limitation may be that the scan analysis is quite time-consuming which is potentially offset by the efficient intervention results. When learning to do the scan analysis, the process takes several hours; however, with experience, the analysis takes about 1 hour to complete (Bernhardt & Stemberger, 2000). There is also a computer program available to assist with the analysis, the CAPES (Masterson & Bernhardt, 2001). Overgeneralization tends not to occur.

Today, clinicians are beginning to perform phonological analyses to use as a basis for selecting treatment objectives, although the scan analysis is not widely used by practicing clinicians in the United States. Some clinicians do use a cycling approach with children, particularly young children, who have multiple articulation errors and select targets that are compatible with nonlinear goals, particularly the segmental objectives.

SUMMARY

Several linguistically based treatment approaches have been developed since the 1970s. The bases for the treatment strategies come from phonological acquisition data and from psycholinguistic theories. These approaches focus on teaching clients with disordered phonologies the phonological rules of their language. However, there is often a phonetic component to the articulatory/phonologic disorder that may need to be addressed with techniques from more traditional phonetic approaches. Many of the treatment strategies use contrasting sounds in various levels of production to teach the client the difference between speech sounds or speech sound/word patterns. These approaches include distinctive features, minimal meaningful contrasting pairs, maximal opposition, and Metaphon. With one exception, these approaches have clients produce contrasting pairs of words that differ only in the phonological feature being targeted. Others, namely the phonological cycling and nonlinear approaches, involve the clients practicing speech sound and word structure patterns that they are not using. The Metaphon treatment is unique in that it explicitly incorporates metaphonology awareness training in addition to production practice. The phonological cycling approach has evolved to incorporate phonological awareness activities into treatment in conjunction with the implementation of the cycling strategy described above (Hodson, 1997, 2004). Some treatment studies have been conducted on all of the approaches described in this chapter, and there are varying degrees of evidence to support the treatment effectiveness of all of them. No one approach has been shown to be superior to the others partially because there is great variability among clients in terms of their phonological systems, cognitive abilities, age levels, linguistic environment, and perceptual abilities, not to mention clinician variables. Practicing speech-language pathologists need to be familiar with various approaches to plan and implement intervention that is efficacious for various clients with articulatory/phonologic disorders.

REVIEW QUESTIONS

1. What is the general focus of phonological or linguistic treatment approaches for articulatory/phonologic disorders?

2. In one or two sentences, characterize each of the following treatment approaches:

   • Distinctive features

   • Phonological cycling

   • Minimal meaningful contrasting pairs

   • Maximal opposition

   • Metaphon

   • Nonlinear

3. Differentiate among the distinctive features, minimal meaningful contrasting pairs, maximal opposition, and Metaphon approaches.

4. Differentiate between the phonological cycling and nonlinear approaches. How do they differ from the approaches listed in question #3?

5. What are the theoretical bases (rationale) for each of the above phonological approaches?

6. What are the advantages and limitations for each of the above phonological approaches?

7. For what types of clients are these phonological approaches suitable?

CHAPTER 10

Implementation of Intervention and Transition to Dismissal

"Speak the speech, I pray you,
as I pronounced it to you."
—William Shakespeare

CHAPTER OBJECTIVES

- Describe structural modes used for artic-ulation/phonological treatment sessions.
- Describe various procedures for the elici-tation of speech sounds.
- Describe techniques for transfer of iso-lated sound production into syllables and words.
- Characterize stimulus generalization and response generalization.

- Describe types of transfer to correct tar-get production into phonemic contexts and situational contexts.
- Characterize what is meant by the terms *maintenance* and *carryover.*
- Discuss factors that potentially affect carryover.

Once the client is assessed and an intervention plan is formulated, articulation/phonological treat-ment is implemented. Many clinicians consider this the *fun* part of their jobs, although often chal-lenging. Unless the client is readily stimulable for the target, the first challenge for the clinician and client is elicitation and production, respectively, of the target sound or pattern. A myriad of techniques are used by clinicians to elicit the target, and many more will be invented in the future. After the client can produce the target successfully, the next step is to transfer that production into other contexts, such as into syllables and words, other sound positions, various phonetic contexts, and more complex lin-guistic units. Transfer can be problematic for some clients. Fortunately, available techniques are help-ful for this transition.

One of the greatest challenges facing clinicians of articulatory/phonologic disorders is the achievement of carryover in their clients. Many clinicians have had the discouraging experience of hearing clients articulate a sound correctly or use an appropriate phonological pattern in conversa-tional speech during several consecutive clinical sessions only to observe those same clients misar-ticulate their target sound pattern outside the clinic room. This frustrating experience not only illus-trates the difficulty in determining progress to-ward carryover, but it also suggests the great chal-lenge involved in deciding when carryover has occurred and when the client is ready to be dis-missed. Unfortunately, much of what clinicians do for carryover is a potpourri of tasks, some of which may be helpful and some of which may not contribute to improved skills. This chapter de-scribes various ways to structure treatment ses-sions, general techniques used to elicit target sounds and patterns, procedures for transferring correct sound production into other contexts, carryover procedures and activities, and ways to measure progress toward generalization and maintenance.

> Describe four structural modes of articulation/phonological treatment sessions.

STRUCTURE OF TREATMENT SESSIONS

The style of articulation/phonological treatment sessions varies on a continuum from highly structured to loosely structured; that is, from a drill approach to a play approach. The structure used by clinicians depends on the client's personality, cognitive level, and linguistic abilities; the particular target; and the stage of treatment, such as elicitation or stabilization practice, and production in isolation and in syllables, words, sentences, or spontaneous speech; as well as the clinician's preference or clinical style. Four structural modes of intervention, as originally described by Shriberg & Kwiatkowski (1982b) are:

• Drill
• Drill play
• Structured play
• Play

In the *drill* mode, treatment is a structured stimulus-response paradigm in which the clinician presents a stimulus or antecedent instructional event that is followed by client responses. Positive reinforcement is given for correct responses, and corrective feedback is given for incorrect responses. Corrective feedback can be in the form of repeat-simplify-modify (Shriberg & Kwiatkowski, 1982b), which represents a sequence of instructional events that many speech-language pathologists seem to do intuitively. When a response is incorrect, the clinician gives the client a second trial by repeating the stimulus. If the response is still incorrect, the clinician simplifies the stimulus and may, for example, go to a lower linguistic level. The final corrective step is to modify the stimulus form by, for example, exaggerating the target in duration or intensity. In the drill mode, the client has no control over the stimulus or presentation rate. When carried out to its fullest, the stimuli are presented in rapid succession. The idea is that drill maximizes efficiency; that is, it results in more responses from the client.

Drill play has the same components as drill, except that a motivational event is incorporated before, during, or after the stimulus is presented. In

this approach, the clinician formally presents the stimuli as in the drill mode, but a "fun" element is added to the activity. Examples of activities used in conjunction with the presentation of stimulus items are card games (such as Go Fish or Concentration), board games, spinning a spinner, and active games (such as throwing a bean bag on stimulus cards or bowling). The rationale for drill play is that it is more fun and thus more motivating for the child even though it is seemingly less efficient than drill.

In *structured play*, the structure of the session is similar to drill play, but the stimuli are presented as part of play activities. Unlike drill and drill play, the clinician has the option of not providing instructional feedback about incorrect responses. Depending on the client, the clinician may choose to continue the play activity without comment about incorrect responses.

In the *play* mode, stimuli and client responses occur as natural components of play activities. The clinician arranges activities so that the target response occurs naturally. The clinician uses techniques such as self-talk and modeling in a natural way in the context of play. Table 10.1 illustrates these four modes of treatment.

Which treatment style is the best practice? Drill and drill play treatment modes were shown to be more effective and more efficient for articulation/phonological intervention than structured play and play modes in three studies conducted by Shriberg & Kwiatkowski (1982b). Drill play was found to be as efficient and as effective as drill. Overall, clinicians in the Shriberg and Kwiatkowski study perceived drill play as the most effective, most efficient, and most preferred of the four modes, ranking the drill mode second. Finally, not surprisingly, the clinicians perceived that children prefer the play, structured play, and drill play modes over the drill mode.

Clinicians have the choice of four modes of articulation/phonological intervention and should use the one they deem most appropriate for individual clients and for the stage of treatment. Often, a drill approach seems suitable for adult clients in the initial stages of treatment while drill play is often preferable for young children. More structured approaches are probably needed during the earlier stages of intervention so that clients develop a clear idea about what the target is and whether they are meeting the target. However, as intervention progresses to conversational speech, it necessarily needs to be more loosely structured to approximate natural communication situations and interactions. In summary, no one mode is effective for all clients and the mode should vary throughout the course of treatment.

TABLE 10.1

Examples of Activities for Each of Four Structural Modes of Articulation/Phonological Treatment

Mode	Stimulus Materials	Antecedent Motivational Event	Antecedent Stimulus	Subsequent Instructional Event	Subsequent Motivational Event
Drill	Picture cards containing the target	None	Clinician holds up each card and says, "What is this?"	Verbal positive reinforcement or corrective feedback	Token for correct responses; tokens traded in for stickers
Drill Play	Picture cards containing the target	Clinician introduces "fishing" game. Client is to fish for the cards using a pole with a magnet. Client names the "fish" caught.	Clinician says, "What did you catch?"	Verbal positive reinforcement or corrective feedback	Client keeps the "fish" produced correctly. Clinician gets the "fish" produced incorrectly
Structured Play	Picture cards containing the target	Clinician introduces "fishing" game and stresses that it's fun; target is secondary	Clinician says, "What did you catch?"	Verbal positive reinforcement. Corrective feedback only if child is receptive	Client keeps all fish
Play	Picture cards containing the target	Clinician introduces "fishing" game and stresses that it's fun; no mention of target	Clinician plays with the child using self talk, modeling, etc. "Look, I caught a _____." "Oh, you caught a _____."	No explicit reinforcement or corrective feedback. Provide model of target only as incorporated in play.	Child keeps the "fish" and talks about what to do with them.

> What are some techniques clinicians use to elicit speech sound targets?

ELICITATION OF SPEECH SOUNDS

No matter which treatment approach is used, often the first task in articulation/phonological treatment is elicitation of the target sound or, in the case of a phonological approach, a sound that contains the target distinctive feature or phonological pattern. When clients do not have the target sound or pattern in their repertoire, it needs to be established; that is, the client first needs to learn to produce the sound and then to produce it voluntarily. The sound is initially elicited in isolation, syllables, or words depending upon the target, the treatment approach, and the client's articulation/phonological skills. It is almost impossible to produce the stops and glides in isolation as they are almost always produced in combination with a vowel (usually /ə/). Fricatives and affricates can be produced in isolation. It has been our experience that it is more effective for transfer purposes to teach the liquids (/l, r/) in the context of vowels, rather than in isolation.

Earlier chapters stressed the importance of eliciting sounds in the simplest way for the client with a minimum of verbal instruction. Over the years, speech-language pathologists and their clients have been quite inventive in devising speech sound elicitation techniques. It is not feasible to present here the innumerable specific elicitation techniques for all speech sounds, but as a starting point, some general methods for eliciting speech sounds are described next. Examples of specific techniques that have been effective for many clients are interspersed (Table 10.2). Keep in mind that many resources are available commercially, including clinical materials and textbooks. Another excellent resource is suggestions from colleagues.

Provide an Auditory-Visual Model

Most of the time, the first sound elicitation method tried by clinicians is to have the client imitate the clinician's auditory-visual model. In this approach, the client focuses visually on the clinician's mouth and auditorily on the isolated sound as the clinician produces it. For example, the clinician might say, "Listen and watch me say the /ʃ/ sound and repeat after me" or "Watch my mouth and say /ʃ/." To further focus attention to the visual part of the model, clinicians draw attention to the mouth area by touching their own face while simultaneously providing the auditory model. To highlight the auditory portion of the modeled sound, clinicians use vocal emphasis, including increased vocal intensity and/or prolonged production, or sound amplification, including the use of an auditory trainer. Modeling is often used in conjunction with other techniques described here. As treatment progresses, modeling is gradually faded; for example, discontinuing vocal emphasis and the auditory portion of the model by mouthing the sound.

Use a Mirror

A mirror can be used to facilitate production of the target sound. In this procedure, the clinician and client are both looking in a mirror. The clinician produces the sound while the client watches in the mirror; then, while watching in the mirror, the client imitates the clinician's production. A variation is for the two to produce the sound in unison while watching themselves in the mirror. They then can compare their articulation postures and movements of the visible articulators, which the client can adjust as needed. This technique can be particularly effective with phonemes whose productions are externally visible, as is the case for the bilabials, labiodentals, dentals, alveolars, and some palatals, including /ʃ/, /tʃ/, /dʒ/.

Use Tactile-Kinesthetic Cues

The clinician's provision of tactile-kinesthetic stimulations is effective in many instances. At least four systems have been developed to use for facilitating speech sounds production:

- Motokinesthetic (Young & Stinchfield-Hawk, 1955)
- Speech facilitation cues (Vaughn & Clark, 1979)
- Touch-cue (Bashir, Grahamjones, & Bostwick, 1984)
- PROMPT (Chumpelik, 1984; Hayden & Square, 1994)

In these systems, the clinician provides tactile-kinesthetic cues to assist the client in speech production. There is a specified tactile-kinesthetic stimulation for each speech sound. In the motokinesthetic approach, these stimulations primarily involve the clinician manipulating the client's articulators on the outside of the face and neck, although sometimes intra-oral devices, such as tongue depressors, are used. Appendix I describes the motokinesthetic standard stimulations for all consonants, vowels, and diphthongs. In the speech facilitation cues approach, intra-oral devices are used extensively such that speech facilitation cues involve both external stimulations and

TABLE 10.2

General Methods and Examples for Eliciting Target Speech Sounds

Speech Sound Elicitation Strategy	Descriptions	Examples
Auditory-visual model	Client instructed to watch clinician's mouth and listen to clinician's model	"Listen and watch my mouth. /tʃ/, /tʃ/, /tʃ/. Say /tʃ/"
Mirror	Client watches clinician produce the target while both look in a mirror. Client imitates clinician's production	"Look in the mirror and watch my mouth—/f/. Now watch yourself in the mirror as you say /f/" Does your mouth look like mine?"
Tactile-kinesthetic cues	Motokinesthetic stimulations Speech facilitation cues Touch-cue PROMPT Touching the two articulator locations Clinician-created cues	1. For /k/, place thumb on one side of the throat under the back of the tongue externally and index finger on opposite side. Press upward, then release quickly. 2. For /s/, using a cotton swab, touch the tongue tip and alveolar ridge. "Touch these two parts together and blow like this—/s/."
Modification of nontarget sounds	Move from a sound (speech or nonspeech) to the target sound	"Say /θ/ and slowly move your tongue back to behind your teeth like this /θ—s/."
Visual illustration of articulator placement	Show the client where the articulators should be placed using pictures or puppets.	1. For /l/, "Look at this picture. Touch the tip of your tongue tip right behind the teeth as shown in the picture and say /l/." 2. For /k/, "Look at this puppet with a tongue. He's making the /k/ sound. Raise the back of your tongue like the puppet and say /k/."
Visual cues	Show oral or nasal airflow with external objects	1. For /m/, "Make this mirror fog up when you say /m/." 2. For /r/, using spectrographic display, "Practice making your /r/ sound until it looks like mine does on this picture (display). See, these two lines (first and second formant) should be close together."
Auditory cues	Amplify the production of the target sound	1. Using an auditory trainer, "Put on these earphones, speak into the mic, and say /s/. How did that sound?" 2. Holding a drinking straw in front of the client's medial incisors, "Say /s/; make the sound come through the straw."
Facilitating phonetic contexts	Identify a phonetic facilitating context, one in which the client produces the sound correctly. Use this as a starting point	"Say /pɑts/" (for the /s/ sound if the context of /t/ is a facilitating context).
Verbal instructions	Provide verbal instructions for where the articulators should be placed for producing the target sound	"Raise the tip of your tongue up to the roof of your mouth; then curl it back; say /ɝ/."
Successive approximation (shaping)	Elicit an attempt of the target sound by modeling and then modify the production to make it closer to correct target production	"Say /s/. Not quite. Move your tongue tip back farther and say /s/. That's better" (assuming that it is).

extensive intra-oral cues. Touch-cue prompts provide tactile cues for the production of eight consonants. The PROMPT stimulations for all speech sounds are applied externally on the mandible, lips, and face, as well as through the mylohyoid muscle for the tongue.

Additionally, clinicians and clients are often inventive and develop their own tactile-kinesthetic cues applied externally or intra-orally. For example, clinicians sometimes manipulate the client's tongue with a tongue depressor. An example would be to use a tongue depressor to push the tongue tip back, which results in the tongue bunching up in the back for production of a "centrally bunched" /r/, or to use a tongue depressor to raise the tongue tip for producing a retroflex /r/. Another effective technique is for the clinician to use a tongue depressor, cotton swab stick, or gloved finger to touch the points of two articulators that should contact each other when the sound is produced and instruct the client to put those two parts together. Examples include touching the tongue tip then the alveolar ridge with a tongue depressor or other device as cues for the production of alveolar sounds and touching the lower lip and upper medial incisors for production of /f/ and /v/.

Modification of Nontarget Sounds

In many instances, target sounds can be elicited by instructing clients to move their articulators from a sound that is in the client's repertoire to the target sound. The starting point can be a speech sound. For example, for /s/, instruct the client to produce /θ/ continuously (to continue the airflow through the oral cavity) and move the tongue tip back to inside the mouth or have the client produce /ʃ/ and retract the lips to a position for /i/ while continuing the oral airflow. /ʃ/ can be elicited by producing /t/ and /j/ in rapid succession, /tʃ/ by producing /t/ and /ʃ/ or /t/ and /j/ in rapid succession, and similarly /dʒ/ by producing /d/ and /ʒ/ or /d/ and /j/ in rapid succession. An effective technique for eliciting /ɝ, ɚ/ is to have the client produce /l/ and move the tongue tip back touching the roof of the mouth until the client must drop the tongue tip, which often results in production of a retroflex /r/ or /ɝ, ɚ/. /l/ can be elicited by having the client say /ə/ with the tongue tip held against the alveolar ridge; then instruct the client to drop the tongue tip resulting in the production of /lə/.

Nonspeech sounds can also serve as a beginning point. Sometimes, /k/ can be elicited by having clients cough or clear their throats and move to /k/. This strategy obviously is to demonstrate the velar position needed for /k/. Another example, is to have the client phonate while moving the tongue

around in the mouth until /ɝ, ɚ/ is produced. In this technique, the clinician can touch the client's hand when /ɝ, ɚ/ is produced, instructing the client to prolong that sound being produced when the hand was touched.

Visual Illustration of Placement of Articulators

It is sometimes helpful to use visual illustrations of where the articulators are to be placed. One way to do this is to show pictures, such as *Form-a-Sound* (Great Ideas for Teaching), of the appropriate placement of the articulators. Another technique is for clinicians to use their hands to demonstrate placement. For example, the hand can be used to show tongue placement and movement for retroflex /r/ production by indicating that the finger tips are the front of the tongue and the palm of the hand is the back of the tongue and illustrate the retroflex movement such that the tongue tip (finger tips) moves up and curls back. A puppet of the mouth, such as *Mouthy Mouth Finger Puppet* (Super Duper Publications), including the jaws, teeth, alveolar ridge, and tongue is a useful device to illustrate production of the velars, alveolars, dentals, and /r/.

Recently, a more sophisticated visual approach has been developed that includes the palatometric instrumentation described in Chapter 8. In this technique, a palatometer provides a graphic representation of how the client produced the target sound, showing the place and pattern of contact of the tongue against the palate, alveolar ridge, and inner margins of the teeth (Fletcher, 1992). The client's placement can be compared to the clinician's palatogram (Figures 8.1 and 8.2).

Provision of Visual Cues

Visual cues can be used to illustrate target sound characteristics such as nasal and oral airflow. Examples include using a cotton ball or feather to show oral airflow for the oral consonants. When placed near the mouth opening, quick movements of these objects demonstrate short oral air bursts of the plosives and affricates, and continuous movements demonstrate continuous oral airflow for the fricatives. A small mirror placed horizontally under the nasal passageways can show nasal air emission (steam on the mirror) or lack of nasal air emission (clear mirror). The See-Scape (Pro-Ed) product can show nasal emission or no nasal emission. Spectrographic displays of speech sound production can sometimes facilitate elicitation of target speech sounds, using instrumentation such as the Visi-Pitch or spectrographic computer software.

Provision of Auditory Cues

Auditory cues can facilitate elicitation of target sounds. One such technique is to amplify the clinician's model and/or the client's production through an auditory trainer. Simpler devices also can be used to amplify the client's productions, such as an auditory feedback loop constructed from PVC pipe or the Toobaloo (Learning Loft, LLC) in which sounds are directed through a tube from the clients' mouth to one of their ears. Another simple device that provides auditory information to the client for correction of a lateral /s/ is a drinking straw. A straw is used to demonstrate where in the dental arch the oral air stream is being directed; for example, one side or both sides of the mouth or between the medial or lateral incisors, bicuspids, cuspids, or molars, followed by the clinician instructing the client to direct the airflow through the straw when it is held directly in front of the medial incisors.

Facilitating Phonetic Contexts

Sometimes, it is easier to elicit sounds in syllables or words that contain facilitative contexts. For instance, because /s/ and /t/ have the same place of production, /s/ can often be elicited in the context of initial /st/ or final /ts/ clusters, especially if the client uses the phonological deficiency of stopping. Velar sounds can facilitate a back tongue position needed for the production of /r/ such that /r/ can sometimes be elicited in words that contain back vowels, /g/ or /k/, or /gr/ or /kr/ blends. Syllables or words containing back vowels tend to facilitate production of the velars /k/ and /g/.

Results of a test for facilitative contexts (such as the *Contextual Test of Articulation*, Aase et al., 2000; *Articulation Consistency Probe*, Tattersall & Dawson, 1997; and *Deep Test of Articulation*, McDonald, 1964a) can help find facilitative contexts. Clinicians can also develop their own criterion-referenced tests for identifying facilitative contexts for individual clients. These facilitative phonetic contexts can then be used as a beginning point for expanding the correct production of the target to other phonetic contexts.

Verbal Instructions

Providing verbal directions for placement of the articulators can be effective when the instructions are not too complex. When a certain instruction has been successful in eliciting the target, the same terminology on subsequent trials should be used each time a description is given so that the client is not confused. The use of clear, simple instructions

is usually best, and unclear, lengthy, and confusing instructions for the client should be avoided.

Successive Approximation (Shaping)

In the successive approximation or shaping strategy, the clinician begins by eliciting a response that the client already has and gradually changes it in small, logically sequenced steps until the target sound is produced. The client is reinforced for each successive step such that earlier steps in the progression are no longer reinforced once the client's productions are closer to the target. Thus, there is a gradual shift from a sound the client can produce to the standard sound. Often, the clinician uses verbal instructions, models, and manipulations of the articulators to change the incorrect sound to the correct sound gradually. An example of the shaping approach is provided in Table 10.3.

> What are some techniques clinicians use to facilitate transfer of the target from production in isolation to production in syllables and words?

TARGET PRODUCTION IN SYLLABLES AND WORDS

After clients consistently produce the target sound in isolation, treatment proceeds to the nonsense syllable or meaningful word level, depending on the treatment approach being used. In some approaches, production does not begin in isolation, but rather production practice begins at the nonsense syllable level (such as in the sensory motor or motokinesthetic approaches) and at the meaningful word level in others (such as in the phonological cycling, contrasting pairs, or nonlinear approaches). Nonetheless, production of target sounds/patterns in combination with a vowel or vowel/consonant or consonant/vowel is sometimes a difficult stage of treatment even though the client can easily produce the target sound in isolation.

Traditionally, clinicians begin the production phase of intervention in the initial or prevocalic position of syllables and words probably because this is what often occurs developmentally. However, the clinician should probe each client's ability to produce the target behavior in all three positions to determine the easier one for the client. Production in syllables and/or words should begin with the position that is easiest for the client, whether it is prevocalic, postvocalic, or intervocalic. For exam-

TABLE 10.3

Steps in Shaping Production of /r/

Step	Instructions
1	Stick your tongue out (model provided).
2	Stick your tongue out and touch the tip of your finger (model provided).
3	Put your finger on the bumpy place right behind your top teeth (model provided).
4	Now put the tip of your tongue lightly on that bumpy place (model provided).
5	Now put your tongue tip there again and say /l/ (model provided).
6	Say /l/ each time I hold up my finger (clinician holds up finger).
7	Now say /l/ for as long as I hold my finger up, like this: (model provided for 5 seconds). Ready, go.
8	Say a long /l/, but this time as you're saying it, drag the tip of your tongue slowly back along the roof of your mouth—so far back that you have to drop it. (Accompany instructions with hand gesture of moving fingertips back slowly, palm up.)

From Shriberg, L. D. (1975). A response evocation program for /ɚ/. *Journal of Speech and Hearing Disorders, 40,* 92–105. Adapted with permission.

ple, fricatives are often most easily elicited in the final position when the misarticulation/phonological deviation is stopping. Clinicians have noted that it is easier for many clients to produce /s/ in clusters rather than as a singleton consonant. After production is mastered in one position, production of the other positions should be probed or tested to determine whether, and how much, practice may need to be done with the untrained positions. Some treatment approaches target sounds only in the initial and final positions, skipping the medial position. If the target sound has generalized to the other positions, the clinician can save treatment time by skipping extensive production practice and move on to the next step of treatment. Conversely, if transfer has not occurred, the sound will need to be taught and practiced in these novel contexts.

The clinician needs to be inventive to assist the client in putting the target sound into the context of a syllable or word. One technique is to have the client produce the target sound separately from the rest of the syllable, such as /s/ /pause/ /i/. At first, the clinician models the syllable/word with the pause then gradually shortens the length of the pause until there is no pause. Simultaneous hand movements can be used to provide additional input for the client, such as moving the left hand as a signal for producing the target sound and moving the right hand as a signal for the rest of the syllable/word. The two hands can be farther apart concomitant with a longer pause and gradually moved closer together showing shorter pauses. Eventually, the clinician's verbal model is discontinued

and the client produces the syllables/words in response to the hand signals. Another technique useful for continuants is to instruct the client to prolong the target sound until a signal is given to produce the rest of the syllable/word. For example, the client and/or clinician prolong the target sound /s/ as they trace along a picture of a snake until the tail is reached or the clinician can slide a finger along the client's arm up to the shoulder whereupon, the rest of the syllable is produced. Another example is for the client to prolong the sound until the clinician gives a signal, such as patting the table, to say the vowel. Sometimes, instructing the client to shadow the clinician's syllable or word production is effective. In this technique, the client does not know ahead of time what the clinician is going to say, but says what the clinician says almost simultaneously.

> Identify and define two primary types of generalization.

TRANSFER OR GENERALIZATION

Transfer and generalization are often used interchangeably with both terms referring to the use of a target behavior in untrained conditions. Unlike the earlier stages of intervention (elicitation or production) in which the target behavior is taught, transfer of the target sound is facilitated by the clinician so that it is used in novel or untrained contexts and situations (Bernthal & Bankson, 2004). Because the client has already learned the motor and/or phonological patterns, the clinician must then set up tasks and situations that facilitate the use of those newly learned patterns in untrained contexts. Correct production of the target sound must transfer to several different contexts, including word position, phonetic context, linguistic unit, situations and settings, and possibly different sounds with similar features (Bernthal & Bankson, 2004; Dunn, 1983; Mowrer, 1989; Secord, 1989). There are two primary types of generalization: stimulus generalization and response generalization. Stimulus generalization occurs when target behaviors that were taught in response to certain stimuli are used in response to different stimuli, such as in new activities, with different people, in new settings, and with different pictures. Response generalization refers to the use of untrained responses based on prior learning of trained responses. The new untrained behavior is similar to, but different from, the trained behavior. For example, in articulation/phonological treatment, if the target speech sound or pattern is produced without training in different word positions, phonetic contexts, linguistic levels, and/or phonemes, response generalization is said to have occurred. It is important to be aware of the various types of generalization and to program intervention so that the target behavior transfers to all of these situations. It is impossible to provide training for correct production of a sound/pattern in every word in which it occurs as well as in every situation in which those words would be used. Basically, generalization needs to occur in various phonemic contexts and situational contexts.

> To what phonemic contexts does target production transfer?

Phonemic Contexts

Transfer of the target behavior to untrained phonemic contexts occurs from one word position to another, from one linguistic level to another, from one phonetic context to another, and from one phoneme to another. Sometimes, such transfer seemingly occurs automatically, but sometimes it must be programmed in the treatment process, depending upon the client and the intervention approach used.

It is important that the client use the target sound in varying word positions. Traditionally, this has meant the initial, medial, and final positions, but some approaches train in the context of the releasing and arresting positions. Some research has shown that transfer occurs from one word position to another, no matter which position was first trained (Elbert & McReynolds, 1975, 1978; Powell & McReynolds, 1969; Weston & Irwin, 1971). Other studies have demonstrated only minimal generalization from one position to another, at least for some subjects (Compton, 1975; McLean, 1970), in which case all positions need to be specifically trained. It should be noted that the McLean study was conducted on children with mental retardation, while the child used in Compton's (1975) study had normal intelligence. Also, there is evidence that children who practice target sounds in all three word positions show more generalization across clinical sessions and in probe (untrained) words (Ruscello, 1975; Weaver-Spurlock & Brasseur, 1988). Finally, it seems likely that the specific target sound affects generalization to other sound positions as shown by Olswang and Bain (1985b) who found that position generalization occurs for /s/, but not for /l/. In any case, the clinician should probe the client's productions throughout the treatment process in all sound positions to determine the positions that need to be trained and how intensely.

A second phonemic context to which the target behavior must transfer is phonetic context, such as production of the target phoneme when preceding or following various vowels and consonants as well as in consonant clusters for some sounds. Children sometimes misarticulate sounds only in certain contexts, which is probably the case for the phonological deviations of assimilation, coalescence, cluster reduction, and some idiosyncratic patterns. For example, a client may misarticulate /k/ and /g/ only in words that also contain alveolars or omit /s/ only in /s/ clusters. The *Deep Test of Articulation* (McDonald, 1964a), the *Contextual Test of Articulation* (Aase et al., 2000), and *Secord Contextual Articulation Test* (Secord & Shine, 1997) were developed to identify contexts in which phonemes may be produced correctly. Those contexts can be used to facilitate correct production in other phonetic environments. Studies have shown that transfer does occur across phonetic contexts, although with varying degrees of success among clients (Elbert & McReynolds, 1978; Elbert, Powell, & Swartzlander, 1991; Weiner, 1981; Zehel, Shelton, Arndt, Wright, & Elbert, 1972). Most clients seem to need only a few exemplars for generalization to occur in other phonetic contexts, but this varies from one client to the next. The clinician needs to probe to determine the contexts that facilitate correct production for each client because it varies somewhat among clients. For example, it is often essential to teach /r/ by controlling and systematically varying the phonetic context, after determining the context that is easiest for the client to produce. Some clients have an easier time with consonantal /r/, while others more easily produce vocalic /ɝ, ɚ/ and still others do better with /r/ clusters. Abilities also vary with the particular vowel that precedes or follows /ɝ, ɚ/ and /r/. The clinician always needs to be cognizant of particular contexts that are facilitative and that are inhibitory for individual clients. Intuitively, one should start with facilitative or easy contexts and gradually progress to those that are more difficult. Sometimes, clinicians need to provide drill or extra practice on specific phonetic contexts that are particularly difficult for an individual client.

A third level of phonemic context transfer is transfer to other linguistic unit levels; that is, isolation, nonsense syllables, words, phrases, sentences, reading, and spontaneous speech. Studies have shown that varying amounts of transfer between linguistic unit levels does occur throughout the course of intervention, such as from nonsense syllables to words (McReynolds & Bennett, 1972; Powell & McReynolds, 1969) and from words to running speech (Elbert, Dinnsen, Swartzlander, & Chin, 1990; Olswang & Bain as cited in Dunn, 1983). Conversely, transfer from isolation to words was not shown in McReynolds and Bennett's study. Transfer from one linguistic level to another seems to occur automatically in some clients, but not for others. The clinician needs to probe or test the client's abilities in more complex linguistic unit levels to determine the need for specific practice of the target in the next treatment level. It may be useful to teach target sounds in nonsense syllables and nonsense words as advocated by Gerber (1973), Van Riper and Erickson (1996), and Winitz (1969, 1975) to eliminate the interference of meaningful words in which the client has been practicing the sound incorrectly. Certainly, such training facilitates the motor patterns needed for correct production, but probably does not contribute to learning the phonological rules of the language. Practice in nonsense contexts is recommended when the client needs to learn the motor or phonetic patterns and shows difficulty producing the targets in meaningful words, but not when the client needs only to learn the phonological rules. The process of transfer across linguistic levels seems to be highly variable from one individual to the next.

Finally, phonemic context transfer occurs in other sounds that have features similar to the target. Clinicians frequently observe that transfer of correct production occurs on the untrained cognate of the target sound, such as the transfer of /s/ to /z/ and /k/ to /g/. Research has verified that this type of transfer does occur, and as a matter of fact, the wedge,

distinctive feature, and phonological treatment approaches are based on this type of generalization. One study (Elbert, Shelton, & Arndt, 1967) showed that children who learned to produce /s/ generalized correct production to the untrained /z/ phoneme, but not to the untrained /r/ which makes sense because /z/ is quite similar to /s/ while /r/ is not. In addition to cognates, research has shown transfer to sounds of the same distinctive feature class such as place and manner features (Dunn & Till, 1982; McReynolds & Bennet, 1972; Mowrer & Case, 1982; Weiner, 1981). For example, a study showed feature generalization of + stridency, + voicing, and + continuancy in individuals, although the transfer was not 100% complete (McReynolds & Bennet, 1972).

As mentioned, some treatment approaches are based on the premise of transfer of correct production to sounds with similar features, particularly the distinctive feature, phonological processes, and wedge approaches. These approaches are designed to take advantage of this type of phonemic context generalization to provide more efficient intervention with quicker results. Some programs use only one phonemic contrasting pair based on the assumption that the correct pattern will generalize to other contrasting pairs. For example, /s/ and /t/ can be used to teach frication and ideally, the /s/ productions will transfer to correct productions of /z, ʃ, ʒ/ and possibly /tʃ, dʒ/ (Ozanich, 1997). Other researchers have recommended using two or more phonemes or contrasts to teach the rules for using certain phonemic features or for decreasing certain inappropriate phonological processes. In their program, Costello and Onstine (1976) used two fricative sounds and a nonfricative sound to teach the manner feature of frication. Others have used multiple sounds, rather than one pair of contrasting sounds, to teach clients to reduce the occurrence of final consonant deletion, stopping of fricatives, and velar fronting (Weiner, 1979, 1981; Fokes, 1982). Similarly, Winitz and Bellerose (1978) suggested that the clinician should teach several sounds at once, sounds that are produced with a similar error pattern. For example, you may want to include /s, z, ʃ, ʒ/ in your intervention program when the client uses stops for sibilants or /k, g, ŋ/ when the client substitutes alveolars for velars. Another strategy is to target dissimilar speech sounds to facilitate use of several phonetic features not in the client's repertoire. For example, /s/, /k/, and /tʃ/ might be selected because they have the fricative, velar, and affricate features, respectively, and perhaps /z, ʃ/, /k, ŋ/, and /dʒ/ will not need to be targeted. Whatever approach you as a clinician use, you should probe to determine whether transfer to other similar sounds is occurring before initiating treatment procedures for those sounds because transfer may very well occur on sounds with similar features. This is the case for motor *and* phonological treatment approaches.

To what situational contexts does target production transfer?

Situational Contexts

The second primary type of transfer has been referred to as situational or response generalization, which refers to transfer of the target behavior to novel situations, such as different materials, clinical activities, settings, and people. Obviously, transfer of the target behavior from the clinical setting to outside settings and from talking with the clinician to talking with others is critical to the carryover process and is really the goal of articulation and phonological treatment. Unfortunately, this is where the intervention often breaks down.

One type of situation that varies and needs to be considered is the materials and activities actually used in the clinical setting. Little research has been conducted to determine how much stimulus variability in the production training is needed to ensure that the target behavior will transfer to other situations, such as different activities, settings, and persons. The clinician must probe for the production of the target sound in untrained words, materials, and activities to determine how much more practice the client will likely need to master the target behavior and eventually to use it in other situations. Some intervention programs use a limited number of words and activities during the establishment phases, but it is not known whether this limitation inhibits generalization of the desired results. Costello and Bosler (1976) found that more generalization to novel environments occurred on trained words as compared with generalization of untrained words. Results such as these suggest that the more variety used in the choice of words in the clinical setting, the greater the transfer to other settings. Dunn (1983) suggested "children with cognitive and linguistic deficits may need more diversity of materials and activities . . . the diversity should be introduced systematically as the children are capable of responding to new stimuli" (p. 48). The stimulus pictures, words, and activities used in clinic should be varied as much as possible to increase the probability of situational generalization. Additionally, words used in the clinical setting should be ones that the client will likely use in spontaneous speech, words that are within the client's vocabulary, and

words that represent various grammatical structures, such as nouns, verbs, adjectives, adverbs, and articles (Dunn, 1983; Hodson & Paden, 1991; McCabe & Bradley, 1975; McDonald, 1964b).

Some transfer does occur from the clinical setting to nonclinical settings; that is, the client sometimes uses the target behavior in places other than the clinic room and with other persons (Bankson & Byrne, 1972; Costello & Bosler, 1976; Koegel, Koegel, & Ingham, 1986; Olswang & Bain, 1985b). One study found that words learned in a home training program transferred to different environments, although more transfer occurred on trained words than on untrained words (Costello & Bosler, 1976). The probes for transfer were at the word linguistic level rather than in conversational speech. The researchers had predicted that a situational hierarchy of transfer might emerge such that one situation would be more conducive to generalization than another situation, but this did not occur. In other words, no "generalization gradient" among the four novel situations appeared from the data, a result that gives further evidence of the great amount of variability among clients.

Several approaches have been studied to determine whether transfer to untrained situations occurs. For example, Bankson and Byrne (1972) found that the target sound transferred to conversational speech in the clinic and at home, with varying degrees of success, after training, which required the clients to produce a word list rapidly. Another approach has been to teach self-monitoring skills. Teaching clients to monitor their own productions has been found to facilitate generalization to conversational speech in nonclinical school settings with persons other than the clinician (Engel, Erickson, & Groth, 1970; Koegel et al., 1986; Koegel, Koegel, Van Voy, & Ingham, 1988; Shriberg & Kwiatkowski, 1987). It should be noted that, in the Koegel et al. (1988) study, the self-monitoring strategy resulted in situational generalization only when clients were required to self-monitor outside the clinical setting; generalization did not occur when self-monitoring was done only in the clinic. Conversely, self-monitoring was not found to be effective in a study conducted by Gray and Shelton (1992) who replicated the Koegel et al. (1988) study. Thus, it remains to be seen whether or not a self-monitoring approach works. Still others have taken the approach of incorporating other persons in the carryover process. The use of persons other than the clinician has been shown to facilitate generalization. Some researchers have incorporated peers to assist or monitor the client's speech (Kalash, 1970; Engel et al., 1970) while several others have shown positive results by incorporating parents (Carrier, 1970; Mowrer,

TABLE 10.4

TABLE 10.4

Rank Order of the Effectiveness of Carryover Procedures as Perceived by Public School Clinicians

Ranking of Effectiveness	Carryover Procedure
1	Client self-evaluation
2	Client practices until responses are automatic
3	Follow a structured behavior modification program
4	Client works with individuals other than the clinician
5	Client works with the clinician outside the clinic room
6	Use auditory discrimination training
7	Client completion of homework assignments
8	Distribute reminders in the client's environment
9	Include creative dramatics in management
10	Integrate management with the language arts program
11	Client develops own homework assignments
12	Client practices under emotional conditions

Baker, & Schutz, 1968; Shelton, Johnson, & Arndt, 1972; Shelton, Johnson, Willis, & Arndt, 1975).

The effectiveness of various carryover approaches was investigated by a survey form completed by 125 public school clinicians (Polson, 1980). In the survey, carryover was defined as "the transfer of newly learned speech skills to all speaking situations outside the clinical setting" (p. 75). The responding clinicians rank ordered the effectiveness of carryover methodologies as shown in Table 10.4. It must be remembered that the effectiveness hierarchy is based upon clinical judgment, not empirical data. There is a paucity of research into generalization to untrained situational contexts, and consequently, most methods used are based upon clinical sense and have not been empirically analyzed.

What occurs during the maintenance phase of treatment?

MAINTENANCE

The last phase of articulation/phonological intervention is maintenance or retention. Maintenance is defined as continued use of the target sound/pattern in all speaking situations over time. Ideally, automatization and habituation occurs along with maintenance, which means that correct production

of the sound occurs without conscious or deliberate effort (Manning, Keappock, & Stick, 1976; Sommers & Kane, 1974). Usually during this stage of intervention, the client has less frequent contact with the clinician and takes more responsibility for the correct productions. The clinician periodically assesses the client's spontaneous speech in various settings either directly or through the reports of others. Appropriate times for these assessments to occur include after breaks in treatment, such as after spring break or summer vacation, when the client is still enrolled actively in a treatment program and when the client is scheduled on a consultative basis. It is critical that the client be followed over time to ensure that maintenance has indeed occurred (Hegde, 1998; McCabe & Bradley, 1975). The measurement or assessment of maintenance is discussed later in this chapter.

What is meant by the term *carryover*?

CARRYOVER

Carryover can be described as the habitual use of target sounds in all speaking situations, including conversational speech in and out of the clinic. It also involves articulation of the target sound without deliberate or conscious effort (Gerber, 1973;

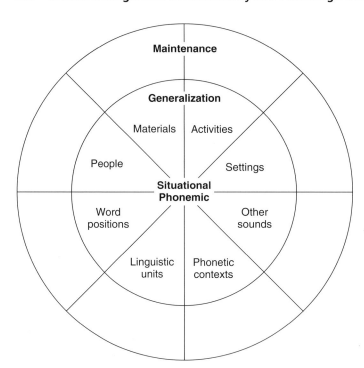

FIGURE 10.1   Components of the carryover process.

Sommers & Kane, 1974) and is part of the final stages of treatment, namely transfer and maintenance. Various terms, such as transfer, generalization, maintenance, retention, automatization, and habituation, are used when describing the carryover process. All of these terms have slightly varying meanings to speech-language pathologists and researchers so that the term *carryover* does not have the same meaning for all clinicians. Some use carryover to connote the conversational stage of intervention in and outside the clinical setting, while others use it to refer to the continued use of the target sound/pattern after treatment on the sound has been terminated. Still others use it to describe any instance in which a client uses the target sound or phonological pattern in an untrained situation or context. Figure 10.1 characterizes the components of carryover. In this chapter, carryover is defined as the habitual use of target sounds and sound patterns in conversational speech in and out of the clinical setting.

> What are potential influential factors on the carryover process?

Influences on Carryover

Carryover occurs at different rates for different individuals, and sometimes is never achieved. Occasionally, a client is dismissed from treatment only to be reenrolled at a later time because carryover did not occur. All the variables that account for successful carryover or for differences in learning rate are unknown, but some are client-related characteristics and others are program-related (Costello & Bosler, 1976; Dunn, 1983; Elbert, Dinnsen, & Powell, 1984; Elbert & McReynolds, 1978; Elbert, Powell, & Swartzlander, 1991; Gierut, Elbert, & Dinnsen, 1987; McReynolds, 1987; Mowrer, 1971). One set of child-related factors is the nature of the disorder, such as severity level, error patterns, consistency of error production, degree of intelligibility, stimulability, and original etiology. Child aptitudes include characteristics such as cognition, communication aptitude, and self-monitoring skills. Environmental factors such as social background, family characteristics, history of reinforcement, and others' reactions may be related. Finally, personal traits of the client including talkativeness, motivation, and personality are likely to be factors influencing carryover. Interestingly, some clients seem to show a sudden insight or "aha" experience (McReynolds, 1987). These clients incorporate their newly acquired targets into spontaneous speech seemingly as a result of internal factors. However, not all clients readily experience this phenomenon and need intervention directed at carryover. Both types of clients are seen in clinical practice—those who achieve carryover automatically and those who achieve it only after direct carryover training.

Program or treatment factors include the nature of the treatment approach, involvement of significant people and settings, relevance of materials used, frequency of practice and treatment sessions, amount of practice, number of responses elicited, and reinforcement during the treatment process. Important factors affecting carryover include the natural occurrence of reinforcement and the presentation of scheduled reinforcement (Dunlap & Plienis, 1988; McReynolds & Spradlin, 1989). In the acquisition phases of intervention, clients typically receive direct reinforcement which might tie the response to the place, time, and stimuli associated with the reinforcement. However, outside the clinical setting, reinforcement generally is unscheduled and noncontingent; that is, clients do not know when or if they will be reinforced for the target. If reinforcement is extremely inconsistent or nonexistent, clients might not learn to produce the target in natural situations outside of the clinical setting. It probably will help if the in-clinic reinforcement is modified to be more naturalistic and/or the frequency of the reinforcement is increased in the natural setting. In-clinic reinforcement can be made more natural by decreasing the amount of reinforcement, increasing the variability of the reinforcement, and using social reinforcement. One strategy used to assist with carryover is to train clients to evaluate their own productions. Some hypothesize that self-evaluations can be self-reinforcing (Ertmer & Ertmer, 1998; Hughes, 1985). Also, clients can be taught to ask for reinforcement if they can accurately discriminate between their correct and incorrect productions (Hughes, 1985; Stokes & Osnes, 1988). Thus, if clients can evaluate their own productions, they can provide themselves with internal reinforcement and can seek reinforcement from people in their environment.

Why does carryover to outside clinical situations not occur even though the target behavior is produced in conversational speech in the clinic? A survey of 125 public school speech-language pathologists regarding their carryover practices and beliefs might provide some insight (Polson, 1980). In an open-ended question—"What do you see as the major problem(s) in attaining carryover?"—64% reported lack of assistance in the carryover process from outside persons such as parents, teachers, and peers; 45% noted client attitude, primarily lack of motivation; and 33% indicated nonconducive clinical management practices including time limitations, caseload size, age of client when treatment is implemented, and shift of emphasis from articulatory to language disorders.

Perhaps, the reason a client produces a sound correctly during word and phrase practice but not in conversational speech is that the error response interferes with the newly acquired sound; that is, what a person has learned previously interferes with retaining and using the new behavior as a substitute for the old behavior (Winitz, 1975). The years of practice a child or adult has had in using the misarticulation (habit strength) intervenes in the ability to remember the newly learned sound (Mowrer, 1971). Also, interference conceivably comes from an activity following newly learned response patterns such as practicing a different sound after practice with the target.

Finally, several others have suggested that the intervention program may be ineffective in facilitating generalization because of lack of systematic planning or not planning appropriate activities (Koegel et al., 1986; Mowrer, 1989). As Secord (1989) explained "the clinician's challenge, then, is to enlarge the therapy situation to include all important settings in the client's life; to expand the learning environment so that the client recognizes cues to correct speech outside the therapy room" (p.150).

> What are some guidelines for achieving carryover?

Guidelines for Carryover

Although the ultimate goal of articulation/phonological treatment is carryover, it is not automatically achieved during the treatment process by every client when little attention is given to it (Bernthal & Bankson, 1998; Costello & Bosler, 1976; Koegel et al., 1986). Some clients do attain carryover with little or no instruction directed toward carryover, others with a moderate amount of instruction, and some need extensive training. Certainly, most treatment programs and approaches are quite effective in establishing correct productions in the client's repertoire; that is, the client can readily produce the target sound upon demand, but many do not include specific programming for the situational transfer and maintenance phases of intervention. To meet the final goal of intervention, maintenance of correct production in all speaking situations, the clinician must systematically program treatment for generalization of the target behavior to nontreatment situations for many clients. This means that the clinician needs to expand the treatment setting to the client's natural environment. In consideration of varying abilities to generalize, certain clinical activities can enhance the probability of transfer (Bernthal and Bankson, 2004). Generally, transfer can be facilitated by providing diverse stimuli for the target response and by developing new responses similar to the original response (Dunn, 1983). In other words, the clinician provides for both types of transfer described above, namely for situational contexts and for phonemic contexts.

Carryover does seem to take a certain period of time and considerable planning, as well as incorporation of generalization activities to the treatment program. Actually, the carryover process begins at the initiation of treatment when the client is learning the correct speech production pattern, but specific procedures may need to be incorporated to facilitate generalization and habituation sometime during the treatment process. Three patterns of timing for initiating generalization training have been identified (DelMoral, 2002):

• Early in the treatment program
• End of the treatment program
• Mixed approach

Many suggest that carryover activities should be initiated at the beginning of the treatment program (Fowler & Baer, 1981; Griffiths & Craighead, 1972; Olswang & Bain, 2004; Ruscello & Shelton, 1979; Smit, 2004). In the mixed approach, carryover activities are incorporated at each production level, including isolation, words, sentences, reading, and connected speech, when clients meet a specified criterion (Bernthal & Bankson, 2004; Eisenson & Ogilvie, 1977; Johnson et al., 1967; Powers, 1971). For instance, after the client reaches a specific criterion at a certain production level, clinicians often make outside clinical assignments, including practicing lists of syllables, words, or sentences at home. Another example is working on self-evaluation early in the treatment program. Lastly, others introduce generalization activities after clients produce the target phoneme or phonological pattern at a stable rate within the clinical setting (Gerber, 1973; Hughes, 1985; Koegel et al., 1986, 1988; McReynolds & Spradlin, 1989). They often wait to incorporate environmental training programs, such as conducting sessions outside the clinic room and talking with people other than the clinician and treatment group members, until the client has reached a specified criterion level in connected speech within the clinical setting.

The amount of treatment necessary for the achievement of carryover has not been determined because it varies greatly from one individual to another. Speech-language pathologists need to probe frequently to assess the amount of phonemic and situational transfer that is occurring. Review of the literature and personal clinical experience lead some to recommend consideration of the guidelines shown in Table 10.5 to facilitate the carryover process. Now that the dimensions of and principles for transfer and maintenance have been considered, it is time to examine specific techniques for facilitating carryover.

CARRYOVER METHODS

Several strategies, techniques, and programs have been suggested and devised for achieving carryover. Some of these procedures have been researched, but many have not. Some involve in-clinical activities with only the clinician and clients participating, whereas others incorporate out-of-clinic (extra-clinic) activities and possibly the assistance of people other than the clinician and client.

> Describe some in-clinic procedures found to be useful for assisting clients with carryover.

In-Clinic Strategies

Nonsense Material

The nonsense material approach to articulation treatment was devised primarily for the purpose of effecting carryover (Gerber, 1973). It is based on the hypothesis that individuals with deviant articulation need to learn to produce target sounds effortlessly and consistently. Use of nonmeaningful verbal material facilitates achievement of this objective in that the old articulation habit patterns do not interfere with the motor patterns necessary to produce the newly learned sound. Old learning does not interfere with new learning. Only after the target sound is produced automatically in non-meaningful contexts is meaning introduced. At this point, real words are easily produced by the client who can then concentrate on the content of the message while attending minimally to the mechanics of articulation. According to Gerber, if meaningful material is introduced too early in the treatment process, the target sound in these words will be deliberately and laboriously produced. Many treatment approaches certainly involve practice of the target phonemes in nonsense material, but not to the extent that Gerber suggested.

A study conducted by Leonard (1973) investigated the effectiveness of using nonsense drill material. One group, the "nonsense" group was taught to produce /s/ in words with nonsense definitions,

TABLE 10.5

General Guidelines for the Carryover Process

- Initially schedule several short sessions, rather than fewer longer sessions.
- Select sounds for intervention that are examples of error patterns in the client's speech to initiate transfer to other sounds with a similar error pattern.
- Begin instruction with positions or contexts that are the most facilitative in producing the target, then transfer productions to other positions and contexts.
- Incorporate production in syllabic contexts as soon as possible because syllable production is more similar to contextual speech than to isolated sounds.
- Use nonsense syllables and words with varying stress patterns to stabilize articulatory productions before using real words. Meaningful words may interfere with learning the motor patterns. (Note: This strategy is not appropriate for most phonological treatment approaches.)
- Use standard stimuli from the client's natural environments.
- Use common verbal antecedents during the treatment program.
- Use materials and activities that are meaningful for the client.
- Use stimuli in the production phases that share features of the stimuli in natural situations.
- Use intermittent reinforcement schedules after production in each linguistic level is established.
- Incorporate the proprioceptive sense to feel correct productions in addition to using the auditory sense.
- Ensure that the client can easily and quickly produce a series of target responses before moving on to the next step.
- Use a wide variety of words, grammatical categories, activities, and such in the treatment program.
- Begin using situational transfer activities when the client can produce the target in meaningful words.
- Use situations in which meanings of correct articulation have pragmatic significance.
- Teach clients to self-evaluate and self-monitor their own speech.
- Vary the physical setting of the sessions to include the client's natural setting.
- Vary the audience.
- See the client less frequently during maintenance.
- Incorporate parents and others, such as teachers and siblings, to reinforce and provide corrective feedback.

and the other group, the "meaningful" group, was taught to produce the same /s/ words in meaningful contexts. The "nonsense" group learned the correct production more effectively; however, the "meaningful" group had better generalization. Leonard suggested that nonsense contexts may facilitate acquisition of the target sound, but may not be as effective for generalization so that possibly one should begin with nonmeaningful words and move to meaningful ones. Gerber's approach (1973) does proceed from nonsense to meaningful material, and the approach is reported to be effective in achieving carryover. This approach is often appropriate for phonetic disorders in which the client needs to learn motor patterns, but usually inappropriate for phonologic disorders in which the client needs to learn phonological rules.

After reviewing research results, Winitz (1975) also recommended the use of nonsense words (alone and in conversation) before practicing the target sounds in meaningful material. Mowrer (1988) pointed out that meaningful words usually are retained longer than nonsense words and cautioned that some practice materials used by speech-language pathologists, such as rhymes, tongue twisters, and poems, are really not meaningful for clients and thus may not contribute much to carryover of the target sound into spontaneous speech. The use of nonsense materials emphasizes the motor or mechanical aspects of articulation; that is, production without the competition of meaning and former negative habit patterns. Later, meaning is added to the motor component of articulation.

Timed Productions

Another motor approach to articulation treatment is to use speech-sound production timed drills or speed drills (Bankson & Byrne, 1972; Smit, 2004). The purpose of this carryover approach is to develop articulation motor skills so that phonemes are produced easily and rapidly. The hypothesis is that carryover may not occur because of inadequate practice of the motor skills used in production of the target sound; therefore, overpractice may be important in maintaining correct production of the target sound rather than reverting to habitual error patterns (Bankson & Byrne, 1972; Byrne & Shervanian, 1977). In Bankson and Byrne's procedure, the client reads a 60-word list 25 times per session in a given time limit. The time limit is reduced by two seconds each time the list is read with 100% accuracy. Ten seconds are added to the time limit at the beginning of each succeeding session, providing a warmup period, and two seconds are taken off with each successful reading. If misarticulations occur, the time limit is expanded by two seconds for five trials. The goal is correct, effortless, automatic articulation. Using this procedure over a 10-day period, 5 of 5 subjects showed improved performance in the training task and 4 of 5 achieved at least some carryover to three different settings. Gerber (1973) also stressed rapid, effortless, and consistent production, suggesting that competition during clinical activities helps fast production and recommended activities requiring responses under a time limit.

Self-Monitoring

A treatment component that may enhance carryover is client self-evaluation and self-monitoring for which auditory perceptual training forms the base (DelMoral, 2002; Ertmer & Ertmer, 1998; Gerber, 1973; Powers, 1971; Ruscello & Shelton, 1979; Scarry & Scarry-Larkin, 1996; Van Riper & Emerick, 1984; Winitz, 1975). In articulation/phonological treatment, self-evaluation refers to the immediate or delayed assessment by clients of their own speech production relative to its correctness. Self-monitoring refers to clients assessing their speech production and immediately changing it on their own when they incorrectly produce speech sounds. Training in self-evaluation can occur throughout the treatment process, primarily through the auditory modality, although visual, tactile, and kinesthetic modes are sometimes incorporated. The rationale is that the clients need to detect their own errors so that they achieve carryover. According to Powers (1971), thorough auditory discrimination training is critical to the achievement of carryover because persons need to be able to identify their own errors to use correct articulation in conversational speech. If generalization to spontaneous speech is not occurring, possibly the clinician should incorporate specific speech sound discrimination procedures into the treatment process, including training in connected speech.

One procedure for teaching self-monitoring is for the client to be trained to do this through a series of steps that are briefly described in Table 10.6 and through positive reinforcement of accurate self-evaluation. A second technique de-

TABLE 10.6

Self-Monitoring Program Developed by Gerber (1973)

Step	Procedure
1	Clinician produces three sounds or syllables or words. Client evaluates the productions by stating that all are correct or all are not correct. If the latter, the client states the ones that were not correct: #1, #2, or #3.
2	Clinician tape-records a group of three productions, either correct or demonstrating errors. Client evaluates production on playback, identifying any errors by numbers.
3	Clinician produces a single utterance, which the client tries to imitate. Both productions are recorded and played back. Client judges whether own production sounded the same as that of the clinician model. At first, clinician rewards client for correct evaluation. Later, both correct production and evaluation are rewarded.
4	Clinician produces a group of three utterances. Client attempts to match them, producing three utterances. Model and imitation are recorded and played back for evaluation by client. At first, client is rewarded for correct evaluation and later for correct evaluation and production.
5	Client records three utterances without a model. During playback, client evaluates own productions, identifying errors by number.
6	Client records three utterances on tape without a model and listens carefully to productions while producing them. Client evaluates the productions *before* playback, identifying any errors by number. Client then listens to the same production during playback and evaluates them. Then, client compares the two evaluations.

scribed by Winitz (1975) is as follows: When a client misarticulates the target sound, the speech-language pathologist initially responds to what the client actually said rather than to the client's misarticulated intent, then eventually responds appropriately by articulating the word correctly several times. Eventually, as a result of this procedure, the client will likely produce the sound correctly. A third self-monitoring procedure requires clients to evaluate their own productions (scanning and self-analysis) before being reinforced. When they produce the sound correctly and identify it as correct, they are reinforced. Engel and Groth (1976) devised a program that required clients to evaluate their articulation after production and before delivery of a reinforcer by the clinician. This procedure was used at the reading level so that when the client produced the target sound correctly and signaled that it was correct, the clinician provided reinforcement. When the client did not say the target word correctly or did not signal when a correct production was used, the client was not reinforced. All six subjects in their study achieved normal articulation in oral reading outside the clinical setting, and persons other than the clinician reported that correct articulations also generalized to conversational speech in various settings. This behavior was maintained throughout the school year. The theory for this approach is that feedback for correct self-evaluation can be established as an internal

reinforcer and, consequently, the rate of correct productions increases.

A program developed by Koegel et al. (1986) requires clients to record correct responses on a data sheet outside the clinic after they learn to record correct responses in the clinic. In their study, the self-monitoring phase of treatment was begun at various linguistic levels for different clients; that is, some clients began recording their own correct productions after using the target in sentences, some after two consecutive sentences, others after short monologues, and still others after unstructured conversation in the clinic. The self-monitoring procedure was effective for all students, no matter when in the treatment program self-monitoring was begun. No generalization to spontaneous speech outside the clinical setting occurred until self-monitoring began and generalization was maintained even when the clients no longer carried the data sheets, and on a 5-month follow-up. The specific steps of the intervention program are shown in Table 10.7. In a follow-up study, carryover of correct production of the targets when self-monitoring procedures were used within the clinical setting was compared with using self-monitoring procedures outside of the clinical setting (Koegel et al, 1988). Clients did not carry over correct production of their targets to nontreatment environments when they only used self-evaluation within the clinical setting; however, they did generalize to other settings after they were

TABLE 10.7

Self-Monitoring Program Developed by Koegel, Koegel, and Ingham (1976)

Step	Procedure
1	Clinician demonstrates a correct and an incorrect target sound. Client produces a correct and incorrect target.
2	Clinician teaches client to record correct responses during conversation. Clinician first produces a few example sentences and demonstrates how to mark a response immediately following each correct response. A counter can be used instead of "paper tracking."
3	Client continues to talk with clinician. Every time the client produces a correct response, client records the response on the data sheet or counter. Clinician provides feedback and has client make corrections in the tracking activity.
4	Client produces and records the target sound correctly all the time in the clinical session. Clinician stresses that the client carry data sheets or counter and record responses in all environments. Clinician explains that points can be earned only for correct productions that occur during reading and conversation with another person, not for drill activities or talking alone.
5	Client self-monitors and records data in clinic in unstructured spontaneous speech. Client exchanges data sheets for positive reinforcers. No reinforcers are given when client does not bring data sheets.
6	Client is no longer required to carry data sheets when there is evidence of at least 70% correct responses on the object probes and positive feedback from subjective parent and teacher reports.

required to self-evaluate their productions outside the clinical setting when the clinician was not present. This approach of self-monitoring outside the clinical setting has the advantage of not being time-consuming or logistically difficult to arrange because only the client and clinician need to be involved directly.

Self-evaluation is included as a part of some computer programs designed for articulation-phonological intervention, such as LocuTour Multimedia Articulation program (Scarry & Scarry-Larkin, 1996). In this computerized program, a picture is shown on the screen and the computer provides an auditory model for clients to repeat. The clients' productions are recorded, and the computer plays back the model and the clients' production of the syllable, word, or sentence. Clients then evaluate their own productions as correct, distorted, or incorrect and the clinician provides feedback to clients about their self-evaluation as well as their production of the target. Two clients (aged 5 years/10 months and 8 years/5 months) who participated in single-subject studies showed improved production for their target sounds (/l/ and /r/, respectively) in conversational speech after 15 days of treatment with the LocuTour computer program (Cook, 1999; MacWilliams, 2001). In one of these two studies, the younger client improved more in his articulation of the target (/l/) treated with the computer program that had a self-evaluation component than on the target (/θ, ð/) treated traditionally without a self-evaluation component. However, the opposite results occurred in the older client who improved more with on the sound (/s/) treated traditionally than with the sound (/r/) treated with the computer program.

Another self-evaluation approach is to use video playback in clinical sessions (DelMoral, 2002). In DelMoral's study, a 12-session treatment program was implemented with two students (aged 7 years and 11 years) who correctly articulated the target sounds at the sentence and conversational levels within the clinical setting but misarticulated their target outside the clinical setting. They each viewed a videotaped playback of themselves in speech activities and evaluated their production of their target as "old" or "new" (Table 10.8). Additionally, the students periodically completed questionnaires about their perceptions of their use of the "old" and "new" sounds and had the opportunity to discuss self-correction and motivation strategies that helped them produce their target phonemes outside the clinical setting. Carryover was measured using an extra-clinic covert procedure in which the students did not know they were being observed by a speech language pathology graduate student or practicing clinician who was not the investigator (clinician). Both students showed a clinically significant generalization gain as well as an ability to self-evaluate. The procedure of using in-clinic video playback of recorded speech samples seems to be a viable procedure for achieving carryover outside the clinical setting.

Self-Regulation

A constructivist approach for articulation/phonological carryover was outlined by Ertmer and Ertmer (1998). "Constructivism defines learning as the creation of meaning from experience . . . That is, learners create their own knowledge through participation in meaningful tasks" (p. 68). In this approach, clients discover the metacognitive processes involved in carryover. The strategy is to increase motivation, increase metacognitive knowledge, and develop metacognitive control of articulation production.

A seven-step program for developing self-regulation for articulation/phonological carryover was described by Ertmer and Ertmer (1998) specifically for clients who are proficient in producing their targets during clinical sessions, but which does not carry over to speech production outside the clinical setting (Fig. 10.2). The first step is to increase motivation for carryover with the goal of increasing the awareness of the benefits of carryover. This step involves clients doing contrastive productions and categorizing their productions without positive or negative labels (e.g., "old sound" and "new sound"). In this way, they discover that misarticulated targets result in nonsense or unintentional words. During this contrastive drill, the clinician might ask clients to identify their preference of the old or the new way of speaking then discuss and make a list of when, where, and with whom they would like to use the target sound. New situations can be added to this list, and it can also be used to evaluate progress toward carryover.

The second step is to increase awareness of barriers to carryover. The clinician can use guiding questions such as "Where do you use your new speech the most?," "How do you feel when you use your new speech sound?," "Why is that?," and "When is it hardest to remember your new speech sounds—when you talk to me, to your friends, or to your teacher—and why?" (Ertmer & Ertmer, 1998, p. 72). If this is hard for the client, clinicians can verbalize their own thoughts as a model ("When I talk with my friends, I have something I want to tell them and I don't think

TABLE 10.8

Activities for a Self-Evaluation Treatment Program for External Clinic Generalization

Session #	Treatment Activities
1	1. Complete self-evaluation questionnaire. 2. Discuss production strategies. 3. Engage in a minimal pairs contrast task. 4. Learn how to operate the VCR. 5. Listen to videotaped productions, identifying the productions as "old" or "new." 6. Discuss the use of self-correction and motivation strategies. 7. Learn how to mark production performance on the chart for which prizes would be awarded at the end of the program.
2–5	1. Engage in a 6- to 10-minute speech activity while being videotaped. 2. Stop and start the video playback of the speech activity when the target production is identified. 3. Evaluate each target as "old" or "new." 4. Discuss strategies used or not used in the videotaped production. 5. Count tokens (correct responses).
6	1. Engage in a 6- to 10-minute speech activity while being videotaped. 2. Complete self-evaluation questionnaire. 3. Review self-evaluation and motivation strategies.
7–11	1. View videotaped production made in the previous session. 2. Evaluate production. 3. Count tokens (correct responses). 4. Engage in a 6- to 10-minute speech activity while being videotaped.
12	1. View videotaped production made in the previous session. 2. Evaluate target productions. 3. Count tokens (correct responses). 4. Complete self-evaluation questionnaire. 5. Trade tokens for prizes.

From DelMoral, S. J. (2002). Self-evaluating video-playback of articulatory productions to promote environmental generalization. Unpublished master's thesis, Portland State University, Portland, OR. Adapted with permission.

about how I'm speaking. Does this happen to you?"). Discussion can evolve from there to help clients identify the barriers for them as individuals. The third step is to increase awareness of personal learning resources. The clinician asks guiding questions about past experiences and strategies for handling similar situations, such as "What do you do when you really want to remember something?" or "If I asked you to give your teacher a message today, what would you do to remember it? (Ertmer & Ertmer, 1998, p. 72).

The metacognitive knowledge gleaned in the first three steps sets the stage for planning, self-monitoring, and self-evaluation of speech targets in everyday speaking situations. The fourth step is to plan strategies for carryover during performances (including telling jokes and riddles, presenting puppet shows, telling stories, giving oral reports, or presenting plays). The clinician can help clients develop strategies by asking guided questions or discussing the benefits and drawbacks of various strategies. Examples of strategies for consideration include "verbal rehearsal (self-talk prior to a performance), visualization (forming mental images of successful carryover in varied situations), speech logs (diaries of written goals and strategies), speech buddies (pairing peers to help each other), and physical reminders (wearing a piece of string on the finger)" (Ertmer & Ertmer, 1998, p. 73). The next step is to increase self-monitoring during rehearsals

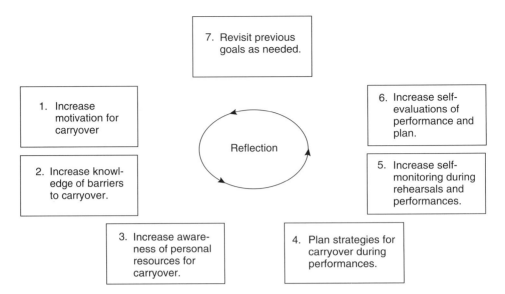

FIGURE 10.2 Sequence of goals for the development of motivation, metacognitive knowledge, and metacognitive control for phonological carryover. From Ertmer, D., Ertmer P. (1998). Constructivist strategies in phonological intervention: Facilitating self-regulation for carryover. *Language, Speech, and Hearing Services in Schools, 29*, 67–75. (Copyright 1998 by American Speech-Language-Hearing Association. Reprinted with permission.)

and performances. At this stage, clinicians and group members model and discuss self-correction behaviors; for example, ignore incorrect targets, but try to remember the correct production at the next opportunity; say "I mean" and repeat the word correctly; use covert self-evaluation. Clients can also view themselves and others in videotaped performances and note and discuss self-monitoring behaviors. The next step is to increase self-evaluation of performance and plan. Here, clients become skilled in assessing their plan, performances, and progress toward carryover. They judge whether their strategies are helping them to say their target sounds during rehearsal and everyday speaking situations. Videotape recordings can be helpful for this as well as guiding questions, such as "Which sound are you using more often?" The last step is reflection and revision. Guiding questions and modeling thought processes facilitate critical reflection. This approach has not been well researched to date. A study conducted by DelMoral (2002) that incorporated some of the techniques resulted in improved carryover in two students.

Comparison of Error and Correct Sounds

For the purpose of generalization, Winitz (1975) suggested using a procedure to develop and strengthen an association between the error and correct sounds. In the clinical session, the clinician articulates words incorrectly and the client responds by producing the word correctly. The child never intentionally produces the word incorrectly; it is only heard incorrectly (a form of **negative practice**). In this way, it is hypothesized that the client associates the incorrect production with the correct production. Later, when misarticulating the sound, clients might associate the error with the standard sound and correct themselves.

Negative practice (deliberate production of the error) is occasionally suggested. Generally when this procedure is used, the client first uses incorrect sound production in words followed by correct production of the target sound in the same word. The purpose is to make the client aware of errors; however, such a procedure may actually strengthen the error pattern. Therefore caution should be exercised when using negative practice.

The use of meaningful contrasts is a similar procedure in that the client produces words that differ in one phonemic feature or phonological pattern; however, unlike negative practice, meaning is attached to each of the two words. The intention is that the client will learn when it is appropriate to use one phoneme and when it is appropriate to use the other phoneme. For example, if a client fronts or substitutes /t/ for /k/, it is useful for the client to produce contrasting pairs such as *tea* and *key* and *make* and *mate* in meaningful contexts that illustrate the appropriate meanings for each of the words. In this case, the client is not merely practicing so-called errors, but is learning when it is correct to use a certain phoneme and when it is not. Theoretically, in negative practice as originally conceived, the client is practicing motor patterns; whereas in contrastive pairs, the client is practicing or using phonological rules.

Paired-Stimuli Approach

Weston and Irwin (in Peña-Brooks & Hegde, 2000) developed the paired-stimuli approach to articulation treatment to assist generalization with the termination criterion set at 15 consecutive correct productions of the target sound in conversation on two successive treatment sessions (Chapter 8). In this approach, the key word (a word the client produces acceptably in at least 9 of 10 trials) serves as a model for the training words and for providing correct auditory and tactile feedback. A study was conducted with 80 experimental subjects who were treated with the paired-stimuli approach and 80 control subjects who were not (Irwin & Weston, 1975). The experimental group performed better on conversational posttests administered immediately following treatment and again one month later, suggesting that such an approach facilitates carryover.

Programmed Approach

Mowrer (1971) preferred using a systematic programmed approach without manipulation of external stimuli. If the program is carefully and logically designed with an emphasis on techniques to facilitate positive transfer, it may not be necessary to plan extra-clinic activities. Mowrer cited one study that showed a programmed approach to be more effective for carryover than a nonprogrammed traditional approach. Another study (Tremblay, 1982) showed that an operant program resulted in relatively more carryover into spontaneous speech outside the clinical setting as compared to a nonoperant intervention program. There was quite a bit of variability among the subjects' posttest performances, however, and no client achieved 100% correct production of the target in spontaneous speech.

Creative Drama

Creative drama and language experiences in activities such as pantomimes, improvised stories and skits, and language-related movement activities have been recommended for the purpose of carryover (Bush, 1978). The use of creative language experiences, including sense awareness activities, communication games, production of videotapes and movies, interviews, and dramatic readings have been effective techniques. Such activities can be used with all age levels and in multiage groups. The rationale is that after the target sound has been established in controlled intervention situations, creative drama provides natural language situations in which the phonemes can be practiced. A side benefit is that such procedures can expand expressive abilities (Bush, 1978). In order for clients to use new speech skills, they must have opportunities to practice them in nearly normal situations. The procedure for creative drama is as follows:

- Clinician tells a story using extensive dialogue.
- Clinical group discusses the characters.
- Individual clients select parts and act out the story.
- Clients change roles and again act out the story.
- If a client is self-conscious, first do the story in pantomime and movement, and then group vocal activities so that no child is pressured to participate.
- Individual clients and clinician can discuss their performance during individual session.
- Group may choose to do live or videotaped performances for others.

The stories are acted out without scripts. Other language experience activities also can be used to assist in the carryover process.

Group Intervention

Group intervention can facilitate carryover by providing the opportunity for more natural conversational situations, although individual treatment sessions may be needed by some clients. In many instances, group treatment is particularly effective in later stages of intervention. Some studies have shown group treatment to be as effective, if not more so, than individual treatment with school-aged clients with articulation deviations (Sommers et al., 1964; Sommers et al., 1966). Group work saves time for the clinician, does not always sacrifice advantages of individual treatment, and has some distinct advantages over individual work. Unique advantages of group work include:

- Clients tend to stimulate and motivate each other.
- Many opportunities are provided for natural speaking situations and interactions.
- Setting provides for socialization and peer interaction.
- Clients realize that others also have communication problems.
- A broader variety of materials and activities can be used.

- Opportunities are provided to learn by observing others.
- Client's dependence on clinician's evaluation is reduced because the clinician is not the sole evaluator.
- Carryover is facilitated.
- Clinician time can be used more economically (Backus & Beasley, 1951; Johnson et al., 1967; McDonald, 1964b; Powers, 1971; Roth & Worthington, 2001).

Naturally, each client likely will receive less attention than in individual sessions. Other disadvantages include fewer opportunities to address specific needs of individual clients, shy or reticent clients may be reluctant to participate, one or two group members may dominate and monopolize the group, and the group's rate of progress may be too fast for some and too slow for others (McDonald, 1964b; Roth & Worthington, 2001). Perhaps, a combination of group and individual treatment is optimum. Certainly, some individual work can be done with those who are not progressing as rapidly as other group members, although such differences in progress rate can be handled effectively within a group framework. Where individual differences exist within the group, 5 or 10 minutes of individual attention prior to or immediately following a group session (such as a pre-clinic or post-clinic session) may be helpful.

Of course, group treatment is not effective if used inappropriately. All too often, such an approach merely involves clients taking turns rather than all actively participating all the time by interacting with each other and through activities involving the whole group. The speech-language pathologist's role is to keep several clients simultaneously and beneficially involved in the treatment process during the entire session. The following criteria should be met when conducting group sessions:

- All clients are continuously active in participation.
- Group members interact with one another.
- Each client receives some individual attention from the clinician.
- Clinical activities serve individual needs and goals for each client.
- Motivation is centered around speech objectives rather than on winning.
- The client is aware of progress toward the objectives (Black, 1964; Roth & Worthington, 2001; Van Riper, 1952).

Various techniques can be used for keeping all clients actively participating (Black, 1964; McDonald, 1964b; Roth & Worthington, 2001). One procedure is to present a stimulus and pause before calling on a client to respond. In this way, all clients listen to the stimulus and prepare to respond since no one knows who will be called. Another technique involves clients listening to one another and evaluating the response verbally or through a tracking procedure. Also, clients can be instructed to respond in unison. One client can produce an articulation pattern for the others to repeat. Additionally, various stations can be set up for individual clients using tape recorders, Language Masters, and so forth. Clients who are in advanced treatment stages can help those in earlier phases, similar to a "buddy" system. During the carryover phase of treatment, clients can participate in role-playing, dramatizations, putting on plays for classrooms, simulated telephone conversations, and other social activities involving spontaneous speech. Whatever procedures are used, group activities should stimulate interest and be enjoyable for the participants.

Group sessions generally are conducted with two to six clients selected on a homogeneous basis. Length of sessions ranges from 20 to 60 minutes, depending on the size of the group, frequency of sessions, and other factors. Bases for grouping include disorder type, articulation proficiency, similarity of misarticulated sounds, age, education or grade level, and cognitive level. Articulation proficiency is an important consideration so that a group can concentrate on any one of several activities such as auditory perception training, sound production, and carryover. The age spread for children and youth probably should be limited to 2 or 3 years because intellectual and social maturity and interests are significant factors for group interaction. Misarticulation of the same sounds may be considered—/s/ and /z/ group, /r/ group—, although it is quite feasible and appropriate for different group members to be working on different sounds that are at the same proficiency level, such as word level, sentence level, and structured conversation level. Backus and Beasley (1951) recommended heterogeneous grouping, but most other approaches prefer homogeneous grouping as described above. Whichever approach is considered, it should be differentially applied to the specific etiologies.

Traditionally, in the schools, individual and group intervention has been conducted in a pullout model in which clinicians work with clients in a separate room from the classroom. Recently, there has been a trend for clients to receive services in the classroom which is a form of group intervention. Classroom-based strategies generally provide less direct instruction and require careful planning (Bernthal & Bankson, 2004). According to Masterson (1993), treatment provided in the classroom may be more useful for working on conceptual or linguistic rule type errors than for motor-based errors. Also, intervention in the classroom is especially useful during the carryover phases of treatment.

A unique group treatment procedure in which older students (14 to 17 years of age) worked with younger students (6 to 8 years of age) on their articulation skills was found to be quite effective (Groher, 1976). The clinician met with the group of older students weekly. Each older student met with a younger student twice a week for half-hour sessions for 4 months. One group of older students had articulation deviancies and received treatment from the clinician once a week, and another group had articulatory disorders, but did not receive treatment. The younger clients who worked with the older group receiving treatment improved the most. Both groups of older students also improved in their articulation skills. Subjectively, speech-language pathologists noted that the older students who were receiving and providing treatment were more receptive to their own individual sessions. All in all, group remediation seems to be an efficient and useful method of administering articulation treatment.

Proprioceptive Feedback

Enhancing proprioceptive feedback has been reported to be effective in facilitating transfer of correct productions (Secord, 1989; Shine, 1989; Van Riper & Erickson, 1996). The most typical approach in this regard is to reduce or eliminate auditory feedback so that the client must rely upon kinesthetic and tactile feedback. Methods for doing this include using speech containing the target in the presence of masking noise, whispering, and speaking while wearing earplugs.

Other In-Clinic Techniques

Other specific techniques for in-clinic carryover activities have been suggested. It is beneficial to practice nucleus words and phrases (for example, greetings, courtesies, names, and frequent requests) in clinical sessions and to encourage the client to articulate correctly these expressions in everyday situations (Johnson et al., 1967; Powers, 1971). Some time should be devoted to such practice every session. Along these same lines, words from classroom subject matter, vocabulary related to holidays and special events, slang words, and core vocabularies (words meaningfully related) can be practiced in and out of clinical sessions.

Calling the client's attention to the errors may result in a decrease in their occurrence. Instructing the

client to track or note errors, write down error words, or tap a foot for incorrect speech sound production can focus clients on their errors. Such a procedure should first be practiced in the clinical setting where the speech-language clinician can monitor the client's self-monitoring accuracy. Later, clients can track themselves outside the clinic.

Motivation certainly seems to be a factor in carryover and every attempt should be made to motivate the client to use target sounds outside the clinical setting. It is often motivating for clients to follow progress of the treatment process so they understand what has been accomplished and what the future goals are. Results can be shown objectively through graphs, charts, and other records. Time should be devoted to the client and clinician conversing with one another and engaging in other activities requiring the client to use connected speech, for example, role playing, storytelling, dramatizations, and puppetry. It is helpful to introduce games, competition, and similar activities in clinical sessions after the target sound is produced in connected speech in ideal conditions to heighten a client's emotional level. Such activities tend to induce excitement and distraction. Such speech productions could be tape-recorded for later analysis by both the client and clinician. Numerous other in-clinic techniques can be used to aid carryover into conversational speech which is limited only by the combined creativity of the clinician and client.

> Describe some out-of-clinic procedures found to be useful for assisting clients with carryover.

Out-of-Clinic Strategies

Assignments

Because the final goal is correct articulation of the standard sound/pattern in all speaking situations, several techniques have been devised to help generalization to extra-clinic settings. Giving speech assignments for clients to complete outside the clinical setting is an approach frequently used. Generally, these assignments should be devised for individual clients in terms of their ability levels and environments, and the clinician should require reports from the client. Speech notebooks may bridge the gap between clinical and outside environments. The client puts pictures or words containing the target sound in the notebook, which is used for home practice. New words are not added until the client demonstrates proficiency in producing them within the clinical session. The purpose is to increase the client's awareness of speech between sessions and to provide stimulus material for the client, teacher, parents, and other key persons. Establishing a weekly quota of words to be produced correctly outside the clinical session could be assigned to the client. Another type of assignment is to set up nucleus situations outside the clinical setting in which correct speech is required. Examples would be at the dinner table, talking with a parent after arriving home from school, and during the end of the day before bedtime. The clinician may want to enlist the support of family for these nucleus situations. Other types of assignments can be given to aid in carryover, but certain cautions should be taken. Assignments should be made for particular times or situations, not for all day everyday. Remember that clients cannot generalize to all words and situations at once. A good rule of thumb is never assign a task for the client to perform outside the clinic until the task is achieved within the clinical setting.

Extra-Clinic Environments

Early in the carryover process, the child and clinician engage in conversational speech in the clinical setting and then in outside environments similar to and near the clinic room. Still later, an unfamiliar clinician or someone trained to detect misarticulations converses with the client in these same environments. Creating discriminative stimuli or reminders in extra-clinic environments should foster carryover (Engel, Brandriet, Erickson, Gronhovd, & Gunderson, 1966; Gerber, 1973). Examples are signs placed in outside environments, books used during clinical sessions and read in other settings, word lists taped to the desk and bedroom door, and so forth.

Enlisting the assistance of interested persons, such as parents, teachers, siblings, classmates, and educational aides, facilitates carryover. In most instances, for such a procedure to be effective, the speech-language pathologist must train the person helping in the treatment process. In the public school setting, classroom teachers are often asked to assist in the treatment process. They can help the client carry out speech assignments, monitor the client's speech during certain activities, provide classroom material to be used during clinical sessions, track the client's errors, and intermittently reinforce correct sound productions. Mowrer (1967) described a procedure in which aides were trained in three half-hour sessions to learn to discriminate between correct and incorrect sound production, provide instruction when clients make errors, and provide group speaking activities to foster correct sound production.

Then, the teacher listened to students in reading class and provided feedback to the clients. This is an example of how to incorporate the classroom teacher, natural speaking situations, and familiar materials to facilitate generalization. We caution, however, that a classroom teacher should be requested to perform only activities that do not demand much time and that are compatible with normal classroom activities. Additionally, instructions should be clear and specific, preferably in written form. Some teachers do not have the time and/or the desire to assist; therefore, demands should not be made on them. Rather, they should be asked if they would like to help.

When the client is a child, parent involvement is frequently solicited by the speech-language clinician for the purpose of facilitating carryover. If feasible, it is helpful for parents to participate in clinical sessions along with the clinician. Many parents can work quite effectively with their child on articulation skills and have good ideas for how the whole family can be involved and assist. Most parents who are interested in assisting must be trained in some way. Merely providing them with instructions is usually not sufficient because they usually do not have the background and skills needed to evaluate and reinforce their child for articulation proficiency. Parents need to learn to discriminate between their child's correct and incorrect sound productions in words, sentences, and conversation, to reinforce positively, to correct misarticulations, and possibly to track articulation performance. Ideally, such training includes explanation by the clinician of the articulation treatment program, parent observation or participation of clinical sessions with the client and clinician working together, verbal and written explanation of the parent role in treatment, and practice by the parent and child in the clinical setting with observation and comment by the clinician.

Research has shown that it is worthwhile to train parents to assist in treatment (Carrier, 1970; Fudala, 1973; Van Hattum, 1985; Wing & Heimgartner, 1973). Care must be taken in selecting parents to provide articulation treatment to their child, because it seems that those who willingly assist will probably produce better results (McCroskey & Baird, 1971). In one study, clients whose parents attended clinical sessions and subsequently worked with their children at home showed three times as much progress as those children whose parents did not attend the sessions (Fudala, 1973). Two training sessions were held with the parents. Parents then observed clinical sessions and were given assignments to complete at home with their child.

This procedure was effective probably because the parents expressed a willingness to participate and observed the clinician using techniques they were to use later in the home assignments.

An articulation carryover program implemented by parents was developed by Wing and Heimgartner (1973). They contended that the final phase of treatment, conversational speech, is too broad for both the clinician and client in that there are varying levels of difficulty in this last step of treatment. Therefore, a five-level carryover program was devised:

- Oral reading within a limited time span (10 minutes)
- Oral reading and oral discussion of the reading with a limited time span (5 minutes of reading and 5 minutes of discussion)
- Structured conversation about preselected topics within a limited time span (10 minutes)
- Unstructured conversational speaking within an increased time span (10 minutes within a certain hour)
- Unstructured conversational speaking within an expanded time span (10 minutes within a day)

Criterion for movement from one step to the next is zero errors for three consecutive practice sessions on at least three different days. The five-step program is carried out by the parent and child with weekly clinician–parent telephone conferences. These telephone conferences serve to monitor progress, answer parent questions, maintain interest, and reinforce the child and parent. Training consists of familiarizing the parent with the child's treatment program, training the parent how to identify and record articulation errors, explaining the five-step carryover program, and training the parent in how to maintain and record data for each home practice session. Results of a pilot study using the program with six subjects showed it to be effective in generalization of correct articulation patterns to other speaking situations as reported by parents, teachers, and speech-language clinicians. It is assumed that this program is effective because home assignments are clearly defined, length of home sessions is specifically prescribed for frequent intervals, realistic achievable objectives are specified, results are recorded daily, and periodic telephone contacts with the parents occur. Similar programs could be developed using other forms of communication such as e-mail and involving siblings, aides, classmates, older students, or other key persons in the client's environment. A critical element involves the clinician and parents, siblings, or key person working together to determine the roles that each will play in a carryover program because not all have the neces-

sary time, desire, or skills to implement it effectively.

A slightly different approach was used by Fudala, England, and Ganoug (1972). No specific training was done with the parents, but they attended and observed their children's clinical sessions. The children whose mothers attended made greater gains in articulation skills than those whose mothers did not attend. The teachers reported similar results. Principals and teachers, as well as parents, expressed overwhelming approval of the program. They noted benefits in areas other than speech. The results show that parents can be involved effectively with a minimum of extra clinician effort.

A simple, clearly written program was devised by Carrier (1970) to be implemented by parents after clients learned to imitate the speech-language pathologist producing the target sound in isolation. Mothers participating in the study effectively administered the program, and at the end of the program the clients were beginning to use the standard sound in conversation. Carrier believed that it was successful because the speech tasks were simple and clearly stated.

Another program has been devised to transfer correct articulation responses to the client's everyday environment after the clinician teaches the target sound in words (Shelton et al., 1972; Shelton, Johnson, Willis, & Arndt, 1975). Parents are trained to make auditory discriminations between sounds. For 3 consecutive days, the parent elicits 10 different words from the child. Then, 30 different words are elicited in conversational speech for a period of 4 weeks. Correct responses are positively reinforced, corrective feedback is given for incorrect responses, and all responses are tracked. The procedure was found to be somewhat, but not totally, effective with preschool and school-aged children.

Peers and older students have also been used to aid with carryover. Marquardt (1959) was one of the first to report on the effectiveness of speech pals. A classmate who has normal articulation is selected to be a client's speech pal and attends the speech sessions with the client once a week. After the clinician determines that the classmate can effectively assist the client and after a conference, the speech pal helps the client practice speech while reading and conversing outside the clinic 15 minutes per day. The parents of the client and of the speech pal, principal, and teachers should approve of the plan before it is implemented. The rationale of the procedure is that peers are powerful reinforcers. Marquardt reported that the procedure is quite effective in achieving carryover.

In addition to classmates, older students in the school can serve as speech pals. Mowrer (1971) also has suggested using peers, but cautions that they must be trained by the speech-language pathologist in order for the procedure to be effective. The peer is trained to discriminate between correct and incorrect productions and to reinforce the client. Also, often it is effective to provide consequences to the peer for the client's performance, for example, to award the peer points for correct productions and take away points for incorrect productions. In this way, the peer has a vested interest in the client's performance and progress. Kalash (1970) devised a procedure in which he spoke to the classrooms of clients and informed them about the client's speech goals and that they could assist by listening for correct sound productions. When they heard enough correct productions from the client, the whole class was rewarded for the client's success. The technique had varying degrees of success for the subjects in his study, but it was quite effective for some of them. From their research, Johnston and Johnston (1972) concluded that peers function well as discriminative stimuli for correct articulation. Two clients were taught to monitor correct and incorrect speech sounds of each other. This monitoring continued in the classroom even when reinforcement was not provided for doing so. Conley (1966) used a procedure in which classroom peers were brought to clinical sessions to listen to the client tell stories. Peers and clients alike were rewarded for the client's correct productions. Because the client had daily contact with these peers, carryover was enhanced. It appears then that peers can be a valuable resource in the carryover process.

MEASURING CARRYOVER

An inherent problem with the final phase of articulation treatment is how to determine whether carryover has been achieved because it is not feasible for the speech-language pathologist to evaluate the client's articulation in all speaking situations (Irwin & Weston, 1975; Johnson, Winney, & Pederson, 1980; Manning et al., 1976). Additionally, the presence of the clinician in various outside speaking environments may serve as a stimulus for the client to use the target sound, whereas the client may use misarticulations when the clinician is not present. Thus, speech observed by the clinician may not be representative. No universal systematic procedure for measuring carryover has been developed. However, it might be helpful to clarify the client's progress by differentiating among three types of generalization and evaluating articulation performance for each type (Costello & Bosler, 1976):

- Intra-therapy generalization occurs within the treatment program in that correct articulation generalizes to different stimuli; for example, in different word positions, levels of production, different stimulus conditions, and different words.
- Carryover is generalization from treatment to spontaneous speech in the clinic.
- Extra-therapy generalization occurs outside the treatment setting in that correct articulation generalizes to different environments.

Often articulation production is evaluated only in the clinical setting, yet accurate evaluation of spontaneous speech within the clinic and outside the clinic is important in determining when to dismiss a client (Manning et al., 1976).

One way to determine whether automatization of articulation production has been achieved is to use an auditory masking procedure (Manning et al., 1976). The accuracy of a client's speech production produced in noisy conditions is measured. The rationale for this procedure is based on Van Riper's theory (Van Riper & Erickson, 1996) that if a person correctly produces words without auditory feedback, the articulation movements are relatively stable. It was thus hypothesized that if correct articulation occurs in the presence of auditory masking, articulation movements have become automatic, but if the masking disrupts correct production, automatization has not yet been achieved. Because auditory masking appears to result in making more accurate estimates of automatization than testing carryover without masking noise, more research needs to be conducted.

Costello and Bosler (1976) took another approach. They trained mothers of children with articulatory disorders to administer a home treatment program. Extra-therapy generalization was measured in the clinical environment because treatment was conducted in the home. The clients were tested on 25 words (20 used in training plus five new words) in four situations:

- Mother and client in a small clinic room
- Experimenter and client in a small clinic room
- Experimenter and client in a large classroom
- A different experimenter and client in the waiting room on a couch

The results did not differ in these four situations, suggesting that the physical dimensions of the evaluation situation do not seem to influence the client's articulatory performance. Although Costello and

Bosler (1976) did evaluate extra-therapy generalization, they did not assess carryover of correct articulation into spontaneous speech.

Much more research needs to be done to determine how to evaluate efficiently and accurately articulation proficiency in spontaneous speech in all situations. In the meantime, to evaluate carryover, one needs to assess the client's articulation proficiencies in spontaneous speech both inside and outside the clinical setting. Winitz (1975) suggested weekly or biweekly probes of 5 to 10 minutes of conversational speech done when the client is achieving some success in words and phrases. This should be done inside and outside the clinical setting. The speech-language pathologist records the percentage of correct productions to track the progress for intra-therapy generalization and carryover. Sometimes, parents, siblings, classroom teachers, aides, and classmates can be trained to be accurate evaluators and to report progress to the clinician. Another way to evaluate articulation carryover is for a clinician not known to the client to interact and assess the client's spontaneous speech in various settings. Additionally, the clinician can unobtrusively observe the client in any of a variety of settings; for example, in the classroom, on the playground, in the lunchroom, with the mother in the clinic room, with friends outside the clinic room, and at home. It is important to be accurate in the assessment of carryover to determine when to dismiss the client. The final test is consistently correct production of the target sound in rapid speech under somewhat stressful or emotional conditions when attention is directed to the meaning of what is being said rather than to the mechanics of articulation.

The measurement of articulation carryover traditionally consists of the percentage of correct production of the target sound in a sample of conversational speech, either in a certain time frame such as 3, 5, or 10 minutes or on a certain number of occurrences in a sample, such as 10, 25, 50, or 100 instances. Another measurement of articulation proficiency is whole word accuracy, or WWA (McCabe & Bradley, 1975; Schmitt, Howard, & Schmitt, 1983). WWA is the percentage of words in conversation that are free of phonemic errors. This is a measurement often used to determine general proficiency in conversational speech in addition to measuring the accuracy of individual phonemes in spontaneous speech.

As has been indicated, research results are rather sparse on the topic of the carryover process. Clinicians must collect data on their clients to provide more insight into transfer and maintenance of sound production.

SUMMARY

Four structural modes used for articulation/phonological treatment sessions have been identified, including drill, drill play, structured play, and play. Each mode may be useful at some point during the treatment process depending upon several factors. Research results show the drill and drill play modes to be more effective and efficient. Elicitation of speech sounds is often difficult, but general procedures are effective for elicitation of speech sounds, such as modeling, using a mirror, tactile-kinesthetic cues, modification of nontarget sounds, visual illustration, visual cues, auditory cues, facilitating phonetic contexts, verbal instructions, and shaping. It can also be difficult to transfer isolated sound production into syllables and words. Fortunately, there are techniques to assist with such transfer. Two types of generalization or transfer are stimulus and response generalization, and both are involved in carryover. In articulation/phonological intervention, treatment is designed for transfer to phonemic and situational contexts. Many client-related and program-related factors seem to influence the success of carryover, and there is great individual variability in achievement of carryover. Several in-clinic and out-of-clinic strategies have been used by clinicians, with varying degrees of effectiveness. Various methods are used for determining whether carryover has been achieved, although clinicians and researchers experience difficulty in measuring carryover.

REVIEW QUESTIONS

1. Compare and contrast each of four structural modes of articulation/phonological treatment: *drill, drill play, structured play,* and *play.*

2. Under what circumstances would you as a clinician use each of four structural modes?

3. What are 10 general techniques for eliciting isolated speech sound production? Briefly describe each technique and provide one example for each.

4. Describe three techniques that can be used to transfer correct isolated speech sound production into syllable or word contexts.

5. What is meant by the terms *carryover, transfer, generalization,* and *maintenance*?

6. Identify and describe two primary types of generalization.

7. Identify four types of phonemic context generalization and provide an example of each.

8. Identify four types of situational context generalization and provide an example of each.

9. Why is it important to probe various types of transfer throughout the course of treatment?

10. How do distinctive feature and phonological process treatment approaches rely upon transfer of the target phoneme to other phonemic contexts?

11. What do research findings indicate about automatic generalization in untrained contexts?

12. What is the clinician's role in maintenance?

13. What are some potential influencing factors on carryover?

14. What are some possible reasons why carryover would not occur?

15. List some guidelines that may assist in successful carryover.

16. What are advantages to in-clinic activities as opposed to extra-clinic activities? Of extra-clinic activities?

17. Describe some in-clinic strategies for facilitating carryover.

18. Describe some extra-clinic strategies for facilitating carryover.

19. How can clinicians determine whether carryover has been achieved? What are some inherent problems in measuring it?

International Phonetic Alphabet (revised to 1993, updated 1996)

APPENDIX A

THE INTERNATIONAL PHONETIC ALPHABET (revised to 1993)

CONSONANTS (PULMONIC)

	Bilabial	Labiodental	Dental	Alveolar	Postalveolar	Retroflex	Palatal	Velar	Uvular	Pharyngeal	Glottal
Plosive	p b			t d		ʈ ɖ	c ɟ	k ɡ	q ɢ		ʔ
Nasal	m	ɱ		n		ɳ	ɲ	ŋ	ɴ		
Trill	ʙ			r					ʀ		
Tap or Flap				ɾ		ɽ					
Fricative	ɸ β	f v	θ ð	s z	ʃ ʒ	ʂ ʐ	ç ʝ	x ɣ	χ ʁ	ħ ʕ	h ɦ
Lateral fricative				ɬ ɮ							
Approximant		ʋ		ɹ		ɻ	j	ɰ			
Lateral approximant				l		ɭ	ʎ	ʟ			

Where symbols appear in pairs, the one to the right represents a voiced consonant. Shaded areas denote articulations judged impossible.

CONSONANTS (NON-PULMONIC)

Clicks		Voiced implosives		Ejectives	
ʘ	Bilabial	ɓ	Bilabial	ʼ	as in:
|	Dental	ɗ	Dental/alveolar	pʼ	Bilabial
!	(Post)alveolar	ʄ	Palatal	tʼ	Dental/alveolar
ǂ	Palatoalveolar	ɠ	Velar	kʼ	Velar
‖	Alveolar lateral	ʛ	Uvular	sʼ	Alveolar fricative

VOWELS

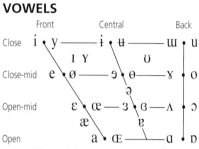

Where symbols appear in pairs, the one to the right represents a rounded vowel.

SUPRASEGMENTALS

ˈ	Primary stress	ˌfoʊnəˈtɪʃən
ˌ	Secondary stress	
ː	Long	eː
ˑ	Half-long	eˑ
˘	Extra-short	ĕ
.	Syllable break	ɹi.ækt
|	Minor (foot) group	
‖	Major (intonation) group	
‿	Linking (absence of a break)	

TONES & WORD ACCENTS

LEVEL		CONTOUR	
e̋ or ˥	Extra high	ě or ˩˥	Rising
é or ˦	High	ê or ˥˩	Falling
ē or ˧	Mid	e᷄ or ˦˥	High rising
è or ˨	Low	e᷅ or ˩˨	Low rising
ȅ or ˩	Extra low	e᷈ or ˧˦˧	Rising-falling
↓ Downstep		↗ Global rise	etc.
↑ Upstep		↘ Global fall	

DIACRITICS   Diacritics may be placed above a symbol with a descender, e.g. ŋ̊

ₒ	Voiceless	n̥ d̥	̈	Breathy voiced	b̤ a̤	̪	Dental	t̪ d̪
ᵥ	Voiced	s̬ t̬	̰	Creaky voiced	b̰ a̰	̺	Apical	t̺ d̺
ʰ	Aspirated	tʰ dʰ	̼	Linguolabial	t̼ d̼	̻	Laminal	t̻ d̻
̹	More rounded	ɔ̹	ʷ	Labialized	tʷ dʷ	̃	Nasalized	ẽ
̜	Less rounded	ɔ̜	ʲ	Palatalized	tʲ dʲ	ⁿ	Nasal release	dⁿ
₊	Advanced	u̟	ˠ	Velarized	tˠ dˠ	ˡ	Lateral release	dˡ
̠	Retracted	i̠	ˤ	Pharyngealized	tˤ dˤ	̚	No audible release	d̚
̈	Centralized	ë	̴	Velarized or pharyngealized	ɫ			
̽	Mid-centralized	ě	̝	Raised	e̝ (ɹ̝ = voiced alveolar fricative)			
̩	Syllabic	ɹ̩	̞	Lowered	e̞ (β̞ = voiced bilabial approximant)			
̯	Non-syllabic	e̯	̘	Advanced Tongue Root	e̘			
˞	Rhoticity	ɚ	̙	Retracted Tongue Root	e̙			

OTHER SYMBOLS

ʍ   Voiceless labial-velar fricative

w   Voiced labial-velar approximant

ɥ   Voiced labial-palatal approximant

ʜ   Voiceless epiglottal fricative

ʢ   Voiced epiglottal fricative

ʡ   Epiglottal plosive

ɕ ʑ   Alveolo-palatal fricatives

ɺ   Alveolar lateral flap

ɧ   Simultaneous ʃ and x

Affricates and double articulations can be represented by two symbols joined by a tie bar if necessary.

k͡p t͡s

Traditional Distinctive Features System (Drexler, 1976)

Syllable Releasing (Initial) Position

	Vowel	Nasal	Glide	Liquid	Lateral	Stop	Fricative	Affricative	Strident	Voiced	Labial	Dental	Alveolar	Palatal	Velar	Glottal
p						+					+					
b						+				+	+					
t						+							+			
d						+				+			+			
k						+									+	
g						+				+					+	
m		+								+	+					
n		+								+			+			
ŋ																
w			+							+	+					
j			+							+				+		
l				+	+					+			+			
r				+						+				+		
f							+		+		+					
v							+		+	+	+					
θ							+					+				
ð							+			+		+				
s							+		+				+			
z							+		+	+			+			
ʃ							+		+					+		
ʒ																
h							+									+
tʃ						+	+	+	+					+		
dʒ						+	+	+	+	+				+		

Note: The empty boxes indicate that the phoneme has a (−) feature.

Syllable Arresting (Final) Position

	Vowel	Nasal	Glide	Liquid	Lateral	Stop	Fricative	Affricative	Strident	Voiced	Labial	Dental	Alveolar	Palatal	Velar	Glottal
p						+					+					
b						+				+	+					
t						+							+			
d						+				+			+			
k						+									+	
g						+				+					+	
m		+								+	+					
n		+								+			+			
ŋ		+								+					+	
w			+							+						
j			+							+				+		
l	+			+	+					+			+			
ɝ, ɚ	+			+						+						
f							+		+		+					
v							+		+	+	+					
θ							+					+				
ð							+			+		+				
s							+		+				+			
z							+		+	+			+			
ʃ							+		+					+		
ʒ							+		+	+				+		
h							+									+
tʃ						+	+	+	+					+		
dʒ						+	+	+	+	+				+		

Note: The empty boxes indicate that the phoneme has a (−) feature.

From Drexler, H. (1976). A simplified application of distinctive feature analysis to articulation therapy. *Journal of the Oregon Speech and Hearing Association, 15*, 2–5. Adapted with permission.

Percentages of Responses Considered "Acceptable" in Single-Word Productions (Data from Smit et al., 1990)

APPENDIX C1

Percentages of Responses Considered "Acceptable" in Single-Word Productions (Data from Smit et al., 1990)

	3:0		3:6		4:0		4:6		5:0		5:6		6:0		7:0	8:0	9:0
	F	M	F	M	F	M	F	M	F	M	F	M	F	M	F/M	F/M	F/M
m	90	95	99	99	96	99	99	99	100	98	98	99	99	95	99	97	98
n	81	93	100	96	94	96	99	94	98	97	100	99	99	95	99	98	99
ŋ	50	72	69	66	70	70	73	66	73	72	82	72	81	75	72	82	88
h	98	90	96	100	96	94	99	98	100	100	100	100	100	99	100	100	100
w	100	94	96	100	99	97	100	99	100	100	100	100	100	99	100	100	100
j	59	68	77	93	95	81	92	84	93	92	100	96	97	94	99	99	100
p	94	92	99	99	98	97	98	99	99	93	100	98	97	98	98	99	98
b	96	97	97	99	99	97	99	97	100	99	100	100	100	99	100	100	100
t	88	82	85	86	93	95	93	96	90	94	93	93	95	92	96	97	96
d	95	91	98	98	98	98	99	99	100	98	100	99	99	98	99	99	100
k	85	86	93	91	100	94	98	97	99	95	100	99	100	99	99	99	100
g	82	85	90	88	98	93	96	95	88	97	97	98	98	96	97	98	99
f	84	68	85	90	91	86	88	92	89	92	97	96	96	94	98	99	100
v	52	54	58	66	82	74	90	78	89	85	95	94	96	92	97	99	99
θ	29	29	52	41	59	46	68	53	71	55	80	69	92	78	91	97	99

Age Levels (Years: Months)

(continued)

APPENDIX C1 (Continued)

Percentages of Responses Considered "Acceptable" in Single-Word Productions (Smit et al., 1990)

	3:0		3:6		4:0		4:6		5:0		5:6		6:0		7:0	8:0	9:0
	F	M	F	M	F	M	F	M	F	M	F	M	F	M	F/M	F/M	F/M
ð	32	20	58	52	76	43	90	64	91	74	98	87	97	83	96	100	100
s	76	47	77	77	71	68	76	70	83	79	79	68	88	79	83	84	90
z	46	40	60	54	57	61	64	67	76	67	73	63	83	75	80	83	89
ʃ	67	44	73	69	87	70	85	73	85	87	86	82	90	88	94	93	98
tʃ	65	40	68	67	79	72	87	76	86	87	90	83	92	89	92	96	97
dʒ	65	48	76	70	78	75	87	77	86	85	88	86	91	88	94	96	96
l-	77	36	79	69	82	58	86	75	93	74	94	86	98	96	97	98	100
-l	36	16	54	39	52	48	74	52	63	65	83	72	89	76	90	95	98
-l-	59	28	73	72	84	69	80	73	87	78	91	87	94	90	95	94	99
r-	25	26	46	52	62	56	67	47	63	71	69	78	79	76	87	92	96
ɚ	45	43	61	68	85	68	71	61	74	84	76	81	85	82	86	96	97
-r-	45	36	46	55	70	54	71	59	71	70	71	79	79	76	87	95	97

Age Levels (Years: Months)

Note: Phonemes were produced in initial and final positions in single words unless otherwise noted.

Data from Smit, A. B., Hand, L., Freilinger, J. J., Bernthal, J. E., & Bird, A. (1990). The Iowa articulation norms project and its Nebraska replication. *Journal of Speech and Hearing Disorders, 55*, 779–798.

Percentage of Correct Usage of Consonants by Age (Irwin & Wong, 1983)

Phonemes	Age (years)				
	1.5	2	3	4	5
/k/	47	71	98	97	100
/g/	49	71	94	99	97
/t/	36	55	98	89	99
/d/	64	64	99	68	77
/p/	56	66	99	98	99
/b/	90	97	100	95	99
/f/	67	65	97	99	100
/v/	13	7	96	76	83
/θ/	0	2	49	81	78
/ð/	5	1	40	64	65
/s/	8	54	98	87	93
/z/	1	33	98	89	94
/ʃ/	2	43	99	95	87
/ʒ/	—	—	100	—	—
/tʃ/	22	35	97	74	100
/dʒ/	9	53	96	75	83
/m/	84	97	100	99	100
/n/	63	75	100	98	99
/ŋ/	3	74	96	46	57
/l/	4	27	93	85	95
/r/	2	20	89	81	82
/h/	68	78	100	97	91
/w/	63	94	100	99	99
/j/	71	55	99	95	98
/ʔ/	—	—	—	—	—
Total	50	63	93	88	92

From Irwin, J., & Wong, S. (1983). *Phonological development in children 16 to 72 months (p. 159)*. Carbondale, IL: Southern Illinois University Press, (p. 159). Reprinted with permission.

Case History Information

QUESTIONNAIRE

The questionnaire is an effective tool for obtaining background information in a relatively short amount of time. It is highly structured and can be used to obtain considerable data from several persons at the same time and provide a record of the information for future reference. It is also a flexible tool—its thoroughness can be modified to address individual needs and specific areas can be stressed and others deleted. The questionnaire can be used as a guide for the oral interview or as a supplement to the oral interview. It can also be completed in advance of diagnostic testing, giving the informant time to think about or research the answers before coming in for the interview and evaluation. Contents generally include any or all of the following: identifying information; statement of the problem; general development; and medical, dental, educational, communication, environmental, social, and daily history.

As with other approaches, the questionnaire has disadvantages, including the possibility that informants may misinterpret the questions, report incompletely or give answers that "sound" best, answer the questions superficially, not answer all of the questions, and assign equal weight to each question because it appeared on the questionnaire. Nevertheless, as a supplement to observing, interviewing, and testing, the questionnaire can provide helpful information. Also, the questionnaire should be accompanied with a release of information form to be signed and returned to the diagnostician. This will help to ensure that human rights are protected.

AUTOBIOGRAPHY

Perhaps less commonly used is the autobiography. It can be very helpful, however, with more severe problems. It can be a narrative or an oral account, depending on the age and abilities of the client. The advantages of a written account include providing a sample of the client's language skills and allowing as much time as necessary for the client to think about the contents. Written accounts provide insights into how clients think and feel about themselves in particular and about life in general. These revelations of self, others, and the world can be helpful in forming accurate concepts of the client. The autobiography can have remedial as well as diagnostic value. Because of the time involved, the autobiography is not routinely used, depending, of course, on the individual problem. Many clients also do not have the skill or the will to write anything that may be significant.

OBSERVATIONS

Many different kinds of observations may be used to collect significant information about the client, family, and home environment. They include *spectator* observation, *participant* observation, and *other informant* observation. Spectator observation usually includes the diagnostician or other invited person observing the client through a one-way window. This method occurs without the client's awareness of being observed and is used in situations in which the client interacts with other children, adults, family members, or others. A good observer documents details, discrepancies between reports and observed behavior, range of behaviors, and various interactions. These observations can be made without influencing or affecting the client's behavior because of the absence of the diagnostician. However, a setting using a one-way observation window is usually somewhat artificial and thus may have inherent limitations and obvious effects on the client's typical behavior.

Participant observation, on the other hand, may preclude typical behavior by the client because of the presence of the diagnostician. This situation can be more structured to obtain more pertinent samples of behavior. The behavior of the client naturally will be affected by the type of rapport previously established and reactions to the presence of the diagnostician. Whether or not a separate situation needs to be established solely for the purpose of having some other informant observe is debatable. After all, the diagnostician is observing and interacting with the client during formal and informal testing procedures. Part of the testing situation is observation of the client's interaction, especially during the less formal activities. Observational data of other observers should be compared, consolidated, and interpreted with other existing information. Observations, including home visitations, are among the most important methods of obtaining needed information about children with communication disorders.

OTHER CLINICAL RECORDS

Medical, dental, communication, educational, psychosocial, nutritional, and other data can provide much needed additional information about the client. Information about illnesses, diseases, tests, hospitalizations, surgeries, and medical treatment can reveal valuable information about the client's communication disorder and potential causes, age of onset, communication intervention procedures, and prognosis. Similarly, dental, educational, nutritional, and other records about the client's historical development should be explored and considered in diagnosis and treatment. Each piece of information helps to complete the historical puzzle of the client. Time spent in obtaining historical and other diagnostic data will greatly facilitate diagnostic and remedial procedures.

With this basic foundation of how background information may be gathered, let us proceed to look at the information that should be collected. The type and extent of necessary information will vary with the age of the client, type of disorder, severity of disorder, age of onset, and other factors. An individualistic approach certainly must be practiced during this phase of clinical management.

AREAS TO ADDRESS

It is helpful to address several areas relative to case history information. Open-ended, general questions and more specific questions can be used to gather needed information. The questions presented below address gathering specific information, but more open-ended questions can also elicit the desired information.

Communication Information

The most important clinical records to a speech-language pathologist are those pertaining to communication. Some basic questions that might be asked include:

1. Excluding crying, was the client a quiet, average, or very vocal infant?
2. What sounds did the client make during the first year? Examples include cooing, gurgling, babbling, pitch inflection, and attempts to imitate sounds of parents.
3. When were the first words, other than "Mommy" and "Daddy," spoken? What were they?
4. Were words added regularly thereafter?
5. When did naming people and objects begin?
6. When did two-word combinations begin to appear?
7. Were the words easy or difficult to understand?
8. Does the client tend to use speech or gestures?
9. Did struggle behavior accompany the speech efforts?
10. Has any progress occurred in the client's speech during the last 6 months?
11. Has the client's speech ever been better than it is now? If so, in what way and when did it change?
12. What percentage of the time is the client understood by other members of the family? By persons who are not often around the client?
13. Is the client aware of a speech difference? If so, how is this awareness shown?
14. Does the speech cause the client to show concern about it?
15. At what age was the client first believed to have an articulatory disorder? By whom?
16. What is the parents' estimate of severity of the speech problem?
17. Have family members or others called attention to the speech problem? If so, in what way?
18. What has been done to help the client talk better?

19. Has the client's speech ever been evaluated? If so, when and by whom?
20. Was speech treatment ever provided? If so, when, how long, for what, and with what degree of success? Who was the clinician?
21. Do other family members have speech problems? Who? What kind?

These questions are directed at some of the information that should be pursued. The list certainly is not exhaustive, but it should provide a core of basic information about communication development. Most of this information must come from parents, but a school speech-language clinician or teacher can also provide some of it.

Hearing Information

Also important to articulation is information pertaining to hearing. Some questions that might be asked include:

1. During the first year of life, did the client startle; blink; turn to search for sound sources; or change immediate activity in response to sudden, loud, or different sounds?
2. Did the client, at a young age, imitate gurgling and cooing sounds or respond to noise-making toys?
3. Did the client respond to his or her own name before 1 year of age?
4. Do people have to raise their voices to get the client's attention?
5. Does the client frequently say "huh" or "what" when someone is speaking?
6. Does the client respond inconsistently to sound?
7. Is the client overly careful to watch the speaker's face?
8. Does the client turn one ear toward the sound source?
9. Does the client consistently talk in an overly soft or overly loud voice?
10. Does hearing ability seem to fluctuate from time to time? If so, how often and to what extent?
11. Does the client have a history of ear infections?
12. Does the client ever complain of his or her ears hurting? How often?
13. Have there been considerable upper respiratory and middle ear infections?
14. Has the client been exposed to considerable loud noise over extended periods?
15. Does the client ever complain of ringing in the ear, dizziness, or nausea? How often?
16. Has there been treatment for otitis media (middle ear infection)? If so, how often and what kind?
17. Did the mother of the client have any problems during pregnancy, such as rubella or Rh blood type incompatibility?
18. Is there a familial history of hearing problems? If so, who, what kind, and what degree of severity was involved?

These and other questions should be asked to determine whether the client has or has had significant hearing problems. Parents usually can provide most of this information, but the client's teacher, speech clinician, clinic records, and family physician may be very helpful.

Developmental Information

Some of the more typical questions that relate to developmental landmarks are:

1. When did the client:
   a. First hold up his head?
   b. First roll over?
   c. First crawl?
   d. First sit without support?
   e. First pull self to a standing position?
   f. Get his first tooth?
   g. First walk unaided?
   h. Gain bowel control?
   i. Gain bladder control?
   j. Dress self?
   k. Feed self?
2. What is/was the client's:
   a. Birth weight?
   b. Weight at age 6 months?
   c. Weight at age 1 year?
   d. Present weight?
   e. Present height?
3. At what age did the client establish handedness? What is the handedness?
4. Does the client have good balance or lose balance easily? If the latter, in what way and how often?
5. Does the client seem coordinated or does he or she seem awkward and uncoordinated?
6. Does the client have good, average, or poor fine motor coordination?
7. Does the client currently have (or is there a history of) difficulty in chewing or swallowing? If so, how often and how severe?
8. Has the client ever drooled, other than when teething?
9. Does the client have difficulty in moving his or her tongue or lips for speech purposes?
10. Did the client ever walk on his or her toes?

Answers to these questions should assist in determining whether the client had any developmental delay that might explain, at least in part, the reason for the articulatory disorder. The family physician and medical records can help provide this information, but most of it usually will come from the parents.

Medical Information

Medical information includes prenatal, natal, and postnatal history including illnesses, diseases, hospitalizations, surgeries, and medications. Some questions to ask include:

1. Did the mother have any illnesses, accidents, or complications or did she take medications during pregnancy with the client? If so, what kind and to what extent?
2. What was the length of the pregnancy with the client, including the birth weight?
3. What was the duration of the delivery?
4. Were there any complications at birth? Any unusual conditions?
5. Were there any unusual conditions shortly after birth?
6. What diseases or serious injuries has the client had and were there any complications?
7. Has the client ever been hospitalized? If so, why, when, and for how long?
8. Did the client ever suffer a severe head injury or high fever? If so, when, what kind, and what was the severity of the injury or extent of the fever?
9. What is the present condition of the client's health?
10. Does the client have any physical problems? If so, what are they?
11. Is the client receiving any medication or is he or she under medical treatment now? If so, what kind and for what reason?
12. What is the name of the family physician?

This kind of medical information can be helpful in specifying etiology and diagnostic and remedial procedures. It can be obtained in several ways, including questionnaire, medical records, school records, interviews with family physician (in person or by telephone), and interviews with parents and client.

Educational Information

Also important in understanding the totality of the client's problem is the educational information. Some questions to include are:

1. Did the client ever attend a day care center or nursery school? What were his or her strong points? What were some problems, if any?
2. Did the client attend kindergarten? What were his or her strong points? What were some problems, if any?
3. At what age did the client begin school?
4. Was the client ever retained a grade in school? If so, which grade? Why?
5. Did the client ever skip a grade? If so, which one?
6. What is the client's history of school attendance? Explain the reasons for frequent absences, if applicable.
7. What are or were the client's poorest subjects? Best subjects?
8. What grades does or did the client achieve?
9. How does or did the client feel about school and the teachers?
10. Currently, what is the client's grade level? If he or she is out of school, what is the highest grade level the client achieved?
11. Has the client ever attended any special classes or received special instruction? If so, why, when, for how long, where, and what were the results?
12. What are the educational levels of the parents? What are the educational levels and performances of the other siblings?

Educational background information can provide helpful data for better understanding the client and for planning communication treatment for the client. It can be obtained by questionnaire or through interviews with school personnel and parents.

Psychosocial Information

This category includes various interpersonal and personal behaviors, home and family relationships, history and environmental conditions, and other social characteristics. Among the questions that can be asked are:

1. With whom does the client interact? How often? What activities are involved?
2. How does the client relate to others?
3. How does the client get along with others at home?
4. What adjectives best describe the client? Does the client seem to be carefree, nervous, fearful, happy, or unhappy? If so, in what ways?
5. Are there any disciplinary problems? If so, in what settings and under what circumstances do these problems manifest themselves?
6. Are there or have there been problems in eating or sleeping?
7. Is the client overactive? Lethargic?

8. What interests, hobbies, or other activities does the client have?
9. What is the neighborhood like?
10. What are leisure time activities of the family?
11. What are the names, ages, and relationships of other family members, including others living in the same household?
12. What are the occupations of the parents?
13. What are the educational levels of the parents?
14. What is the health of the parents and siblings?
15. What ethnic, social, or other related aspects of the family need to be considered?
16. What other psychosocial information might be helpful in better understanding the client?

Many more questions could be asked regarding the psychosocial aspects of the client. The number and range of questions should be determined individually. Most of this information can be obtained from the parents through interviews, questionnaires, or both, but school records and interviews with teachers are often helpful.

Dental Information

Occasionally, past and present dental information is related to the client's communication problem. However, relating dental history and status to disordered articulation should be done with caution. It might be well to pursue the following questions:

1. Has the client had any unusual dental treatment or oral surgery?
2. Have any dental prostheses ever been worn? If so, did they affect the client's speech? How?
3. Has the client ever undergone orthodontic treatment? If so, for what kind of teeth alignment problem?
4. Has the term *tongue thrust* ever been used in reference to the client? If so, by whom?
5. Are any dental problems present now?
6. Are any other mouth structural deviations present?

Dental information usually can be obtained from the parents. Additional information may be obtained from the client's dentist. A rating scale may be useful in determining whether the particular dental information, or any other specific historical information for that matter, is significantly related to the present speech disorder. The higher the numeric rating, the more likely the dental or other data are relevant to disordered articulation. The following rating scale could be used:

0—Insignificant: The information probably is unrelated to the problem.

1—Possibly significant: The information may be, but probably is not, related to the problem.
2—Mildly significant: The information appears to be related somewhat to the problem and should be considered in managing the client.
3—Significant: The information definitely appears to be related to the problem and must be considered in managing the client.

Nutritional Information

The awareness of the role of nutrition in normal development has increased considerably during the past few years. Its importance should not be overlooked when gathering historical data. Some of the questions that might be included are:

1. What are the nutritional habits in the home? Regularity of meals? Type of diet?
2. What are the parental attitudes toward nutrition?
3. Do the nutritional needs of the client appear to be met? If not, what is lacking?
4. Have the parents ever received nutritional counseling?
5. Does nutrition seem to be related to the client's communication problem? If so, in what way?

The diagnostician should be aware of the potential problems resulting from inappropriate diet and should carefully explore the nutritional habits of the client. Parents must be relied on for most of this kind of information. The nutritionist, school nurse, teacher, and family physician or clinic records may be of help.

Identifying Information

The following information should be collected for future reference and correspondence and for obtaining a more complete idea about the client:

1. Date
2. Name
3. Age
4. Date of birth
5. Gender
6. Address
7. Telephone number
8. Grade level
9. Parents' names and addresses
10. Statement of problem
11. Marital status
12. Occupation
13. Referral source and reason for the referral
14. Name of physician
15. Name of school

Guidelines for Effective Interviewing

BEGINNING THE INTERVIEW

The interview with the client or others should begin with general (open-ended) questions, rather than specific ones. Specificity at the outset can motivate the informant to become passive, rather than active, in responding to interview questions (McNamara, 2002). An appropriate way to begin the interview is by asking why the client came or was brought for an evaluation. Sometimes, a simple "How can I help you today?" can be very effective. In this way, the interviewer releases some control to the interviewee, "leading to increased trust and willingness to share information about sensitive and important issues" (McNamara, 2002, p. 189). Answers to these beginning general questions should guide the diagnostician during the interview and throughout testing.

Establish Mutual Respect

An effective way of establishing an appropriate atmosphere for interviewing is to achieve a feeling of mutual respect. An attitude of mutual concern, genuine sincerity, honesty, acceptance, empathy, and humility can greatly assist the feeling of mutual respect. An open, relaxed setting should be the goal. Attitudes of superiority, rigidity, aloofness, condemnation, and superficiality definitely should be avoided. The interviewer must delve beneath the superficial and routine when asking questions.

Avoid Excessive Probing

Excessive probing in the interview process should be avoided. An in-depth psychoanalytic approach by an unqualified interviewer can cause resentment, defensiveness, and lack of cooperation. The limits on exactly how far to probe to obtain the necessary information seem to be related to the interviewer's clinical knowledge, sensitivity, and experience. No specific rules or guidelines are applicable in every instance. A sense of when to stop and when to proceed further in questioning appears to evolve with experience and with a knowledge of one's own professional and personal limitations. At times, it may be best to stop informants from revealing sensitive, unrelated information that they may later regret having shared. If mutual respect and understanding are not gained at the outset, the interview is in danger of failing.

EXPLAIN THE PURPOSE OF THE INTERVIEW

The informant should be told that many specific questions will be asked for the purpose of achieving a better understanding of the client's problems and potential solutions. It is also helpful to explain the reason for seeking certain information or for asking questions in such detail. The informant should be encouraged to talk freely and openly, and an opportunity should be provided for the informant to ask questions of the interviewer and to interrupt for purposes of clarification. If the informant is convinced that the interview is one of the most important and necessary aspects of the diagnostic work-up, then relevant information will come more easily.

BE A GOOD LISTENER

The importance of good listening is so obvious that mention of it hardly seems necessary. Yet, most of us could benefit from improving our listening skills

(Nichols, 1955). One of the major roadblocks to good listening skills is that some people talk too much (Weiss & Lillywhite, 1981). People overly verbalize for many reasons. They are talk oriented, or they grow up with a fear of being silent in the presence of others—attitudes that can carry over into the interview. Mark Twain wryly observed that we have two ears and only one mouth, and his admonition to listen twice as much as we talk should be remembered and followed in any interview. A good interviewer listens not only to what the informant says but also to what the informant does not say. "Listening between the lines" is an art that comes with much experience. It requires sensitivity, humility, patience, and perceptive listening skills.

ASK QUESTIONS APPROPRIATELY

The interview topics should be pursued in an orderly, sequential way with the interviewer using statements that transition from one topic to another and that may refer back to something the informant previously said. A cardinal rule in any interview is to state the questions carefully. If a binary question is asked, the client will give a binary response. A vague question will probably be answered with a vague response. Likewise, asking leading questions may elicit biased information. For some types of information, open-ended questions are most appropriate while closed questions can be effectively used to elicit specific information, such as age, birth date, number of siblings, and percent of intelligibility. It may also be helpful to provide a range of possible answers such as numbers and percentages or degrees ranging from never to always or from mild to very severe. In any case, the interviewer should understand why a particular question is being asked. A student diagnostician once asked an adult who stuttered to tell about his birth and state when he said his first word. Although the intent may have been good, the questions were inappropriate for this particular informant/client.

Effective questioning implies well-stated and specific sentences, an understandable vocabulary, and possible examples of answers being searched for. Avoid technical jargon whenever possible and define or give examples of technical terms that cannot be avoided unless it is clear that the informant is familiar with this type of terminology. Carefully worded questions can be effectively used to encourage the listener to elaborate on the answer, to invite participation, and to develop an attitude of being fully involved in a search for a solution to the problem. This may be done by prefacing the questions with such phrases as, "Do you think it might be . . . ?," "Is it possible that . . . ?," and "I wonder if it could have been . . . ?" Although blunt, direct questions may sometimes be necessary in the interview, the interviewer should be aware that such an approach can limit information and possibly result in the informant becoming nonresponsive.

MINIMIZE ANXIETY

Even though anxiety in interviews cannot always be avoided, it can be minimized. The interviewer should assume that the informant has some concerns and that these concerns frequently are accompanied by anxiety. Rapport, relaxed environment, understanding, and arranging the interview sequence so that it progresses from low to high emotional content can limit the informant's level of anxiety. An empathic attitude by the interviewer can also help to minimize the anxiety of the informant.

CONDUCT AN EFFICIENT INTERVIEW

Efficiency in interviewing can be achieved in several ways: by phrasing questions economically, avoiding unnecessary verbal digression and editorializing, asking relevant questions, preparing and individualizing many of the interview questions in advance, and guiding the informant back to the original question in the event digression occurs. The rate at which questions are asked is also important. The interviewer should not tarry, spend unnecessary time rephrasing and clarifying questions, pause excessively, or slow the speaking to an exaggerated rate to improve the eloquence and preciseness of articulation. For best results, the rate of questions and comments should be geared to the interviewer's perceptions of the informant's ability to receive and process verbal messages.

MAINTAIN EYE CONTACT

The interviewer should not only look at the informant, but should also be interested, sincere, and understanding. Eye contact is especially important during moments when tension, emotion, and guilt are related by the informant. To look away or to look at the informant too intently at these times could be misinterpreted as negative judgments of the informant's behavior and may cause embarrassment, uneasiness, or lack of interest. Intermittent, natural eye contact should be maintained for fostering effective communication and interaction and should always be practiced in interviews.

TAKE NOTES DURING THE INTERVIEW

Because of the vast amount of information that can be conveyed during an interview, it is wise to take notes. Develop some system of shorthand; otherwise, it will be impossible to write down the important points shared by the informant. If too much time is spent in writing, however, eye contact and rapport potentially may suffer. If necessary, the informant should be asked to repeat an answer, but the number of times repetition is requested should be limited. Another approach may be to record the interview on audiotape or videotape, provided the informant has no objection. The presence of a tape recorder can sometimes thwart open communication and curtail the sharing of valuable, personal information by some informants, although most persons tend to adjust readily to it. Discretion should be used regarding the extent of note taking and whether or not to record the interaction, but some degree of documenting should always occur.

ASK PERSONAL QUESTIONS IN A STRAIGHTFORWARD MANNER

If the informant has been told the reasons why he or she will be asked a range of casual and personal questions, there should be no problem. Personal questions should be asked matter-of-factly and directly. If the interviewer seems awkward, evasive, and uneasy in asking the questions, the interviewee may likewise feel uncomfortable. The interviewer must be certain about the need for certain questions to be asked and must be able to explain or justify their importance in obtaining the requested information. Sometimes, questions are asked without sufficient reason or a clear understanding as to why they are being asked (Emerick & Hatten, 1986). If the information being requested does not relate to the overall management of the client, obtaining it may not be necessary.

USE TACT IN EMOTIONAL SITUATIONS

Not uncommonly during an interview, some questions may relate to very emotional, personal experiences or may trigger memories of sorrowful or overwhelming experiences. Such questions can elicit unexpected emotional behavior. Apologizing in such situations is not necessary, but patience and understanding are. Usually after a moment or two, the informant will regain composure and the interview can proceed, though perhaps in a somewhat different direction. If emotionality persists, the interviewer may express understanding (empathy), may excuse himself or herself from the room for a little while, or can seek other (hopefully less emotional) information. The interviewer should be careful not to express disapproval, show embarrassment, or exhibit other emotional reactions.

PROBE SUPERFICIAL RESPONSES

Occasionally, an informant will provide a cursory or superficial answer to an important question. For example, the interviewer may ask what activities have been employed in the home to help the child learn to talk. Supposing the response to this question is "nothing," the response should be pursued by providing ideas of what some teaching activities could be before probing the original, superficial answer. It may be necessary to rephrase the question. Curt responses by the informant may indicate a lack of understanding of the question or a lack of awareness of the subject or its importance. Answers to important questions should be pursued to the interviewer's satisfaction, but specific points or topics should not be belabored.

CLARIFY DISCREPANCIES

It is entirely possible that discrepancies (or what appear to be discrepancies) will be observed. These should be clarified before the interview is concluded. The apparent discrepancy may be a misunderstanding either by the informant or by the interviewer and may indicate uncertainty, ambivalence, confusion, or untruthfulness. In any event, clarification should be sought, if not to get a better understanding of the client's history, then to get a better understanding of the informant if it is someone other than the client. Whatever the reason, it is important not to reach conclusions prematurely or to pass judgments hastily.

ASK FOR INTERPRETATION OF INFORMATION

In addition to clarifying answers, it may also be necessary to seek interpretations. How does the informant perceive the different events? By asking, "Can you give an example of that?" or "What do you mean?," "How do you feel about that?," and "How do you see the problem?," the diagnostician can obtain significant interpretations. Not all information should be accepted at face value; some interpretations are occasionally more revealing and more valuable than the actual statement that preceded them.

KEEP THE PURPOSE IN MIND

At all times, the purpose of the interview should be clear: to obtain the information necessary for better understanding the client, the etiology, and the possible treatment and management procedures that will be most effective. An interview is not primarily for venting feelings; neither is it intended to be therapeutic, although both of these functions may occur. The goal of obtaining answers to relevant questions should be accomplished by keeping the interview on course. Additional needs of the informant can be dealt with at another time and place. It sometimes may be necessary, however, to let the informant express strong feelings before getting back to the purpose of the interview.

ANSWER QUESTIONS

The informant should be encouraged to ask questions during the interview. The interviewer should be prepared for questions and should answer them as accurately as possible. If the interviewer does not know the answer, the informant should be told that the answer will be found and provided at a later time. Situations should be handled honestly. If the answer to a question might jeopardize the interviewer–interviewee relationship, the answer should be deferred to another person or held for another time. Most questions can usually be answered at the time they are asked, provided the diagnostician is knowledgeable. Also, when a response is an opinion, a personal bias, or something other than fact, this should be indicated. It is generally a good idea to terminate the interview by asking the informant whether he or she has any additional questions.

BE AWARE OF POSSIBLE LANGUAGE OR CLASS DIFFERENCES

It is important to remember that language, social level, education, occupation, and other differences may exist between the interviewer and the interviewee. These differences tend to be more obvious when the informant and interviewer come from different ethnic, social, or age groups. The competent interviewer recognizes possibilities for misunderstanding in these situations and adjusts quickly to them by using language and other behaviors appropriate to the situation. Less obvious barriers to communication may exist even when there are no clear ethnic, age, or social differences. In these situations, both parties are likely to assume that they "speak the same language"; that is, that their concepts of the problem and of each other are accurate. Such assumptions are rarely accurate, and as a consequence, the interview may proceed with many false assumptions and inaccurate interpretations being made. In any case, whether or not the differences are obvious, the responsibility lies with the interviewer to interpret concepts and understandings as accurately as possible and to use language that is subject to minimal misunderstanding; in other words, to see that the "map–territory" relationships of the situation are as accurate as they can be (Weiss & Lillywhite, 1976). The interviewer should ensure that the relationships between the word map (verbal representation of a message) that an individual tries to draw and the territory (information, thoughts, ideas, opinions, and feelings) that the map is supposed to represent are compatible.

TERMINATE THE INTERVIEW EFFECTIVELY

This step of the interview is not always easy to achieve. The interview should be concluded with an expression of appreciation and thanks toward the informant for cooperating and providing helpful information. If additional information comes to mind or if other questions arise later, subsequent communication should be encouraged. It should be explained that the overall findings and impressions about the client will be discussed with the informant following diagnostic testing and interpretation. The timetable of events should be indicated at the close of the interview. If important information was not available at the time of the interview, the informant should be asked to provide it, by telephone or other means, as soon as it can be located (Emerick & Hatten, 1986). Sometimes, it is beneficial to ask a parent to bring to the interview a baby book or other source of documented information. Also, the informant should sign a release of information form when information is being requested from another source or when information from the diagnostic work-up is being sent elsewhere.

Practicing these guidelines will help to ensure an effective interview. In addition, the diagnostician must be careful not to provide information too soon in the interview. It is also important to remember that methods other than the oral interview are available to the diagnostician, some of which are discussed in Appendix D.

Short Test of Sound Discrimination

EXAMPLES

te–de ere–ere os–og

A	B	C	D
1. te–te	1. ne–ne	1. fo–θo	1. pe–ke
2. hwe–we	2. dʒe–tʃe	2. vo–ðo	2. tʃo–ʃo
3. ne–me	3. ʃe–tʃe	3. zo–zo	3. ki–ti
4. ðe–de	4. im–iŋ	4. ʃe–ʒe	4. eb–eb
5. fi–vi	5. hwi–wi	5. fi–θi	5. ewhe–ewe
6. he–pe	6. ge–ge	6. ze–ze	6. en–em
7. se–ze	7. dʒi–tʃi	7. maɪ–naɪ	7. eð–ed
8. θe–θe	8. faɪ–faɪ	8. θe–θe	8. ehe–epe
9. ʒe–dʒe	9. ðe–ve	9. he–he	9. ov–ov
10. vo–bo	10. pe–pe	10. dʒi–ʒi	10. eθ–eθ

E	F	G
1. eʒ–edʒ	1. eð–ev	1. if–iθ
2. ov–ob	2. et–ep	2. aɪm–aɪn
3. ed–ed	3. ep–ep	3. eθ–eθ
4. en–en	4. of–oθ	4. ini–iɲi
5. edʒ–etʃ	5. ov–oð	5. ef–ep
6. eʃ–etʃ	6. ed–eg	6. eð–eð
7. imi–iɲi	7. em–em	7. idʒ–iʒ
8. ihwi–iwi	8. eð–ez	8. ep–ek
9. eg–eg	9. aɪraɪ–aɪwaɪ	9. otʃ–oʃ
10. is–iz	10. eʃ–eʒ	10. ez–eð

KEY

All D except:
A. 1, 8
B. 1, 6, 8, 10
C. 3, 6, 8, 9
D. 4, 9, 10
E. 3, 4, 9
F. 3, 7
G. 3, 6

NORMS BASED ON 30 NORMAL-SPEAKING CHILDREN FROM EACH OF GRADES 2 THROUGH 6 (PORTLAND STATE UNIVERSITY SPEECH–LANGUAGE AND HEARING CLINIC, UNKNOWN DATE)

Grade	Average Number of Errors
2	14.2
3	11.8
4	10.1
5	10.2
6	10.1

From Templin, M. C. (1943). A study of the sound discrimination ability of elementary school pupils. *Journal of Speech Disorders, 8,* 127–132. Copyright 1943 by American Speech-Language-Hearing Association. Adapted with permission.

Farquar–Bankson In-Depth Test of Auditory Discrimination—/s/

SUBTEST A

Shield mouth while presenting stimulus items.

Say to the child: "I want you to listen for this sound—/s/. Now listen again—/s/. Each time you hear me say /s/, raise your hand. Let's practice—/s/; good, you remembered to raise your hand when I said /s/. Let's try it once more—/b/. That's right. You didn't raise your hand. Let's begin now to listen carefully and raise your hand each time you hear me say /s/."

SUBTEST B

Shield mouth while presenting stimulus items.

Say to the child: "This time I am going to say two words. I want you to listen to the two words and tell me if they are the same. If I say 'man–man', are they the same or different? That's right, they are the same."

SUBTEST C

Shield mouth while presenting stimulus items.

Say to the child: "I am going to say the names of some pictures the right way and others the wrong way. If I say the word the right way, raise your hand. If I say the word the wrong way, don't raise your hand. If I said that you are a dirl/–oy, did I say the word right? No I didn't, and you didn't raise your hand. Let's begin."

SUBTEST D

Say to the child: "Now I want you to look at this picture and tell me if there should be a /s/ in it. Do this for each of the pictures and tell me if there should be a /s/ in the word."

SUBTEST E

Say to the child: "I am going to say some words. I want you to repeat each word after me and tell me if you said the /s/ in each word the same way that I did."

SUBTEST F

Say to the child: "I am going to show you some pictures. Each picture is of a word that has a /s/ in it. Tell me the names of the pictures and if you said the /s/ in each word right."

Farquar–Bankson In-Depth Test of Auditory Discrimination—/s/

NAME_____

AGE_____

DATE_____

EXAMINER_____

SCORE SUMMARY

PART I_____

  A_____

  B_____

  C_____

PART II_____

  D_____

  E_____

  F_____

TOTAL _____ / 90

PART I—External Monitoring. Draw a line through those items answered incorrectly.

Subtest A

1. a	6. t	11. θ
2. ε	7. s	12. f
3. u	8. tʃ	13. s
4. s	9. k	14. ʃ
5. i	10. p	15. θ

Total_____ / 15

Subtest B

1. sun–bun	6. cat–sat	11. saw–saw
2. bus–bug	7. bus–bus	12. nice–nice
3. bustle–bustle	8. tackle–tassel	13. loft–lost
4. fun–fuss	9. mass–map	14. mouse–mouth
5. sum–sum	10. sat–sat	15. sink–think

Total_____ / 15

Subtest C

Use the child's exact articulation error on those items shown with an asterisk (*).

1. seal	4. ice skate	7. sock	10. rooster	*13. glass
*2. fence	*5. desk	*8. cross	*11. whistle	*14. motorcycle
*3. seven	6. mouse	9. stove	12. star	15. grapes

Total_____ / 15

PART II—Internal Monitoring. Draw a line through those items answered incorrectly.

Subtest D

1. soup	6. shirt	11. sandwich
2. sled	7. fish	12. thumb
3. three	8. spoon	13. saw
4. thrush	9. pencil	14. fishing pole
5. mixer	10. teeth	15. house

Total_____ / 15

Subtest E

1. sack	6. mess	11. sink
2. face	7. last	12. police
3. goose	8. rollerskate	13. nest
4. sand	9. nice	14. lettuce
5. silly	10. dancing	15. nurse

Total_____ / 15

Subtest F

1. soap	6. horse	11. bicycle
2. school	7. baseball	12. Santa
3. stop	8. dress	13. mask
4. salt	9. ice	14. popsicle
5. face	10. ice cream cone	15. blocks

Total_____ / 15

From Bernthal, J. E., & Bankson, N. W. (1981). *Articulation disorders* (pp. 202–203). Englewood Cliffs, NJ: Prentice-Hall. Reprinted with permission.

Sample Individualized Education Plan (IEP)

Part B: Oregon Standard Individualized Education Program

To be used in conjunction with Individualized Education Program, Part A: IEP Guidelines for Completionz

Student: Johnny Smith   District: ABC Public School District   Grade: 01

Gender: M F Birth Date: 05/26/1999   Home School: George Washington   IEP Meeting Date: 03/21/2005

State Student ID: 123456   Attending School: George Washington   Reevaluation Due: 03/21/2006

District Student ID: 123456   Disability Code: 50   Case Manager: Mr. Bender, SLP

IEP Meeting Participants

Mr. & Mrs. Smith	Ms. Soliday	
Parent(s)	Regular Education Teacher	Other

	Student	Other
Special Education Teacher/Provider		

Ms. Carter-Anderson, School Psychologist	Mr. Bender, SLP	
District Representative	Individual Interpreting Evaluations	Other

Service Summary (continue on next page if necessary)

	Anticipated Amount/Frequency	Anticipated Location	Starting Date	Ending Date	Provider: e.g. LEA ESD, Regional, LEA
Specially Designed Instruction					
Speech Articulation/Phonology	90 minutes per month	SPED/SLP Room	03/21/2005	03/21/2006	LEA

Related Services

_____ _____ _____

Supplementary Aids/Services; Modifications & Accommodations

_____ _____ _____

Supports for School Personnel

3:1 Model Consultation with Teacher/Parent	30 minutes per month	General Ed. Class	03/21/2005	03/21/2006	LEA

123456

Page ___ of ___

IEP Form Revised 2/02

Student: <u>Johnny Smith</u>   Date: <u>03/21/2005</u>

Consideration of Special Factors

A. Does the student need assistive technology devices or services?

☐ Yes, services/devices addressed in IEP   ☒ No

B. Does the student have communication needs?

☒ Yes, addressed in IEP   ☐ No

C. Does the student exhibit behavior that impedes his/her learning or the learning of others?

☐ Yes   ☒ No

(If yes, the IEP Team must consider strategies, positive behavioral interventions, and supports to address the behavior(s).)

D. Does the student have limited English proficiency?

☐ Yes   ☒ No

(If yes, the IEP Team must consider the language needs of the student as those needs relate to the IEP.)

E. Is the student blind or visually impaired?

☐ Yes   ☒ No

(If yes, Braille needs are addressed in the IEP, or evaluation of reading/writing needs is completed and a determination is made that Braille is not appropriate.)

F. Is the student deaf or hard of hearing?

☐ Yes   ☒ No

(If yes, the IEP addresses the student's language and communication needs, opportunities for direct communication mode, academic level, and full range of needs, including opportunities for direct instruction in the student's language and communication mode.)

Nonparticipation Justification

Does the student need to be removed from participation with nondisabled students in general education classes, extracurricular activities, and nonacademic activities?

☒ Yes   ☐ No

If yes, describe the extent of the removal, and provide justification.

<u>For 90 mintues per month, Johnny will receive direct intervention from the SLP</u>
<u>targeting the improvement of his speech intelligibility.</u>

Extended School Year (ESY) Services

ESY services will be provided for this student:

☐ Yes   ☒ No

☐ To be considered   Will meet to consider by: _____ (Date)

If yes, ESY services to be provided must be included in the Service Summary of the IEP.

District: ABC Public School District

Transition

Is the student age 14 or older?

    ☐ Yes   ☒ No

If yes, the IEP must describe the student's **Transition Service Needs**. The anticipated course of study is:

_____

_____

Is the student age 16 or older?

    ☐ Yes   ☒ No

If yes, the IEP must describe the student's **Transition Services.** Does the student need:

A.   instruction, included as goals and objectives, related services, and/or activities?

      ☐ Yes, addressed in IEP   ☐ Not needed

B.   community experiences that will be addressed in goals and objectives, related services, and/or activities?

      ☐ Yes, addressed in IEP   ☐ Not needed

C.   employment and other post-school adult living objectives, addressed in goals and objectives, related services, and/or activities?

      ☐ Yes, addressed in IEP   ☐ Not needed

D.   daily living skills addressed in goals and objectives, related services, and/or activities, if appropriate?

      ☐ Yes, addressed in IEP   ☐ Not needed

E.   a functional vocational evaluation, if appropriate?

      ☐ Yes, addressed in IEP   ☐ Not needed

Agency Participation

If the representative from any other agency likely to be responsible for providing or paying for transition services did not attend, document the information received for consideration in planning transition services.

_____

_____

Graduation   Anticipated graduation date: <u>2016</u>

                    ☒ With regular diploma

                    ☐ With alternate document (describe) _____

Transfer of Rights

The student has been informed of his/her rights under Part B of IDEA that will transfer to the student at the age of majority.

      ☐ Yes   Date student was informed   _____

The district must also provide written notice of the transfer of rights to the student and the parent when the student reaches the age of majority.

IEP Form Revised 2/02

Student: Johnny Smith _____ Date: 3/21/2005 _____ District: ABC Public School District

Present Levels of Educational Performance

The Present Levels statement must identify how the student's disability affects involvement and progress in the general curriculum.

In developing the Present Levels of Educational Performance Statement, the IEP team should consider:

- the strengths of the student;
- the concerns of the parents for enhancing the education of their child;
- the results of the initial or most recent evaluation (including functional and developmental information);
- as appropriate, the results of performance on State or district-wide assessment;
- for students age 14 and older, consider the student's preferences, needs, interests, and post-school outcomes.

Johnny is a very motivated student who wants to improve his speech. Mr. and Mrs. Smith feel that treatment is important and do not want his articulation delay to impact his social, educational, or vocational interests in the future. An updated articulation screening and conversational sample concurred with ongoing treatment data that Johnny can now produce the phonemes /k/ and /g/ in all word positions, sentences, and conversational speech. He can also produce the /s/ and /z/ phonemes in isolation. However, he continues to distort the /s/ and /z/ sounds in CV, VC blends and monosyllabic words. Johnny is able to self-correct production errors when provided either a verbal or tactile cue. During the 3:1 model consultation week, the SLP consults with the general education teacher regarding cuing strategies to help facilitate articulation carryover and generalization within the classroom and with Johnny's parents regarding a regular homework program.

Continue on additional page(s) if necessary

Page ___ of ___

123456

IEP Form Revised 2/02

Student: _Johnny Smith_   Date: _3/21/2005_   District: _ABC Public School District_

Goals/Objectives: For Students Through Age 15
Measurable Annual Goal:
Speech & Language: Articulation—Phonological Processes

Johnny will improve his intelligibility by accurately producing /s/ and /z/ phonemes during a 5-minute conversational sample.

Progress will be measured as indicated below:

Criteria	Evaluation Procedures
80 % Accuracy (with at least 10 opportunities) without a cue.	SLP treatment data and quarterly progress monitoring using a conversational sample.

How will progress be reported to parents:

On a quarterly basis aligned with the general education report cards.

Progress Notes:

March 2004: Johnny is able to produce the /k/ and /g/ sounds in the initial and final positions of monosyllabic words with 100% accuracy.

June 2004: Johnny is able to produce the /k/ and /g/ sounds in phrases and simple sentences with 80% accuracy according to a spontaneous conversational sample. The classroom teacher also reports improvement in Johnny's intelligibility.

November 2005: Johnny's intelligibility did not regress over the summer, and he continues to make improvement with his production of /k/ and /g/ in conversation. However, on multisyllabic words, he continues to substitute /d/ for /g/.

January 2006: Johnny continues to make great progress. His substitutions in multisyllabic words have reduced, and he is producing the /k/ and /g/ in conversational speech with 80% accuracy without a cue provided.

Measurable Short-Term Objectives:

1) Johnny will produce the /s/ and /z/ sounds within CV / VC syllables, with 90% accuracy, without a cue, during a speech activity.

2) Johnny will produce the /s/ and /z/ sounds in the initial and final positions of monosyllabic words, with 90% accuracy and without a cue, during a speech activity.

3) Johnny will produce the /s/ and /z/ sounds in initial and final positions of monosyllabic words in short and complex sentences, with 90% accuracy and without a cue, during a speech activity.

4) Johnny will produce the /s/ and /z/ sounds while engaged in an age-appropriate choral reading activity, with 90% accuracy and without a cue.

5) Johnny will produce the /s/ and /z/ sounds during a 3-minute conversational sample, with 90% accuracy utilizing a verbal / visual cue, during a speech activity.

Page __ of __

123456

IEP Form Revised 2/02

Student: _Johnny Smith_ Date: _3/21/2005_ District: _ABC Public School District_

Will the student participate in Statewide Assessment during this IEP period?

☐ Yes ☒ No, assessment participation not required at this grade level.

If yes, describe participation decisions below. Continue on additional page(s) if necessary.

	Benchmark (indicate 1, 2, 3, or CIM; Also indicate challenging up or down, as appropriate)	Standard Administration (with or without accommodations) List any accommodations to be provided:	Juried (Standard Administration)	Modifications to be provided:	Extended Assessment	CLRAS	Exempt (only parent may exempt)
Reading/ Literature							
Math							
Math Problem Solving							
Writing							
Science							
dfd							
Social Science							

123456

Page _ of _

IEP Form Revised 2/02

Student: ___Johnny Smith___   Date: ___3/21/2005___   District: ___ABC Public School District___

Participation in Districtwide Assessment(s): (applies only if Districtwide Assessment(s) are administered in the District)

Will the student participate in Districtwide Assessment(s) during this IEP period?
- ☐ Yes, describe participation below:
- ☒ No, assessment participation not required at this grade level.

1. Will the student participate in the standard administration or Districtwide Assessment(s)?
   - ☐ Yes
   - ☐ No, go to question #2 below.

2. Will the student participate in Districtwide assessment(s) with modifications?
   - ☐ Yes, describe the modifications:
   - ☐ No

3. The parent requests an exemption from **all** Districtwide assessment(s)?
   - ☐ Yes
   - ☐ No

The parent requests an exemption from **parts** of Districtwide assessment(s)?
- ☐ Yes, describe the exemption(s):
- ☐ No

123456

Page ___ of ___

IEP Form Revised 2/02

Student: Johnny Smith   Date: 3/21/2005   District: ABC Public School District

Special Education Placement Determination

Placement Team (name and title):

Ms. Soliday, General Education Teacher   Mr. Bender, SLP   Ms. Carter-Anderson, School Psychologist
Person Knowledgeable About the Child   Person Knowledgeable About Evaluation Data   Person Knowledgeable about Placement Options

Mr. and Mrs. Smith
Parent   Other   Other

This placement is based on:

☒ attached IEP, dated: 03/21/2005
☐ attached evaluation information
☐ evaluation information listed here:

Below, document discussions regarding placement option(s), and indicate selected placement

Placement Options(s) Considered	Benefits	Possible Harmful Effects on the Child and/or the Services to be Provided	Modification/Supplementary Aids & Services Considered to Reduce Harmful Effects	Indicate Whether Option is Selected and Reason(s) Rejected or Selected
General Education with Special Education Support	Johnny will receive individualized support for his articulation/phonological delay.	Johnny will miss 90 minutes per month of general education instruction.	Cuing from his general education teacher was not enough to remediate Johnny's articulation delay.	**Selected:** General Education with Special Education Support

Page ___ of ___   123456   IEP Form Revised 2/02

Motokinesthetic Sound Stimulations

VOICELESS CONSONANTS

/h/ Push on diaphragm while moving the lower jaw downward into the next vowel.

/p/ Using the thumb and middle finger below the lower lip placed about half of the distance between the midline and mouth corners, move the lower jaw up then downward quickly.

/t/ Using the index finger, touch center of region midway between the nose and mouth (philtrum) and quickly move the finger downward to just above the midline of the upper lip.

/k/ Place the index and middle fingers on each side of the throat under the back of the tongue; press upward and inward, then release quickly.

/f/ Use the thumb, middle finger, and index finger. Place the thumb and middle finger below the lower lip about half the distance between the midline and mouth corners while pushing inward with the index finger below the midline of the lower lip so that the upper teeth contact the lower lip.

/θ/ Curve the index finger above the upper lip and push inward.

/s/ Place the thumb and index finger above the midline of the upper lip and press inward. Do not pinch.

/ʃ/ Place thumb and middle finger outside the corners of the mouth slightly above the upper lip and move the lips toward the center so that the lips are rounded (but not like a fish).

/tʃ/ Placement and movement is the same as /ʃ/ but with a quick release.

VOICED CONSONANTS

/b/ Place thumb and middle finger of one hand above the upper lip and those of the other hand below the lower lip and bring lips together with pressure then separate (pull apart) immediately.

/d/ Same placement and movement as /t/ but more firmly.

/g/ Same placement and movement as /k/ but more firmly.

/v/ Same placement and movement as /f/ but with firmer contact with the edges of the upper teeth.

/ð/ Same placement and movement as /θ/ but with firmer contact.

/z/ Same placement and movement as /s/ but with firmer contact.

/ʒ/ Same placement and movement as /ʃ/ but with firmer contact.

/dʒ/ Same placement and movement as /tʃ/ but with firmer contact.

/m/ Place thumb and middle finger below lower jaw about halfway between the midline and the mouth corners (same placement as /p/); move lower jaw up until the lower lip touches the upper lip. Place the index finger of the other hand firmly on the bridge of the nose.

/n/ Place the index finger at midpoint above upper lip on the philtrum (same placement as /t, d/) while placing the index finger of the other hand firmly on the bridge of the nose.

/ŋ/ Place the index and middle fingers on each side of the throat under the back of the tongue (same placement as for /k, g/); press upward and inward and hold while placing index finger of the other hand firmly on the bridge of the nose.

/l/   Place thumb and middle finger one-third of the way between midline and mouth corners above upper lip, pressing inward; place thumb and middle finger of the other hand in the same position below the lower lip, pulling slightly downward and laterally.

/r, ɝ, ɚ/   Place the thumb and middle finger above upper lip about halfway between mouth corners and midline, pushing laterally slightly (to prevent lip rounding) with a similar placement with the other hand below the lower lip, pushing slightly inward and downward. Alternatively, use the same placement for upper jaw and place the index finger of the lower hand on the throat below the base of the tongue and push up.

/w/   Place thumb and middle finger of one hand above lips about three-quarters of the way between midline and mouth corners and place the other hand similarly below the lips. Move the lips from the corners toward the midline to round the lips moving to the following vowel.

/j/   Start with the stimulation for /i/ and move the jaws quickly into the next vowel.

VOWELS

/i/   Place middle finger and thumb above the upper lip and the lower lip about halfway between the midline and mouth corners. Retract the lips with both hands. Alternatively, do the retracting movement using only the upper hand.

/ɪ/   Place the index finger below the midline of the lower lip and pull the lip down slightly.

/ɛ/   Place the index finger below the midline of the lower lip and pull the lip down farther than for /ɪ/.

/æ/   Place thumb and middle finger about halfway between the midline and mouth corners below lower lip, pulling down on the lower jaw, lower than for /ɛ/. Then press against the jaw while moving laterally from the midline.

/ʌ, ə/   Place thumb and middle finger about halfway between the midline and mouth corners below lower lip, pulling straight down on the lower jaw.

/ɑ/   Place thumb and middle finger about halfway between the midline and mouth corners below lower lip, pulling down on the lower jaw lower than for /ʌ/.

/ʊ/   Place thumb and middle finger of one hand above upper lip toward corners of mouth and place the other hand in a similar position below lower lip, moving the lips toward the midline with both hands simultaneously, rounding the lips and releasing quickly.

/u/   Place thumb and middle finger of one hand above upper lip toward corners of mouth and place the other hand in a similar position below lower lip, moving the lips toward the midline with both hands simultaneously, rounding the lips without a quick release.

/o/   Place thumb and forefinger below lower lip about three-quarters of the distance between the midline and mouth corners and lower the jaw; then move jaw upward and lips inward while using the other hand above the upper lip to move upper lip into a rounded position.

DIPHTHONGS

/eɪ/   Place thumb and forefinger below lower lip about halfway between midline and mouth corners. Press against lower jaw and bring it downward at the same time. Then, immediately move jaw upward and slightly toward corners without lifting them as for /i/.

/aɪ/   Use the /ɑ/ stimulation to lower the jaw followed by the /i/ stimulation using both hands.

/aʊ/   Use the /ɑ/ stimulation to lower the jaw followed by the /u/ stimulation using both hands to round the lips.

/ɔɪ/   Place middle finger and thumb near mouth corners above and below lips. Bring lips to a rounded position (/o/) followed by retracting the lips as for /i/.

From Young, E. H., & Stinchfield-Hawk, S. (1955). *Motokinesthetic speech training therapy.* Stanford, CA: Stanford University Press.

Sample Clinician Verbal Instructions for Palatometric Instrumental System

STEP 1: FOCUSING

Watch the screen closely (point to upper, central location on the screen where the [s] groove will appear when you say "ahs"). I'm going to show you how the [s] is made in the word "ahs." You will see that it is different from the [t] in "beet." I'll say "beet" first then "ahs" three times. Notice exactly how the points on the screen light up when my tongue touches the palate to make each word. (p. 258)

STEP 2: IMAGING

Now I'm going to say the words "ahs" and "beet" again. During "ahs," you will be able to see how the [s] looks because the tongue doesn't touch the palate during "ah." Notice the groove right here (point to the top, central part of the screen) for the air to pass through for the [s]. During the [t] in "beet," the tongue touches all around the edges of the palate (touch around the outer margins of the sensor display on the video screen). No groove is formed, and air can't pass through. Try to form a picture in your mind of exactly what the pattern should look like on the screen for the [s] and for the [t] sounds. Then, try to imagine air flowing through the groove for the [s]. (p. 259)

STEP 3: REHEARSING

Now I'll say the number "1" then the words "beet" then "ahs" three times each. The number "1" will alert you to notice *exactly* how the points on the screen light up when my tongue touches the palate to make each word. Then, I'll say the number "2."

When I do that, close your eyes and try to see an image in your mind of just what the screen should look like in "beet" and in "ahs." When I say "3," think about how it *should feel* in your mouth when you actually say "beet" and "ahs," but don't say anything yet. Just concentrate on what the sounds should feel like inside your mouth when you make them correctly. (p. 260)

STEP 4: EXECUTING

Now we are going to add another new task. At the count of "1," watch closely to what happens when I say "beet" then "ahs" three times each. At the count of "2," close your eyes and picture in your mind exactly what appears on the screen as each word is spoken. Focus particularly on the patterns for the [t] and the [s] sounds. At the count of "3," rehearse in your mind how it *should feel* in your mouth when you say each word, but don't say anything yet. Rehearse especially the differences in how the [t] and [s] should feel when they are spoken correctly. At the count of "4," say "beet" then "ahs" three times each. Don't think about what is happening inside your mouth this time. Just watch the patterns on the screen and notice how close they are to the patterns when I say them. (p. 262)

STEP 5: VERIFYING

Now I'm going to teach you how to judge your success in learning how to say words correctly. At the count of "1," watch exactly what happens when I say "beet" then "ahs" three times each. At the count of "2," close your eyes and picture in your mind what you saw on the video screen. At the count of "3," rehearse in your mind how it *should feel* in your mouth when you actually say the words, but don't say anything out loud. Just rehearse what it should feel like as you say each word. At the count of "4," say the words three times each. Don't think about what is happening inside your mouth as you say them though. Just watch the pattern on the screen and try to make the words so they are closer to my model each time you say them. At the count of "5," we will judge how well you did in matching my model. If the patterns are *exactly* like mine, we will give you a "10." If they look almost like mine, we will give you an "8" or a "9." If one word is right on target but the other word isn't, the score will be about "5." If neither word is close, the score should be "2" or "3." After we have assigned scores, I'll replay both patterns so we see just how close my pattern and yours match. We will also decide what needs to be changed to improve. The goal is to have all "10s." You should try for a "10" every time you imitate what I say. (p. 263)

From Fletcher, S. G. (1992). *Articulation: A physiological approach* (pp. 258–263). San Diego: Singular Publishing Group, Inc. (pp. 258–263).

Sample Goal, Behavioral Objectives, and Procedures

GENERAL GOAL

Client will produce developmental age-level sounds in spontaneous speech.

BEHAVIORAL TERMINAL OBJECTIVES

1. Client will produce /k/ in the initial, final, and medial positions in connected speech with 90% accuracy in 20 trials for each position.
2. Client will produce /l/ in the initial and medial positions in connected speech with 90% accuracy in 20 trials for each position.
3. Client will produce syllable-initial /l/ blends (/bl, pl, kl, gl/) in connected speech with 90% accuracy in 10 trials for each blend.
4. Client will produce /s/ in the initial, final, and medial positions in connected speech with 90% accuracy in 20 trials for each position.

PROCEDURES

The wedge approach was used to select the targets with a velar (/k/), a liquid (/l/), and a strident sound (/s/) being used as exemplars for these phonetic sound classes. The production phases of the stimulus (traditional) approach will be used in working on these sounds. Speech sound discrimination training will be not be incorporated in the initial phase. Speech discrimination work will be used as needed throughout the production phases. Treatment will begin at the isolation level for /s/ and /k/ and move to nonsense syllables, words, phrases, sentences, and connected speech. Various elicitation techniques will be used as needed. Treatment for singleton /l/ will begin at the nonsense syllable level in the initial position. A criterion of correct phoneme production in 18/20 times for two consecutive trials must be met before proceeding to the next step. Clinician models along with pictures, objects, and games will be used to elicit client responses. Initially, the activities will be drill and drill play and will move on to structured play and play. Clinician models will gradually be faded from direct to indirect to partial models and finally to no model. Token reinforcement will be incorporated along with social praise. Initially, the reinforcement schedule will be 1:1 and gradually faded to 1:10.

Sample Group Approach Lesson

UNIT II, LESSON 3

1. *Interpersonal situation*: obtaining and giving information
2. *Speaking aspects of situation*: asking and answering questions
3. *Particular speech patterns*:

"Yes." "No." "Right here."
"Guess again." "Is this right?"

Street addresses "Can you find my birthday?"
Age "I'm thinking of a birthday."
Birth date "When is your birthday?"
Telephone number "Is that your birthday?"
  "Where is your birthday?"
  "Show me your birthday."

4. *Sounds emphasized*: s θ ∫ r ð k
5. *Equipment*: chalkboard and chalk

Procedures	Notes

Clinician: If you go to the doctor or the dentist, or enroll in a new school, or ask for a package to be sent, what are some questions you are usually asked?

Children: *(Individually)* They ask your name, your address, how old you are, when your birthday is, and sometimes what your telephone number is.

Clinician: Today you are going to be working on speech you use in getting information about other people or giving information about yourself, particularly birthdays. Try the word "birthday." It has a /θ/ sound in it like "thank you" and "think."

Children: *(Individually)* "Birthday." *(Clinician gives help where it is indicated.)*

Clinician: Do you like having a birthday? I'm going to ask you some questions about birthdays. Some of the questions will require "yes" for an answer, some of them "no." Let's see how well you can make the word "yes" today. It is getting easier for some of you.

Children: *(Individually)* Yes. *(The clinician may require their giving this response fairly rapidly, singling out those who need help.)*

Clinician: As I ask these questions, you may think of some questions to ask, too. "Do you sometimes have ice cream on your birthday?"

Child: Yes.

The speech clinician will usually have this data available in his or her records and should have it accessible in this lesson in case a child needs help.

The word "birthday" (containing /r/ and /θ/ is more difficult phonetically for some children and should be stressed only with children able to handle it, but can be used by all.

The clinician may ask questions similar to those suggested. In many groups, the children will be able to do the asking. A few leading words on the board such as cake, spanking, presents, party, and the like may give them ideas around which to construct their questions.

The word sometimes is essential in phrasing the questions.

(continued)

Procedures	Notes
Clinician: Do you sometimes have cake on your birthday? **Child:** Yes. *(May continue by asking the next question.)* *(Other suggestions: Do you sometimes have presents, a spanking, a party, a surprise, a picnic, birthday cards, special fun, etc. on your birthday? Do you sometimes eat the cake, open the presents, hurt from the spanking, see friends at the party, get surprised, have fun, cut the cake, blow out the candles, and read the birthday cards on your birthday?)*	The clinician should guide this question-and-answer period so that chief emphasis is placed on the response "yes." This may be done by stopping the conversation for a moment and asking, "Why are you asking each other questions? Yes, to get practice on the words 'yes' and 'birthday.' Keep that in mind as you go along."
Clinician: Let's find out when your birthdays are. That is a question you often ask a new friend. Listen: "When is your birthday?" Try asking it, with the /θ/ especially. **Children:** *(Individually)* When is your birthday?	The response "your" may be used for work on the /r/ if it is appropriate for the area in which the child lives.
Clinician: As you give us information about your birthday, I will write it with your name on the board. I'm going to suggest that we begin on this side of the circle and go directly around. It will be easier to keep the dates straight that way. I will ask the first question; you can go on from there.	The ordinals are somewhat difficult for children who have deficient sounds. It is suggested that the clinician help individual children as they show a need for it, but not go on giving particular work on it at this time.
Clinician: When is your birthday? **Child:** On August 7th. *(Continues with questioning.)*	
Clinician: Take a look at each of the birthdays that are listed here. I'm going to erase the names soon and see if you remember whose birthday comes at each date. If you have difficulty, you can count around the group and figure it out that way. *(Erases names after children have studied list.)*	
Clinician: Can you find my birthday? **Child:** Yes. Is this right? or is it right here? **Clinician:** Yes.	
Clinician: Before we go on, let's give the people who are having difficulty with /r/ some work on the speech response, "Is this right?" or "Right here?" *(Gives help as indicated.)*	
(Continue with above pattern and guide the children to check themselves on the /ð/, /s/, /r/. Other patterns may be worked out in connection with the list on the board.)	
Child: Show me your birthday. **Child:** That one. *(Continue)* **Child:** Ann, is that your birthday? **Child:** Yes. *(Continue)*	
Child: I'm thinking of a birthday. **Child:** That one? **Child:** No. Guess again. **Child:** That one? **Child:** Yes. *(Continue)*	A similar lesson can be worked out dealing with street addresses and telephone numbers. Such lessons can be used to help children with the ways in which they say numbers, which is important in various phases of school work as well as in furnishing the above information.
Clinician: Can you erase your birthday? **Child:** Yes. **Child:** Should I erase my birthday? **Child:** I think so. **Clinician:** What have you worked on saying better today? Why?	

From Backus, O., & Beasley, J. (1951). *Speech therapy with children*. Boston: Houghton Mifflin. Adapted with permission.

Example HAPP-3 Assessment Results and Cycle 1 and Cycle 2 Projected Targets

CLIENT: C. F.

Birth date: 8/7/2000

HAPP-3 Results

Phonological Deviations	Percentage of Occurrence 9/6/2004 (Initial Assessment)	Percentage of Occurrence 1/5/2005 (After Cycle 1)	Percentage of Occurrence 5/27/2005 (After Cycle 2)
Word/Syllable Structures (Omissions)			
Syllables	69	13	6
Consonant Sequences/Clusters	107	100	70
Prevocalic Singletons	36	14	4
Intervocalic Singletons	7	7	0
Postvocalic Singletons	34	31	0
Consonant Category Deficiencies (Omissions and Specified Substitutions)			
Prevocalic /l/	90	80	60
Prevocalic /r/	78	55	22
Nasals	23	33	5
Glides	70	50	40
Stridents	76	67	50
Velars	91	91	91
Anterior Nonstridents (backing)	0	0	0
Severity Level	Severe	Severe	Moderate

Cycle 1 Projection

Phonological Deviation Patterns	Target Patterns	Sound/Sound Context Targets
Syllable Omission	Syllables	Bisyllable spondees Trisyllable spondees
Glide Deficiency	Glides	Initial /w/ /tw/
Consonant Sequence Omission Strident Deficiency	Consonant Sequences/Stridents (through /s/ clusters)	Initial /sp/ Initial /st/ Initial /sm/ Final /ts/
Velar Deficiency	Velar Obstruents	Initial /k/ Final /k/
Liquid Deficiency	Prevocalic /l/ Prevocalic /r/	Initial /l/ Initial /r/ (non-lip rounding)

Cycle 2 Projection

Phonological Deviation Patterns	Target Patterns	Sound/Sound Context Targets
Consonant Sequence Omission Strident Deficiency	Consonant Sequences/Stridents (through /s/ clusters)	Initial /sp/ and /st/ Initial /sn/ and /sm/ Initial /sw/ Final /ps/
Velar Deficiency	Velar Obstruents	Initial /g/ Medial /k/
Liquid Deficiency	Prevocalic /l/ Prevocalic /r/	/pl/ Medial /l/ (prevocalic) Initial /r/

Glossary

Abutting consonants: Adjacent consonants; two consonants that are side by side.

Accent modification: Training for persons who are native speakers of a language other than English for the purpose of improving their speech production of English so that it more closely resembles the speech production of native speakers.

Accent reduction: Another term for accent modification.

Addition: Insertion of an unnecessary sound such as /ə/ between the consonants in the consonant blend in the word "green" (gərin).

Adducted: Parts of the body have pulled toward each other, such as the vocal folds moving toward approximation or closure. Note: Vocal folds are adducted or closed during phonation.

Affricate: Consonant whose production begins as a stop, then ends as a fricative (/tʃ, dʒ/).

Affrication: Stop feature added to a continuant consonant, most commonly a fricative.

Aglossia: Partial or complete absence of the tongue; partial absence of the tongue sometimes is referred to as dysglossia.

Air turbulence: Air passing through the vocal folds or oral cavity but being affected by the oral structure in such a manner that a "noisy" sound is created.

Allophone: Noncontrastive variant form of a phoneme that does not change the meaning of a word; variations in pronunciation of a phoneme such that the variation remains part of the phoneme family.

Alveolar ridge: Part of the maxilla that is directly behind the upper front teeth; anterior part of the hard palate.

Alveolar sound: Consonant produced with tongue tip contacting the alveolar ridge (/t, d, s, z, n, l/).

Ankyloglossia: A lingual frenulum that is too short or one that is attached too far forward on the inferior portion the tongue; commonly referred to as tongue-tie.

Approximants: Consonants produced with the air stream directed through the oral cavities with the articulators approaching one another, but not to the extent that air turbulence is produced; includes the glide and liquid phonemes.

Apraxia: Disruption of the voluntary or purposive movement in a specific modality while involuntary muscle movements remain intact; some types include verbal apraxia, oral apraxia, and limb apraxia.

Apraxia of speech: An impaired capacity to position the vocal tract structures and to sequence muscle movements (respiratory, laryngeal, articulation, and resonation) for volitional speech production in the absence of motor impairments for other actions using the same musculature; synonymous with verbal apraxia and verbal dyspraxia. The term dyspraxia sometimes refers to a less severe form of the disorder.

Articulation: The vocal tract and speech structure movements and adjustments of positions to produce speech sounds.

Aspirated: A characteristic of sounds, usually stops, that are produced with audible friction because of airflow from the oral cavity. For example, the /p/ in pole is produced with aspiration.

Assimilation: The influence of one speech sound upon another sound in which one (or more) of the features change to become more like the influencing sound. Phonological deviation or process in which a sound or syllable is changed to become more similar respective to another sound or syllable in the word; the sounds or syllables of a word become more alike; synonymous with harmony.

Auditory discrimination: Process of distinguishing among various sounds that may be speech or nonspeech sounds.

Auditory perception: Identification, selection, interpretation, or organization of auditory sensory information received through the ear. Meaningful awareness of auditory stimuli; differs from auditory sensitivity (acuity).

Auditory perceptual: Referring to auditory perception.

Auditory training: In articulation/phonological treatment programs, a process of training a person to listen to speech utterances ranging from sounds in isolation to connected speech and then to identify sounds, discriminate between sounds, indicate the placement of a sound in a word, evaluate sound productions, and such; also termed speech perception training and ear training.

Behavior modification: A system for modifying, shaping, or changing behavior based on principles of positive and negative reinforcement and punishment; target responses are behaviorally defined and programmed in small sequential steps. Improving or modifying speech or any segment of speech can be considered behavior in this context.

Bidialectal: Characteristic of a person with the ability to speak two dialects with equal facility and to code switch appropriately.

Bilabial: Consonant produced with the upper and lower lips (/p, b, m, w, hw/).

Bilateral: Pertaining to two sides.

Blend: Two or more consonants positioned next to one another with no intervening vowel in the same syllable; sometimes synonymous with cluster.

Canonical babbling: Comprised of consonant-vowel syllables that are produced with a true consonant and a fully resonant vowel.

Cardinal vowels: High, mid, and low front and back vowels; also called anchor vowels (/i, e, æ, u, o, ɑ/).

Carryover: Habitual use of newly learned skills. In articulation/phonological disorders, carryover connotes the habitual use of target sounds and sound patterns in conversational speech in and out of the clinical setting. Other terms used for carryover or different stages of it are automatization, generalization, habituation, maintenance, retention, and transfer.

Central auditory processing disorder (CAPD): Impaired ability to attend, discriminate, recognize, or interpret auditory input even though hearing and intelligence are within normal limits; breakdown in a person's auditory skills that results in diminished learning through hearing even though hearing sensitivity is normal. Auditory processing is a term used to describe the brain's ability to recognize and interpret the sounds in the immediate area; synonymous with auditory processing disorder.

Cerebral palsy: A neuromuscular disability caused by damage to the brain characterized by muscular weakness, paralysis, rigidity, lack of muscular control, poor coordination, or any combination of the preceding; occurs prenatally, at birth, or postnatally before maturation of the neurological system.

Childhood apraxia of speech: Speech disorder in childhood characterized by difficulty positioning and sequencing muscle movements for speech production resulting in multiple and inconsistent articulation errors and atypical prosody in the absence of weakness, paralysis, spasticity, or incoordination of the speech musculature; also termed developmental verbal dyspraxia, developmental apraxia of speech, and childhood dyspraxia of speech.

Cleft palate: Failure of the two sides of the palate to unite or fuse at the midline resulting in an opening in the roof of the mouth that may extend through the uvula, soft palate, and hard palate; may or may not occur with cleft lip.

Cluster reduction: Omission of one or more consonants from a consonant cluster.

Clusters: Two or more consonants positioned next to one another with no intervening vowel that may or may not be in the same syllable; sometimes used synonymously with blend such that the two consonants must be in the same syllable.

Coalescence: The replacement of two consonants in a cluster with a different consonant that contains phonetic features of the two target consonants of a cluster; also, omission of one or more syllables from a multisyllabic word with segments from both syllables being retained.

Coarticulation: Articulation movements for one speech sound carried over into the production of previous or subsequent phonemes that do not affect the primary place of articulation, such as rounding the lips on the /t/ sound when saying the word "to"; influence of one phoneme in the production of another phoneme (Nicolosi et al., 2004).

Code switch: Use of one dialect or language and changing to another dialect or language during one event or from one situation to another.

Cognate: Consonant produced with the same phonetic placement and manner but differs in the voicing feature; cognate pairs have the same place and manner of production, but one is voiced and the other is voiceless (/p-b/, /t-d/, /k-g/, /f-v/, /θ-ð/, /s-z/, /ʃ-ʒ/, /tʃ-dʒ/).

Conductive hearing loss: Hearing impairment resulting from an obstruction or lesion in the outer ear or the middle ear; hearing impairment caused by the failure of sound waves to reach the cochlea through the outer and middle ear.

Consonant: A speech sound produced by modification, interruption, or obstruction of the voiced or unvoiced breath stream; phoneme produced by a partially or completely constricted vocal tract.

Continuant: A speech sound that can be prolonged for a period of time through either the oral or nasal passageway; a distinctive feature of a sound produced with incomplete obstruction so that air flows through the vocal tract without being blocked.

Contrasting pairs approach: Treatment approach in which phonological patterns are targeted in contrasting word pairs, one of which contains the targeted pattern and the other does not.

Creole: A language that develops from contact between two languages; of or pertaining to a language that originates from contact between two other languages and has features of both.

Deaffrication: Replacement of an affricate speech sound with a nonaffricate; changing an affricate to a continuant or a stop.

Denasality: Insufficient nasal resonance during speech; synonym is hyponasality.

Denasalization: Occurs when a nasal speech sound is replaced by a nonnasal sound, often a stop that has the same articulation placement.

Dental: Pertaining to the teeth. Characterization of a speech sound produced by the tongue or lip contacting the teeth; /f, v/ are classified as labiodentals; /θ, ð/ are classified as dentals, interdentals, or linguadentals.

Dentalization: Occurs when speech sounds are produced with the tongue touching the front teeth. Articulation errors caused by placing the tongue too far forward so that it contacts the front teeth, often occurring on the production of alveolar speech sounds.

Depalatalization: Occurs when a palatal consonant is replaced by a nonpalatal.

Developmental apraxia of speech (DAS): Synonymous with childhood apraxia of speech.

Developmental verbal dyspraxia (DVD): Synonymous with childhood apraxia of speech.

Diadochokinesis: Execution of rapid repetitive movements of the articulators.

Diadochokinetic: Pertaining to rapid repetition of articulator movements.

Dialect: A variation of a language spoken by a group specific to a geographical region, socioeconomic environment, class, ethnicity, or educational background; variation of a language differing sufficiently from the larger language community to be considered distinct, but not sufficiently different to be regarded as a separate language.

Differential reinforcement: Procedure in which one response is reinforced and another response is not reinforced or ignored; procedure in which a combination of reinforcement and extinction is used. Desired result is to increase the frequency of occurrence of the target response and decrease the frequency of the undesired response.

Diminutization: Adding an /i/ or /ɪ/ or consonant plus /i/ or /ɪ/ to the end of a word.

Diphthong: A speech sound in which two vowels are produced consecutively within the same syllable to bring two vowels together to form one sound unit as the nucleus of a syllable. Examples: /aɪ, aʊ, ɔɪ/).

Distinctive features: Phonetic attributes of phonemes that differentiate one phoneme from another in a given language. Distinctive features are based on a binary system with each characteristic or feature being either present or absent in a given phoneme.

Distinctive features approach: Articulation treatment approach in which distinctive features of sounds are targeted through the production of contrasting exemplar phonemes, one of which contains the feature and the other that does not contain the feature.

Distocclusion: A malocclusion in which the mandibular dental arch is posterior to (behind) the maxillary dental arch resulting in protrusion of the maxillary front teeth (incisors) and possibly creating an overbite.

Distortion: A misarticulation error in which the standard phoneme is modified so that it is approximated, although incorrect.

Doubling: Repetition of a word, usually a monosyllabic word, resulting in a multisyllabic word.

Dysarthria: A motor speech disorder manifested as disorders of phonation, articulation, resonation, and/or prosody resulting from impairment of the central nervous system, peripheral nervous system, or muscular system.

Dyslalia: An articulation disorder resulting from faulty learning or abnormality of the external speech organs and not from neuromuscular impairment.

Dyspraxia: Often referring to a lesser form of apraxia; sometimes used synonymously with childhood apraxia of speech.

Ellipsis: Omission of an element of a linguistic unit (such as a phoneme, syllable, word, phrase, or sentence); missing element is understood and may be subconsciously supplied.

Epenthesis: Addition of a sound to a word.

Extinction: Procedure in which reinforcement is terminated and the behavior is allowed to occur until it disappears; technique of ignoring a certain behavior.

Flap: Consonant produced by a single bounce of the tongue tip to contact the alveolar ridge, teeth, or hard palate and returned to the floor of the mouth along the same path (/r/); sometimes used as medial /t, d, r/; synonymous with tap.

Focused auditory input: A method in the phonological cycling treatment approach in which the major phonological patterns are stimulated and the client interacts with the clinician, but the client is not required to say anything.

Foreign accent: Pronunciation of an individual's first (native) language carried over into the individual's second (nonnative) language.

Formants: Frequency regions of vowels and sonorant consonants "in which a relatively high degree of acoustic energy is concentrated" (Nicolosi et al., 2004); peak resonant frequencies.

Frenulum: A slip of connective tissue from the floor of the mouth attached to the midline undersurface of the tongue; synonymous with lingual frenum.

Fricative: Consonant produced with partial blockage of the breath stream forcing the air stream through a narrow channel with considerable intraoral breath pressure causing turbulence or friction (/f, v, θ, ð, s, z, ʃ, ʒ, h/).

Fronting: Replacement of a target phoneme with another phoneme whose articulation placement is anterior to the target sound.

Generalization: Use of a target behavior in untrained conditions; sometimes used synonymously with transfer.

Glides: Consonants produced with continued movement of the articulators, providing a rapid transition to or from a vowel (/w, j/).

Gliding: Replacing a nonglide consonant with a glide; often occurs on liquid consonants.

Glossectomy: Surgical removal of part or all of the tongue.

Glottal: Pertaining to the glottis, the opening between the vocal folds. Glottal consonants are produced at the level of the larynx (/h, ʔ/).

Glottal replacement: The substitution of a glottal stop for a consonant.

Glottal stop: Consonant produced by stopping and releasing the breath stream at the level of the glottis; not a phoneme in standard American English, but does occur in some English dialects.

Habituation: The process of making the use of the target sound/pattern automatic, used without conscious effort both outside and inside the clinic; synonymous with automatization.

Harmony: Phonological deviation or process in which a sound or syllable is changed to become more similar respective to another sound or syllable in the word; the sounds or syllables of a word becoming more alike; synonymous with assimilation.

Heterogeneous group approach: An old treatment approach that incorporates all types of communication problems in a group setting, targeting sounds from whole to part to whole.

Homorganic: Sounds produced with the same placement of the articulators, but differing in one or more phonetic features such as voicing and manner.

Hypernasality: Excessive amount of perceived nasal resonance during phonation.

Hyponasality: Insufficient nasal resonance during speech; synonymous with denasality.

Idioglossia: Unique speech code used by an individual that differs markedly from the linguistic community and is generally not understandable to others; type of language and speech often used by twins for communication with each other and not understandable to others.

Idiolect: Speech characteristic of an individual that results from the speech history of that individual; phonological deviations that are unique to an individual's phonological system.

Integral stimulation: Articulation treatment approach that involves imitation of the clinician's multisensory models in stimulable sounds.

Intelligibility: Understandability; often expressed as a percentage of contextual speech understood by the listener; degree of understandability of one's utterances by listeners.

Interdental: Consonant produced with the tongue tip contacting the back of the front teeth or placed between the upper and lower front teeth (/θ, ð/); also referred to as dental and linguadental sounds. Also, type of lisp in which the tongue touches or protrudes between the anterior front teeth.

Intervocalic: Pertaining to a consonant positioned between two vowels; also referred to as the medial position.

Isolation: Pertaining to a single phoneme that is presented alone for production or discrimination; a phoneme that is not a part of a syllable or word, but stands alone.

Kinesthetic: Relating to the muscle sense. In speech, pertaining to awareness of the movement or position of the speech muscles and structures; involved in proprioception.

Labial: Pertaining to the lips. Speech sounds produced involving the lips; labial consonants including /p, b, m, w, f, v/.

Labiodental: Consonants produced with contact between the lips and teeth (/f, v/).

Lateral: Consonant produced with breath stream directed around one or both sides of the tongue (/l/); type of lisp in which breath stream passes over the side of the tongue referred to as a lateral lisp. The side of the body or structure.

Lingua-alveolar: Contact between the tongue and alveolar ridge acting in conjunction to produce sounds; sometimes, a label given to specific sounds produced by contact between the tongue and alveolar ridge; more frequently referred to as an alveolar consonant.

Linguadental: Contact between the tongue and teeth to produce sounds; sometimes, a label given to consonants produced with the tongue tip contacting the back of the front teeth or placed between the upper and lower front teeth (/θ, ð/). Also referred to as dental or interdental sounds.

Lingual: Pertaining to the tongue.

Linguistic interference: Phenomenon that occurs when a person's underlying linguistic patterns of the first language are applied incorrectly to a second language.

Lip incompetence: " . . . a lips-apart resting posture or the inability to achieve a lips-together resting posture without muscle strain" (ASHA, 1993, p. 22).

Liquid: A generic term used for classifying the /l/ and /r/ sonorant consonants.

Lisp: Misarticulation of one or more of the sibilant sounds (/s, z, ʃ, ʒ, tʃ, dʒ/). Lingual, frontal, dental, and interdental lisps occur when the tongue is placed too far forward in the mouth. A lateral lisp occurs when the air stream is directed over one or both sides of the tongue. A nasal lisp occurs when part or all of the air stream is directed through the nasal cavity. A strident lisp results in a high-frequency whistle or hissing sound caused by grooving the tongue tip too much or by the breath stream passing between the tongue and a hard surface. An occluded or dentalized lisp does not have a sibilant quality, resulting from occluding the breath stream in the oral cavity, usually by placing the tongue too far forward or not allowing for a narrow, grooved passageway for the breath stream to pass between the tongue and alveolar ridge.

Macroglossia: Atypically enlarged tongue.

Maintaining causes: Conditions (factors) that continue to cause or maintain articulation problems.

Maintenance: Continuing use of learned behavior in all settings and situations over time.

Malocclusions: Deviations from normal teeth occlusion; irregularities in dental and jaw alignment.

Maximal opposition approach: Phonological treatment approach that involves production of contrasting word pairs differing in multiple phonetic features with the goal of increasing the phonetic inventory and complexity level of the phonological system.

Mesioclusion: A malocclusion in which the mandibular dental arch is too far anterior to (forward of) the maxillary arch resulting in the protrusion of the mandibular front teeth (incisors) and creating an underbite.

Metalinguistics: Aspect of language that is the "conscious awareness and use of language as a tool" (Nicolosi et al., 2004, p. 170); ability to think about and reflect on language and its usage.

Metaphon treatment approach: Phonological treatment approach that targets phonological rule systems (phonological processes) through phonological awareness training, communication awareness training, and production of contrasting word pairs.

Metaphonology: "The ability to pay attention to and reflect upon the phonological structure of the language" (Howell & Dean, 1994, p. 65).

Metathesis: Transposing or reversing consonants in a word.

Microglossia: Atypically small tongue.

Migration: Phonological pattern in which a phoneme is moved from one position in the word to another position.

Misarticulation: Articulation error; any speech sound produced incorrectly, such as a phoneme produced with insufficient accuracy and precision.

Morpheme: Smallest meaningful unit of language.

Morphology: Branch of language that deals with words and word forms; "study of how morphemes are put together to form words . . . indicates how words are formed" (Nicolosi et al., 2004, p. 173).

Morphophonemics: The change in the sound structure of morphemes; sound changes resulting from combining morphemes. "Rules of pronunciation . . . indicate how words in a sentence are to be pronounced" (Nicolosi et al., 2004, p. 173).

Motokinesthetic articulation treatment: Articulation treatment approach that involves manipulation by the clinician of the articulators externally on the face and neck to guide an articulation mechanism in speech sound production.

Motokinesthetic stimulations: Specific manipulations, such as touching and moving the client's tongue, lips, and jaw on the outside of the face, that the clinician uses for each speech sound for the purpose of eliciting the sound from the client.

Multiple phonemic approach: Articulation treatment approach that targets production of all error sounds at a time (with each progressing at its own rate) and uses a traditional/instructional programming strategy.

Nasal: Pertaining to the nose or nasal passages. Nasals are sounds produced by the breath stream passing through the nose (/m, n, ŋ/).

Negative practice: Deliberate production of the incorrect behavior or incorrect speech sound usually for the purpose of making the client more aware of the incorrect behavior and thus helping to eliminate it.

Neutralization: Several different phonemes are replaced by one phoneme.

Neutroclusion: A malocclusion in which the mandibular and maxillary dental arches are in correct anterior–posterior relationship, but individual teeth may be crowded, missing, in wrong position, at atypical size, or in an open bite relationship.

Nonlinear approach: Phonological treatment in which various segmental and syllable/word structure levels are targeted through the production of exemplar words for a specified time period.

Nonsense material approach: Articulation treatment approach in which simultaneous auditory training and speech production is provided and sounds are targeted in nonmeaningful material at all levels prior to meaningful material.

Nonsense syllables: Sequences of sounds that have no meaning; used as stimulus material to elicit sound responses.

Obstruents: Consonants in which the vocal tract air stream is partially or completely blocked causing air turbulences; stops, fricatives, and affricates.

Offglide: "A transition from a vowel of longer duration to one of shorter duration" (Edwards, 2003, p. 373).

Omissions: Deletions of a speech sound from a word.

Onglide: "A transition from a preceding sound into a vowel of longer duration" (Edwards, 2003, p. 373).

Open bite: A malocclusion in which the upper anterior teeth (incisors) do not reach the midline.

Oral apraxia: Impairment in performing nonspeech tasks using the articulation structures on command or in imitation; difficulty in voluntarily moving the articulators for nonspeech activities in the absence of structural or functional abnormalities of the articulators.

Orofacial myofunctional disorder: "Any pattern involving oral and/or orofacial musculature that interferes with normal growth, development, or function of structures, or calls attention to itself" (ASHA, 1993, p. 22).

Orthographic transcription: A written out, traditionally spelled version of the words spoken by a speaker.

Otitis media: Inflammation of the middle ear.

Overjet: Malocclusion in which the upper teeth extend toward the lips past the normal line of occlusion.

Paired stimuli approach: Articulation treatment approach that uses key words paired with words in which the target sound is produced incorrectly at the word, sentence, and conversational levels.

Palatal: Pertaining to the palate. Consonant produced by the tongue contacting or approaching the hard palate (/ʃ, ʒ, tʃ, dʒ, j, r/).

Palatalization: Occurs when a palatal consonant replaces a nonpalatal consonant.

Palatometric instrument approach: Articulation approach that uses a pseudopalate to provide visual feedback.

Paresis: Partial or incomplete paralysis.

Phonation: Production of voice or voiced sounds through vocal fold vibration.

Phoneme: A family, class, or group of phonetically similar sounds that are perceived to be the same sound. H. T. Edwards describes a phoneme as an " . . . abstract speech sound found in the phonological system of a particular language" (Edwards, 2003, p. 374).

Phones: Speech sounds; sounds produced by the human vocal tract without regard to a particular language.

Phonetic placement approach: Articulation treatment approach in which instruction is given in specific placement of the articulators to produce speech sounds. A technique for eliciting speech sounds by providing instruction in the placement of the articulators.

Phonological awareness: "The ability to reflect on and manipulate the structure of an utterance (e.g., into words, syllables, or sounds) as distinct

from the meaning" Stackhouse, 1997, p. 157); "the awareness of aspects related to the sounds of one's language, including blending, segmenting, and manipulating sounds and syllables" (Hodson & Edwards, 1997, p. 229).

Phonological cycling approach: Phonological treatment approach in which phonological patterns are targeted in words containing exemplar sounds and sound contexts for a specified time through the production of words.

Phonological processes: Differences between (or alterations of) speech sounds actually produced and those present in the adult standard production; statement of a rule that accounts for errors in speech sound production. Strategy children use to simplify speech when attempting to utter adult words.

Phonology: The study of the sound system of language.

Phonotactics: Study of the rules for how sounds can be combined and sequenced to formulate syllables and words of a particular language.

Pidgin: Simplified language used by individuals speaking different languages often with features of both languages; an abbreviated language form that occurs when a dominant culture needs to communicate for trade purposes with a second subjugated culture.

Plosive: Consonant produced by momentarily stopping and releasing the breath stream by the articulators; consonant produced by complete blockage of airflow through the oral cavity; also called a stop and stop-plosive consonant.

Postvocalic: Pertaining to a consonant positioned after a vowel; also referred to as the syllable or word *final* position.

Pragmatics: Branch of language that deals with the use of language in context; "study of linguistic acts and the contexts in which they are performed" (Nicolosi et al., 2004).

Precipitating causes: Conditions (factors) that originally caused the articulation problems and may or may not continue to be operative in maintaining the disorder.

Prevocalic: Pertaining to a consonant positioned before a vowel; also referred to as the syllable or word *initial* position.

Programmed instruction approach: Articulation treatment approach in which stimuli, client responses, and consequences (such as reinforcement, punishment, and differential reinforcement) are specified in small sequential steps; analogous to operant conditioning, behavior modification, behavior therapy, and (sometimes) learning theory.

Progressive approximation: A procedure in which the client starts with a sound he or she already produces and progresses by stimulus and response through a series of sounds gradually more closely approximating the target sound; sometimes called successive approximation or shaping.

Progressive assimilation: A sound in a word that is influenced by a preceding sound.

Proprioceptive: Pertaining to body information regarding the sense of touch, as well as body movements and body position provided by sensory nerve terminals within muscles, tendons, joints, and the labyrinth; proprioception includes kinesthesia (awareness of body movements and position) and taction (sense of touch or contact).

Prosody: Melody of speech resulting from stress, pitch inflection, intonation, rhythm, and duration; suprasegmental components of speech.

Punishment: Consequence following a behavior or response that decreases the frequency of that behavior or response.

Reduplication: Occurs when all or part of a syllable in a multisyllabic word is repeated; can occur in complete and partial forms—complete reduplication (/wɑwɑ/ for water) and partial reduplication (/wɑtɑ/ for water).

Register: A language style that is used to accommodate the perceived needs of the listener; varies on a continuum from informal to formal.

Regressive assimilation: A sound in a word that is influenced by a later-occurring sound in the word.

Reinforcement: Consequence following a behavior or response which increases the frequency of that behavior or response. Positive reinforcement involves the presentation of a desirable event after a response is made. Negative reinforcement involves the removal of, reduction in, postponement of, or prevention of an aversive event in response to a desired behavior (Hegde, 1998).

Resonation: Amplification of the voiced air stream moving upward from the larynx, by the pharyngeal, oral, and nasal cavities; vibration of the air in the cavities above the larynx in response to the air stream moving upward from the larynx.

Respiration: The process of breathing consisting of inhalation and exhalation; exhaled air stream is the source of energy for speech.

Response generalization: One stimulus elicits several different responses; occurrence of an untrained speech behavior that is similar to, but different from, the trained behavior.

Rhotic: Pertaining to the /r/ family of speech sounds including the /r/-colored vowels (/ɝ, ɚ/). Distinctive feature characterizing /r/-colored vowels.

Segments: Speech sounds; phonemes.

Self-evaluation: Client judgment of own speech productions regarding whether they are produced correctly or incorrectly.

Self-monitoring: Occurs when a client evaluates own sound productions and corrects incorrect productions.

Semantics: Branch of language pertaining to the meanings of words and other linguistic units.

Semivowel: A consonant that has vowel-like quality, including the nasals, liquids, and glides.

Sensorineural hearing loss: Hearing loss resulting from impairment in the inner ear, in the cochlea, or in cranial nerve VIII.

Sensory-motor approach: Articulation treatment approach that includes bisyllable and trisyllable drill for multisensory awareness of speech sound patterns and production of error sounds in facilitating phonetic contexts that gradually are expanded.

Shaping: A procedure in which the client starts with a sound that he or she already produces and progresses by stimulus and response through a series of sounds that gradually more closely approximate the target sound; sometimes called progressive or successive approximation.

Sibilant: Consonant produced with mid to high frequency range characterized by a "hissing" quality as the breath stream is forced between articulators (/s, z, ʃ, ʒ, tʃ, dʒ/).

Singleton: Consonant that is preceded by or followed by a vowel; consonant not preceded by nor followed by another consonant.

Sonorant: Speech sound produced with no obstruction in the vocal tract; includes vowels, diphthongs, and semivowels (including nasals, glides, and liquids).

Speech perception training: In articulation/phonological treatment programs, a process of training a person to listen to speech utterances ranging from sounds in isolation to connected speech and to identify sounds, discriminate between sounds, indicate the placement of a sound in a word, evaluate sound productions, and such; also called auditory training and ear training.

Speech sound discrimination: A process of distinguishing among speech sounds; ability to sort and differentiate speech sounds from one another and the ability to distinguish between two speech sounds.

Stereognosis: The ability to discriminate various geometric shapes placed inside the mouth with the tongue.

Stimulability: The ability of a client to imitate speech sounds when given vocal-visual model; ability to produce a misarticulated sound correctly by imitation.

Stimulability enhancement approach: Articulation treatment approach in which the client is taught to produce a consonant (or consonant-vowel) in isolation to increase the number of stimulable sounds.

Stimulus: An external or internal event that elicits a response or behavior from an individual. In treatment, it is the antecedent behavior by the clinician for the purpose of eliciting a correct response from the client.

Stimulus approach: Articulation treatment approach that involves auditory training and production practice of target sounds in progressively increasing levels of linguistic complexity; often called the traditional approach.

Stimulus generalization: Occurrence of target behaviors that were taught in response to certain stimuli and used in response to different stimuli.

Stopping: Producing a stop consonant in place of a nonstop consonant; often occurs on fricatives.

Stop-plosives: Consonants produced by a momentary stopping and releasing of the breath stream by the articulators; consonants produced by the complete blockage of airflow through the oral cavity; also called plosive and stop consonants.

Stops: Consonants produced by a momentary stopping and releasing of the breath stream by the articulators; consonants produced by the complete blockage of airflow through the oral cavity; also called plosive and stop-plosive consonants.

Strident: Consonant produced with a high frequency of air turbulence by directing airflow against a hard surface (/s, z, ʃ, ʒ, f, v, tʃ, dʒ/).

Substitution: A phoneme used incorrectly as a replacement for another.

Successive approximations: Procedure in which the client starts with a sound he or she already produces and progresses by stimulus and response through a series of sounds gradually more closely approximating the target sound; sometimes called progressive approximation or shaping.

Suprasegmental: Prosodic elements of speech; melody of speech including stress intonation, duration, rate, and juncture; synonymous with prosody.

Syllabic: Having the features of a syllable; a sound that functions as the nucleus of a syllable, including vowels, diphthongs, and vowel-like consonants (such as liquids and nasals).

Syllable deletion: Omission of one or more syllables in a multisyllabic word; also called syllable omission and syllable reduction. Weak or unstressed syllable deletion refers to omission of an unstressed syllable in a multisyllabic word.

Syllable structure deviations: Phonological deviations or processes that are changes in the consonant/vowel (CV) makeup of the syllables of standard adult word forms; the number and sequence of vowels and consonants in the surface form differs from those in the adult standard form of the target word.

Syntax: Branch of language regarding the way words are sequenced in a sentence to convey meaning. "The internal structure of language, including the order in which the elements of a language can occur and the relationships among the elements in an utterance." (Nicolosi et al., 2004, p. 269)

Tactile: The sense of touch; perception through touch.

Tap: Consonant produced by a single bounce of the tongue tip to contact the alveolar ridge, teeth, or hard palate and returned to the floor of the mouth along the same path (/ɾ/); sometimes used as medial /t, d, r/; synonymous with flap (Edwards, 2003).

Tongue thrust: The "inappropriate or excessive lingual contacts against or between the teeth at rest or during vegetative or communicative functions" (ASHA, 1993, p. 22).

Transfer: Use of a target behavior in untrained conditions; sometimes used synonymously with generalization.

Unaspirated: Characteristic of sounds, usually stops, that are produced without audible friction of airflow from the oral cavity; for example, the /p/ in spot is produced without aspiration.

Unilateral: Pertaining to one side; single-sided function or activity.

Velar: Pertaining to the soft palate or velum. Consonant sound produced with contact between the back of the tongue and the soft palate (/k, g, ŋ/).

Velopharyngeal closure: Closure of the nasal cavity from the oral cavity by the synergistic action of the velum and the upper pharynx to direct the air stream into the oral cavity.

Velopharyngeal port: Opening or gateway between the oral and nasal cavities.

Velum: Soft palate.

Verbal apraxia: An impaired capacity to position the vocal tract structures and to sequence muscle movements (respiratory, laryngeal, articulation, and resonation) for volitional speech production in the absence of motor impairments for other actions using the same musculature; synonymous with apraxia of speech and verbal dyspraxia.

Verbal dyspraxia: An impaired capacity to position the vocal tract structures and to sequence muscle movements (respiratory, laryngeal, articulation, and resonation) for volitional speech production in the absence of motor impairments for other actions using the same musculature; synonymous with verbal apraxia and apraxia of speech; sometimes refers to a lesser form of apraxia of speech.

Vocal tract: In speech, the pharyngeal, oral, and nasal cavities and their structures; the part of the speech mechanism above the vocal folds that modify speech sounds generated by the vocal folds.

Vocalization: Using the vocal folds to produce voice. A phonological deviation in which a vowel replaces a consonant, often a syllabic or postvocalic consonant; synonymous with vowelization.

Voiced: Sound produced with vibration of the vocal folds.

Voiceless: Consonant produced without vocal fold vibration (/p, t, k, f, θ, s, ʃ, tʃ/); also called unvoiced.

Vowelization: A phonological deviation in which a vowel replaces a consonant, often a syllabic or postvocalic consonant; synonymous with vocalization.

Vowels: Voiced phonemes produced without obstruction of the air stream; vowels form the nucleus of nearly all syllables.

Weak syllable deletion: Omission of an unstressed syllable in a multisyllabic word; also referred to as unstressed syllable deletion.

Wedge approach: Articulation treatment approach that targets two or more speech sounds at a time using sounds that have dissimilar phonetic features generally using the stimulus or traditional approach.

Bibliography

Aase, D., Hovre, C., Krause, K., Schelfhout, S. Smith, J., & Carpenter, L. (2000). *Contextual Test of Articulation*. Eau Claire, WI: Thinking Publications.

Air, D. H., Wood, A. S., & Neils, J. R. (1989). Considerations for organic disorders. In N. A. Creaghead, P. W. Newman, & W. A. Secord. *Assessment and remediation of articulatory and phonological disorders* (2nd ed., pp. 265–301). Columbus, OH: Merrill Publishing Company.

American Association on Mental Retardation (AAMR). (2002). Mental retardation: Definition, classification, and systems of supports (10th ed.). Washington, DC: Author.

American Speech-Language-Hearing Association (ASHA) (1983). Social dialects. *ASHA, 25*, 23–24.

American Speech-Language-Hearing Association (ASHA) (1989). Bilingual speech-language pathologists and audiologists. *ASHA, 30*, 93.

American Speech-Language-Hearing Association (ASHA). (1989, November). Report: Ad hoc committee on labial-lingual posturing function. *ASHA, 31*, 92–94.

American Speech-Language-Hearing Association (ASHA). (1991). The role of the speech-language pathologist in assessment and management of oral myofunctional disorders. *ASHA, 33*, (Suppl. 5), 7.

American Speech-Language-Hearing Association (ASHA). (1993). Orofacial myofunctional disorders: Knowledge and skills. *ASHA, 35*, (Suppl. 10), 21–23.

American Speech-Language-Hearing Association Panel on Audiologic Assessment 1996 (1997). Rockville, MD: Author.

American Speech-Language-Hearing Association (ASHA) (1998). Provision of English-as-a-second language instruction by speech-language pathologists in school settings; position statement and technical report. *ASHA, 40* (Suppl. 18), 24–27.

American Speech-Language-Hearing Association (ASHA) (2003). Technical report: American English dialects. *ASHA Supplement 23*, 45–46.

Andrews, J. (1996). Theory and practice in speech-language pathology: A review of systemic principles. *Seminar in Speech and Language, 17*, 97–106.

Andrews, J., & Andrews, M. (2000). *Family based treatment in communicative disorders: A systemic approach* (2nd ed.). DeKalb, IL: Janelle Publications.

Arlt, P. B., & Goodban, M. T. (1976). A comparative study of articulation acquisition as based on a study of 240 normals, aged three to six. *Language, Speech, and Hearing Services in Schools, 7*, 173–180.

Arndt, W., Elbert, M., & Shelton, R. (1970). Standardization of a test of oral stereognosis. In J. Bosma (Ed.), *Second symposium on oral sensation and perception*. Springfield, IL: Charles C Thomas.

Arndt, J., & Healey, E. C. (2001). Concomitant disorders in school-age children who stutter. *Language, Speech, and Hearing Services in Schools, 32*, 68–78.

Aungst, L., & Frick, J. (1964). Auditory discrimination ability and consistency of articulation of /r/. *Journal of Speech and Hearing Disorders, 29*, 76–85.

Backus, O. (1957). Group structure in speech therapy. In L. Travis (Ed.), *Handbook of speech pathology and audiology*. New York: Appleton-Century-Crofts.

Backus, O., & Beasley, J. (1951). *Speech therapy with children*. Boston: Houghton Mifflin.

Bacon, V. J. (1995). Validity and efficiency of the check-slash transcription method for measuring intelligibility. Unpublished master's thesis, Portland State University, Portland, OR.

Bain, B. A. (1994). A framework for dynamic assessment in phonology: Stimulability revisited. *Clinics in Communication Disorders, 4*, 12–22.

Baker, R. D., & Ryan, B. P. (1971). *Programmed conditioning for articulation*. Monterey, CA: Monterey Learning Systems.

Ball, E. W. (1993). Assessing phoneme awareness. *Language, Speech, and Hearing Services in Schools, 24*, 130–139.

Bankson, N. W., & Bernthal, J. E. (1990a). *Bankson-Bernthal Test of Phonology*. Chicago: Riverside Press.

Bankson, N. W., & Bernthal, J. E. (1990b). *Quick Screen of Phonology*. Chicago: Riverside Press.

Bankson, N. W., & Byrne, M. (1962). The relationship between missing teeth and selected consonant sounds. *Journal of Speech and Hearing Disorders, 27*, 341–348.

Bankson, N. W., & Byrne, M. (1972). The effect of a timed correct sound production task on carryover. *Journal of Speech and Hearing Research, 15*, 160–168.

Barlow, J. A., & Gierut, J. A. (1999). Optimality theory in phonological acquisition. *Journal of Speech, Language, and Hearing Research, 42*, 1482–1498.

Bashir, A. S. (1980). A touch cue method of therapy with developmentally apraxic children. Special videotape forum. American Speech-Language-Hearing Association Annual Convention, Detroit, MI.

Bashir, A. S., Grahamjones, F., & Bostwick, R. Y. (1984). The touch-cue method of therapy for developmental verbal apraxia. *Seminars in Speech and Language, 5,* 127–137.

Bates, E., & MacWhinney, B. (1987). Competition, variation, and language learning. In B. MacWhinney (Ed.), *Mechanisms of language acquisition* (pp. 157–194). Hillsdale, NJ: Lawrence Erlbaum.

Bennet, C. W., & Runyan, C. M. (1982). Educators' perceptions of the effects of communication disorders upon educational performance. *Language, Speech, and Hearing Services in Schools, 13,* 260–263.

Bern, S. A. (1999). Comparison of two intelligibility measures using elementary teachers as listeners. Unpublished master's thesis, Portland State University, Portland, OR.

Bernhardt, B. (1990). Application of nonlinear phonological theory to intervention with six phonologically disordered children. Unpublished doctoral dissertation, University of British Columbia, Vancouver, BC, Canada.

Bernhardt, B. (1992). The application of nonlinear phonological theory to intervention with one phonologically disordered child. *Clinical Linguistics and Phonetics, 6,* 283–316.

Bernhardt, B., & Stemberger, J. P. (1998). *Handbook of phonological development: From the perspective of constraint-ba*sed *nonlinear phonology.* San Diego: Academic Press.

Bernhardt, B., & Stoel-Gammon, C. (1994). Nonlinear phonology: Introduction and clinical application. Tutorial. *Journal of Speech and Hearing Research, 37,* 123–143.

Bernhardt, B., & Stoel-Gammon, C. (1997). Grounded phonology: Application to the analysis of disordered speech. In M. J. Ball & R. D. Kent, *The new phonologies: Developments in clinical linguistics* (pp. 163–210). San Diego: Singular Publishing Group, Inc.

Bernhardt, B., & Stemberger, J. P. (2000). *Workbook in nonlinear phonology for clinical application.* Austin, TX: Pro-Ed.

Bernstein, M. (1956). The relation of speech defects and malocclusion. *Alpha Omega, 150,* 90–97.

Bernthal, J. E., & Bankson, N. W. (1981). *Articulation disorders.* Englewood Cliffs, NJ: Prentice-Hall.

Bernthal, J. E., & Bankson, N. W. (2004). *Articulation and phonological disorders* (5th ed.). Boston: Allyn & Bacon.

Bernthal, J. E., & Beukelman, D. (1978). Intraoral air pressure during the production of /p/ and /b/ by children, youths, and adults. *Journal of Speech and Hearing Research, 21,* 361–371.

Bird, J., & Bishop, D. V. M. (1992). Perception and awareness of phonemes in phonologically impaired children. *European Journal of Disorders of Communication, 27,* 289–311.

Bird, J., Bishop, D. V. M., & Freeman, N. H. (1995). Phonological awareness and literacy development in children with expressive phonological impairments. *Journal of Speech and Hearing Research, 38,* 446–462.

Blache, S. E. (1982). Minimal word pairs and distinctive feature training. In M. Crary (Ed.), *Phonological intervention: Concepts and procedures* (pp.61–96). San Diego: College-Hill Press.

Blache, S. E., Parsons, C. L., & Humphreys, J. M. (1981). A minimal-word-pair model for teaching the linguistic significance of distinctive feature properties. *Journal of Speech and Hearing Disorders, 46,* 291–296.

Black, M. (1964). *Speech correction in the schools.* Englewood Cliffs, NJ: Prentice-Hall.

Blakeley, R. W. (1972). *The practice of speech pathology.* Springfield, IL: Charles C Thomas.

Blakeley, R. W. (1983). Treatment of developmental apraxia of speech. In W. H. Perkins (Ed.), *Dysarthria and apraxia* (pp. 25–33). New York: Thieme-Stratton.

Blakeley, R. W. (2001). *Screening Test for Developmental Apraxia of Speech* (2nd ed.). Austin, TX: Pro-Ed.

Bleile, K. M. (1989). A note on vowel patterns in two normally developing children. *Clinical Linguistics & Phonetics, 3,* 203–212.

Bloodstein, O. (1979). *Speech pathology: An introduction.* Boston: Houghton Mifflin.

Bloomer, H. (1971). Speech defects associated with dental malocclusions and related abnormalities. In L. Travis (Ed.), *Handbook of speech pathology and audiology* (pp. 715–766). New York: Appleton-Century-Crofts.

Bloomer, H., & Hawk, A. (1973). Speech considerations: Speech disorders associated with ablative surgery of the face, mouth and pharynx—Ablative approaches to learning. In *ASHA Report #8: Orofacial Anomalies.* Washington, DC: American Speech-Language-Hearing Association.

Boothroyd, A. (1985). Evaluation of speech production of the hearing impaired: Some benefits of forced-choice testing. *Journal of Speech and Hearing Research, 28,* 185–196.

Bopp, K. (1995, April). *The effects of phonological intervention on morphosyntactic development in preschool children with phonological and morphosyntactic disorders.* Unpublished master's thesis. University of British Columbia, Vancouver, BC, Canada.

Boshart, C. A. (1998). *Oral-motor analysis and remediation techniques.* Temecula, CA: Speech Dynamics Incorporated.

Boshart, C. A. (1999). *Treatise on the tongue. Analysis and treatment of tongue abnormalities.* Temecula, CA: Speech Dynamics Incorporated.

Bountress, N., & Richards, I. J. (1979). Speech, language, and hearing disorders in an adult penal institution. *Journal of Speech and Hearing Disorders, 44,* 293–300.

Bradley, D. P. (1989). A systematic multiple-phoneme approach. In N. A. Creaghead, P. W. Newman, & W. A. Secord. *Assessment and remediation of articulatory and phonological disorders* (2nd ed., pp. 305–322). Columbus, OH: Merrill Publishing Company.

Braley, R., & Stoudt, R. (1977). A five-year longitudinal study of development of articulation proficiency in elementary school children. *Language, Speech, and Hearing Services in Schools 8,* 176–180.

Brinton, B., & Fujiki, M. (1993). Language, social skills, and socioemotional behavior. *Language, Speech, and Hearing Services in Schools, 24,* 194–198.

Brown, I., Timm, K., & Evans, E. (1978). *Universal articulation program.* Boston: Teaching Resources, Inc.

Buckendorf, G. R., & Gordon, C. J. (2002). Speech-mechanism assessment. In R. Paul (Ed.), *Introduction to clinical methods in communication disorders.* Baltimore: Paul H. Brookes Publishing Co.

Bush, C. (1978). Creative drama and language experiences: Effective clinical techniques. *Language, Speech and Hearing Services in Schools, 9,* 254–258.

Byrne, M., & Shervanian, C. (1977). *Introduction to communicative disorders.* New York: Harper & Row.

Bzoch, K. R. (Ed.) (1997). *Communicative disorders related to cleft lip and palate* (4th ed.). Austin, TX: Pro-Ed.

Calvert, D. R. (1982). Articulation and hearing impairments. In N. Lass, J. Northern, D. Yoder, & L. McReynolds (Eds.), *Speech, Language and Hearing* (Volume 2). Philadelphia: W. B. Saunders.

Cantwell, D., & Baker, L. (1991). *Psychiatric and developmental disorders in children with communication disorders.* Washington, DC: American Psychiatric Press.

Carrell, J. (1968). *Disorders of articulation.* Englewood Cliffs, NJ: Prentice-Hall.

Carrier, J. (1970). A program of articulation therapy administered by mothers. *Journal of Speech and Hearing Disorders, 35,* 344–353.

Carpenter, M. (1983). *Human Neuroanatomy* (8th ed.). Baltimore: Williams & Wilkins.

Carter, E., & Buck, M. (1958). Prognostic testing for functional articulation disorders among children in the first grade. *Journal of Speech and Hearing Disorders, 23,* 124–133.

Caruso, A. J., & Strand, E. A. (1999). Motor speech disorders in children: Definitions, background, and a theoretical framework. In A. J. Caruso & E. A. Strand (Eds.), *Clinical management of motor speech disorders in children* (pp. 1–27), New York: Thieme.

Carver, R. (1997). A comparison of two phonological-based treatment approaches. Unpublished master's thesis, Portland State University, Portland, OR.

Catts, H. (1991). Facilitating phonological awareness: Role of speech-language pathologists. *Language, Speech, and Hearing Services in Schools, 22,* 196–203.

Cave, M. R. (1999). Interrater agreement for the Weiss check-slash method of measuring intelligibility. Unpublished master's thesis, Portland State University, Portland, OR.

Chappell, G. (1973). Childhood verbal apraxia and its treatment. *Journal of Speech and Hearing Disorders, 38,* 362–368.

Chapman, R., Streim, N., Crais, E., Salmon, D., Strand, E., & Negri, N. (1992). Child talk: Assumptions of a developmental process model for early language learning. In R. Chapman (Ed.), *Processes in language acquisition and disorders* (pp. 3–19). St. Louis: Mosby-Year Book, Inc.

Cheng, L. L. (1989). Service delivery to Asian/Pacific LEP children: A cross-cultural framework. *Topics in Language Disorders, 9,* 1–14.

Cheng, L. L. (1991). *Assessing Asian language performance* (2nd ed.). Oceanside, CA: Academic Communication Associates.

Chomsky, N. (1957). *Syntactic structures.* The Hague: Mouton.

Chomsky, N. (1965). *Aspects of the theory of syntax.* Cambridge, MA: MIT Press.

Chomsky, N. (1981). *Lectures on government and binding.* Dordrecht, Holland: Foris.

Chomsky, N., & Halle, M. (1968). *The sound pattern of English.* New York: Harper & Row, Publishers.

Chumpelik, D. (1984). The PROMPT system of therapy. *Seminars in Speech and Language, 5,* 139–156.

Churchill, J. D., Hodson, B. W., Jones, B. W., & Novak, R. E. (1988). Phonological systems of speech disordered clients with positive/negative histories of otitis media. *Language, Speech, and Hearing Services in Schools, 19,* 100–106.

Clarke, H. G. (1997). Gross estimation: A study of the clinical validity of measuring intelligibility. Unpublished master's thesis, Portland State University, Portland, OR.

Clarke-Klein, S., & Hodson, B. (1995). A phonologically based analysis of misspellings by third graders with disordered-phonology histories. *Journal of Speech and Hearing Research, 38,* 839–849.

Collins, P., & Cunningham, G. (1976). *Writing individualized programs: A workbook for speech pathologists.* Gladstone, OR: CC Publications.

Compton, A. (1970). Generative studies of children's phonological disorders. *Journal of Speech and Hearing Disorders, 35,* 315–339.

Conley, D. (1966). The effects of using standardized instructions to evaluate speech correction procedures. Unpublished master's thesis, Arizona State University, Tempe, AZ.

Connolly, J. H. (1986). Intelligibility: A linguistic view. *British Journal of Disorders of Communication, 21,* 371–376.

Cook, J. (1999). Clinical application of two articulation treatment approaches: Traditional and computer-based interventions. Unpublished special project, Portland State University, Portland, OR.

Cornick, C. M., & Thomas, T. M. (1986). Oral language in the classroom. In J. M. Creighton, & C. A. Weiner (Eds.), *Practical strategies: Successful programs in public school speech/language pathology* (pp. 91–101). Phoenix, AZ: Syndactic, Inc.

Costello, J. (1975). Articulation instruction based on distinctive features theory. *Language, Speech, and Hearing Services in Schools, 6,* 61–71.

Costello, J. (1977). Programmed instruction. *Journal of Speech and Hearing Disorders, 42,* 3–28.

Costello, J., & Bosler, S. (1976). Generalization and articulation instruction. *Journal of Speech and Hearing Disorders, 41,* 359–373.

Costello, J., & Onstine, J. (1976). The modification of multiple articulation errors based on distinctive feature therapy. *Journal of Speech and Hearing Disorders, 41,* 199–215.

Creaghead, N. A., & Newman, P. W. (1989). Articulatory phonetics and phonology. In N. A. Creaghead, P. W. Newman, & W. A. Secord. *Assessment and remediation of articulatory and phonological disorders* (2nd ed., pp. 9–33). Columbus, OH: Merrill Publishing Company.

Creaghead, N. A., Newman, P. W., & Secord, W. A. (1989). *Assessment and remediation of articulatory and phonological disorders* (2nd ed.). Columbus, OH: Merrill Publishing Company.

Crow Hall, B. J. C. (1991). Attitudes of fourth and sixth graders toward peers with mild articulation disorders. *Language, Speech, and Hearing Services in Schools, 22,* 334–340.

Crowe, T. A., Byrne, M. E., & Henry, A. N. (1999). Prison services: The Parchman project. *ASHA, 41,* 50–54.

Crumrine, L., & Lonegan, H. (1999). *Pre-Literacy Skills Screening.* Austin, TX: Pro-Ed.

Crumrine, L., & Lonegan, H. (2000). *Phonemic Awareness Skills Screening.* Austin, TX: Pro-Ed.

Crystal, D. (1985). *A dictionary of linguistics and phonetics* (2nd ed.). Oxford: Basil Blackwell.

Cullinan, W. L., Brown, C. S., & Blalock, P. D. (1986). Ratings of intelligibility of esophageal and tracheoesophageal speech. *Journal of Communication Disorders, 19,* 185–195.

Cummins, J. (1992). The role of primary language development in promoting educational success for language minority students. In C. Leyba (Ed.), *Schooling and language minority students: A theoretical framework.* California State University, Los Angeles.

Dale, P. S. (1972). *Language development structure and function.* Hinsdale, IL: Dryden Press.

Darley, F., Aronson, A., & Brown, J. (1975). *Motor speech disorders*. Philadelphia: W. B. Saunders.

Darley, F., & Spriestersbach, D. (1978). *Diagnostic methods in speech pathology* (2nd ed.). New York: Harper & Row.

Davis, B., & Bedore, L. M. (2000). Articulatory and phonological disorders. In R. B. Gillam, T. P. Marquardt, & F. N. Martin, *Communication sciences and disorders. From science to clinical practice* (pp. 25–61), San Diego: Singular Publishing Group.

Davis, B., & MacNeilage, P. (1990). Acquisition of correct vowel production: A quantitative case study. *Journal of Speech and Hearing Research, 33*, 16–27.

Davis, B., & Velleman, S. L. (2000). Differential diagnosis and treatment of developmental apraxia of speech in infants and toddlers. *Infant-Toddler Intervention, 10*, 177–192.

Davis, E. (1937). The development of linguistic skills in twins, singletons with siblings, and only children from age five to ten years. University of Minnesota *Institute of Child Welfare Monograph Series, 14*, Minneapolis, MN: University of Minnesota.

Dawson, J., & Tattersall, P. J. (2001). *Structured Photographic Articulation Test II*. DeKalb, IL: Janelle Publications.

Dawson, L. (1929). A study of the development of the rate of articulation. *Elementary School Journal, 29*, 610–615.

Dean, E. C., Howell, J., Hill, A., & Waters, D. (1990). *Metaphon Resource Pack*. Windsor, Berks: NFER Nelson.

Dean, E. C., Howell, J., Waters, D., & Reid, J. (1995). Metaphon: A metalinguistic approach to the treatment of phonological disorder in children. *Clinical Linguistics & Phonetics, 9*, 1–58.

DelMoral, S. J. (2002). Self-evaluating video-playback of articulatory productions to promote environmental generalization. Unpublished master's thesis, Portland State University, Portland, OR.

Denes, P. B., & Pinson, E. N. (1993). *The speech chain. The physics and biology of spoken language* (2nd. ed.). New York: W. H. Freeman and Company.

Dinnsen, D. (1992). Variation in developing and fully developed phonetic inventories. In C. A Ferguson, L. Menn, & C. Stoel-Gammon (Eds.), *Phonological development: Models, research, implications* (pp. 191–210). Timonium, Md: York Press.

Dinnsen, D., Chin, S. B., Elbert, M., & Powell, T. W. (1990). Some constraints on functionally disordered phonologies: Phonetic inventories and phonotactics. *Journal of Speech and Hearing Research, 33*, 28–37.

Dodd, B. (1995). *The differential diagnosis and treatment of children with speech disorder*. London: Whurr Publishers.

Donegan, P. J., & Stampe, D. (1979). The study of natural phonology. In D. A. Dinnsen (Ed.), *Current approaches to phonological theory* (pp. 126–173). Bloomington, IN: Indiana University Press.

Drexler, H. (1976). A simplified application of distinctive feature analysis to articulation therapy. *Journal of the Oregon Speech and Hearing Association, 15*, 2–5.

Duder, C., Camarata, S., Camarata, M., Koegel, R., & Koegel, L. (1998, Novemter). *No free lunch? Language change during phonological treatment of children*. Presented at the Annual Convention of the American Speech-Language-Hearing Association, San Antonio, TX.

Dukart, C. J. (1996). A comparison of speech intelligibility measures between unsophisticated listener judgments and orthographic transcription. Unpublished master's thesis, Portland State University, Portland, OR.

Dunlap, G., & Plienis, A. J. (1988). Generalization and maintenance of unsupervised responding via remote contingencies. In R. H. Horner, G. Dunlap, & R. L. Koegel (Eds.), *Generalization and maintenance: Lifestyle changes in applied settings* (pp. 121–142). Baltimore: Paul H. Brookes.

Dunn, C. (1983). A framework for generalization in disordered phonology. *Journal of Childhood Communication Disorders, 7*, 46–58.

Dunn, C., & Till, J. (1982). Morphophonemic rule learning in normal and articulation-disordered children. *Journal of Speech and Hearing Research, 25*, 322–333.

Dworkin, J. P. (1978). Protrusive lingual force and lingual diadochokinetic rates: A comparative analysis between normal and lisping speakers. *Language, Speech, and Hearing Services in Schools, 9*, 8–16.

Dworkin, J. P. (1980). Characteristics of frontal lispers clustered according to severity. *Journal of Speech and Hearing Disorders, 45*, 37–44.

Dworkin, J. P. (1991). *Motor speech disorders. A treatment guide*. St. Louis: Mosby-Year Book.

Dworkin, J. P., & Culatta, R. A. (1980). Tongue strength: Its relationship to tongue thrusting, open-bite, and articulatory proficiency. *Journal of Speech and Hearing Disorders, 45*, 227–282.

Dworkin J. P., & Culatta, R. A. (1985). Oral structural and neuromuscular characteristics in children with normal and disordered articulation. *Journal of Speech and Hearing Disorders, 50*, 150–156.

Dworkin, J. P., & Culatta, R. A. (1996). *Dworkin-Culatta Oral Mechanism & Treatment System*. Nicholasville, KY: Edgewood Press.

Dyson, A. (1988). Phonetic inventories of 2- and 3-year-old children. *Journal of Speech and Hearing Disorders, 53*, 89–93.

Dyson, A. & Paden, E. (1983). Some phonological acquisition strategies used by two-year-olds. *Journal of Childhood Communication Disorders, 7*, 6–18.

Ebert, K. A., & Prelock, P. A. (1994). Teachers' perceptions of their students with communication disorders. *Language Speech, and Hearing Services in Schools, 25*, 211–214.

Edwards, H. T. (2003). *Applied phonetics: The sounds of American English* (3rd ed.). Clifton, NY: Delmar Learning.

Edwards, M. L. (1986). *Introduction to applied phonetics*. San Diego: College-Hill Press.

Edwards, M. L., & Shriberg, L. (1983). *Phonology: applications in communicative disorders*. San Diego: College-Hill Press.

Eisenson, J., & Ogilvie, M. (1977). *Speech correction in the schools* (4th ed.). New York: Macmillan, 1977.

Elbert, M., Dinnsen, D. A., & Powell, T. (1984). On the prediction of phonologic generalization learning patterns. *Journal of Speech and Hearing Disorders, 49*, 309–317.

Elbert, M., Dinnsen, D. A., Swartzlander, P., & Chin, S. B. (1990). Generalization to conversational speech. *Journal of Speech and Hearing Disorders, 55*, 694–699.

Elbert, M., & Gierut, J. A. (1986). *Handbook of clinical phonology: Approaches to assessment and treatment*. San Diego: College-Hill Press.

Elbert, M., & McReynolds, L. V. (1975). Transfer of /r/ across contexts. *Journal of Speech and Hearing Disorders, 40*, 380–387.

Elbert, M., & McReynolds, L. V. (1978). An experimental analysis of misarticulating children's generalization. *Journal of Speech and Hearing Research, 21*, 136–149.

Elbert, M., Powell, T. W., & Swartzlander, P. (1991). Toward a technology of generalization: How many exemplars are sufficient? *Journal of Speech and Hearing Research, 34*, 81–87.

Elbert, M., Shelton, R., & Arndt, W. (1967). A task for evaluation of articulation change: 1. Development of methodology. *Journal of Speech and Hearing Research, 10*, 281–288.

Emerick, C., & Hatten, J. (1986). *Diagnosis and evaluation in speech pathology* (3rd ed.). Englewood Cliffs, NJ: Prentice-Hall.

Enderby, P. M. (1983). *Frenchay Dysarthria Assessment.* San Diego: College-Hill Press.

Engel, D., Brandriet, S., Erickson, K., Grunhovd, K. D., & Gunderson, G. (1966). Carryover. *Journal of Speech and Hearing Disorders, 31*, 227–233.

Engel, D., Erickson, K., & Groth, L. (1970). *Two approaches to articulation carryover therapy which can be done in the school setting.* Paper presented at the ASHA Annual Convention, New York.

Engel, D., & Groth, L. (1976). Reinforcing postarticulation responses based on feedback. *Language, Speech, and Hearing Service in Schools, 7*, 93–101.

Ertmer, D., & Ertmer, P. (1998). Constructivist strategies in phonological intervention: Facilitating self-regulation for carryover. *Language, Speech, and Hearing Services in Schools, 29*, 67–75.

Everhart, R. (1953). The relationships between articulation and other developmental factors in children. *Journal of Speech and Hearing Disorders, 18*, 332–338.

Everhart, R. (1956). Paternal occupational classification and the maturation of articulation. *Speech Monographs, 23*, 75–77.

Fadiman, A. (1997). *The spirit catches you and you fall down: A Hmong Child, her American doctors, and the collision of two cultures.* New York: Farrar, Straus and Giroux.

Fairbanks, G., & Bebout, B. (1950). A study of minor organic deviations of articulation: 3. Tongue, *Journal of Speech and Hearing Disorders, 15*, 348–352.

Fairbanks, G., & Green, E. (1950). A study of minor organic deviations in "functional" disorders of articulation. 2. Dimension and relationship of the lips. *Journal of Speech and Hearing Disorders, 15*, 165–168.

Fairbanks, G., & Lintner, M. (1951). A study of minor organic deviations in functional disorders of articulation. *Journal of Speech and Hearing Disorders, 16*, 273–279.

Fantini, A. E. (1978). Bilingual behavior and social cues: Case studies of two bilingual children. In M. Paradis (Ed.), *Aspects of bilingualism.* Columbia, SC: Hornbeam Press.

Farquhar, M. S. (1961). Prognostic value of imitative and auditory discrimination tests. *Journal of Speech and Hearing Disorders, 26*, 342–347.

Felsenfeld, S., McGue, M., & Broen, P. A. (1995). Familial aggregation of phonological disorders: Results from a 28-year follow-up. *Journal of Speech and Hearing Research, 38*, 1091–1107.

Felsenfeld, S., & Plomin, R. (1997). Epidemiological and offspring analyses of developmental speech disorders using data from the Colorado adoption project. *Journal of Speech and Hearing Research, 40*, 778–791.

Ferguson, C. A., & Garnica, O. K. (1975). Theories of phonological development. In E. H. Lenneberg & E. Lenneberg (Eds.), *Foundations of language development.* New York: Academic Press.

Ferrier, L. (1991). Pronunciation training for foreign teaching assistants. *ASHA 33*, 65–71.

Fey, M. E. (1992). Articulation and phonology: Inextricable constructs in speech pathology. *Language, Speech, and Hearing Services in Schools, 23*, 225–232.

Fey, M. E., Cleave, P. L., Ravida, A. I., Long, S. H., Dejmal, A. E., & Easton, D. L. (1994). Effects of grammar facilitation on the phonological performance of children with speech and language impairments. *Journal of Speech and Hearing Research, 37*, 594–607.

Fillmore, C. (1968). The case for case. In E. Bach & R. Harmas (Eds.), *Universals in linguistic theory* (pp. 1–88). New York: Holt, Rinehart & Winston.

Fisher, H. B., & Logemann, J. A. (1971). *Fisher-Logemann Test of Articulation Competence.* Boston: Houghton Mifflin.

Fitzsimmons, R. (1958). Developmental, psychosocial and educational factors in children with nonorganic articulation problems. *Child Development, 29*, 481–489.

Fletcher, S. G. (1992). *Articulation: A physiological approach.* San Diego: Singular Publishing Group, Inc.

Fletcher, S., Casteel, R., & Bradley, D. (1961). Tongue thrust swallow, speech articulation and age. *Journal of Speech and Hearing Disorders, 26*, 201–208.

Fletcher, S., & Meldrum, J. (1968). Lingual function and relative length of the lingual frenulum. *Journal of Speech and Hearing Disorders, 11*, 382–390.

Fluharty, N. B. (2000). *Fluharty Preschool Speech and Language Screening Test-Second Edition.* Austin, TX: Pro-Ed.

Flynn, P., & Byrne, M. (1970). Relationship between reading and selected auditory abilities of third-grade children. *Journal of Speech and Hearing Research, 13*, 731–740.

Fokes, J. (1982). Problems confronting the theorist and practitioner in child phonology. In M. Crary (Ed.), *Phonological intervention: Concepts and procedures* (pp. 13–34). San Diego: College-Hill Press.

Fowler, S. A., & Baer, D. M. (1981). "Do I have to be good all day?" The timing of delayed reinforcement as a factor in generalization. *Journal of Applied Behavior Analysis, 14*, 13–24.

Freeby, N., & Madison, C. L. (1989). Children's perceptions of peers with articulation disorders. *Child Study Journal, 19*, 133–144.

Fudala, J. B. (1973). Using parents in public school speech therapy. *Language, Speech, and Hearing Services in Schools, 4*, 91–94.

Fudala, J. B. (2000). *Arizona Articulation Proficiency Scale, Third Revision.* Los Angeles: Western Psychological Services.

Fudala, J. B., England, G., & Ganoug, L. (1972). Utilization of parents in a speech correction program. *Exceptional Children, 38*, 407–412.

Gallagher, T. M., & Shriner, T. H. (1975a). Articulatory inconsistencies in the speech of normal children. *Journal of Speech and Hearing Research, 18*, 168–175.

Gallagher, T. M., & Shriner, T. H. (1975b). Contextual variables related to inconsistent /s/ and /z/ production. *Journal of Speech and Hearing Research, 18*, 623–633.

Gammon, S., Smith, P., Daniloff, R., & Kim, C. (1971). Articulation and stress juncture production under oral anesthetization and masking. *Journal of Speech and Hearing Research, 14*, 271–282.

Gardner, E. (1975). *Fundamentals of neurology* (6th ed.). Philadelphia: W. B. Saunders.

Garn-Nunn, P. G., & Lynn, J. M. (2004). *Descriptive phonetics* (3rd ed.). New York: Thieme.

Gelfer, M. P. (1996). *Survey of communication disorders: A social and behavioral perspective.* New York: The McGraw-Hill Companies, Inc.

Genesee, F. (1989). Early bilingual development: One language or two? *Journal of Child Language, 16*, 161–179.

Gerber, A. (1973). *Goal: Carryover an articulation manual and program.* Philadelphia: Temple University Press.

Gerber, A. (1977). Programming for articulation modification. *Journal of Speech and Hearing Disorders, 26*, 29–43.

Gierut, J. A. (1989). Maximal opposition approach to phonological treatment. *Journal of Speech and Hearing Disorders, 54,* 9–19.

Gierut, J. A. (1990). Differential learning of phonological oppositions. *Journal of Speech and Hearing Research, 33,* 540–549.

Gierut, J. A. (1992). The conditions and course of clinically-induced phonological change. *Journal of Speech and Hearing Research, 35,* 1049–1063.

Gierut, J. A., Elbert, M., & Dinnsen, D. (1987). A functional analysis of phonological knowledge and generalization learning in misarticulating children. *Journal of Speech and Hearing Research, 39,* 462–479.

Gierut, J. A., Morrisette, M. L., Hughes, M. T., & Rowland, S. (1996). Phonological treatment efficacy and developmental norms. *Language, Speech, and Hearing Services in Schools, 27,* 215–230.

Gilham, R. B., & Bedore, L. M. (2000). Communication across the lifespan. In R. B. Gillam, T. P. Marquardt, & F. N. Martin (Eds.), *Communication sciences and disorders. From science to clinical practice* (pp. 25–61), San Diego: Singular Publishing Group.

Gleason, J. B. (2005). *The development of language* (6th ed.). New York: Allyn & Bacon.

Goldman, R., & Fristoe, M. (1986). *Goldman-Fristoe Test of Articulation-Second Edition.* Circle Pines, MN: American Guidance Service, Inc.

Goldman, R., & Fristoe, M. (2000). *Goldman-Fristoe Test of Articulation—Second Edition.* Circle Pines, MN: American Guidance Service, Inc.

Goldman, R., Fristoe, M., & Woodcock, R. W. (1976). *Goldman-Fristoe-Woodcock Test of Auditory Discrimination.* Circle Pines, MN: American Guidance Service, Inc.

Goldsworthy, C. (1996). *Developmental reading disabilities: A language-based treatment approach.* San Diego: Singular Publishing Group.

Gordon-Brannan, M. (1993). Speech intelligibility assessment of young children with varying levels of phonological proficiency/deficiency. Unpublished doctoral dissertation, Wichita State University, Wichita, KS.

Gordon-Brannan, M. (1994). Assessing intelligibility in children. *Topics in Language Disorders, 14,* 17–25.

Gordon-Brannan, M., & Hodson, B. (2000). Intelligibility/severity measurements of prekindergarten children's speech. *American Journal of Speech-Language Pathology, 9,* 141–150.

Gordon-Brannan, M., Hodson, B., & Wynn, M. (1992). Remediating unintelligible utterances of a child with a mild hearing loss. *American Journal of Speech-Language Pathology, 1,* 28–38.

Gray, S. I., & Shelton, R. L. (1992). Self-monitoring effects on articulation carryover in school-age children. *Language, Speech, and Hearing Services in Schools, 23,* 334–342.

Griffiths, H., & Craighead, W. E. (1972). Generalization in operant speech therapy for misarticulation. *Journal of Speech and Hearing Disorders, 37,* 485–494.

Groher, M. (1976). The experimental use of cross-age relationships in public school remediation. *Language, Speech, and Hearing Services in Schools, 7,* 250–258.

Gross, G. H., St. Louis, K. O., Ruscello, D. M., & Hull, F. M. (1985). Language abilities of articulatory-disordered school children with multiple or residual errors. *Language, Speech, and Hearing Services in Schools, 16,* 171–186.

Grossman, H. (Ed.) (1983). *Classification in mental retardation.* Washington, DC: American Association on Mental Deficiency.

Grunwell, P. (1987). *Clinical phonology* (2nd ed.). Baltimore: Williams & Wilkins.

Grunwell, P. (1997). Natural phonology. In M. J. Ball & R. D. Kent, *The new phonologies: Developments in clinical linguistics* (pp. 35–75). San Diego: Singular Publishing Group, Inc.

Hadley, P. A., & Rice, M. L. (1991). Conversational responsiveness in speech and language-impaired preschoolers. *Journal of Speech and Hearing Research, 34,* 1308–1317.

Haelsig, P. C., & Madison, C. L. (1986). A study of phonological processes exhibited by 3-, 4-, and 5-year-old children. *Language, Speech, and Hearing Services in Schools, 17,* 107–114.

Hall, B. J., Oyer, H. J., & Haas, W. H. (2001). Speech, language, and hearing disorders: A guide for the teacher (3rd ed.). Boston: Allyn & Bacon.

Hall, M. (1938). Auditory factors in functional articulatory speech defects. *Journal of Experimental Education, 7,* 110–132.

Hall, P. K. (1994). The oral mechanism. In J. B. Tomblin, H. L. Morris, & D. C. Spriestersbach, *Diagnosis in speech-language pathology* (pp. 67–98). San Diego: Singular Publishing Group, Inc.

Hall, P. K., Jordon, L. S., & Robin, D. A. (1993). *Developmental apraxia of speech: Theory and clinical practice.* Austin, TX: Pro-Ed.

Halle, M. (1964). On the bases of phonology. In J. Fodor & J. Katz (Eds.), *The structure of language: Readings in the philosophy of language* (pp. 324–333). Englewood Cliffs, NJ: Prentice-Hall.

Ham, R. (1958). Relationship between misspelling and misarticulation. *Journal of Speech and Hearing Disorders, 23,* 294–297.

Hanson, M. L. (1994). Oral myofunctional disorders and articulatory patterns. In J. Bernthal & N. Bankson (Eds.), *Child Phonology: Characteristics, assessment, and intervention with special populations* (pp. 29–53). New York: Thieme Medical Publishers.

Hayden, D. (1999). *The P.R.O.M.P.T. System Level 1: Manual.* Santa Fe, NM: PROMPT Institute, Inc.

Hayden, D., & Square, P. (1994). Motor speech treatment hierarchy: A systems approach. *Clinics in Communication Disorders, 4,* 151–161.

Hayden, D., & Square, P. (1999). *Verbal Motor Production Assessment for Children.* San Antonio, TX: Psychological Corporation.

Haynes, W. O., & Pindzola, R. H. (2004). *Diagnosis and evaluation in speech pathology* (6th ed.). Boston: Allyn & Bacon.

Heffner, R. (1952). *General phonetics.* Madison, WI: University of Wisconsin Press.

Hegde, M. N. (1998). *Treatment procedures in communicative disorders* (3rd ed.). Austin, TX: Pro-Ed.

Hickman, L. A. (1997). *The Apraxia Profile.* San Antonio, TX: Communication Skill Builders.

Hocket, C. (1960). The origin of speech. *Scientific American, 203,* 89–97.

Hodge, M., & Hancock, H. R. (1994). Assessment of children with developmental apraxia of speech: A procedure. *Clinics in Communication Disorders, 4,* 102–118.

Hodson, B. W. (1986a). *The Assessment of Phonological Processes-Revised.* Austin, TX: Pro-Ed.

Hodson, B. W. (1986b). *Assessment of Phonological Processes - Spanish.* San Diego: Los Amigos Research Associates.

Hodson, B. W. (1994). Helping individuals become intelligible, literate, and articulate: The role of phonology. *Topics in Language Disorders, 14,* 1–16.

Hodson, B. W. (1997). Disordered phonologies: What have we learned about assessment and treatment? In B. W. Hodson & M. L. Edwards (Eds.), *Perspectives in applied phonology* (pp. 197–224). Gaithersburg, MD: Aspen Publishers, Inc.

Hodson, B. W. (2003). *Hodson Computerized Analysis of Phonological Patterns.* Wichita, KS: PhonoComp Software.

Hodson, B. W. (2004). *Hodson Assessment of Phonological Patterns* (3rd ed.). Austin, TX: Pro-Ed.

Hodson, B. W., Chin, L., Redmond, B., & Simpson, R. (1983). Phonological evaluation and remediation of speech deviations of a child with a repaired cleft palate: A case study. *Journal of Speech and Hearing Disorders, 48,* 93–98.

Hodson, B. W., & Edwards, M. L. (Eds.) (1997). *Perspectives in applied phonology.* Gaithersburg, MD: Aspen Publishers Inc.

Hodson, B. W., & Gordon-Brannan, M. (1992). *Phonological assessment and remediation: Expediting intelligibility gains.* Conference sponsored by Portland Center for Hearing and Speech, Beaverton, OR.

Hodson, B. W., & Paden, E. P. (1981). Phonological processes that characterize unintelligible and intelligible speech in early childhood. *Journal of Speech and Hearing Disorders, 46,* 369–373.

Hodson, B. W., & Paden, E. P. (1991). *Targeting intelligible speech.* Austin, TX: Pro-Ed.

Hodson, B. W., Scherz, J. A., & Strattman, K. H. (2002). Evaluating communicative abilities of a highly unintelligible preschooler. *American Journal of Speech-Language Pathology, 11,* 236–242.

Hoffman, P. R., & Norris, J. A. (1989). On the nature of phonological development: Evidence from normal children's spelling errors. *Journal of Speech and Hearing Research, 32,* 787–794.

Hoffman, P. R., Norris, J. A., & Monjure, J. (1990). Comparison of process targeting and whole language treatments of phonologically delayed children. *Language, Speech, and Hearing Services in Schools, 21,* 102–109.

Holm, A., & Dodd, B. (1999). An intervention case study of a bilingual child with a phonological disorder. *Child Language Teaching & Therapy, 15,* 139–158.

Howell, J., & Dean, E. (1994). *Treating phonological disorders in children (2nd ed.).* London: Whurr Publishers Ltd.

Hughes, D. L. (1985). *Language treatment and generalization: A clinician's handbook.* San Diego: College-Hill Press.

Hulit, L. M., & Howard, M. R. (2002). *Born to talk: An introduction to speech and language development* (3rd ed.). Boston: Allyn & Bacon.

Hull, F., Mielke, P., Timmons, R., & Willeford, J. (1971). The national speech and hearing survey: Preliminary results. *ASHA, 13,* 501–509.

Hummel, L. J., & Prizant, B. M. (1993). A socioemotional perspective for understanding social difficulties of school-age children with language disorders. *Language, Speech, and Hearing Services in Schools, 24,* 216–224.

Iglesias, A., & Goldstein, B. (2004). Language and dialectal variations. In J. Bernthal and N. Bankson (Eds.), *Articulation and phonological disorders* (5th ed., pp.348–375). Boston: Pearson Education, Inc.

Individuals with Disabilities Education Act Amendments of 1997 (IDEA) (1997), 20 USC § 1400 *et seq.*

Ingham, J. C., & Parks, D. R. (1989). *Accuracy and reactivity of self-monitoring of correct and incorrect articulation responses.* Paper presented at the Annual convention of the American Speech-Language-Hearing Association, San Antonio, TX.

Ingram, D. (1981). *Procedures for the phonological analysis of children's language.* Baltimore: University Park Press.

Ingram, D. (1989). *Phonological disability in children* (2nd ed.). San Diego: Singular Publishing Group, Inc.

Ingram, D. (1997). Generative phonology. In M. J. Ball & R. D. Kent, *The new phonologies: Developments in clinical linguistics* (pp. 7–33). San Diego: Singular Publishing Group, Inc.

Irwin, J., & Weston, A. (1971–1975). *Paired stimuli kit.* Milwaukee, WI: Fox Point.

Irwin, J., & Weston, A. (1975). The paired stimuli. *ASHA Monograph, 6,* 1–76.

Irwin, J., & Wong, S. (1983). *Phonological development in children 16 to 72 months.* Carbondale, IL: Southern Illinois University Press.

Jakobson, R. (1968). *Child language, aphasia and phonological universals.* (A. R. Keiler, translator). The Hague: Mouton. (From *Kindersprache, aphasie und allgemeine lautgestze,* Uppsala, Sweden: 1941).

Jakobson, R. (1971). The sound laws of child language and their place in general phonology. In A. Bar-Adon & W. F. Leopold (Eds.), *Child language: A book of readings* (pp. 75–82). Englewood Cliffs, NJ: Prentice-Hall.

Jakobson, R., Fant, G., & Halle, M. (1952). *Preliminaries to speech analysis.* Cambridge, MA: MIT Press.

Jakobson, R., & Halle, M. (1956). *Fundamentals of language.* The Hague: Mouton.

James, S. L. (1990). *Normal language acquisition.* Austin, TX: Pro-Ed.

Jamieson, D. G., & Rvachew, S. (1992). Remediation of speech production errors with sound identification training. *Journal of Speech-Language Pathology and Audiology, 16,* 519–521.

Jann, B., Ward, M., & Jann, H. (1964). A longitudinal study of articulation, deglutition and malocclusion. *Journal of Speech and Hearing Disorders, 29,* 424–435.

Jelm, J. (2002). *Verbal Dyspraxia Profile.* DeKalb, IL: Janelle Publications.

Johnson, D. D. (1975). Communication characteristics of NTID students. *Journal of the Academy of Rehabilitative Audiology, 8,* 17–32.

Johnson W., Brown, S. F., Curtis, J. F., Edney, C. W., & Keaster, J. (1967). *Speech handicapped school children* (3rd ed.). New York: Harper & Row.

Johnson, J., Whinney, B., & Pederson, O. (1980). Single word versus connected speech articulation testing. *Language, Speech, and Hearing Services in Schools, 11,* 175–179.

Johnston, J., & Johnston, G. (1972). Modification of consonant speech-sound articulation in young children. *Journal of Applied Behavior Analysis, 5,* 233–246.

Judson, L., & Weaver, A. (1965). *Voice science* (2nd ed.). New York: Appleton-Century-Crofts.

Kalash, S. (1970). *A study of carryover techniques for articulation therapy.* Paper presented at the ASHA Annual Convention, New York.

Kaufman, N. (1995). *Kaufman Speech Praxis Test for Children.* Detroit, MI: Wayne State University Press.

Kemper, K. V. (1996). Comparison of two phonological treatment procedures for a child with phonological disorders. Unpublished master's thesis, Portland State University, Portland, OR.

Kenney, K. W., & Prather, E. M. (1986). Articulation development in preschool children: Consistency of productions. *Journal of Speech and Hearing Research, 29,* 29–36.

Kent, R. D. (1990). *The emergence of pediatric phonetic science: Implications for the 0–3 population.* Paper presented at the American Speech-Language-Hearing Association convention, Seattle, WA.

Kent, R. D. (1996). Hearing and believing: Some limits to the auditory-perception assessment of speech and voice disorders. *American Journal of Speech-Language Pathology, 5,* 7–23.

Kent, R. D., Kent, J. F., Weismer, G., Sufit, T. L., Rosenbek, J. C., Martin, R. E., & Brooks, B. R. (1990). Impairment of speech intelligibility in men with amyotrophic lateral sclerosis. *Journal of Speech and Hearing Disorders, 55,* 721–728.

Kent, R. D., Miolo, G., & Bloedel, S. (1992, November). *Measuring and assessing intelligibility.* Miniseminar presented at the annual meeting of the American Speech-Language-Hearing Association, San Antonio, TX.

Kent, R. D., Miolo, G., & Bloedel, S. (1994). The intelligibility of children's speech: A review of evaluation procedures. *American Journal of Speech-Language Pathology, 3,* 81–95.

Khan, L. M. (1982). A review of 16 major phonological processes. *Language, Speech, and Hearing Services in Schools, 13,* 77–85.

Khan, L. M. (1985). *Basics of phonological analysis: A programmed learning text.* San Diego: College-Hill Press.

Khan, L. M. (2002). The sixth view: Assessing preschoolers' articulation and phonology from the trenches. *American Journal of Speech-Language Pathology, 11,* 250–254.

Khan, L. M., & Lewis, N. P. (2002). *Khan-Lewis Phonological Analysis 2.* Circle Pines, MN: American Guidance Service, Inc.

Kinzler, M. C. (1992). *Joliet 3-Minute Preschool Speech and Language Screen.* San Antonio, TX: Harcourt Assessment, Inc.

Kinzler, M. C., & Johnson, C. C. (1993). *Joliet 3-Minute Speech and Language Screen* (Revised). San Antonio, TX: Harcourt Assessment, Inc.

Kisatsky, T. (1967). The prognostic value of Carter-Buck tests in measuring articulation skills in selected kindergarten children. *Exceptional Children, 34,* 81–85.

Koch, H. (1956). Sibling influence on children's speech. *Journal of Speech and Hearing Disorders, 21,* 322–328.

Koegel, L. K., Koegel, R. L., & Ingham, J. C. (1986). Programming rapid generalization of correct articulation through self-monitoring procedures. *Journal of Speech and Hearing Disorders, 51,* 24–32.

Koegel, R. L., Koegel, L. K., Von Voy, K., & Ingham, J. C. (1988). Within-clinic versus outside-of-clinic self-monitoring of articulation to promote generalization. *Journal of Speech and Hearing Disorders, 19,* 335–338.

Krashen, S. (1992). Bilingual education and second language acquisition theory. In C. Leyba (Ed.), *Schooling and language minority students: A theoretical framework.* California State University, Los Angeles.

Kuhl, P. K. (1994). Learning and representation in speech and language. *Current Opinion in Neurobiology, 4,* 812–822.

Kwiatkowski, J., & Shriberg, L. D. (1992). Intelligibility assessment in developmental phonological disorders: Accuracy of caregiver gloss. *Journal of Speech and Hearing Research, 35,* 1095–1104.

Ladefoged, P. (2001). *A course in phonetics* (7th ed.). Orlando, FL: Harcourt, Inc.

Langdon, H. W. (1992). Speech and language assessment of LEP/bilingual Hispanic students. In H. W. Langdon, & L. L. Cheng, (Eds.), *Hispanic children and adults with communication disorders: Assessment and intervention* (pp. 201–271). Gaithersburg, MD: Aspen Publishers, Inc.

Langdon H.W., & Cheng, L. (2002). *Collaborating with interpreters and translators: A guide for communication disorders professionals.* Eau Claire, WI: Thinking Publications.

Langdon, H. W., & Merino, B. J. (1992). Acquisition and development of a second language in the Spanish Speaker. In H. W. Langdon, & L. L. Cheng, (Eds.), *Hispanic children and adults with communication disorders: Assessment and intervention* (pp. 132–167). Gaithersburg, MD: Aspen Publishers, Inc.

Lanphere, T. (1998). *Test of Articulation in Context.* Austin, TX: Pro-Ed.

Lapko, L., & Bankson, N. W. (1975). Relationship between auditory discrimination, articulation stimulability and consistency of misarticulation. *Perceptual and Motor Skills, 40,* 171–177.

LaPointe, L., & Wertz, R. (1974). Oral-movement abilities and articulatory characteristics of brain-injured adults. *Perceptual Motor Skills, 39,* 39–46.

Larrivee, L. S., & Catts, H. W. (1999). Early reading achievement in children with expressive phonological disorders. *American Journal of Speech-Language Pathology, 8,* 118–128.

Lehman, W. (1973). *Historical linguistics: An introduction* (2nd ed.). New York: Holt, Rinehart & Winston, Inc.

Lenneberg, E. H. (1967). *Biological foundations of language.* New York: John Wiley.

Leonard, L. (1973). The nature of deviant articulation. *Journal of Speech and Hearing Disorders, 38,* 156–161.

Leonard, R. J. (1994). Characteristics of speech in speakers with oral/oralpharyngeal ablation. In J. E. Bernthal, & N. W. Bankson (Eds.), *Child phonology: Characteristics, assessment, and intervention with special populations* (pp. 54–78). New York: Thieme Medical Publishers.

Leopold, W. (1970). *Speech development of a bilingual child.* New York: AMS Press.

Lewis, B. A., Ekelman, B. L., & Aram, D. M. (1989). A familial study of severe phonological disorders. *Journal of Speech and Hearing Research, 32,* 713–724.

Lewis, B. A., & Freebairn, L. (1993). A clinical tool for evaluating the familial basis of speech and language disorders. *American Journal of Speech-Language Pathology, 2,* 38–43.

Lillywhite, H. (1948). Make mother a clinician. *Journal of Speech and Hearing Disorders, 13,* 61–66.

Lippke, B. A., Dickey, S. E., Selmar, J. W., & Soder, A. L. (1997). *Photo Articulation Test-Third Edition.* Austin, TX: Pro-Ed.

Locke, J. L. (1968). Oral perception and articulation learning. *Perceptual and Motor Skills, 26,* 1259–1264.

Locke, J. L. (1980). The inference of speech perception in the phonologically disordered child. Part I: A rationale, some criteria, the conventional tests. *Journal of Speech and Hearing Disorders, 4,* 431–444.

Locke, J. & Mather, P. (1987). *Genetic factors in phonology. Evidence from monozygotic and dizygotic twins.* Paper presented at the annual convention of the American Speech-Language-Hearing Association, New Orleans, LA.

Lof, G. L. (1996). Factors associated with speech-sound stimulability. *Clinics in Communication Disorders, 29,* 255–278.

Lof, G. L. (2002). Two comments on this assessment series. *Journal of Speech-Language Pathology, 11,* 255–256.

Lof, G. L. (2003). Oral motor exercises and treatment outcomes. *Language Learning and Education, 10,* 7–11.

Louko, L., Edwards, M. E., & Conture, E. (1990). Phonological characteristics of young stutterers and their normally fluent peers: Preliminary observations. *Journal of Fluency Disorders, 15,* 93–106.

Lowe, R. J. (1994). *Phonology. Assessment and intervention applications in speech pathology.* Baltimore: Williams & Wilkins.

Lowe, R. J., Knutson, P. J., & Monson, M. (1985). Incidence of fronting in preschool children. *Language, Speech, and Hearing Services in Schools, 16*, 119–123.

Luchsinger, R., & Arnold, G. (1965). *Voice, speech, language.* Belmont, CA: Wadsworth.

MacWilliams, S. M. (2001). A comparison of the effectiveness of a computer-based versus a traditional articulation intervention in remediating articulation errors. Unpublished master's thesis, Portland State University, Portland, OR.

Madison, C. L. (1992). Attitudes toward mild misarticulation-disordered peers. *Language, Speech, and Hearing Services in Schools, 23*, 188.

Manning, W., Keappock, N., & Stick, S. (1976). The use of auditory masking to estimate automatization of correct articulatory productions. *Journal of Speech and Hearing Disorders, 41*, 143–149.

Marquardt, E. (1959). Carry-over with speech pals. *Journal of Speech and Hearing Disorders, 24*, 154–157.

Marquardt, T., & Saxman, J. (1972). Language comprehension and auditory discrimination in articulation deficient kindergarten children. *Journal of Speech and Hearing Research, 15*, 382–389.

Marshala, P. (2001). *Oral-motor techniques in articulation & phonological therapy.* Temecula, CA: Speech Dynamics, Incorporated.

Martin, F. N., & Noble, B. E. (2002). Hearing and hearing disorders. In G. H. Shames, & N. B. Anderson (Eds.), *Human Communication Disorders* (6th ed., pp. 303–348). Boston: Allyn & Bacon.

Maskarinec, A. S., Cairns, G. F., Butterfield, E. C., & Weamer, D. K. (1981). Longitudinal observations of individual infants' vocalizations. *Journal of Speech and Hearing Disorders, 46*, 267–273.

Mason, M., Smith, M., & Hinshaw, M. (1976). *Medida Española de Articulación (Measurement of Spanish Articulation).* San Ysidro, CA: San Ysidro School District.

Mason, R., & Proffit, W. (1974). The tongue thrust controversy: Background and recommendations. *Journal of Speech and Hearing Disorders, 39*,115–132.

Massengill, R., Maxwell, S., & Picknell, K. (1970). An analysis of articulation following partial and total glossectomy. *Journal of Speech and Hearing Disorders, 35*, 170–173.

Masterson, J. (1993). Classroom-based phonological intervention. *American Journal of Speech-Language Pathology, 2*, 5–9.

Masterson, J., & Bernhardt, B. (2001). *Computerized Articulation & Phonology Evaluation System.* San Antonio, TX: The Psychological Corporation.

Matheny, A., & Bruggeman, C. (1973). Children's speech: Heredity components and sex differences. *Folia Phoniatrica, 25*, 442–449.

Matheny, N., & Panagos, J. (1978). Comparing the effects of articulation and syntax programs on syntax and articulation improvement. *Language, Speech, and Hearing Services in Schools, 9*, 57–61.

Mattes, L. J. (1995). *Spanish Articulation Measures* (Rev. ed.). Oceanside, CA: Academic Communication Associates.

Mattes, L. J., & Omark, D. (1991). *Speech and language assessment for the bilingual handicapped.* (2nd ed.). Oceanside, CA: Academic Communication Associates.

McCabe, R., & Bradley, D. P. (1975). Systematic multiple phonemic approach to articulation therapy. *Acta Symbolica, 61*, 1–18.

McCroskey, R., & Baird, V. (1971). Parent education in a public school program of speech therapy. *Journal of Speech and Hearing Disorders, 36*, 449–505.

McDonald, E. (1964a). *A Deep Test of Articulation.* Pittsburgh, PA: Stanwix House.

McDonald, E. (1964b). *Articulation testing and treatment: A sensory-motor approach.* Pittsburgh, PA: Stanwix House.

McEnery, E, & Gaines, F. (1941). Tongue-tie in infants and children. *Journal of Pediatrics, 18*, 252–255.

McLaughlin, S. (1998). *Introduction to language development.* San Diego: Singular Publishing Group.

McLean, J. E. (1970). Extending stimulus control of phoneme articulation by operant techniques. *ASHA Monographs No. 14*, 24–47.

McNamara, K. M. (2002). Interviewing, counseling, and clinical communication. In R. Paul (Ed.), *Introduction to clinical methods in communication disorders* (pp. 183–217). Baltimore: Brookes.

McNeil, M. R., Robin, D. A., & Schmidt, R. A. (1997). Apraxia of speech: Definition, differentiation, and treatment. In M. R. McNeil (Ed.), *Clinical management of sensorimotor speech disorders* (pp. 311–344). New York: Thieme.

McNutt, J. (1977). Oral sensory and motor behaviors of children with /s/ or /r/ misarticulations. *Journal of Speech and Hearing Research, 20*, 694–703.

McReynolds, L. V. (1987). A perspective on articulation generalization. *Seminars in Speech and Language, 8*, 217–239.

McReynolds, L. V., & Bennett, S. (1972). Distinctive feature generalization in articulation training. *Journal of Speech and Hearing Disorders, 37*, 462–470.

McReynolds, L. V., & Engmann, D. (1975). *Distinctive feature analysis of misarticulations.* Baltimore: University Park Press.

McReynolds, L. V., & Spradlin, J. E. (1989). *Generalization strategies in the treatment of communication disorders.* Philadelphia: B. C. Decker.

Metz, D. E., Samar, V. J., Schiavetti, N., Sitler, R. W., & Whitehead, R. L. (1985). Acoustic dimensions of hearing-impaired speakers' intelligibility. *Journal of Speech and Hearing Research, 28*, 345–355.

Metz, D. E., Schiavetti, N., Samar, V. J., & Sitler, R. W. (1990). Acoustic dimensions of hearing-impaired speakers' intelligibility: Segmental and suprasegmental characteristics. *Journal of Speech and Hearing Research, 33*, 476–487.

Meyer, S. M. (1998). *Survival guide for the beginning speech-language clinician.* Gaithersburg, MD: Aspen Publishers, Inc.

Miccio, A. W. (2002). Clinical problem solving: Assessment of phonological disorders. *American Journal of Speech-Language Pathology, 11*, 221–229.

Miccio, A. W., & Elbert, M. (1996). Enhancing stimulability: A treatment program. *Journal of Communication Disorders, 29*, 335–352.

Miccio, A. W., Elbert, M., & Forrest, K. (1999). The relationship between stimulability and phonological acquisition in children with normally developing and disordered phonologies. *American Journal of Speech-Language Pathology, 8*, 347–363.

Miccio, A. W., Gallagher, E., Grossman, C. B., Yont, K. M., & Vernon-Feagans, L. (2001). Influence of chronic otitis media on phonological acquisition. *Clinical Linguistics & Phonetics, 15*, 47–51.

Milisen, R. (1954). A rationale for articulation disorders. *Journal of Speech and Hearing Disorders, Monograph Supplement 4*, 4–17.

Milisen, R., & Associates (1954). The disorder of articulation: A systematic clinical and experimental approach. *Journal of Speech and Hearing Disorders, Monograph Supplement 4.*

Minifie, F., Hixon, T., & Williams, F. (Eds.) (1973). *Normal aspects of speech, hearing, and language.* Englewood Cliffs, NJ: Prentice-Hall.

Monsen, R. B. (1981). A usable test for the speech intelligibility of deaf talkers. *American Annals of the Deaf, 126,* 845–852.

Moore-Brown, B., & Montgomery, J. (2001). *Making a difference for America's children: Speech-language pathologists in public schools.* Eau Claire, WI: Thinking Publications.

Morehead, D., & Morehead, A. (Eds.) (1976). *Normal and deficient child language.* Baltimore: University Park Press.

Morley, M. (1970). *Cleft palate and speech.* London: E & S Livingstone.

Mowe, K. M. (1997). Comparison of intelligibility estimation and orthographic transcription methods by preprofessional speech-language pathologists. Unpublished master's thesis, Portland State University, Portland, OR.

Mowrer, D. E. (1967). Programmed speech therapy–A field test. *ASHA, 9,* 369.

Mowrer, D. E. (1971). Transfer of training in articulation therapy. *Journal of Speech and Hearing Disorders, 36,* 427–446.

Mowrer, D. E. (1988). *Methods of modifying speech behaviors* (2nd ed.). Prospect Heights, IL: Waveland Press, Inc.

Mowrer, D. E. (1989). The behavioral approach to treatment. In N. A. Creaghead, P. W. Newman, & W. A. Secord. *Assessment and remediation of articulatory and phonological disorders* (2nd ed., pp. 159–192). Columbus, OH: Merrill Publishing Company.

Mowrer, D. E., Baker, R., & Schutz, R. (1968). *S-Programmed Articulation Control Kit.* Tempe, AZ: Educational Psychological Research Associates.

Mowrer, D. E., & Case, J. (1982). *Clinical management of speech disorders.* Rockville, MD: Aspen Publishers, Inc.

Mowrer, D. E., Wahl, P., & Doolan, S. J. (1978). Effect of lisping on audience evaluation of male speakers. *Journal of Speech and Hearing Disorders, 43,* 140–148.

Mowrer, O. H. (1952). Speech development in the young child: The autism theory of speech development and some clinical applications. *Journal of Speech and Hearing Disorders, 17,* 263–268.

Muter, V., Hulme, C., & Snowling, M. (1997). *Phonological Abilities Test.* San Antonio, TX: The Psychological Corporation.

Nation, J. E., & Aram, D. M. (1977). *Diagnosis of speech and language disorders.* St. Louis: C. V. Mosby.

Nelson, L. K. (1995). Establishing production of speech sound contrast using minimal "triads." *The Clinical Connection, 8,* 16–19.

Nemoy, E., & Davis, S. (1954). *The correction of defective consonant sounds.* Magnolia, MA: Expression Co.

Newman, P. W., & Creaghead, N. A. (1989). Assessment of articulatory and phonological disorders. In N. A. Creaghead, P. W. Newman, & W. A. Secord. *Assessment and remediation of articulatory and phonological disorders* (2nd ed., pp. 69–126). Columbus, OH: Merrill Publishing Company.

Nichols, R. (1955). Ten components of effective listening. *Education, 75,* 292–302.

Nicolosi, L., Harryman, E., & Kresheck, J. (2004). *Terminology of communication disorders. Speech-language-hearing* (4th ed.). Baltimore: Williams & Wilkins.

Nippold, M. A. (1990). Concomitant speech and language disorders in stuttering children: A critique of the literature. *Journal of Speech and Hearing Disorders,* 55, 51–60.

Nippold, M. A. (2001). Phonological disorders and stuttering in children: What is the frequency of co-occurrence? *Clinical Linguistics & Phonetics, 15,* 219–228.

Oller, D. K. (1973). Regularities in abnormal child phonology. *Journal of Speech and Hearing Disorders, 38,* 36–47.

Oller, D. K. (1980). The emergence of the sounds of speech in infancy. In G. Yeni-Komshian, J. Kavanaugh, & C. A. Ferguson (Eds.), *Child Phonology* (Volume 1, pp. 93–112). New York: Academic Press.

Oller, D. K., & Delgado, R. (1990). *Logical international phonetic programs: Version 1.03* (MS DOS Computer Program). Intelligent Hearing Systems.

Oller, D. K., Eilers, R., Bull, D., & Carney, A. (1985). Prespeech vocalizations of a deaf infant: A comparison with normal metaphonological development. *Journal of Speech and Hearing Research, 28,* 47–63.

Olmstead, D. (1966). A theory of the child's learning of phonology. *Language, 42,* 531–535.

Olmstead, D. (1971). *Out of the mouths of babes.* The Hague: Mouton.

Olswang, L. B., & Bain, B. A. (1985a). Monitoring phoneme acquisition for making treatment withdrawal decisions. *Applied Psycholinguistics, 6,* 17–37.

Olswang, L. B., & Bain, B. A. (1985b). The natural occurrence of generalization articulation treatment. *Journal of Communication Disorders, 18,* 109–129.

Ortíz, A. A., & García, S. G. (1988). A prereferral process for preventing inappropriate referrals of Hispanic students to special education. In A. A. Ortíz & B. Ramírez (Eds.), *Schools and the culturally exceptional student: Promising practices and future directions* (pp. 6–18). Reston, VA: Council for Exceptional Children.

Otomo, K., & Stoel-Gammon, C. (1992). The acquisition of unrounded vowels in English. *Journal of Speech and Hearing Research, 35,* 604–616.

Owens, R. E. (2002). Development of communication, language, and speech. In G. H. Shames & N. B. Anderson (Eds.), *Human communication disorders: An introduction* (6th ed.). Boston: Allyn & Bacon.

Ozanich, K. A. (1997). The generalization of stridency from treated to untreated misarticulated phonemes. Unpublished master's thesis, Portland State University, Portland, OR.

Paden, E. P., Matthies, M. L., & Novak, M. A. (1989). Recovery from OME-related phonologic delay following tube placement. *Journal of Speech and Hearing Disorders, 54,* 94–100.

Paden, E. P., Novak, M. A., & Beiter, A. L. (1987). Predictors of phonological inadequacy in young children prone to otitis media. *Journal of Speech and Hearing Disorders, 52,* 232–242.

Paden, E. P., Yairi, E., & Ambrose, N. G. (1999). Early stuttering II: Initial status of phonological abilities. *Journal of Speech, Language, and Hearing Research, 42,* 1113–1124.

Palmer, J. (1962). Tongue-thrusting: A clinical hypothesis. *Journal of Speech and Hearing Disorders, 27,* 323–333.

Panagos, J., & Prelock, P. (1982). Phonological constraints on the sentence productions of language disordered children. *Journal of Speech and Hearing Research, 25,* 171–176.

Panagos, J., Quine, M., & Klich, R. (1979). Syntactic and phonological influences on children's articulation. *Journal of Speech and Hearing Research, 22,* 841–848.

Pannbacker, M. D., & Lass, N. J. (2003). *Effectiveness of oral motor treatment in SLP.* Poster presented at the ASHA Annual Convention, Chicago, IL.

Peña-Brooks, A., & Hegde, M. N. (2000). *Assessment and treatment of articulation and phonological disorders in children.* Austin, TX: Pro-Ed.

Perkins, W. H. (1977). *Speech pathology: An applied behavioral science.* St. Louis: C. V. Mosby.

Perkins, W. H. (1978). *Human perspectives in speech and language disorders.* St. Louis: CV Mosby.

Petinou, K., Schwartz, R. G., Mody, M., & Gravel, J. S. (1999). The impact of otitis media with effusion on early phonetic inventories: A longitudinal investigation. *Clinical Linguistics & Phonetics, 13*, 351–367.

Piaget, J. (1962). *Play, dreams and imitation in childhood.* New York: W. W. Norton.

Platt, L. J., Andrews, G., Young, M., & Quinn, P. T. (1980). Dysarthria of adult cerebral palsy: I. Intelligibility and articulatory impairment. *Journal of Speech and Hearing Research, 23*, 28–40.

Pollack, E., & Rees, N. (1972). Disorders of articulation: Some clinical applications of distinctive feature theory. *Journal of Speech and Hearing Disorders, 37*, 451–461.

Pollock, K. E. (1991). The identification of vowel errors using traditional articulation or phonological process test stimuli. *Language, Speech, and Hearing Services in Schools, 22*, 23–27.

Pollock, K. E., & Schwartz, R. G. (1988). Structural aspects of phonological development: Case study of a disordered child. *Language, Speech, and Hearing Services in Schools, 19*, 5–16.

Polson, J. (1980). A survey of carryover practices of public school clinicians in Oregon. Unpublished master's thesis, Portland State University, Portland, OR.

Poole, E. (1934). Genetic development of articulation of consonant sounds in speech. *Elementary English Review, 11*, 159–161.

Powell, T. W. (2003). Stimulability and treatment outcomes. *Language Learning and Education, 10*, 3–6.

Powell, T. W., Elbert, M., & Dinnsen, D. A. (1991). Stimulability as a factor in the phonological generalization of misarticulating preschool children. *Journal of Speech and Hearing Research, 34*, 1318–1328.

Powell, T. W., & McReynolds, L. V. (1969). A procedure for testing position generalization from articulation training. *Journal of Speech and Hearing Research, 12*, 625– 645.

Powell, T. W., & Miccio, A. W. (1996). Stimulability: A useful clinical tool. *Journal of Communication Disorders, 29*, 237–254.

Powers, M. (1971). Functional disorders of articulation symptomatology and etiology. In L. Travis, *Handbook of speech pathology* (pp. 837–875). New York: Appleton-Century-Crofts.

Prather, E., Hedrick, D., & Kern, C. (1975). Articulation development in children aged two to four years. *Journal of Speech and Hearing Research, 40*, 179–191.

Prather, E., Miner, A., Addicott, M. A., & Sunderland, L. (1971). *Washington Speech Sound Discrimination Test.* Danville, IL: Printers & Publishers, Inc.

Preisser, D. A., Hodson, B. W., & Paden, E. P. (1988). Developmental phonology: 18–29 months. *Journal of Speech and Hearing Disorders, 53*, 125–130.

Prins, D. (1962). Analysis of correlations among various articulatory deviations. *Journal of Speech and Hearing Research, 5*, 152–160.

Prizant, B., Audet, L., Burke, G., Hummel, L., Maher, S., & Theadore, G. (1990). Communication disorders and emotional/behavioral disorders in children. *Journal of Speech and Hearing Disorders, 55*, 179–192.

Prizant, B., & Meyer, E. C. (1993). Socio-emotional aspects of communication disorders in young children and their families. *American Journal of Speech-Language Pathology, 2*, 56–71.

Prosek, R., & House, A. (1975). Intraoral air pressure as a feedback cue in consonant production. *Journal of Speech and Hearing Research, 18*, 133–147.

Ratner, N. B. (1995). Treating the child who stutters with concomitant language or phonological impairment. *Language, Speech, and Hearing Services in Schools, 26*, 180–186.

Ray, J. (2002). Treating phonological disorders in a multilingual child: A case study. *American Journal of Speech-Language Pathology, 11*, 305–315.

Rheault, B. (2002). Generalization characteristics using the phonological cycling approach. Master's clinical research project, Portland State University, Portland, OR.

Rice, M. L., Sell, M. A., & Hadley, P. A. (1991). Social interactions of speech- and language-impaired children. *Journal of Speech and Hearing Research, 31*, 1299–1307.

Riley, G. D. (1966). *Riley Articulation and Language Test, Revised.* Los Angeles: Western Psychological Services.

Ringel, R., House, A., Burk, K., Dolinsky, J., & Scott, C. (1970). Some relations between orosensory discrimination and articulatory aspects of speech production. *Journal of Speech and Hearing Disorders, 35*, 3–11.

Robb, M. P., Bauer, H., & Tyler, A. (1994). A quantitative analysis of the single-word stage. *First Language, 14*, 37–48.

Robb, M. P., & Bleile, K. M. (1994). Consonant inventories of young children from 8 to 25 months. *Clinical Linguistics & Phonetics, 8*, 295–320.

Roberts, J. E., Burchinal, M. R., Koch, M. A., Footo, M. M., & Henderson, F. W. (1988). Otitis media in early childhood and its relationship to later phonological development. *Journal of Speech and Hearing Disorders, 53*, 424–432.

Roberts, J. E., & Clarke-Klein, S. (1994). Otitis media. In J. Bernthal and N. Bankson (Eds.), *Child phonology: Characteristics, assessment, and intervention with special populations* (pp. 182–198). New York: Thieme Medical Publishers.

Robertson, C., & Salter, W. (1997). *The Phonological Awareness Test.* East Moline, IL: LinguiSystems, Inc.

Rochester Hearing and Speech Center. (2000). *Articulation Severity Index (ASI).* Rochester, NY: Rochester Hearing and Speech Center, Inc.

Roe, V., & Milisen, R. (1942). The effect of maturation upon defective articulation in elementary grades. *Journal of Speech and Hearing Disorders, 7*, 37–50.

Romans, E. F., & Milisen, R. (1954). Effect of latency between stimulation and response on reproduction of sounds. *Journal of Speech and Hearing Disorders, Monograph Supplement 4*, 71–78.

Roseberry-McKibbin, C. (2002). *Multicultural students with special language needs: Practical strategies for assessment and intervention* (2nd ed.). Oceanside, CA: Academic Communication Associates, Inc.

Rosenbek, J. C. (1985). Treating apraxia of speech. In D. Johns (Ed.), *Clinical management of neurogenic communicative disorders* (pp. 267–312). Boston: Little, Brown & Co.

Rosenbek, J. C., Hansen, R., Baughman, C. H., & Lemme, M. (1974). Treatment of developmental apraxia of speech: A case study. *Language, Speech, and Hearing Services in Schools, 5*, 13–21.

Rosenbek, J. C., Kent, R. D., & LaPointe, L. L. (1984). Apraxia of speech: An overview and some perspectives. In J. C. Rosenbek, M. R. McNeil, & A. E. Aronson (Eds.), *Apraxia of speech: Physiology, acoustics, linguistics, management.* San Diego: College-Hill Press.

Rosenbek, J. C., & LaPointe, L. (1985). The dysarthrias: Description, diagnosis and treatment. In D. Johns (Ed.), *Clinical management of neurogenic communicative disorders* (pp. 97–152). Boston: Little, Brown & Co.

Rosenbek, J. C., Lemme, M. L., Ahern, M. B., Harris, E. H., & Wertz, R. T. (1973). A treatment of apraxia of speech in adults. *Journal of Speech and Hearing Disorders, 38*, 462–472.

Rosenfeld-Johnson, S. (2004). *Oral-motor exercises for speech clarity.* Tucson, AZ: Innovative Therapists International.

Roth, F. P., & Worthington, C. K. (2001). *Treatment resource manual for speech-language pathology* (2nd ed.). Albany, NY: Singular Thomson Learning.

Royer, H. K. (1995). Clinical application of two phonological-based treatment approaches. Unpublished master's thesis, Portland State University, Portland, OR.

Ruder, K. F., & Bunce, B. H. (1981). Articulation therapy using distinctive feature analysis to structure the training program: Two case studies. *Journal of Speech and Hearing Disorders, 46,* 59–65.

Ruscello, D. M. (1975). The importance of word position in articulation therapy. *Language, Speech, and Hearing Services in Schools, 6,* 190–196.

Ruscello, D. M., & Shelton, R. L. (1979). Planning and self-assessment in articulatory training. *Journal of Speech and Hearing Disorders, 44,* 504–512.

Ruscello, D. M., St. Louis, K. O., & Mason, N. (1991). School-age children with phonologic disorders: Co-existence with other speech-language disorders. *Journal of Speech and Hearing Research, 34,* 236–242.

Rvachew, S. (1994). Speech perception training can facilitate sound production learning. *Journal of Speech and Hearing Research, 37,* 347–357.

Rvachew, S., & Nowak, M. (2001). The effect of target selection strategy on sound production learning. *Journal of Speech-Language and Hearing Research, 44,* 610–623.

Rvachew, S., Rafaat, S., & Martin, M. (1999). Stimulability, speech perception skills, and treatment of phonological disorders. *American Journal of Speech-Language Pathology, 8,* 33–43.

Saben, C. B., & Ingham, J. C. (1991). The effects of minimal pairs treatment on the speech-sound production of two children with phonologic disorders. *Journal of Speech and Hearing Research, 34,* 1023–1040.

Salter, W., & Robertson, C. (2001). *Phonological Awareness & Reading Profile-Intermediate.* East Moline, IL: LinguiSystems, Inc.

Sample, M., Montague, J., & Buffalo, M. (1989). Variables related to communicative disorders in an adult prison sample. *Journal of Criminal Justice, 17,* 457–470.

Sander, E. (1972). When are speech sounds learned? *Journal of Speech and Hearing Disorders, 37,* 55–63.

Scarry, J., & Scarry-Larkin, M. (1996). *LocuTour multimedia articulation manual.* San Luis Obispo, CA: LocuTour Multimedia.

Schiavetti, N. (1992). Scaling procedures for the measurement of speech intelligibility. In R. D. Kent (Ed.), *Intelligibility in speech disorders* (pp. 11–34). Philadelphia: John Benjamins Publishing.

Schmauch, V., Panagos, J., & Klich, R. (1978). Syntax influences the accuracy of consonant production in language-disordered children. *Journal of Communication Disorders, 11,* 315–323.

Schmitt, L., Howard, B., & Schmitt, J. (1983). Conversational speech sampling in the assessment of articulation proficiency. *Language, Speech, and Hearing Services in Schools, 14,* 210–214.

Schuckers, G. H. (1978). *A coarticulation-based treatment program for phonemic/articulatory disorders.* Short Course presented at the Annual Convention of the American Speech and Hearing Convention, San Francisco, CA.

Scott, C., & Ringel, R. (1971). Articulation without oral sensory control. *Journal of Speech and Hearing Research, 14,* 804–818.

Scott, D. A., & Milisen, R. (1954). The effectiveness of combined visual-auditory stimulation in improving articulation. *Journal of Speech and Hearing Disorders, Monograph Supplement 4,* 51–56.

Scripture, E. (1923). *Stuttering, lisping and correction of the speech of the deaf.* New York: Macmillan.

Scripture, M., & Jackson, E. (1927). *A manual of exercises for the correction of speech disorders.* Philadelphia: F A Davis.

Secord, W. A. (1989). The traditional approach to treatment. In N. A. Creaghead, P. W. Newman, & W. A. Secord. *Assessment and remediation of articulatory and phonological disorders* (2nd ed., pp. 129–157). Columbus, OH: Merrill Publishing Company.

Secord, W. A., & Donohue, J. S. (2002). *Clinical Assessment of Articulation and Phonology.* Greenville, SC: Super Duper Publications.

Secord, W. A., & Shine, R. E. (1997). *Secord Contextual Articulation Tests (S-CAT).* Sedona, AZ: Red Rock Educational Publications, Inc.

Seikel, J. A., King, D. W., & Drumright, D. G. (2005). *Anatomy and physiology for speech, language, and hearing* (3rd ed.). Clifton Park, NY: Delmar Learning.

Selby, J. C., Robb, M. P., & Gilbert, H. R. (2000). Normal vowel articulations between 15 and 36 months of age. *Clinical Linguistics & Phonetics, 14,* 255–265.

Shelton, R. L. (1978). Disorders of articulation. In P. Skinner, & R. L. Shelton. *Speech, Language and Hearing.* Reading, MA: Addison-Wesley.

Shelton, R. L., Johnson, A. F., & Arndt, W. B. (1972). Monitoring and reinforcement by parents as a means of automating articulatory responses. *Perceptual Motor Skills, 35,* 759–767.

Shelton, R. L., Johnson, A. F., & Arndt, W. B. (1977). Delayed judgment speech sound discrimination and /r/ or /s/ articulation status and improvement. *Journal of Speech and Hearing Research, 20,* 704–717.

Shelton, R. L., Johnson, A. F., Ruscello, D. M., & Arndt, W. B. (1978). Assessment of parent-administered listening training for preschool children with articulation deficits. *Journal of Speech and Hearing Disorders, 43,* 242–254.

Shelton, R. L., Johnson, A. F., Willis, V., & Arndt, W. B. (1975). Monitoring and reinforcement by parents as a means of automating articulatory responses: II. Study of pre-school children. *Perceptual and Motor Skills, 40,* 599–610.

Shelton, R. L., Willis, V., Johnson, A. F., & Arndt, W. B. (1973). Oral form recognition training and articulation change. *Perceptual Motor Skills, 36,* 523–531.

Shine, R. E. (1989). Articulatory production training: A sensory-motor approach. In N. A. Creaghead, P. W. Newman, & W. A. Secord. *Assessment and remediation of articulatory and phonological disorders* (2nd ed., pp. 335–358). Columbus, OH: Merrill Publishing Company.

Shriberg, L. D. (1975). A response evocation program for /ɚ/. *Journal of Speech and Hearing Disorders, 40,* 92–105.

Shriberg, L. D. (1982). Diagnostic assessment of developmental phonological disorders. In M. Crary (Ed.), *Phonological intervention: Concepts and procedures.* San Diego: College-Hill Press.

Shriberg, L. D. (1986). *Program to examine phonetic and phonological evaluation records: Version 4.0* (Ms-DOS Computer Program). Hillsdale, NJ: Erlbaum.

Shriberg, L. D. (1997). Developmental phonological disorder(s): One or many? In B. W. Hodson, & M. L. Edwards (Eds.), *Perspectives in applied phonology* (pp. 105–127). Gaithersburg, MD: Aspen Publishers, Inc.

Shriberg, L. D., Aram, D. M., & Kwiatkowski, J. (1997). Developmental apraxia of speech: A subtype marked by inappropriate stress. *Journal of Speech, Language, and Hearing Research, 40,* 286–312.

Shriberg, L. D., & Austin, D. (1998). Comorbidity of speech-language disorder: Implications for a phenotype marker for speech delay. In R. Paul (Ed.), *The speech-language connection* (pp. 73–117). Baltimore: Paul H. Brookes.

Shriberg, L. D., Austin, D., Lewis, B. A., McSweeny, J. L., & Wilson, D. L. (1997). The percentage of consonants correct (PCC) metric: Extensions and reliability data. *Journal of Speech and Hearing Research, 40,* 708–722.

Shriberg, L. D., Flipsen, P., Thielke, H., Kwiatkowski, J., Kertoy, M. K., Catcher, M. L., Nellis, R. A., & Block, M. G. (2000a). Risk for speech disorder associated with recurrent otitis media with effusion: Two retrospective studies. *Journal of Speech, Language, and Hearing Research, 43,* 79–99.

Shriberg, L. D., Friel-Patti, S., Flipsen, P., & Brown, R. L. (2000b). Otitis media, fluctuant hearing loss, and speech-language outcomes: A preliminary structural equation model. *Journal of Speech, Language, and Hearing Research, 43,* 100–120.

Shriberg, L., & Kwiatkowski, J. (1980). *Natural process analysis: A procedure for phonological analysis of continuous speech samples.* New York: John Wiley.

Shriberg, L., & Kwiatkowski, J. (1982a). Phonological disorders I: A diagnostic classification system. *Journal of Speech and Hearing Disorders, 47,* 226–241.

Shriberg, L., & Kwiatkowski, J. (1982b). Phonological disorders II: A conceptual framework for management. *Journal of Speech and Hearing Disorders, 47,* 242–256.

Shriberg, L., & Kwiatkowski, J. (1982c). Phonological disorders III: A procedure for assessing severity of involvement. *Journal of Speech and Hearing Disorders, 47,* 256–270.

Shriberg, L., & Kwiatkowski, J. (1987). Retrospective study of spontaneous generalization in speech-delayed children. *Language Speech, and Hearing Services in Schools, 18,* 144–158.

Shriberg, L., & Kwiatkowski, J. (1994). Developmental phonological disorders I: A clinical profile. *Journal of Speech and Hearing Research, 37,* 1100–1126.

Shriberg, L. D., Kwiatkowski, J., Best, S., Hengst, J., & Terselic-Weber, B. (1986). Characteristics of children with phonological disorders of unknown origin. *Journal of Speech and Hearing Disorders, 51,* 140–160.

Shriberg, L. D., & Smith, A. J. (1983). Phonological correlates of middle-ear involvement in speech-delayed children: A methodological note. *Journal of Speech and Hearing Research, 26,* 293–297.

Shriberg, L. D., Tomblin, J. G., & McSweeny, J. L. (1999). Prevalence of speech delay in 6-year-old children and comorbidity with language impairment. *Journal of Speech, Language, and Hearing Research, 42,* 1461–1481.

Shriberg, L. D., & Widder, C. (1990). Speech and prosody characteristics of adults with mental retardation. *Journal of Speech and Hearing Research, 33,* 627–653.

Silverman, E. M. (1976). Listeners' impressions of speakers with lateral lisps. *Journal of Speech and Hearing Disorders, 41,* 547–552.

Silverman, F. H., & Falk, S. M. (1992). Attitudes of teenagers toward peers who have a single articulation error. *Language, Speech, and Hearing Services in Schools, 23,* 187.

Silverman, F. H., & Paulus, P. G. (1989). Peer relations to teenagers who substitute /w/ for /r/. *Language, Speech, and Hearing Services in Schools, 20,* 219–221.

Simon, C. (1957). The development of speech. In L. Travis, *Handbook of speech pathology* (pp. 3–43). New York: Appleton-Century-Crofts.

Singh, S., & Polen, S. (1972). Use of a distinctive feature model in speech pathology. *Acta Symbolica, 3,* 17–25.

Singh, S., & Singh, K. (1972). A self-generating distinctive model for diagnosis, prognosis, and therapy. *Acta Symbolica, 3,* 89–99.

Skelly, M., Spector, D., Donaldson, R., Brodeur, A., & Paletta, F. (1971). Compensatory physiologic phonetics for the glossectomee. *Journal of Speech and Hearing Research, 36,* 101–114.

Skinner P., & Shelton R. (1978). *Speech, language and hearing: Normal processes and disorders.* Reading, MA: Addison-Wesley.

Small, L. H. (2005). *Fundamentals of phonetics. A practical guide for students* (2nd ed.). Boston: Allyn & Bacon.

Smit, A. B. (1986). Ages of speech sound acquisition: Comparisons and critiques of several normative studies. *Language, Speech, and Hearing Services in Schools, 17,* 175–186.

Smit, A. B. (1993a). Phonologic error distributions in the Iowa-Nebraska articulation norms project: Consonant singletons. *Journal of Speech and Hearing Research, 36,* 533–547.

Smit, A. B. (1993b). Phonologic error distributions in the Iowa-Nebraska articulation norms project: Word-initial consonant clusters. *Journal of Speech and Hearing Research, 36,* 931–947.

Smit, A. G. (2004). *Articulation and phonology resource guide for school-age children and adults.* Clifton Park, NY: Thomson Delmar Learning.

Smit, A. B., & Hand, L. (1997). *Smit-Hand Articulation and Phonology Evaluation.* Los Angeles: Western Psychological Services.

Smit, A. B., Hand, L., Freilinger, J. J., Bernthal, J. E., & Bird, A. (1990). The Iowa articulation norms project and its Nebraska replication. *Journal of Speech and Hearing Disorders, 55,* 779–798.

Smith, B. L., & Oller, D. K. (1981). A comparative study of pre-meaningful vocalizations produced by normally developing and Down's syndrome infants. *Journal of Speech and Hearing Disorders, 46,* 46–51.

Snow, K. (1961). Articulation proficiency in relation to certain dental abnormalities. *Journal of Speech and Hearing Disorders, 26,* 209–212.

Sommers, R. K., Furlong, A. K., Rhodes, F. H., Fichter, G. R., Bowser, D. C., Copetas, F. H., & Saunders, Z. G. (1964). Effects of maternal attitudes upon improvement in articulation when mothers are trained to assist in speech correction. *Journal of Speech and Hearing Disorders, 29,* 126–132.

Sommers, R. K., & Kane, A. (1974). Nature and remediation of functional articulation disorders. In S. Dickson (Ed.), *Communication disorders: Remedial principles and practices.* Glenview, IL: Scott Foresman.

Sommers, R. K., Leiss, R., Delp, M., Gerber, A., Fundrella, D., Smith, R., Revucky, M., Ellis, D., & Haley, V. (1967). Factors related to the effectiveness of articulation therapy for kindergarten, first- and second-grade children. *Journal of Speech and Hearing Research, 10,* 428–437.

Sommers, R. K., Schaeffer, M. H., Leiss, R. H., Gerber, A. J., Bray, M. A., Fundrella, D., Olson, J. K., & Tomkins, E. R. (1966). The effectiveness of group and individual therapy. *Journal of Speech and Hearing Research, 9,* 219–225.

Speech Assessment and Interactive Learning System (SAILS) (2004). Developed by the Software Development and Information Technology Utilization Group. http://sdg.cllrnet.ca/SAILS.

Speech-Ease (1985). *Speech-Ease Screening Inventory (K-1)*. Austin, TX: Pro-Ed.

Spriestersbach, D. (1956). Research in articulation disorders and personality. *Journal of Speech and Hearing Disorders, 21*, 329–335.

Spriestersbach, D., & Sherman, 0. (1968). *Cleft palate and communication*. New York: Academic Press.

Square-Storer, P., & Hayden, D. (1989). Prompt treatment. In P. Square-Storer (Ed.), *Acquired apraxia of speech in aphasic adults*. New York: Taylor and Francis.

St. Louis, K. O., Hansen, G. G. R., Buch, J. L., & Oliver, T. L. (1992). Voice deviations and coexisting communication disorders. *Language, Speech, and Hearing Services in Schools, 23*, 82–87.

St. Louis, K. O., & Ruscello, D. M. (2000). *Oral Speech Mechanism Screening Examination*. Austin, TX: Pro-Ed.

Stackhouse, J. (1997). Phonological awareness: Connecting speech and literacy problems. In B. W. Hodson, & M. L. Edwards (Eds.), *Perspectives in applied phonology* (pp. 105–127). Gaithersburg, MD: Aspen Publishers, Inc.

Stampe, D. (1969). *The acquisition of phonetic representation*. Papers from the Fifth Regional Meeting of the Chicago Linguistic Circle. Chicago: University of Chicago Department of Linguistics.

Stampe, D. (1979). *A dissertation on natural phonology*. New York: Garland Publishing Inc.

Stemberger, J. P., & Bernhardt, B. H. (1997). Optimality theory. In M. J. Ball, & R. D. Kent, *The new phonologies: Developments in clinical linguistics* (pp. 211–245). San Diego: Singular Publishing Group, Inc.

Stern, D. (1992). *The sound & style of American English* (2nd ed.). Lyndonville, VT: Dialect Accent Specialists, Inc.

Stetson, R. (1951). *Motor phonetics* (2nd ed.). Amsterdam: North Holland Publishing Co.

Stevens, N., & Isles, D. (2001). *Phonological Screening Assessment*. Bicester, Oxfordshire, UK: Speechmark Publishing.

Stoel-Gammon, C. (1985). Phonetic inventories, 15–24 months: A longitudinal study. *Journal of Speech and Hearing Research, 28*, 505–512.

Stoel-Gammon, C. (1987). Phonological skills of 2-year-olds. *Language, Speech, and Hearing Services in Schools, 18*, 323–329.

Stoel-Gammon, C. (1991). Theories of phonological development and their implications for phonological disorders. In M. Yavas (Ed.), *Phonological disorders in children: Theories, research and treatment* (pp. 16–36). London: Routledge.

Stoel-Gammon, C., & Dunn, C. (1985). *Normal and disordered phonology in children*. Baltimore: University Park Press.

Stoel-Gammon, C., & Herrington, P. B. (1990). Vowel systems of normally developing and phonologically disordered children. *Clinical Linguistics & Phonetics, 4*, 145–160.

Stoel-Gammon, C., & Otomo, K. (1986). Babbling development of hearing-impaired and normally hearing subjects. *Journal of Speech and Hearing Disorders, 51*, 33–41.

Stokes, T. F., & Osnes, P. G. (1988). The developing applied technology of generalization and maintenance. In R. H. Horner, G. Dunlap, & R. L. Koegel (Eds.), *Generalization and maintenance: Lifestyle changes in applied settings* (pp. 5–21). Baltimore: Paul H. Brookes.

Strand, E. A., & McCauley, R. J. (1999). Assessment procedures for treatment planning in children with phonologic and motor speech disorders. In A. J. Caruso, & E. A. Strand (Eds.), *Clinical Management of motor speech disorders in children* (pp. 73–107). New York: Thieme.

Strand, E. A., & Skinder, E. A. (1999). Treatment of developmental apraxia of speech: Integral stimulation methods. In A. J. Caruso, & E. A. Strand (Eds.), *Clinical Management of motor speech disorders in children* (pp. 109–148). New York: Thieme.

Subtelny, J., Mestre, C., & Subtelny, J. (1964). Comparative study of normal and defective articulation of /s/ as related to malocclusion and deglutition. *Journal of Speech and Hearing Disorders, 29*, 269–285.

Sugarman, N. K. (1994). A comparison of trained ear estimation and orthographic transcription when measuring speech intelligibility in young children. Unpublished master's thesis, Portland State University, Portland, OR.

Sullivan, M., Gaebler, C., Beukelman, D., Mahanna, G., Marshall, J., Lydiatt, D., & Lydiatt, W. (2002). Impact of palatal prosthodontic intervention on communication performance of patients' maxillectomy defects: A multilevel outcome study. *Head and Neck, 244*, 530–538.

Swank, L., & Catts, H. (1994). Phonological awareness and written word decoding. *Language, Speech, and Hearing Services in Schools, 25*, 9–14.

Tade, W. J., & Slosson, S. W. (Ed.). (1986). *Slosson Articulation Language Test with Phonology*. East Aurora, NY: Slosson Educational Publications, Inc.

Tattersall, M. A., & Dawson, J. (1997). *Articulation Consistency Probe*. DeKalb, IL: Janelle Publications, Inc.

Taylor, J. (1969). Incidence of communication disorders among prisoners. Unpublished doctoral dissertation, University of Missouri, Columbia, MO.

Taylor, O. (1986). *Treatment of communications disorders in culturally and linguistically diverse populations*. San Diego: College-Hill Press.

Templin, M. C. (1943). A study of the sound discrimination ability of elementary school pupils. *Journal of Speech Disorders, 8*, 127–132.

Templin, M. C. (1957). *Certain language skills in children: Their development and interrelationships*. Institute of Child Welfare, Monograph 26. Minneapolis, MN: The University of Minnesota Press.

Templin, M. C. (1963). Development of speech. *Journal of Pediatrics, 62*, 11–14.

Templin, M. C., & Darley, F. L. (1969). *The Templin-Darley Tests of Articulation*. Iowa City, IA: Bureau of Educational Research and Service, University of Iowa.

Terrell, S., & Terrell, F. (1983). Distinguishing linguistic differences from disorders: The past, present, and future of non-biased assessment. *Topics in Language Disorders, 3*, 1–7.

Thompson, J. R., Bryant, B., Campbell, E. M., Craig, E. M., Hughes, C., Schalock, R. L., Silverman, W., & Tasse, M. J. (2003). *Supports intensity scale*. Washington, DC: AAMR.

Throneburg, R. N., Yairi, E., & Paden, E. (1994). Relation between phonologic difficulty and the occurrence of disfluencies in the early stage of stuttering. *Journal of Speech and Hearing Research, 37*, 504–509.

Tiffany, W., & Carrell, J. (1977). *Phonetics, theory and application* (2nd ed.). New York: McGraw-Hill.

Tomblin, J. B. (2002). Perspectives on diagnosis. In J. B. Tomblin, H. L. Morris, & D. C. Spriestersbach (Eds.), *Diagnosis in speech-language pathology* (2nd ed.). San Diego: Singular Publishing Group.

Torgesen, J. K., & Bryant, B. R. (1994). *Test of Phonological Awareness*. Austin, TX: Pro-Ed.

Trapp, P. E., & Evans, J. (1960). Functional articulatory defect and performance on a nonverbal task. *Journal of Speech and Hearing Disorders, 25*, 176–180.

Tremblay, M. (1982). A comparison of the effects of non-operant and operant carryover techniques of /l/. Unpublished master's thesis, Portland State University, Portland, OR.

Tsugawa, L. (2001). *The Spanish Preschool Articulation Test.* Portland, OR: Spanish Communication Disorders Press.

Turnbull, A., Turnbull, R., Shank, M., & Smith, S. J. (2004). *Exceptional lives. Special education in today's schools* (4th ed.). Upper Saddle River, NJ: Pearson Education, Inc.

Turton, L., & Clark, M. (1971). Linguistic theory and the child. *Acta Symbolica, 2,* 42–47.

Twain, M. (1960). *The adventures of Huckleberry Finn.* New York: Washington Square Press.

Tyler, A. A., Edwards, M. L., & Saxman, J. (1987). Clinical application of two phonologically based treatment procedures. *Journal of Speech and Hearing Disorders, 52,* 393–409.

Tyler, A. A., & Figurski, G. R. (1994). Phonetic inventory changes after treating distinctions along an implicational hierarchy. *Clinical Linguistics & Phonetics, 8,* 91–107.

Tyler, A. A., Lewis, K. E., Haskill, A., & Tolbert, L. C. (2002). Efficacy of cross-domain effects of a morphosyntax and a phonology intervention. *Language, Speech, and Hearing Services in Schools, 33,* 52–66.

Tyler, A. A., Lewis, K. E., & Welch, C. M. (2003). Predictions of phonological change following intervention. *American Journal of Speech-Language Pathology, 12,* 289–298.

Tyler, A. A., Sandoval K. T. (1994). Preschoolers with phonological and language disorders: Treating different linguistic domains. *Language, Speech, and Hearing Services in Schools, 25,* 215–234.

Tyler, A. A., & Tolbert, L. C. (2002). Speech-language assessment in the clinical setting. *American Journal of Speech-Language Pathology, 11,* 215–220.

Tyler, A. A., & Watterson, K. (1991). Effects of phonological versus language intervention in preschoolers with both phonological and language impairment. *Child Language Teaching and Therapy, 7,* 141–160.

U.S. Bureau of the Census (2000). Statistical abstract of the United States, 2000 (120th ed.). Washington, DC: U.S. Department of Commerce.

U.S. Department of Education (1977). *To assure the free appropriate education of all children with disabilities. Nineteenth annual report to Congress on the implementation of the Individuals with Disabilities Act.* Washington, D.C.: Author

Van Hattum, R. J. (1985). *Organization of speech-language services in schools.* San Diego: College-Hill Press.

Van Riper, C. (1951). The revision of public school speech correction. Unpublished paper.

Van Riper, C., & Emerick, L. (1990). *Speech correction: An introduction to speech pathology and audiology* (8th ed.). Englewood Cliffs, NJ: Prentice-Hall, Inc.

Van Riper, C., & Erickson, R. (1996). *Speech correction: An introduction to speech pathology and audiology* (9th ed.). Englewood Cliffs, NJ: Prentice-Hall, Inc.

Vaughn, G., & Clark, R. (1979). *Speech facilitation.* Springfield, IL: Charles C Thomas.

Vihman, M. M. (1985). Language differentiation by the bilingual infant. *Journal of Child Language, 12,* 297–324.

Vihman, M. M. (2004). Early phonological development. In J. E. Bernthal & N. W. Bankson, *Articulation and phonological disorders* (5th ed., pp. 63–104). Boston: Pearson Education, Inc.

Vihman, M. M., Ferguson, C., & Elbert, M. (1986). Phonological development from babbling to speech: Common tendencies and individual differences. *Applied Psycholinguistics, 7,* 3–40.

Vihman, M. M., & Greenlee, M. (1987). Individual differences in phonological development: Ages one and three years. *Journal of Speech and Hearing Research, 30,* 503–521.

Vihman, M. M., Macken, M. A., Miller, R., Simmons, H. & Miller, J. (1985). From babbling to speech: A reassessment of the continuity issue. *Language, 61,* 397–445.

Vitali, G. J. (1986). *Test of Oral Structures and Functions.* East Aurora, NY: Slosson Educational Publications, Inc.

Volterra, V., & Taeschner, T. (1978). The acquisition and development of language by bilingual children. *Journal of Child Language, 5,* 311–326.

Wadsworth, S. D., Maul, C. A., & Stevens, E. J. (1998). The prevalence of orofacial myofunctional disorders among children identified with speech and language disorders in grades kindergarten through six. *International Journal of Orofacial Myology, 24,* 1–19.

Wagner, C., Gray, L., & Potter, R. (1983). Communicative disorders in a group of adult female offenders. *Journal of Communication Disorders, 55,* 269–277.

Wagner, R., Torgesen, J. K., & Rashotte, C. (1999). *Comprehensive Test of Phonological Processing.* Austin, TX: Pro-Ed.

Weaver, C., Furbee, C., & Everhart, R. (1960). Paternal occupational class and articulatory defects in children. *Journal of Speech and Hearing Disorders, 25,* 171–175.

Weaver-Spurlock, S., & Brasseur, J. (1988). Position training on the generalization training of /s/. *Language, Speech, and Hearing Services in Schools, 19,* 259–271.

Webb, J. C., & Duckett, B. (1990). *RULES Phonological Evaluation.* Vero Beach, FL: The Speech Bin.

Webb, J. C., & Duckett, B. (1996). *RULES Phonological Inventory.* Vero Beach, FL: The Speech Bin, Inc.

Webster, P., & Plante, A. (1992). Effects of phonological impairment on word, syllable, and phoneme segmentation and reading. *Language, Speech, and Hearing Services in Schools, 23,* 176–182.

Weiner, F. (1979). *Phonological Process Analysis.* Baltimore: University Park Press.

Weiner, F. (1981). Treatment of phonological disability using the method of meaningful minimal contrast: Two case studies. *Journal of Speech and Hearing Disorders, 46,* 97–103.

Weiner, P. (1967). Auditory discrimination and articulation. *Journal of Speech and Hearing Disorders, 32,* 19–28.

Weiss, C. E. (1968). The relationships between maximum articulatory rate and articulatory disorders among children. *Central States Speech Journal, 19,* 185–187.

Weiss, C. E. (1970). Orofacial musculature imbalance among mentally retarded children. *British Journal of Disordered Communication, 5,*141–147.

Weiss, C. E. (1980). *Weiss Comprehensive Articulation Test.* Austin, TX: Pro-Ed.

Weiss, C. E. (1982). *Weiss Intelligibility Test.* Tigard, OR: CC Publications.

Weiss, C. E., Gordon, M. E., & Lillywhite, H. W. (1987). *Clinical management of articulatory and phonologic disorders* (2nd ed.). Baltimore: Williams & Wilkins.

Weiss, C. E., & Lillywhite, H. S. (1981). *Communication disorders: A handbook for prevention and early intervention* (2nd ed.). St. Louis: C. V. Mosby.

Wellman, B., Case, I., Mengert, I., & Bradbury, D. (1931). Speech sounds of young children. *University of Iowa Studies in Child Welfare, 5,* 2.

Wepman, J. M., & Reynolds, W. M. (1987). *Wepman's Auditory Discrimination Test-Second Edition.* Austin, TX: Pro-Ed. Los Angeles: Western Psychological Services.

Westby, C. (1990). Ethnographic interviewing: Asking the right questions to the right people in the right ways. *Journal of Childhood Communication Disorders, 13*, 101–111.

Weston, A. J., & Irwin, J. V. (1971). Use of paired stimuli in modification of articulation. *Perceptual and Motor Skills, 32*, 947–957.

Weston, A., & Shriberg, L. D. (1992). Contextual and linguistic correlates of intelligibility in children with developmental phonological disorders. *Journal of Speech and Hearing Research, 35*, 1316–1332.

Wilcox, K., & Morris, S. (1995). Speech outcomes of the language-focused curriculum. In M. Rice & K. Wilcox (Eds.), *Building a language-focused curriculum for the preschool classroom: A foundation for lifelong communication* (pp. 73–79). Baltimore: Brookes.

Wilcox, K., & Morris, S. (1999). *Children's Speech Intelligibility Measure.* San Antonio, TX: The Psychological Corporation.

Wilhelm, C. L. (1971). The effects of oral form recognition training on articulation in children. Unpublished doctoral dissertation, University of Kansas, Lawrence, KS.

Williams, A. L. (2003). Target selection and treatment outcomes. *Perspectives on Language Learning and Education, 10*, 12–16.

Williams, G., & McReynolds, L. (1975). The relationship between discrimination and articulation training in children with misarticulations. *Journal of Speech and Hearing Research, 18*, 401–412.

Wing, D., & Heimgartner, L. (1973). Articulation carryover procedure implemented by parents. *Language, Speech, and Hearing Services in Schools, 6*, 182–195.

Winitz, H. (1969). *Articulatory acquisition and behavior.* New York: Appleton-Century-Crofts.

Winitz, H. (1975). *From syllable to conversation.* Baltimore: University Park Press.

Winitz, H. (1984). Auditory considerations in articulation training. In H. Winitz (Ed.), *Treating articulation disorders: For clinicians by clinicians.* Baltimore: University Park Press.

Winitz, H. (1989). Auditory considerations in treatment. In N. A. Creaghead, P. W. Newman, & W. A. Secord. *Assessment and remediation of articulatory and phonological disorders* (2nd ed., pp. 243–264). Columbus, OH: Merrill Publishing Company.

Winitz, H., & Bellerose, B. (1967). Relation between sound discrimination and sound learning. *Journal of Communication Disorders, 1*, 215–235.

Witt, J. C., Elliott, S. N., Kramer, J. J., & Gresham, F. M. (1994). *Assessment of children: Fundamental methods and practices.* Madison, WI: Brown & Benchmark.

Wolfe, V., & Irwin, R. (1973). Sound discrimination ability of children with misarticulation of the /r/ sound. *Perceptual and Motor Skills, 37*, 415–420.

Wood K. (1971). Terminology and nomenclature. In L. Travis (Ed.), *Handbook of speech pathology and audiology* (pp. 3–26). New York: Appleton-Century-Crofts.

Wood, V. B. (1974). The frequency of retroflex /r/ production in elementary school children. Unpublished master's thesis, Portland State University, Portland, OR.

Yavas, M. (1995). Phonological selectivity in the first fifty words of a bilingual child. *Language and Speech, 38*, 189–202.

Yorkston, K. M., & Beukelman, D. R. (1981). *Assessment of Intelligibility of Dysarthric Speech.* Austin, TX: Pro-Ed.

Yorkston, K. M., Beukelman, D. R., Strand, E. A., & Bell, K. R. (1999). *Management of motor speech disorders in children and adults* (2nd ed.). Austin, TX: Pro-Ed.

Yorkston, K. M., Beukelman, D. R., & Traynor, C. D. (1984). *Computerized Assessment of Intelligibility of Dysarthric Speech.* Austin, TX: Pro-Ed.

Yoss, K., & Darley, F. (1974). Therapy in developmental apraxia of speech. *Speech, Language and Hearing Services in Schools, 5*, 23–31.

Young, E., & Hawk, S. (1938). *Moto-kinesthetic speech training.* Stanford, CA: Stanford University Press.

Young, E. H., & Stinchfield-Hawk, S. (1955). *Moto-kinesthetic speech training therapy.* Stanford, CA: Stanford University Press.

Zehel, Z., Shelton, R., Arndt, W., Wright, V., & Elbert, M. (1972). Item context and /s/ phone articulation results. *Journal of Speech and Hearing Research, 15*, 852–860.

Zemlin, W. (1998). *Speech and hearing science. Anatomy & physiology* (4th ed.). New York: Allyn & Bacon.

Zimmerman, I., Steiner, V. & Pond, R. (2005). *PLS-4 Screening Test Kit.* San Antonio, TX: Harcourt Assessment, Inc.

Index